Nurse's Pocket Guide

Diagnoses, Prioritized Interventions, and Rationales

Nurse's Pocket Guide

Diagnoses, Prioritized Interventions, and Rationales

Marilynn E. Doenges, APRN, BC—Retired
Clinical Specialist—Adult Psychiatric/Mental Health Nursing,
   Retired Adjunct Faculty
Beth-El College of Nursing and Health Sciences, UCCS
Colorado Springs, Colorado

Mary Frances Moorhouse, RN, MSN, CRRN, LNC
Nurse Consultant
TNT-RN Enterprises
Adjunct Faculty
Pikes Peak Community College
Colorado Springs, Colorado

Alice C. Murr, BSN, RN—Retired
Collins, Mississippi

EDITION 12

F. A. DAVIS COMPANY • Philadelphia

F. A. Davis Company
1915 Arch Street
Philadelphia, PA 19103
www.fadavis.com

Publisher, Nursing: Joanne Patzek DaCunha, RN, MSN
Project Editor: Kim DePaul
Design and Illustrations Manager: Carolyn O'Brien

As new scientific information becomes available through basic and clinical research, recommended treatments and drug therapies undergo changes. The author(s) and publisher have done everything possible to make this book accurate, up to date, and in accord with accepted standards at the time of publication. The author(s), editors, and publisher are not responsible for errors or omissions or for consequences from application of the book, and make no warranty, expressed or implied, in regard to the contents of the book. Any practice described in this book should be applied by the reader in accordance with professional standards of care used in regard to the unique circumstances that may apply in each situation. The reader is advised always to check product information (package inserts) for changes and new information regarding dose and contraindications before administering any drug. Caution is especially urged when using new or infrequently ordered drugs.

Library of Congress Cataloging-in-Publication Data

Doenges, Marilynn E., 1922-
Nurse's pocket guide : diagnoses, prioritized interventions, and rationales / Marilynn E. Doenges, Mary Frances Moorhouse, Alice C. Murr.—12th ed.
    p. ; cm.
  Includes bibliographical references and index.
  ISBN-13: 978-0-8036-2234-0
  ISBN-10: 0-8036-2234-1
1. Nursing diagnosis—Handbooks, manuals, etc. 2. Nursing care plans—Handbooks, manuals, etc. I. Moorhouse, Mary Frances, 1947- II. Murr, Alice C., 1946- III. Title.
  [DNLM: 1. Nursing Diagnosis—Handbooks. 2. Nursing Care—classification—Handbooks. 3. Patient Care Planning—Handbooks. WY 49 D651n 2010]
  RT48.6.D64 2010
  616.07'5—dc22
                                                                    2009043345

DEDICATION

This book is dedicated to:

Our families, who helped with the mundane activities of daily living that allowed us to write this book and who provide us with love and encouragement in all our endeavors.

Our friends, who support us in our writing, put up with our memory lapses, and love us still.

Bob Martone, Publisher, Nursing, who asks questions from afar that stimulate thought and discussion, and who maintains good humor throughout. Joanne DaCunha and Kimberly De-Paul who provided direct support and kept us focused. The F. A. Davis production staff who coordinated and expedited the project through the editing and printing processes, meeting unreal deadlines, and sending pages to us with bated breath.

Robert H. Craven, Jr., and the F. A. Davis family.

And last and most important:

The nurses we are writing for, to those who have found the previous editions of the *Pocket Guide* helpful, and to other nurses who are looking for help to provide quality nursing care in a period of transition and change, we say, "Nursing Diagnosis is the way."

CONTRIBUTOR

Sheila Marquez
Formerly Executive Director
Vice President/Chief Operating Officer
The Colorado SIDS Program, Inc.
Denver, Colorado

ACKNOWLEDGMENTS

A special acknowledgment to Marilynn's friend, the late Diane Camillone, who provoked an awareness of the role of the patient and continues to influence our thoughts about the importance of quality nursing care, and to our late colleague, Mary Jeffries, who introduced us to nursing diagnosis.

To our colleagues in NANDA International, who continue to formulate and refine nursing diagnoses to provide nursing with the tools to enhance and promote the growth of the profession.

Marilynn E. Doenges
Mary Frances Moorhouse
Alice C. Murr

CONTENTS

Health Conditions and Client Concerns with Associated Nursing Diagnoses appear on pages 925–1063.

How to Use the Nurse's Pocket Guide xiii

CHAPTER 1
The Nursing Process 1

CHAPTER 2
Application of the Nursing Process 7

CHAPTER 3
Putting Theory Into Practice: Sample Assessment Tools, Plan of Care, Mind Mapping, and Documentation 18

> **SECTION 1**
> Assessment Tools for Choosing Nursing Diagnoses 21
> *Adult Medical/Surgical Assessment Tool 22*
> *Excerpt From Psychiatric Assessment Tool 34*
> *Excerpt From Prenatal Assessment Tool 36*
> *Excerpt From Intrapartal Assessment Tool 38*
>
> **SECTION 2**
> Diagnostic Divisions: Nursing Diagnoses Organized According to a Nursing Focus 40
>
> **SECTION 3**
> Client Situation and Prototype Plan of Care 46
> *Plan of Care for Client With Diabetes Mellitus 54*
> *Another Approach to Planning Client Care—Mind Mapping 62*
>
> **SECTION 4**
> Documentation Techniques: SOAP and Focus Charting® 64

CHAPTER 4
Nursing Diagnoses in Alphabetical Order 69
For each nursing diagnosis, the following information is provided:

Taxonomy II, Domain, Class, Code, Year Submitted/Revised
Diagnostic Division
Definition
Related/Risk Factors, Defining Characteristics: Subjective/Objective
Desired Outcomes/Evaluation Criteria
Actions/Interventions
Nursing Priorities
Documentation Focus

Sample Nursing Outcomes & Interventions Classifications
(NOC/NIC)

CHAPTER 5
Health Conditions and Client Concerns With Associated Nursing
Diagnoses 925

APPENDIX 1
NANDA-I's Taxonomy II 1064

APPENDIX 2
Definitions of Taxonomy II Axes 1068

BIBLIOGRAPHY 1070

INDEX 1111

Contents

HOW TO USE THE NURSE'S POCKET GUIDE

The American Nurses Association (ANA) *Social Policy Statement* of 1980 was the first to define nursing as the diagnosis and treatment of human responses to actual and potential health problems. This definition, when combined with the ANA *Standards of Practice*, has provided impetus and support for the use of nursing diagnosis. Defining *nursing* and its effect on client care supports the growing awareness that nursing care is a key factor in client survival and in the maintenance, rehabilitative, and preventive aspects of healthcare. Changes and new developments in healthcare delivery in the last decade have given rise to the need for a common framework of communication to ensure continuity of care for the client moving between multiple healthcare settings and providers. Evaluation and documentation of care are important parts of this process.

This book is designed to aid the practitioner and student nurse in identifying interventions commonly associated with specific nursing diagnoses as proposed by NANDA International (NANDA-I). These interventions are the activities needed to implement and document care provided to the individual client and can be used in varied settings from acute to community/home care.

Chapters 1 and 2 present brief discussions of the nursing process, data collection, and care plan construction. Chapter 3 contains the Diagnostic Divisions, Assessment Tool, a sample plan of care, mind map, and corresponding documentation and charting examples. For more in-depth information and inclusive plans of care related to specific medical or psychiatric conditions (with rationale and the application of the diagnoses), the nurse is referred to the larger works, all published by the F. A. Davis Company: *Nursing Care Plans: Guidelines for Individualizing Client Care Across the Life Span*, ed. 8 (Doenges, Moorhouse, & Murr, 2010); *Psychiatric Care Plans: Guidelines for Individualizing Care*, ed. 3 (Doenges, Townsend, & Moorhouse, 1998); and *Maternal/Newborn Plans of Care: Guidelines for Individualizing Care*, ed. 3 (Doenges & Moorhouse, 1999) with updated versions included on the CD-ROM provided with *Nursing Care Plans*.

Nursing diagnoses are listed alphabetically in Chapter 4 for ease of reference and include the diagnoses accepted for use by NANDA-I through 2009–2011. Each diagnosis approved for testing includes its definition and information divided into the

NANDA-I categories of Related or Risk Factors and Defining Characteristics. Related/Risk Factors information reflects causative or contributing factors that can be useful for determining whether the diagnosis is applicable to a particular client. Defining Characteristics (signs and symptoms or cues) are listed as subjective and/or objective and are used to confirm actual diagnoses, aid in formulating outcomes, and provide additional data for choosing appropriate interventions. The authors have not deleted or altered NANDA-I's listings; however, on occasion, they have added to their definitions or suggested additional criteria to provide clarification and direction. These additions are denoted with brackets [ ].

With the development and acceptance of Taxonomy II following the biennial conference in 2000, significant changes were made to better reflect the content of the diagnoses within the taxonomy. Taxonomy II was designed to reduce miscalculations, errors, and redundancies. The framework is organized in Domains and Classes, with 13 domains, 47 classes, and 206 diagnoses. (Six diagnoses have been retired from the NANDA-I taxonomy but remain in this edition to allow for possible revision and resubmission.) Although clinicians will use the actual diagnoses, understanding the taxonomic structure will help the nurse to find the desired information quickly. Taxonomy II is designed to be multiaxial with 7 axes (see Appendix 2). An *axis* is defined as a dimension of the human response that is considered in the diagnostic process. Sometimes an axis may be included in the diagnostic concept, such as ineffective community Coping, in which the unit of care (e.g., community) is named. Some are implicit, such as Activity Intolerance, in which the individual is the unit of care. Sometimes an axis may not be pertinent to a particular diagnosis and will not be a part of the nursing diagnosis label or code. For example, the time axis may not be relevant to each diagnostic situation. The Taxonomic Domain and Class are noted under each nursing diagnosis heading.

The ANA, in conjunction with NANDA-I, proposed that specific nursing diagnoses currently approved and structured according to Taxonomy I Revised be included in the International Classification of Diseases (ICD) within the section "Family of Health-Related Classifications." While the World Health Organization did not accept this initial proposal because of lack of documentation of the usefulness of nursing diagnoses at the international level, the NANDA-I list has been accepted by SNOMED (Systemized Nomenclature of Medicine) for inclusion in its international coding system and is included in the Unified Medical Language System of the National Library of Medicine. Today, nurse researchers from around the world have submitted new nursing diagnoses and are validating current diagnoses in support for resubmission and acceptance of the NANDA-I list in future editions of the ICD.

The authors have chosen to categorize the list of nursing diagnoses approved for clinical use and testing into Diagnostic Divisions, which is the framework for an assessment tool (Chapter 3) designed to assist the nurse to readily identify an appropriate nursing diagnosis from data collected during the assessment process. The Diagnostic Division label follows the Taxonomic label under each nursing diagnosis heading.

Desired Outcomes/Evaluation Criteria are identified to assist the nurse in formulating individual client outcomes and to support the evaluation process.

Interventions in this pocket guide are primarily directed to adult care settings (although general age-span considerations are included) and are listed according to nursing priorities. Some interventions require collaborative or interdependent orders (e.g., medical, psychiatric), and the nurse will need to determine when this is necessary and take the appropriate action. In general, interventions that address specialty areas outside the scope of this book are not routinely presented (e.g., obstetrics). For example, when addressing acute Pain, the nurse is directed to administer analgesics as indicated; however, specific direction regarding epidural block is not listed.

The inclusion of Documentation Focus suggestions is to remind the nurse of the importance and necessity of recording the steps of the nursing process.

Finally, in recognition of the ongoing work of numerous researchers over the past 20 years, the authors have referenced the Nursing Interventions and Outcomes labels developed by the Iowa Intervention Projects (Bulechek, Butcher, & Dochterman; Moorhead, Johnson, Mass, & Swanson). These groups have been classifying nursing interventions and outcomes to predict resource requirements and measure outcomes, thereby meeting the needs of a standardized language that can be coded for computer and reimbursement purposes. As an introduction to this work in progress, sample NIC and NOC labels have been included under the heading Sample Nursing Interventions & Outcomes Classifications at the conclusion of each nursing diagnosis section. The reader is referred to the various publications by Joanne C. McCloskey and Marion Johnson for more in-depth information.

Chapter 5 presents 440 disorders/health conditions reflecting all specialty areas, with associated nursing diagnoses written as client diagnostic statements that include the "related to" and "evidenced by" components. This section will facilitate and help validate the assessment and problem or need identification steps of the nursing process.

As noted, with few exceptions, we have presented NANDA-I's recommendations as formulated. We support the belief that practicing nurses and researchers need to study, use, and evaluate the diagnoses as presented. Nurses can be creative as they use the standardized language, redefining and sharing information as the diagnoses are used with individual clients. As new nursing diagnoses are developed, it is important that the data they encompass are added to assessment tools and current database. As part of the process by clinicians, educators, and researchers across practice specialties and academic settings to define, test, and refine nursing diagnosis, nurses are encouraged to share insights and ideas with NANDA-I online at http://www.nanda.org or at the following address: NANDA International, PO Box 157, Kaukauna, WI 54130–0157.

CHAPTER 1

The Nursing Process

Nursing is both a science and an art concerned with the physical, psychological, sociological, cultural, and spiritual concerns of the individual. The science of nursing is based on a broad theoretical framework; its art depends on the caring skills and abilities of the individual nurse. In its early developmental years, nursing did not seek or have the means to control its own practice. In more recent times, the nursing profession has struggled to define what makes nursing unique and has identified a body of professional knowledge unique to nursing practice. In 1980, the American Nurses Association (ANA) developed the first *Social Policy Statement* defining nursing as "the diagnosis and treatment of human responses to actual or potential health problems." Along with the definition of nursing came the need to explain the method used to provide nursing care.

Years before, nursing leaders had developed a problem-solving process consisting of three steps—assessment, planning, and evaluation—patterned after the scientific method of observing, measuring, gathering data, and analyzing findings. This method, introduced in the 1950s, was called *nursing process*. Shore (1988) described the nursing process as "combining the most desirable elements of the art of nursing with the most relevant elements of systems theory, using the scientific method." This process incorporates an interactive/interpersonal approach with a problem-solving and decision-making process (Peplau, 1952; King, 1971; Yura & Walsh, 1988).

Over time, the nursing process expanded to five steps and has gained widespread acceptance as the basis for providing effective nursing care. Nursing process is now included in the conceptual framework of all nursing curricula, is accepted in the legal definition of nursing in the *Nurse Practice Acts* of most states, and is included in the ANA *Standards of Clinical Nursing Practice*.

The five steps of the nursing process consist of the following:

1. *Assessment* is an organized dynamic process involving three basic activities: (a) systematically gathering data, (b) sorting and organizing the collected data, and (c) documenting the data in a retrievable fashion. Subjective and objective data are collected from various sources, such as the client interview and physical assessment. Subjective data are what the client or

significant others report, believe, or feel; and objective data are what can be observed or obtained from other sources, such as laboratory and diagnostic studies, old medical records, or other healthcare providers. Using a number of techniques, the nurse focuses on eliciting a profile of the client that supplies a sense of the client's overall health status, providing a picture of the client's physical, psychological, sociocultural, spiritual, cognitive, and developmental levels; economic status; functional abilities; and lifestyle. The profile is known as the *client database*.

2. *Diagnosis/need identification* involves the analysis of collected data to identify the client's needs or problems, also known as the nursing diagnosis. The purpose of this step is to draw conclusions regarding the client's specific needs or human responses of concern so that effective care can be planned and delivered. This process of data analysis uses diagnostic reasoning (a form of clinical judgment) in which conclusions are reached about the meaning of the collected data to determine whether or not nursing intervention is indicated. The end product is the *client diagnostic statement* that combines the specific client need with the related factors or risk factors (etiology), and defining characteristics (or cues) as appropriate. The status of the client's needs are categorized as *actual* or currently existing diagnoses and potential or *risk* diagnoses that could develop due to specific vulnerabilities of the client. Ongoing changes in healthcare delivery and computerization of the client record require a commonality of communication to ensure continuity of care for the client moving from one setting or level of healthcare to another. The use of standardized terminology or NANDA International (NANDA-I) nursing diagnosis labels provides nurses with a common language for identifying client needs. Furthermore, the use of standardized nursing diagnosis labels also promotes identification of appropriate goals, provides acuity information, is useful in creating standards for nursing practice, provides a base for quality improvement, and facilitates research supporting evidence-based nursing practices.

3. *Planning* includes setting priorities, establishing goals, identifying desired client outcomes, and determining specific nursing interventions. These actions are documented as the *plan of care*. This process requires input from the client/significant others to reach agreement regarding the plan to facilitate the taking of responsibility by the client for his or her own care and the achievement of the desired outcomes and goals. Setting priorities for client care is a complex and dynamic challenge that helps ensure that the nurse's attention and subsequent actions are properly focused. What is perceived today to be the number-one client care need or appropriate nursing intervention could change tomorrow, or, for

that matter, within minutes, based on changes in the client's condition or situation. Once client needs are prioritized, goals for treatment and discharge are established that indicate the general direction in which the client is expected to progress in response to treatment. The goals may be short term—those that usually must be met before the client is discharged or moved to a lesser level of care—and/or long term, which may continue even after discharge. From these goals, desired outcomes are determined to measure the client's progress toward achieving the goals of treatment or the discharge criteria. To be more specific, outcomes are client responses that are achievable and desired by the client that can be attained within a defined period, given the situation and resources. Next, nursing interventions are chosen that are based on the client's nursing diagnosis, the established goals and desired outcomes, the ability of the nurse to successfully implement the intervention, and the ability and the willingness of the client to undergo or participate in the intervention, and they reflect the client's age, situation, and individual strengths, when possible. Nursing interventions are direct-care activities or prescriptions for behaviors, treatments, activities, or actions that assist the client in achieving the measurable outcomes. Nursing interventions, like nursing diagnoses, are key elements of the knowledge of nursing and continue to grow as research supports the connection between actions and outcomes (McCloskey & Bulechek, 2000). Recording the planning step in a written or computerized plan of care provides for continuity of care, enhances communication, assists with determining agency or unit staffing needs, documents the nursing process, serves as a teaching tool, and coordinates provision of care among disciplines. A valid plan of care demonstrates individualized client care by reflecting the concerns of the client and significant others, as well as the client's physical, psychosocial, and cultural needs and capabilities.

4. *Implementation* occurs when the plan of care is put into action and the nurse performs the planned interventions. Regardless of how well a plan of care has been constructed, it cannot predict everything that will occur with a particular client on a daily basis. Individual knowledge and expertise and agency routines allow the flexibility that is necessary to adapt to the changing needs of the client. Legal and ethical concerns related to interventions also must be considered. For example, the wishes of the client and family/significant others regarding interventions and treatments must be discussed and respected. Before implementing the interventions in the plan of care, the nurse needs to understand the reason for doing each intervention, its expected effect, and any potential hazards that can occur. The nurse must also be sure that the interventions are: (a) consistent with the established plan of care,

(b) implemented in a safe and appropriate manner, (c) evaluated for effectiveness, and (d) documented in a timely manner.

5. *Evaluation* is accomplished by determining the client's progress toward attaining the identified outcomes and by monitoring the client's response to and effectiveness of the selected nursing interventions for the purpose of altering the plan as indicated. This is done by direct observation of the client, interviewing the client/significant other, and/or reviewing the client's healthcare record. Although the process of evaluation seems similar to the activity of assessment, there are important differences. Evaluation is an ongoing process, a constant measuring and monitoring of the client status to determine: (a) appropriateness of nursing actions, (b) the need to revise interventions, (c) development of new client needs, (d) the need for referral to other resources, and (e) the need to rearrange priorities to meet changing demands of care. Comparing overall outcomes and noting the effectiveness of specific interventions are the clinical components of evaluation that can become the basis for research for validating the nursing process and supporting evidenced-based practice. The external evaluation process is the key for refining standards of care and determining the protocols, policies, and procedures necessary for the provision of quality nursing care for a specific situation or setting.

When a client enters the healthcare system, whether as an acute care, clinic, or home-care client, the steps of the process noted above are set in motion. Although these steps are presented as separate or individual activities, the nursing process is an interactive method of practicing nursing, with the components fitting together in a continuous cycle of thought and action.

To effectively use the nursing process, the nurse must possess, and be able to apply, certain skills. Particularly important is a thorough knowledge of science and theory, as applied not only in nursing but also in other related disciplines, such as medicine and psychology. A sense of caring, intelligence, and competent technical skills are also essential. Creativity is needed in the application of nursing knowledge as well as adaptability for handling constant change in healthcare delivery and the many unexpected happenings that characterize the everyday practice of nursing.

Because decision making is crucial to each step of the process, the following assumptions are important for the nurse to consider:

• The client is a human being of worth and dignity. This entitles the client to participate in his or her own healthcare decisions and delivery. It requires a sense of the personal in each individual and the delivery of competent healthcare.

• There are basic human needs that must be met, and when they are not, problems arise that may require interventions by others until and if the individual can resume responsibility for self. This challenges healthcare providers to anticipate and initiate actions necessary to save another's life or to secure the client's return to health and independence.

- The client has the right to quality health and nursing care delivered with interest, compassion, competence, and with a focus on wellness and prevention of illness. The philosophy of caring encompasses all of these qualities.
- The therapeutic nurse-client relationship is important in this process, providing a milieu in which the client can feel safe to disclose and talk about his or her deepest concerns.

In 1995, ANA acknowledged that since the release of the original statement, nursing has been influenced by many social and professional changes as well as by the science of caring. Nursing integrated these changes with the 1980 definition to include treatment of human responses to health and illness (*Nursing's Social Policy Statement,* ANA, 1995). The revised statement provided four essential features of today's contemporary nursing practice:

- Attention to the full range of human experiences and responses to health and illness without restriction to a problem-focused orientation (in short, clients may have needs for wellness or personal growth that are not "problems" to be corrected)
- Integration of objective data with knowledge gained from an understanding of the client's or group's subjective experience
- Application of scientific knowledge to the process of diagnosis and treatment
- Provision of a caring relationship that facilitates health and healing

In 2003, the definition of nursing was further expanded to reflect nursing's role in wellness promotion and responsibility to its clients, wherever they may be found. Therefore, "nursing is the protection, promotion, and optimization of health and abilities, prevention of illness and injury, alleviation of suffering through the diagnosis and treatment of human responses, and advocacy in the care of individuals, families, communities, and populations" (*Social Policy Statement,* ANA, 2003, p. 6).

Our understanding of what nursing is, and what nurses do continues to evolve. Whereas nursing actions were once based on variables such as diagnostic tests and medical diagnoses, use of the nursing process and nursing diagnoses provide a uniform method of identifying and dealing with specific client needs or responses in which the nurse can intervene. The nursing diagnosis is thus helping to set standards for nursing practice and should lead to improved care delivery.

Nursing and medicine are interrelated and have implications for each other. This interrelationship includes the exchange of data, the sharing of ideas, and the development of plans of care that include all data pertinent to the individual client as well as the family/significant others. Although nurses work within medical and psychosocial domains, nursing's phenomena of concern are the patterns of human response, not disease processes. Thus, the written plan of care should contain more than just nursing actions in response to medical orders and may reflect plans of care encompassing all involved disciplines to provide holistic care for the individual/family.

Summary

Because the nursing process is the basis of all nursing action, it is the essence of nursing. It can be applied in any healthcare or educational setting, in any theoretical or conceptual framework, and within the context of any nursing philosophy. In using nursing diagnosis labels as an integral part of the nursing process, the nursing profession has identified a body of knowledge that contributes to the prevention of illness as well as the maintenance or restoration of health (or the relief of pain and discomfort when a return to health is not possible). Subsequent chapters in this book help the nurse applying the nursing process to review the current NANDA-I list of nursing diagnoses, their definition, related/risk factors (etiology), and defining characteristics. Aware of desired outcomes and commonly used interventions, the nurse can develop, implement, and document an individualized plan of care.

CHAPTER 2

Application of the Nursing Process

Because of their hectic schedules, many nurses believe that time spent writing a plan of care is time taken away from client care. Plans of care have been viewed as "busy work" to satisfy accreditation requirements or the whims of supervisors. In reality, quality client care must be planned and coordinated. Properly written and applied plans of care can save time by providing direction and continuity of care and by facilitating communication among nurses and other caregivers. They also provide guidelines for documentation and tools for evaluating the care provided.

The components of a plan of care are based on the nursing process presented in the first chapter. Creating a plan of care begins with the collection of data (assessment). The client database consists of subjective and objective information encompassing the various concerns reflected in the current NANDA International (NANDA-I) list of nursing diagnoses (NDs) (Table 2.1). Subjective data are those that are reported by the client (and significant others [SOs]) in the individual's own words. This information includes the individual's perceptions and what he or she wants to share. It is important to accept what is reported because the client is the "expert" in this area. Objective data are those that are observed or described (quantitatively or qualitatively) and include findings from diagnostic testing and physical examination and information from old medical records and other healthcare providers.

Analysis of the collected data leads to the identification or diagnosis of problems or areas of concern or need (including health promotion) specific to the client. These problems or needs are expressed as nursing diagnoses. The diagnosis of client needs has been determined by nurses on an informal basis since the beginning of the profession. The term *nursing diagnosis* came into formal use in the nursing literature during the 1950s (Fry, 1953), although its meaning continued to be viewed in the context of medical diagnosis. In 1973, a national conference was held to identify client needs that fall within the scope of nursing, to label them, and to develop a classification system that could be used by nurses throughout the world. They called the labels *nursing*

TABLE 2.1—Nursing Diagnoses Accepted for Use and Research (2009–2011)

Activity Intolerance [specify level]
Activity Intolerance, risk for
+Activity Planning, ineffective
Airway Clearance, ineffective
Allergy Response, latex
Allergy Response, risk for latex
Anxiety [specify level: mild, moderate, severe, panic]
Anxiety, death
Aspiration, risk for
Attachment, risk for impaired (formerly risk for impaired parent/child Attachment)
Autonomic Dysreflexia
Autonomic Dysreflexia, risk for

*Behavior, risk-prone health (formerly impaired, Adjustment)
+Bleeding, risk for
Body Image, disturbed
Body Temperature, risk for imbalanced
Bowel Incontinence
Breastfeeding [Learning Need], effective
Breastfeeding, ineffective
Breastfeeding, interrupted
Breathing Pattern, ineffective

Cardiac Output, decreased
Caregiver Role Strain
Caregiver Role Strain, risk for
+Childbearing Process, readiness for enhanced
+Comfort, impaired
Comfort, readiness for enhanced
Communication, impaired verbal
Communication, readiness for enhanced
Conflict, decisional [specify]
Conflict, parental role
Confusion, acute
Confusion, chronic
Confusion, risk for acute
Constipation
Constipation, perceived
Constipation, risk for

+New ND
*Revised ND

TABLE 2.1—*(continued)*

Contamination
Contamination, risk for
Coping, compromised family
*Coping, defensive
Coping, disabled family
Coping, ineffective
Coping, ineffective community
Coping, readiness for enhanced
Coping, readiness for enhanced community
Coping, readiness for enhanced family

Death Syndrome, risk for sudden infant
Decision Making, readiness for enhanced
Denial, ineffective
Dentition, impaired
Development, risk for delayed
Diarrhea
Dignity, risk for compromised human
Distress, moral
Disuse Syndrome, risk for
Diversional Activity, deficient

+Electrolyte Imbalance, risk for
Energy Field, disturbed
Environmental Interpretation Syndrome, impaired

Failure to Thrive, adult
Falls, risk for
Family Processes, dysfunctional (formerly dysfunctional Family Process: alcoholism)
Family Processes, interrupted
Family Processes, readiness for enhanced
Fatigue
Fear [specify focus]
Feeding Pattern, ineffective infant
Fluid Balance, readiness for enhanced
[Fluid Volume, deficient hyper/hypotonic]
Fluid Volume, deficient [isotonic]
Fluid Volume, excess
Fluid Volume, risk for deficient
*Fluid Volume, risk for imbalanced

(table continues on page 10)

+New ND
*Revised ND

TABLE 2.1—Nursing Diagnoses Accepted for Use and Research (2009–2011) *(continued)*

Gas Exchange, impaired
Glucose Level, risk for unstable blood
Grieving
Grieving, complicated
Grieving, risk for complicated
Growth, risk for disproportionate
Growth and Development, delayed

Health Maintenance, ineffective
*Health Management, ineffective self (formerly ineffective Therapeutic Regimen Management)
Health Management, readiness for enhanced self (formerly readiness for enhanced Therapeutic Regimen Management)
Home Maintenance, impaired
Hope, readiness for enhanced
Hopelessness
Hyperthermia
Hypothermia

*Identity, disturbed personal
Immunization Status, readiness for enhanced
Infant Behavior, disorganized
Infant Behavior, readiness for enhanced organized
Infant Behavior, risk for disorganized
Infection, risk for
Injury, risk for
Injury, risk for perioperative positioning
Insomnia
Intracranial Adaptive Capacity, decreased

+Jaundice, neonatal

Knowledge [Learning Need] (specify), deficient
Knowledge (specify), readiness for enhanced

Lifestyle, sedentary
*Liver Function, risk for impaired
Loneliness, risk for

+Maternal/Fetal Dyad, risk for disturbed
Memory, impaired

+New ND
*Revised ND

TABLE 2.1—*(continued)*

Mobility, impaired bed
Mobility, impaired physical
Mobility, impaired wheelchair
+Motility, dysfunctional gastrointestinal
+Motility, risk for dysfunctional gastrointestinal

Nausea
+Neglect, self
Neglect, unilateral
Noncompliance [ineffective Adherence] [specify]
Nutrition: less than body requirements, imbalanced
Nutrition: more than body requirements, imbalanced
Nutrition: more than body requirements, risk for imbalanced
Nutrition, readiness for enhanced

Oral Mucous Membrane, impaired

Pain, acute
Pain, chronic
Parenting, impaired
Parenting, readiness for enhanced
Parenting, risk for impaired
+Perfusion, ineffective peripheral tissue
+Perfusion, risk for decreased cardiac tissue
+Perfusion, risk for ineffective cerebral tissue
+Perfusion, risk for ineffective gastrointestinal
+Perfusion, risk for ineffective renal
Peripheral Neurovascular Dysfunction, risk for
Poisoning, risk for
Post-Trauma Syndrome [specify stage]
Post-Trauma Syndrome, risk for
Power, readiness for enhanced
Powerlessness [specify level]
Powerlessness, risk for
Protection, ineffective

Rape-Trauma Syndrome
(Rape-Trauma Syndrome: compound reaction—retired 2009)
(Rape-Trauma Syndrome: silent reaction—retired 2009)
+Relationship, readiness for enhanced
Religiosity, impaired

(table continues on page 12)

+New ND
*Revised ND

Religiosity, readiness for enhanced
Religiosity, risk for impaired
Relocation Stress Syndrome
Relocation Stress Syndrome, risk for
+Resilience, impaired individual
+Resilience, readiness for enhanced
+Resilience, risk for compromised
Role Performance, ineffective

Self-Care, readiness for enhanced
Self-Care Deficit, bathing
Self-Care Deficit, dressing
Self-Care Deficit, feeding
Self-Care Deficit, toileting
Self-Concept, readiness for enhanced
*Self-Esteem, chronic low
Self-Esteem, situational low
Self-Esteem, risk for situational low
Self-Mutilation
Self-Mutilation, risk for
Sensory Perception, disturbed (specify: visual, auditory, kinesthetic, gustatory, tactile, olfactory)
Sexual Dysfunction
Sexuality Pattern, ineffective
+Shock, risk for
Skin Integrity, impaired
Skin Integrity, risk for impaired
Sleep, readiness for enhanced
Sleep Deprivation
*Sleep Pattern, disturbed
Social Interaction, impaired
Social Isolation
Sorrow, chronic
Spiritual Distress
Spiritual Distress, risk for
Spiritual Well-Being, readiness for enhanced
Stress Overload
Suffocation, risk for
Suicide, risk for
Surgical Recovery, delayed
Swallowing, impaired

+New ND
*Revised ND

TABLE 2.1—*(continued)*

(Therapeutic Regimen Management, effective—retired 2009)
(Therapeutic Regimen Management, ineffective community—
   retired 2009)
Therapeutic Regimen Management, ineffective family
Thermoregulation, ineffective
(Thought Processes, disturbed—retired 2009)
Tissue Integrity, impaired
Transfer Ability, impaired
Trauma, risk for
+Trauma, risk for vascular

Urinary Elimination, impaired
Urinary Elimination, readiness for enhanced
Urinary Incontinence, functional
Urinary Incontinence, overflow
Urinary Incontinence, reflex
Urinary Incontinence, stress
(Urinary Incontinence, total—retired 2009)
Urinary Incontinence, urge
Urinary Incontinence, risk for urge
Urinary Retention [acute/chronic]

Ventilation, impaired spontaneous
Ventilatory Weaning Response, dysfunctional
Violence, [actual/]risk for other-directed
Violence, [actual/]risk for self-directed

Walking, impaired
Wandering [specify sporadic or continuous]

+New ND
*Revised ND

Used with permission from NANDA International: Definitions and Classification, 2009–2011. NANDA, Philadelphia, 2009.

Information in brackets added by authors to clarify and enhance the use of nursing diagnoses.

Please also see the NANDA diagnoses grouped according to Gordon's Functional Health Patterns on the inside front cover.

diagnoses, which represent clinical judgments about an individual's, family's, or community's responses to actual or potential health problems and life processes. Therefore, a nursing diagnosis (ND) is a decision about a need or problem that requires nursing intervention and management. The need may be anything that interferes with the quality of life the client is used to and/or desires. It includes concerns of the client, SOs, and/or nurse. The ND focuses attention on a physical or behavioral response, either a current need or a problem at risk for developing.

The identification of client needs and selection of an ND label involve the use of experience, expertise, and intuition. A six-step diagnostic reasoning or critical thinking process facilitates an accurate analysis of the client assessment data to determine specific client needs. First, data are reviewed to identify cues (signs and symptoms) reflecting client needs that can be described by ND labels. This is called *problem-sensing.* Next, alternative explanations are considered for the identified cues to determine which ND label may be the most appropriate. As relationships among data are compared, etiological factors are identified based on the nurse's understanding of biological, physical, and behavioral sciences, and possible ND choices are *ruled out* until the most appropriate label remains. Next, a comprehensive picture of the client's past, present, and potential health status is *synthesized,* and the suggested nursing diagnosis label is combined with the identified related (or risk) factors and cues to create a hypothesis. *Confirming the hypothesis* is achieved by reviewing the NANDA-I definition, defining characteristics (cues), and determining related factors (etiology) for the chosen ND to ensure the accuracy and objectivity in this diagnostic process. Now, based on the synthesis of the data (step 3) and evaluation of the hypothesis (step 4), the *client's needs are listed* and the correct ND label is combined with the assessed etiology and signs/symptoms to finalize the client diagnostic statement. Once all the NDs are identified, the problem list is *reevaluated,* assessment data are reviewed again, and the client is consulted to ensure that all areas of concern have been addressed.

When the ND label is combined with the individual's specific related or risk factors and defining characteristics (as appropriate), the resulting client diagnostic statement provides direction for nursing care. It is important to remember that the affective tone of the ND can shape expectations of the client's response and/or influence the nurse's behavior toward the client.

The development and classification of NDs have continued through the years spurred on by the need to describe what nursing does in conjunction with changes in healthcare delivery and reimbursement, the expansion of nursing's role, and the evolution of the computer age. The advent of alternative healthcare settings (e.g., outpatient surgery centers, home health, rehabilitation or subacute units, extended or long-term care facilities, hospice services) increases the need for a commonality of communication to ensure continuity of care for the client, who moves from one setting or level of care to another. The efficient documentation of the client encounter, whether that is a single office visit or a lengthy hospitalization, and the movement toward a paperless (computerized or electronic) client record have strengthened the need for standardizing nursing language to better demonstrate what nursing is and what nursing does.

NANDA-I nursing diagnosis is one of the standardized nursing languages recognized by the American Nurses Association (ANA) as providing clinically useful terminology that supports nursing practice. NANDA-I has also established a liaison with the International Council of Nursing to support and contribute to the global effort to standardize the language of healthcare with the goal that NANDA-I NDs will be included in the International Classification of Diseases. In the meantime, they are included in the United States version of International Classification of Diseases—Clinical Modifications (ICD-10CM). The NANDA-I nursing diagnosis labels have also been combined with Nursing Interventions Classification (NIC) and Nursing Outcomes Classification (NOC) to create a complete nursing language that has been coded into the Systematized Nomenclature of Medicine (SNOMED). Inclusion in an international coded terminology such as SNOMED is essential if nursing's contribution to healthcare is to be recognized in the computer database. Indexing of the entire medical record supports disease management activities, research, and analysis of outcomes for quality improvement for all healthcare disciplines. Coding also supports telehealth (the use of telecommunications technology to provide healthcare information and services over distance) and facilitates access to healthcare data across care settings and various computer systems.

The key to accurate diagnosis is collection and analysis of data. In Chapter 3, the NDs have been categorized into divisions (Diagnostic Divisions: Nursing Diagnoses Organized According to a Nursing Focus, Section 2), and a sample assessment tool designed to assist the nurse to identify appropriate NDs as the data are collected is provided. Nurses may feel at risk in committing themselves to documenting an ND for fear they might be wrong. However, unlike medical diagnoses, NDs can change as the client progresses through various stages of illness or maladaptation to resolution of the condition or situation.

Desired outcomes are then formulated to give direction to, as well as to evaluate, the care provided. These outcomes emerge from the diagnostic statement and are what the client hopes to achieve. They serve as the guidelines to evaluate progress toward resolution of needs or problems, providing impetus for revising the plan as appropriate. In this book, outcomes are stated in general terms to permit the practitioner to individualize them by adding timelines and other data according to specific client circumstances. Outcome terminology needs to be concise, realistic, measurable, and stated in words the client can understand, because the terms that are used indicate what the client is expected to do or accomplish. Beginning the outcome statement with an action verb provides measurable direction: for example, "Verbalizes relationship between diabetes mellitus and circulatory changes in feet within 2 days" or " Performs procedure for home glucose monitoring correctly within 48 hours."

Interventions are the activities taken to achieve the desired outcomes and, because they are communicated to others, they must be clearly stated. A solid nursing knowledge base is vital to this process because the rationale for interventions needs to be sound and feasible with the intention of providing effective, individualized care. The actions may be independent or collaborative and may encompass specific orders from nursing, medicine, and other disciplines. Written interventions that guide ongoing client care need to be dated and signed. To facilitate the planning process, specific nursing priorities have been identified in this text to provide a general ranking of interventions. This ranking would be altered according to individual client situations. The seasoned practitioner may choose to use these as broad-based interventions. The student or beginning practitioner may need to develop a more detailed plan of care by including the appropriate interventions listed under each nursing priority. It is important to remember that because each client usually has a perception of individual needs or problems he or she faces and an expectation of what could be done about the situation, the plan of care must be congruent with the client's reality or it will fail. In short, the nurse needs to plan care with the client, because both are accountable for that care and for achieving the desired outcomes.

The plan of care is the end product of the nursing process and documents client care in areas of accountability, quality assurance, and liability. Therefore, the plan of care is a permanent part of the client's healthcare record. The format for recording the plan of care is determined by agency policy and may be handwritten, standardized forms or clinical pathways, or computer-generated documentation. Before implementing the plan of care, it should be reviewed to ensure that:

- It is based on accepted nursing practice, reflecting knowledge of scientific principles, nursing standards of care, and agency policies.
- It provides for the safety of the client by ensuring that the care provided will do no harm.
- The client diagnostic statements are supported by the client data.
- The goals and outcomes are measurable, observable, and can be achieved.

- The interventions can benefit the client, family, or significant others in a predictable way in achieving the identified outcomes, and they are arranged in a logical sequence.
- It demonstrates individualized client care by reflecting the concerns of the client and significant others, as well as their physical, psychosocial, and cultural needs and capabilities.

Once the plan of care is put into action, changes in the client's needs must be continually monitored because care is provided in a dynamic environment, and flexibility is required to allow changing circumstances. Periodic review of the client's response to nursing interventions and progress toward attaining the desired outcomes helps determine the effectiveness of the plan of care. Based on the findings, the plan may need to be modified or revised; referrals to other resources may be required; or the client may be ready for discharge from the care setting.

Summary

Healthcare providers have a responsibility for planning with the client and family for continuation of care to the eventual outcome of an optimal state of wellness or a dignified death. Today, the act of diagnosing client problems or needs is well established and the use of standardized nursing language to describe what nursing does is rapidly becoming an integral part of an effective system of nursing practice. Although not yet comprehensive, the current NANDA-I list of diagnostic labels defines and refines professional nursing activity. With repeated use of NANDA-I NDs, strengths and weaknesses of the NDs can be identified, promoting research and further development.

Planning, setting goals, and choosing appropriate interventions are essential to the construction of a plan of care and delivery of quality nursing care. These nursing activities constitute the planning phase of the nursing process and are documented in the plan of care for a particular client. As a part of the client's permanent record, the plan of care not only provides a means for the nurse who is actively caring for the client to be aware of the client's needs (NDs), goals, and actions to be taken, but also substantiates the care provided for review by third-party payers and accreditation agencies, while meeting legal requirements.

CHAPTER 3

Putting Theory Into Practice: Sample Assessment Tools, Plan of Care, Mind Mapping, and Documentation

The client assessment is the foundation on which identification of individual needs, responses, and problems is based. To facilitate the steps of assessment and diagnosis in the nursing process, an assessment tool (Assessment Tools for Choosing Nursing Diagnoses, Section 1) has been constructed using a nursing focus instead of the medical approach of "review of systems." This has the advantage of identifying and validating nursing diagnoses (NDs) as opposed to medical diagnoses.

To achieve this nursing focus, we have grouped the NANDA International (NANDA-I) NDs into related categories titled Diagnostic Divisions (Section 2), which reflect a blending of theories, primarily Maslow's Hierarchy of Needs and a self-care philosophy. These divisions serve as the framework or outline for data collection and clustering that focuses attention on the nurse's phenomena of concern—the human responses to health and illness—and directs the nurse to the most likely corresponding NDs.

Because the divisions are based on human responses and needs and not specific "systems," information may be recorded in more than one area. For this reason, the nurse is encouraged to keep an open mind, to pursue all leads, and to collect as much data as possible before choosing the ND label that best reflects the client's situation. For example, when the nurse identifies the cue of restlessness in a client, the nurse may infer that the client is anxious, assuming that the restlessness is psychologically based and thus overlooking the possibility that it is physiologically based.

From the specific data recorded in the database, an individualized client diagnostic statement can be formulated using the problem, etiology, signs and symptoms (PES) format to accurately represent the client's situation. Whereas a medical diagnosis of diabetes mellitus is the same label used for all individuals with this condition, the diagnostic statement developed by the nurse is individualized to reflect a specific client need. For example, the diagnostic statement may read, "deficient Knowledge regarding diabetic care, related to misinterpretation of information and/or lack of recall, evidenced by inaccurate follow-through of instructions and failure to recognize signs and symptoms of hyperglycemia."

Desired client outcomes are identified to facilitate choosing appropriate interventions and to serve as evaluators of both nursing care and client response. These outcomes also form the framework for documentation.

Interventions are designed to specify the action of the nurse, the client, and/or significant others (SOs). Interventions need to promote the client's movement toward health and independence in addition to achievement of physiological stability. This requires involvement of the client in his or her own care, including participation in decisions about care activities and projected outcomes.

Section 3, Client Situation and Prototype Plan of Care, contains a sample plan of care formulated on data collected in the nursing model assessment tool. Individualized client diagnostic statements and desired client outcomes (with timelines added to reflect anticipated length of stay and individual client and nurse expectations) have been identified. Interventions have been chosen based on concerns or needs identified by the client and nurse during data collection, as well as by physician orders.

Although not normally included in a written plan of care, rationales are included in this sample for the purpose of explaining or clarifying the choice of interventions to enhance the nurse's learning.

Another way to conceptualize the client's care needs is to create a *Mind Map*. This technique was developed to help visualize the linkages between various client symptoms, interventions, or problems as they impact each other. The parts that are great about traditional care plans (problem solving and categorizing) are retained, but the linear or columnar nature of the plan is changed to a design that uses the whole brain—a design that brings left-brain, linear problem-solving thinking together with the free-wheeling, interconnected, creative right brain. Joining mind mapping and care planning enables the nurse to create a holistic view of a client, strengthening critical thinking skills and facilitating the creative process of planning client care.

Finally, to complete the learning experience, samples of documentation based on the client situation are presented in Section 4, Documentation Techniques. The plan of care provides documentation of the planning process and serves as a framework or outline for charting of administered care. The primary nurse needs to periodically review the client's documentation of progress evaluating effectiveness of the treatment plan. Other care providers can also read the notes and obtain a clear picture of what occurred with the client and make appropriate judgments regarding client management. The best way to ensure clarity of the progress notes is through the use of descriptive (or observational) statements. Observations of client behavior and response to therapy provide invaluable information. Through this communication it can be determined if any of the client's current interventions can be eliminated or altered to achieve desired outcomes. Progress notes are an integral component of the overall medical record and should include all significant events that occur in the daily life of the client. They reflect implementation of the treatment plan and document that appropriate actions have been carried out, precautions taken, and so forth. It is important that both the implementation of interventions and progress toward the desired outcomes be documented. The notes need to be written in a clear and objective fashion, specific as to date and time, and signed by the person making the entry.

Use of clear documentation helps the nurse individualize client care. Providing a picture of what has happened and is happening promotes continuity of care and facilitates evaluation. This reinforces each person's accountability and responsibility for using the nursing process to provide individually appropriate and cost-effective client care.

SECTION 1

Assessment Tools for Choosing Nursing Diagnoses

The following are suggested guidelines or tools for creating assessment databases reflecting Doenges & Moorhouse's Diagnostic Divisions of Nursing Diagnoses. They are intended to provide a nursing focus and should help the nurse think about planning care with the client at the center (following mind-mapping theory, see page 63). Although the divisions are alphabetized here for ease of presentation, they can be prioritized or rearranged to meet individual needs. In addition, the assessment tool can be adapted to meet the needs of specific client populations. Excerpts of assessment tools adapted for psychiatric and obstetric settings are included at the end of this section.

ADULT MEDICAL/SURGICAL ASSESSMENT TOOL

General Information

Name: _____ ❑ Age: _____ ❑ DOB: _____
Gender: _____ Race: _____
Admission: Date: _____ ❑ Time: _____ ❑ From: _____
Reason for this visit (primary concern): _____
Cultural concerns (relating to healthcare decisions, religious concerns, pain, childbirth, family involvement, communication, etc.): _____
Source of information: _____ ❑ Reliability (1–4 with 4 = very reliable): _____

Activity/Rest

Subjective (Reports)
Occupation: _____ ❑ Able to participate in usual activities/hobbies: _____
Leisure time/diversional activities: _____
Ambulatory: _____ ❑ Gait (describe): _____
Activity level (sedentary to very active): _____ ❑ Regular exercise/type: _____
Muscle mass/tone/strength (e.g., normal, increased, decreased): _____
History of problems/limitations imposed by condition (e.g., immobility, can't transfer, weakness, breathlessness): _____
Feelings (e.g., exhaustion, restlessness, can't concentrate, dissatisfaction): _____
Developmental factors (e.g., delayed/age): _____
Sleep: Hours: _____ ❑ Naps: _____
Insomnia: _____ ❑ related to: _____ ❑ Difficulty falling asleep: _____
Difficulty staying asleep: _____ ❑ Rested on awakening: _____
❑ Excessive grogginess: _____
Bedtime rituals: _____
Relaxation techniques: _____
Sleeps on more than one pillow: _____
Oxygen use (type): When used: _____
Medications or herbals for/affecting sleep: _____

Objective (Exhibits)
Observed response to activity: Heart rate: _____
Rhythm (reg/irreg): _____ ❑ Blood pressure: _____ ❑ Respiration rate: _____ ❑ Pulse oximetry: _____
Mental status (i.e., cognitive impairment, withdrawn/lethargic): _____

Muscle mass/tone: ___ ❑ Posture (e.g., normal, stooped, curved spine): _____

    Tremors: _____ ❑ Location: _____
    ROM: _____
    Strength: _____ ❑ Deformity: _____
Uses mobility aid (list): _____

Circulation

Subjective (Reports)
History of/treatment for (date): High blood pressure: _____
    Brain injury: _____ ❑ Stroke: _____
    Heart problems/surgery: _____
    Palpitations: _____ ❑ Syncope: _____
    Cough/hemoptysis: _____ ❑ Blood clots: _____
    Bleeding tendencies/episodes: _____ ❑ Pain in legs w/activity: _____
    Extremities: Numbness: _____
    ❑ (location): _____
    Tingling: _____ ❑ (location): _____
Slow healing/describe: _____
Change in frequency/amount of urine: _____
History of spinal cord injury/dysreflexia episodes: _____
Medications/herbals: _____

Objective (Exhibits)
Color (e.g., pale, cyanotic, jaundiced, mottled, ruddy): _____
    Skin: _____
    Mucous membranes: _____ ❑ Lips: _____
    Nailbeds: _____ ❑ Conjunctiva: _____
    Sclera: _____
Skin moisture: (e.g., dry, diaphoretic): _____
BP: Lying: **R** _____ **L** _____ ❑ Sitting: **R** _____ **L** _____
    Standing: **R** _____ **L** _____ ❑ Pulse pressure: _____
    Auscultatory gap: _____
Pulses (palpated 1–4 strength): Carotid: ___ ❑ Temporal: ___
    Jugular: _____ ❑ Radial: _____ ❑ Femoral: _____
    Popliteal: _____ ❑ Post-tibial: _____ ❑ Dorsalis pedis: ___
Cardiac (palpation): Thrill: _____ ❑ Heaves: _____
Heart sounds (auscultation): Rate: _____ ❑ Rhythm: _____
    Quality: _____ ❑ Friction rub: _____
    Murmur (describe location/sounds): _____
Vascular bruit (location): _____
Jugular vein distention: _____
Breath sounds (location/describe): _____
Extremities: Temperature: _____ ❑ Color: _____
    Capillary refill (1–3 sec): _____
    Homans' sign: _____ ❑ Varicosities (location): _____
    Nail abnormalities: _____

Edema (location/severity +1–+4): _____

Distribution/quality of hair: _____

Trophic skin changes: _____

Ego Integrity

Subjective (Reports)

Relationship status: _____

Expression of concerns (e.g., financial, lifestyle, or role changes):

_____

Stress factors: _____

Usual ways of handling stress: _____

Expression of feelings: Anger: _____ ❑ Anxiety: _____

Fear: _____ ❑ Grief: _____

Helplessness: _____ ❑ Hopelessness: _____

Powerlessness: _____

Cultural factors/ethnic ties: _____

Religious affiliation: _____ ❑ Active/practicing: _____

Practices prayer/meditation: _____

Religious/spiritual concerns: _____ ❑ Desires clergy visit: _____

Expression of sense of connectedness/harmony with self and others: _____

Medications/herbals: _____

Objective (Exhibits)

Emotional status (check those that apply): Calm: _____

Anxious: _____ Angry: _____ Withdrawn: _____

Fearful: _____ Irritable: _____ Restive: _____

Euphoric: _____

Observed body language: _____

Observed physiological responses (e.g., palpitations, crying, change in voice quality/volume): _____

Changes in energy field: Temperature: _____

Color: _____ Distribution: _____

Movement: _____

Sounds: _____

Elimination

Subjective (Reports)

Usual bowel elimination pattern: _____ ❑ Character of stool (e.g., hard, soft, liquid): _____ ❑ Stool color (e.g., brown, black, yellow, clay colored, tarry): _____

Date of last BM and character of stool: _____

History of bleeding: _____ ❑ Hemorrhoids/fistula: _____

Constipation acute: _____ ❑ or chronic: _____

Diarrhea: acute: _____ ❑ or chronic: _____

Bowel incontinence: _____

Laxative: _____ ❑ how often: _____

Enema/suppository: _____ ❑ how often: _____

Usual voiding pattern and character of urine: _____
  Difficulty voiding: Urgency: _____
  Frequency: _____
  Retention: _____ ❑ Bladder spasms: _____ ❑ Burning: _____
Urinary incontinence (type/time of day usually occurs): _____
History of kidney/bladder disease: _____
Diuretic use: _____ ❑ Herbals: _____

Objective (Exhibits)

Abdomen (palpation): Soft/firm: _____
  Tenderness/pain (quadrant location): _____
  Distention: _____ ❑ Palpable mass/location: _____
  Size/girth: _____
  Abdomen (auscultation): Bowel sounds (location/type): _____
CVA tenderness: _____
Bladder palpable: _____ ❑ Overflow voiding: _____
Rectal sphincter tone (describe): _____
Hemorrhoids/fistulas: Stool in rectum: Impaction: ___ ❑ Occult
  blood (+ or −): _____
Presence/use of catheter or continence devices: _____
Ostomy appliances (describe appliance and location): _____

Food/Fluid

Subjective (Reports)

Usual diet (type): _____
Calorie/carbohydrate/protein/fat intake (g/day): _____ ❑ # of
  meals daily: _____ ❑ Snacks (number/time consumed): _____
Dietary pattern/content:
  B: _____ L: _____ D: _____
  Snacks: _____
Last meal consumed/content: _____
Food preferences: _____
Food allergies/intolerances: _____
Cultural or religious food preparation concerns/prohibitions: ___
  _____Usual appetite: _____ ❑ Change in appetite: _____
Usual weight: _____
Unexpected/undesired weight loss or gain: _____
Nausea/vomiting: ___ ❑ related to: ___ ❑ Heartburn, indiges-
  tion: _____ ❑ related to: _____ ❑ relieved by: _____
Chewing/swallowing problems: _____
  Gag/swallow reflex present: _____
  Facial injury or surgery: _____
  Stroke/other neurological deficit: _____
Teeth: Normal: _____ ❑ Dentures (full/partial): _____
  Loose/absent teeth/poor dental care: _____
Sore mouth/gums: _____
Diabetes: _____ ❑ Controlled with diet/pills/insulin: _____
Vitamin/food supplements: _____

Medications/herbals: _____

Current weight: ___ ❑ Height: ___ ❑ Body build: ___ ❑ Body
   fat %: _____
Skin turgor (e.g., firm, supple, dehydrated): _____ ❑ Mucous
   membranes (moist/dry): _____
Edema: Generalized: ___ ❑ Dependent: ___ ❑ Feet/ankles: ___
   ❑ Periorbital: _____ ❑ Abdominal/ascites: _____
Jugular vein distention: _____
Breath sounds (auscultate)/location: Faint/distant: _____
   Crackles: _____
   Wheezes: _____
Condition of teeth/gums: _____
Appearance of tongue: _____
   Mucous membranes: _____
Abdomen: Bowel sounds (quadrant location/type): _____
   Hernia/masses: _____
Urine S/A or Chemstix: _____
Serum glucose (Glucometer): _____

Hygiene

Subjective (Reports)
Ability to carry out activities of daily living: Independent/depen-
   dent (level 1 = no assistance needed to 4 = completely depen-
   dent):
Mobility: _____ ❑ Assistance needed (describe): _____
   Assistance provided by: _____
   Equipment/prosthetic devices required: _____
Feeding: _____ ❑ Can prepare food: _____
   Can feed self/use eating utensils: _____
   Equipment/prosthetic devices required: _____
Hygiene: _____ ❑ Get supplies: _____
   Wash body or body parts: _____
   Can regulate bath water temperature: _____
   Get in and out alone: _____
   Preferred time of personal care/bath: _____
Dressing: _____ ❑ Can select clothing and dress self: _____
   Needs assistance with (describe): _____
   Equipment/prosthetic devices required: _____
Toileting: _____ ❑ Can get to toilet or commode alone: _____
   Needs assistance with (describe): _____

Objective (Exhibits)
General appearance: Manner of dress: _____
   Grooming/personal habits: _____ ❑ Condition of hair/
   scalp: _____ ❑ Body odor: _____
   Presence of vermin (e.g., lice, scabies): _____

Neurosensory

Subjective (Reports)

History of brain injury, trauma, stroke (residual effects): _____

_____

Fainting spells/dizziness: _____

Headaches (location/type/frequency): _____

Tingling/numbness/weakness (location): _____

Seizures: _____ ❏ History or new onset seizures: _____

   Type (e.g., grand mal, partial): _____

   Frequency: _____ ❏ Aura: _____ ❏ Postictal state: _____

   How controlled: _____

Vision: Loss or changes in vision: _____

   Date last exam: _____ ❏ Glaucoma: _____

   Cataract: _____ ❏ Eye surgery (type/date): _____

Hearing: Loss or change: _____ ❏ Sudden or gradual: _____

   Date last exam: _____

Sense of smell (changes): _____

Sense of taste (changes): _____ ❏ Epistaxis: _____

Other: _____

Objective (Exhibits)

Mental status: (note duration of change): _____

   Oriented: Person: _____ ❏ Place: _____ ❏ Time: _____

   Situation: _____

Check all that apply: Alert: _____ ❏ Drowsy: _____ ❏ Lethar-

   gic: _____ ❏ Stuporous: _____ ❏ Comatose: _____

   Cooperative: _____ ❏ Agitated/Restless: _____

   Combative: _____

   Follows commands: _____

Delusions (describe): _____ ❏ Hallucinations (describe): _____

Affect (describe): _____ ❏ Speech: _____

Memory: Recent: _____ ❏ Remote: _____

Pupil shape: _____ ❏ Size/reaction: R/L: _____

Facial droop: _____ ❏ Swallowing: _____

Handgrasp/release: R: _____ L: _____

Coordination: _____ ❏ Balance: _____

   Walking: _____

Deep tendon reflexes (present/absent/location): _____

   Tremors: _____ ❏ Paralysis (R/L): _____

   Posturing: _____

Wears glasses: _____ ❏ Contacts: _____ ❏ Hearing aids: _____

Pain/Discomfort

Subjective (Reports)

Primary focus: Location: _____

   Intensity (use pain scale or pictures): _____

   Quality (e.g., stabbing, aching, burning): _____

   Radiation: _____ ❏ Duration: _____

Frequency: _____
Precipitating factors: _____
Relieving factors (including nonpharmaceuticals/therapies): ___
_____
Associated symptoms (e.g., nausea, sleep problems, crying): ___
_____

 Effect on daily activities: _____
 Relationships: _____ ❑ Job: _____ ❑ Enjoyment of life: _____
Additional pain focus/describe: _____
Medications: _____ ❑ Herbals: _____

Objective (Exhibits)
Facial grimacing: _____ ❑ Guarding affected area: _____
 Emotional response (e.g., crying, withdrawal, anger): _____
 Narrowed focus: _____
Vital sign changes (acute pain): BP: _____ ❑ Pulse: _____
 Respirations: _____

Respiration

Subjective (Reports)
Dyspnea/related to: _____
 Precipitating factors: _____
 Relieving factors: _____
Airway clearance (e.g., spontaneous/device): _____
Cough/describe (e.g., hard, persistent, croupy): _____
 Produces sputum (describe color/character): _____
 Requires suctioning: _____
History of (year): Bronchitis: _____ ❑ Asthma: _____
 Emphysema: _____ ❑ Tuberculosis: _____
 Recurrent pneumonia: _____
Exposure to noxious fumes/allergens, infectious agents/diseases,
 poisons/pesticides: _____
Smoker: _____ ❑ Packs/day: _____ ❑ # of years: _____
Use of respiratory aids: _____
 Oxygen (type/frequency): _____
Medications/herbals: _____

Objective (Exhibits)
Respirations (spontaneous/assisted): _____ ❑ Rate: _____
 Depth: _____
 Chest excursion (e.g., equal/unequal): _____
 Use of accessory muscles: _____
 Nasal flaring: _____ ❑ Fremitus: _____
Breath sounds (presence/absence; crackle, wheezes): _____
 Egophony: _____
Skin/mucous membrane color (e.g., pale, cyanotic): _____
Clubbing of fingers: _____
Sputum characteristics: _____

Mentation (e.g., calm, anxious, restless): _____
Pulse oximetry: _____

Safety

Subjective (Reports)
Allergies/sensitivity (medications, foods, environment, latex):
_____
Type of reaction: _____
Exposure to infectious diseases (e.g., measles, influenza, pink
eye): _____
Exposure to pollution, toxins, poisons/pesticides, radiation (de-
scribe reactions): _____
Geographic areas lived in/visited: _____
Immunization history: Tetanus: _____ ❑ Pneumonia: _____
Influenza: ___ ❑ MMR: ___ ❑ Polio: ___ ❑ Hepatitis: ___
HPV: _____
Altered/suppressed immune system (list cause): _____
History of sexually transmitted disease (date/type): _____
Testing: _____
High-risk behaviors: _____
Blood transfusion/number: _____ ❑ Date: _____
Reaction (describe): _____
Uses seat belt regularly: _____ ❑ Bike helmets: _____
Other safety devices: _____
Workplace safety/health issues (describe): _____
Currently working: _____
Rate working conditions (e.g., safety, noise, heating, water,
ventilation): _____
History of accidental injuries: _____
Fractures/dislocations: _____
Arthritis/unstable joints: _____
Back problems: _____
Skin problems (e.g., rashes, lesions, moles, breast lumps, en-
larged nodes)/describe: _____
Delayed healing (describe): _____
Cognitive limitations (e.g., disorientation, confusion): _____
Sensory limitations (e.g., impaired vision/hearing, detecting
heat/cold, taste, smell, touch): _____
Prostheses: _____ ❑ Ambulatory devices: _____
Violence (episodes or tendencies): _____

Objective (Exhibits)
Body temperature/method (e.g., **o**ral, **r**ectal, **t**ympanic): _____
Skin integrity (e.g., scars, rashes, lacerations, ulcerations,
bruises, blisters, burns [degree/%], drainage)/mark location on
diagram below:

Musculoskeletal: General strength: _____
   Muscle tone: _____ ❏ Gait: _____
   ROM: _____ ❏ Paresthesia/paralysis: _____
Results of testing (e.g., cultures, immune function, TB, hepatitis): _____

Sexuality [Component of Social Interaction]

Subjective (Reports)
Sexually active: _____ ❏ Birth control method: _____
   Use of condoms: _____
Sexual concerns/difficulties (e.g., pain, relationship, role problems): _____
_____
   Recent change in frequency/interest: _____

Female: Subjective (Reports)
Menstruation: Age at menarche: _____
   Length of cycle: _____ ❏ Duration: _____
   Number of pads/tampons used/day: _____
   Last menstrual period: ____ ❏ Bleeding between periods: ___
Reproductive: Infertility concerns: _____
   Type of therapy: _____
   Pregnant now: _____ ❏ Para: _____ ❏ Gravida: _____
   Due date: _____
Menopause: Last period: _____
   Hysterectomy (type/date): _____
   Problem with: Hot flashes: _____ ❏ Other: _____
   Vaginal lubrication: _____ ❏ Vaginal discharge: _____
Hormonal therapies: _____

Osteoporosis medications: _____
Breasts: Practices breast self-exam: _____
 Last mammogram, biopsy or surgery date: _____
Last Pap smear: _____ ❑ Results: _____

Objective (Exhibits)
Breast examination: _____
Genitalia: Warts/lesions: _____
Vaginal bleeding/discharge: _____
STD test results: _____

Male: Subjective (Reports)
Circumcised: _____ ❑ Vasectomy (date): _____
Prostate disorder: _____
Practice self-exam: Breast: _____ ❑ Testicles: _____
Last proctoscopic/prostate exam: _____
 Last PSA/date: _____
Medications/herbals: _____

Objective (Exhibits)
Genitalia: Penis: Circumcised: _____ ❑ Warts/lesions: _____
 Bleeding/discharge: _____
 Testicles (e.g., lumps): _____ ❑ Vasectomy: _____
Breast examination: _____
STD test results: _____

Social Interactions

Subjective (Reports)
Relationship status (check): Single: _____ ❑ Married: _____
 Living with partner: ___ ❑ Divorced: ___ ❑ Widowed: ___
 Years in relationship: ___ ❑ Perception of relationship: ___
 Concerns/stresses: _____
Role within family structure: _____
Number/age of children: _____
Perception of relationship with family members: _____
Extended family: _____ ❑ Other support person(s): _____
Ethnic/cultural affiliations: _____
 Strength of ethnic identity: _____
 Lives in ethnic community: _____
Feelings of (describe): Mistrust: _____
 Rejection: _____ ❑ Unhappiness: _____
 Loneliness/isolation: _____
Problems related to illness/condition: _____
Problems with communication (e.g., speech, another language,
 brain injury): _____
 Use of speech/communication aids (list): _____
 Is interpreter needed: _____
 Primary language: _____

Genogram: Diagram on separate page

Objective (Exhibits)

Communication/speech: Clear: _____ ❏ Slurred: _____

   Incomprehensible: _____ ❏ Aphasic: _____

   Unusual speech pattern/impairment: _____

   Laryngectomy present: _____

Verbal/nonverbal communication with family/SO(s): _____

   Family interaction (behavioral) pattern: _____

Teaching/Learning

Subjective (Reports)

Communication: Dominant language (specify): _____

   Second language: _____ ❏ Literate (reading/writing): _____

   Education level: _____

   Learning disabilities (specify): _____

   Cognitive limitations: _____

Culture/ethnicity: Where born: _____

   If immigrant, how long in this country: _____

Health and illness beliefs/practices/customs: _____

Which family member makes healthcare decisions/is spokesperson for client: _____

Presence of Advance Directives: _____ ❏ Code status: Durable

   Medical Power of Attorney: _____ ❏ Designee: _____

Health goals: _____

Current health problem: Client understanding of problem: _____

Special healthcare concerns (e.g., impact of religious/cultural practices): _____

Familial risk factors (indicate relationship): _____

   Diabetes: _____ ❏ Thyroid (specify): _____

   Tuberculosis: _____ ❏ Heart disease: _____

   Stroke: _____ ❏ Hypertension: _____

   Epilepsy/seizures: _____ ❏ Kidney disease: _____

   Cancer: _____ ❏ Mental illness: _____

   Depression: _____ ❏ Other: _____

Prescribed medications: _____

   Drug: _____ ❏ Dose: _____

   Times (circle last dose): _____

   Take regularly: _____ ❏ Purpose: _____

   Side effects/problems: _____

Nonprescription drugs/frequency: OTC drugs: _____

   Vitamins: _____ ❏ Herbals: _____

   Street drugs: _____

   Alcohol (amount/frequency): _____

   Tobacco: _____ ❏ Smokeless tobacco: _____

Admitting diagnosis per provider: _____

Reason for hospitalization per client: _____

History of current problem: _____

Expectations of this hospitalization: _____

Will admission cause any lifestyle changes (describe): _____

Previous illnesses and/or hospitalizations/surgeries: _____

Evidence of failure to improve: _____

Last complete physical exam: _____

Discharge Plan Considerations

Projected length of stay (days or hours): _____

Anticipated date of discharge: _____

Date information obtained: _____

Resources available: Persons: _____

    Financial: _____ ❑ Community supports: _____

    Groups: _____

Areas that may require alteration/assistance:

    Food preparation: _____ ❑ Shopping: _____

    Transportation: _____ ❑ Ambulation: _____

    Medication/IV therapy: _____

    Treatments: _____

    Wound care: _____

    Supplies/DME: _____

    Self-care (specify): _____

    Homemaker/maintenance (specify): _____

    Socialization: _____

    Physical layout of home (specify): _____

Anticipated changes in living situation after discharge: _____

    Living facility other than home (specify): _____

Referrals (date/source/services): Social services: _____

    Rehab services: _____ ❑ Dietary: _____

    Home care/hospice: _____ ❑ Resp/O_2: _____

    Equipment: _____

    Supplies: _____

Other: _____

EXCERPT FROM PSYCHIATRIC NURSING ASSESSMENT TOOL

Ego Integrity

Subjective (Reports)

What kind of person are you (positive/negative, etc.)? _____

What do you think of your body? _____

How would you rate your self-esteem (1–10; with 10 the highest)? _____

What are your problematic moods? Depressed: _____

    Guilty: _____ ❑ Unreal: _____

    Ups/downs: _____ ❑ Apathetic: _____

    Separated from the world: _____

    Detached: _____

Are you a nervous person? ___ ❑ Are your feelings easily hurt?

    _____ Report of stress factors: _____

    Previous patterns of handling stress: _____

Financial concerns: _____

Relationship status: _____

Work history/military service: _____

Cultural/ethnic factors: _____

Religion: _____ ❑ Practicing: _____

Lifestyle: _____ ❑ Recent changes: _____

    Significant losses/changes (dates): _____

Stages of grief/manifestations of loss: _____

Feelings of (check those that apply): Helplessness: _____

    Hopelessness: _____ ❑ Powerlessness: _____

    Restive: _____ ❑ Passive: _____ ❑ Dependent: _____

    Euphoric: ___ ❑ Angry/hostile: ___ ❑ Other (specify): ___

Objective (Exhibits)

Emotional status (check those that apply): Calm: _____

    Friendly: _____ Cooperative: _____ Evasive: _____

    Fearful: ___ Anxious: ___ Irritable: ___ Withdrawn: ___

Defense mechanisms: _____

    Projection: _____ ❑ Denial: _____ ❑ Undoing: _____

    Rationalization: _____ ❑ Repression: _____

    Regression: _____

    Passive/aggressive: _____ ❑ Sublimation: _____

    Intellectualization: _____ ❑ Somatization: _____

    Identification: _____ ❑ Introjection: _____

    Reaction formation: _____

    Isolation: _____ ❑ Displacement: _____

    Substitution: _____

Consistency of behavior: Verbal: _____ ❑ Nonverbal: _____

Characteristics of speech: _____

    Slow/rapid: _____ ❑ Pressured: _____

    Volume: _____ ❑ Impairments: _____

    Aphasia: _____

Motor behaviors: _____ ❑ Posturing: _____
   Restless: _____
   Underactive/overactive: _____
   Stereotypical: _____ ❑ Tics/tremors: _____
   Gait patterns: _____
Observed physiological response(s): _____

Neurosensory

Subjective (Reports)
Dreamlike states: _____ ❑ Walking in sleep: _____
   Automatic writing: _____
Believe/feel you are another person: _____
Perception different than others: _____
Ability to follow directions: _____
   Perform calculations: _____
   Accomplish ADLs: _____
Fainting spells/dizziness: _____ ❑ Blackouts: _____
   Seizures: _____

Objective (Exhibits)
Mental status (note duration of change): _____
Oriented: Person: _____ ❑ Place: _____ ❑ Time: _____
Check all that apply: Alert: _____ ❑ Drowsy: _____
   Lethargic: _____
   Stuporous: _____ ❑ Comatose: _____ ❑ Cooperative: _____
   Combative: _____ ❑ Delusions: _____ ❑ Hallucinations: _____
Memory: Immediate: _____ ❑ Recent: _____ ❑ Remote: _____
   Comprehension: _____
Thought processes (assessed through speech): Patterns of speech
   (e.g., spontaneous/sudden silences): _____
   Content: _____ ❑ Change in topic: _____
   Delusions: _____ ❑ Hallucinations: _____
   Illusions: _____
   Rate or flow: _____ ❑ Clear, logical progression: _____
   Expression: _____ ❑ Flight of ideas: _____
   Ability to concentrate: _____ ❑ Attention span: _____
Mood: Affect: _____ ❑ Appropriateness: _____
   Intensity: _____
   Range: _____
Insight: _____ ❑ Misperceptions: _____
Attention/calculation skills: _____
   Judgment: _____
   Ability to follow directions: _____
   Problem solving: _____
Impulse control: Aggression: _____ ❑ Hostility: _____
   Affection: _____
Sexual feelings: _____

EXCERPT FROM PRENATAL ASSESSMENT TOOL

Safety

Subjective (Reports)

Allergies/sensitivity: _____

    Reaction: _____

Previous alteration of immune system: _____

    Cause: _____

History of sexually transmitted diseases/gynecological infections (date/type): _____

    Testing/date: _____

High-risk behaviors: _____

Blood transfusion/number: _____ ❑ When: _____

    Reaction: _____

    Describe: _____

Childhood diseases: _____

    Immunization history/date: Tetanus: _____

    Pneumonia: _____

    Influenza: _____ ❑ Hepatitis: _____ ❑ MMR: _____

    Polio: _____ ❑ HPV: _____

Recent exposure to German measles: _____

    Other viral infections: _____

    X-ray/radiation: _____ ❑ House pets: _____

Previous obstetric problems: PIH: _____ ❑ Kidney: _____

    Hemorrhage: _____ ❑ Cardiac: _____

    Diabetes: _____ ❑ Infection/UTI: _____ ❑ ABO/Rh sensitivity: _____ ❑ Uterine surgery: _____

    Anemia: _____ ❑ Explain "yes" responses: _____

Length of time since last pregnancy: _____

    Type of previous delivery: _____

History of accidental injuries: Fractures/dislocations: _____

    Physical abuse: _____

    Arthritis/unstable joints: _____

    Back problems: _____

Changes in moles: _____ ❑ Enlarged nodes: _____

Impaired vision: _____ ❑ Hearing: _____

Prostheses: _____ ❑ Ambulatory devices: _____

Objective (Exhibits)

Temperature: _____ ❑ Diaphoresis: _____

Skin integrity: _____ ❑ Scars: _____ ❑ Rashes: _____

    Ecchymosis: _____ ❑ Genital warts/lesions: _____

General strength: _____ ❑ Muscle tone: _____

    Gait: _____

    ROM: _____ ❑ Paresthesia/paralysis: _____

Fetal: Heart rate: _____ ❑ Location: _____

    Method of auscultation: _____ ❑ Fundal height: _____

    Estimated gestation (weeks): _____ ❑ Movement: _____

Ballottement: _____

Fetal testing: Date: _____ ❑ Test: _____ ❑ Result: _____
AFT: _____

Screenings: Serology: _____ ❑ Syphilis: _____
Sickle cell: _____ ❑ Rubella: _____
Hepatitis: _____ ❑ HIV: _____ ❑ AFP: _____

Results of cultures (cervical/rectal): _____
Immune system testing: _____

Blood type: Maternal: _____ ❑ Paternal: _____

Sexuality (Component of Social Interactions)

Subjective (Reports)

Sexual concerns: _____

Menarche: _____ ❑ Length of cycle (days): _____
Duration (days): _____

First day of last menstrual period: _____ ❑ Amount: _____
Bleeding/cramping since LMP: _____
Vaginal discharge: _____

Client's belief of when conception occurred: _____

Estimated date of delivery: _____

Last Pap smear: _____ ❑ Practices breast self-examination: _____

Recent contraceptive method: _____

OB history (GPTPAL): Gravida: ___ ❑ Para: ___ ❑ Term: ___
Preterm: _____ ❑ Abortions: _____ ❑ Living: _____ ❑ Multiple
births: _____

Delivery history: Year: _____ ❑ Place of delivery: _____
Length of gestation (weeks): _____
Length of labor (hours): _____ ❑ Type of delivery: _____
Born (alive): _____ ❑ Weight: _____ ❑ Apgar scores: _____

Complications (maternal/fetal): _____

Objective (Exhibits)

Pelvic: Vulva: _____ ❑ Perineum: _____ ❑ Vagina: _____
Cervix: _____ ❑ Uterus: _____ ❑ Adnexal: _____
Diagonal conjugate: _____
Transverse: _____ ❑ Diameter: _____ ❑ Outlet (cm): _____
Shape of sacrum: _____ ❑ Arch: _____ ❑ Coccyx: _____
SS notch: _____
Ischial spines: _____
Adequacy of inlet: _____ ❑ Mid: _____ ❑ Outlet: _____

Prognosis for delivery: _____

Breast exam: _____ ❑ Nipples: _____

Pregnancy test: _____ ❑ Serology test (date): _____

Pap smear results: _____

EXCERPT FROM INTRAPARTAL ASSESSMENT TOOL

Pain/Discomfort

Subjective (Reports)
Uterine contractions began: _____ ❑ Became regular: _____
   Character: ____ ❑ Frequency (minutes): ____ ❑ Duration: ____
Location of contractile pain (check): Front: ____ Sacral area: ____
Degree of discomfort (check): Mild: _____ Moderate: _____
   Severe: _____
How relieved: Breathing/relaxation techniques: _____
   Positioning: _____ ❑ Sacral rubs: _____ ❑ Effleurage: _____
   Other: _____

Objective (Exhibits)
Facial expression: _____ ❑ Narrowed focus: _____
Body movement: _____ ❑ Change in BP: _____ ❑ Pulse: _____

Safety

Subjective (Reports)
Allergies/sensitivity: _____
   Reaction (specify): _____
History of STD (date/type): _____
Month of first prenatal visit: _____
Previous/current obstetric problems/treatment:
   PIH: ____ ❑ Kidney: ____ ❑ Hemorrhage: ____ ❑ Cardiac: ____
   Diabetes: _____ ❑ Infection/UTI: _____
   ABO/Rh sensitivity: _____ ❑ Anemia: _____
   Uterine surgery: _____
Length of time since last pregnancy: _____
Type of previous delivery: _____
Health status of living children: _____
Blood transfusion: _____ ❑ When: _____
   Reaction (describe): _____
Maternal stature/build: _____
   Pelvis: _____
Fractures/dislocations: _____ ❑ Arthritis/unstable joints: _____
Spinal problems/deformity: Kyphosis: _____ ❑ Scoliosis: _____
   Trauma: _____
   Surgery: _____
Prosthesis: _____ ❑ Ambulatory devices: _____

Objective (Exhibits)
Temperature: _____
Skin integrity: _____ ❑ Rashes: _____ ❑ Sores: _____
   Bruises: _____ ❑ Scars: _____
Paresthesia/paralysis: _____

Fetal status: Heart rate: _____ ❑ Location: _____
   Method of auscultation: _____
   Fundal height: _____ ❑ Estimated gestation (weeks): _____
   Activity/movement: _____
   Fetal assessment/testing: Test: _____
   Date: _____ ❑ Results: _____
Labor status: Cervical dilation: _____ ❑ Effacement: _____
   Fetal descent: _____ ❑ Engagement: _____
   Presentation: _____ ❑ Lie: _____ ❑ Position: _____
Membranes: Intact: _____ ❑ Ruptured/time: _____
   Nitrazine test (+/−): _____
   Amount of drainage: _____ ❑ Character: _____
Blood type/Rh: Maternal: _____ ❑ Paternal: _____
Screens (check): Sickle cell: _____ ❑ Rubella: _____
   ❑ Hepatitis: _____ ❑ HIV: _____ ❑ TB: _____ ❑ HPV: _____
Serology: Syphilis (+/−): _____ ❑ Cervical/rectal culture
   (+/−): _____
Vaginal warts/lesions: _____ ❑ Perineal varicosities: _____

SECTION 2

Diagnostic Divisions: Nursing Diagnoses Organized According to a Nursing Focus

After data are collected and areas of concern or need identified, the nurse is directed to the Diagnostic Divisions to review the list of nursing diagnoses that fall within the individual categories. This will assist the nurse in choosing the specific diagnostic label to accurately describe the data. Then, with the addition of etiology or related/risk factors and signs and symptoms or cues (defining characteristics) when present, the client diagnostic statement emerges.

ACTIVITY/REST—Ability to engage in necessary or desired activities of life (work and leisure) and to obtain adequate sleep or rest

Activity Intolerance [specify level]
Activity Intolerance, risk for
Activity Planning, ineffective
Disuse Syndrome, risk for
Diversional Activity, deficient
Fatigue
Insomnia
Lifestyle, sedentary
Mobility, impaired bed
Mobility, impaired wheelchair
Sleep, readiness for enhanced
Sleep Deprivation
Sleep Pattern, disturbed
Transfer Ability, impaired
Walking, impaired

CIRCULATION—Ability to transport oxygen and nutrients necessary to meet cellular needs

Autonomic Dysreflexia
Autonomic Dysreflexia, risk for
Bleeding, risk for
Cardiac Output, decreased
Intracranial Adaptive Capacity, decreased
Perfusion, ineffective peripheral tissue

Perfusion, risk for decreased cardiac tissue
Perfusion, risk for ineffective cerebral tissue
Perfusion, risk for ineffective gastrointestinal
Perfusion, risk for ineffective renal
Shock, risk for

EGO INTEGRITY—Ability to develop and use skills and behaviors to integrate and manage life experiences*

Anxiety [specify level: mild, moderate, severe, panic]
Anxiety, death
Behavior, risk-prone health
Body Image, disturbed
Conflict, decisional [specify]
Coping, defensive
Coping, ineffective
Coping, readiness for enhanced
Decision Making, readiness for enhanced
Denial, ineffective
Dignity, risk for compromised human
Distress, moral
Energy Field, disturbed
Fear
Grieving
Grieving, complicated
Grieving, risk for complicated
Hope, readiness for enhanced
Hopelessness
Identity, disturbed personal
Post-Trauma Syndrome [specify stage]
Post-Trauma Syndrome, risk for
Power, readiness for enhanced
Powerlessness [specify level]
Powerlessness, risk for
Rape-Trauma Syndrome
[Rape-Trauma Syndrome: compound reaction]
[Rape-Trauma Syndrome: silent reaction]
Relationship, readiness for enhanced
Religiosity, impaired
Religiosity, readiness for enhanced
Religiosity, risk for impaired
Relocation Stress Syndrome
Relocation Stress Syndrome, risk for
Resilience, impaired individual
Resilience, readiness for enhanced
Resilience, risk for compromised
Self-Concept, readiness for enhanced
Self-Esteem, chronic low
Self-Esteem, situational low
Self-Esteem, risk for situational low

Sorrow, chronic
Spiritual Distress
Spiritual Distress, risk for
Spiritual Well-Being, readiness for enhanced

ELIMINATION—Ability to excrete waste products*

Bowel Incontinence
Constipation
Constipation, perceived
Constipation, risk for
Diarrhea
Motility, dysfunctional gastrointestinal
Motility, risk for dysfunctional gastrointestinal
Urinary Elimination, impaired
Urinary Elimination, readiness for enhanced
Urinary Incontinence, functional
Urinary Incontinence, overflow
Urinary Incontinence, reflex
Urinary Incontinence, risk for urge
Urinary Incontinence, stress
[Urinary Incontinence, total]
Urinary Incontinence, urge
Urinary Retention [acute/chronic]

FOOD/FLUID—Ability to maintain intake of and utilize nutrients and liquids to meet physiological needs*

Breastfeeding [Learning Need], effective
Breastfeeding, ineffective
Breastfeeding, interrupted
Dentition, impaired
Electrolyte Imbalance, risk for
Failure to Thrive, adult
Feeding Pattern, ineffective infant
Fluid Balance, readiness for enhanced
[Fluid Volume, deficient hyper/hypotonic]
Fluid Volume, deficient [isotonic]
Fluid Volume, excess
Fluid Volume, risk for deficient
Fluid Volume, risk for imbalanced
Glucose Level, risk for unstable blood
Liver Function, risk for impaired
Nausea
Nutrition: less than body requirements, imbalanced
Nutrition: more than body requirements, imbalanced
Nutrition: more than body requirements, risk for imbalanced
Nutrition, readiness for enhanced
Oral Mucous Membrane, impaired
Swallowing, impaired

HYGIENE—Ability to perform activities of daily living

Neglect, self
Self-Care, readiness for enhanced
Self-Care Deficit, bathing
Self-Care Deficit, dressing
Self-Care Deficit, feeding
Self-Care Deficit, toileting

NEUROSENSORY—Ability to perceive, integrate, and respond to internal and external cues

Confusion, acute
Confusion, risk for acute
Confusion, chronic
Infant Behavior, disorganized
Infant Behavior, readiness for enhanced organized
Infant Behavior, risk for disorganized
Memory, impaired
Neglect, unilateral
Peripheral Neurovascular Dysfunction, risk for
Sensory Perception, disturbed (specify: visual, auditory, kinesthetic, gustatory, tactile, olfactory)
Stress Overload
[Thought Processes, disturbed]

PAIN/DISCOMFORT—Ability to control internal and external environment to maintain comfort

Comfort, impaired
Comfort, readiness for enhanced
Pain, acute
Pain, chronic

RESPIRATION—Ability to provide and use oxygen to meet physiological needs

Airway Clearance, ineffective
Aspiration, risk for
Breathing Pattern, ineffective
Gas Exchange, impaired
Ventilation, impaired spontaneous
Ventilatory Weaning Response, dysfunctional

SAFETY—Ability to provide safe, growth-promoting environment

Allergy Response, latex
Allergy Response, risk for latex
Body Temperature, risk for imbalanced
Contamination
Contamination, risk for
Death Syndrome, risk for sudden infant
Environmental Interpretation Syndrome, impaired
Falls, risk for

Health Maintenance, ineffective
Home Maintenance, impaired
Hyperthermia
Hypothermia
Immunization Status, readiness for enhanced
Infection, risk for
Injury, risk for
Injury, risk for perioperative positioning
Jaundice, neonatal
Maternal/Fetal Dyad, risk for disturbed
Mobility, impaired physical
Poisoning, risk for
Protection, ineffective
Self-Mutilation
Self-Mutilation, risk for
Skin Integrity, impaired
Skin Integrity, risk for impaired
Suffocation, risk for
Suicide, risk for
Surgical Recovery, delayed
Thermoregulation, ineffective
Tissue Integrity, impaired
Trauma, risk for
Trauma, risk for vascular
Violence, [actual/]risk for other-directed
Violence, [actual/]risk for self-directed
Wandering [specify sporadic or continual]

SEXUALITY—[Component of Ego Integrity and Social Interaction] Ability to meet requirements/characteristics of male/female role*

Childbearing Process, readiness for enhanced
Sexual Dysfunction
Sexuality Pattern, ineffective

SOCIAL INTERACTION—Ability to establish and maintain relationships*

Attachment, risk for impaired
Caregiver Role Strain
Caregiver Role Strain, risk for
Communication, impaired verbal
Communication, readiness for enhanced
Conflict, parental role
Coping, compromised family
Coping, disabled family
Coping, ineffective community
Coping, readiness for enhanced community
Coping, readiness for enhanced family
Family Processes, dysfunctional
Family Processes, interrupted

Family Processes, readiness for enhanced
Loneliness, risk for
Parenting, impaired
Parenting, readiness for enhanced
Parenting, risk for impaired
Role Performance, ineffective
Social Interaction, impaired
Social Isolation

TEACHING/LEARNING—Ability to incorporate and use information to achieve healthy lifestyle/optimal wellness*

Development, risk for delayed
Growth, risk for disproportionate
Growth and Development, delayed
Health Management, ineffective self
Health Management, readiness for enhanced self
Knowledge [Learning Need] (specify), deficient
Knowledge, readiness for enhanced
Noncompliance [ineffective Adherence] [specify]
[Therapeutic Regimen Management, effective]
[Therapeutic Regimen Management, ineffective community]
Therapeutic Regimen Management, ineffective family

Please also see the NANDA-I diagnoses grouped according to Gordon's Functional Health Patterns on the inside front cover.

*Information that appears in brackets has been added by authors to clarify and enhance the use of nursing diagnoses.

Client Situation and Prototype Plan of Care

Client Situation

Mr. R. S., a client with type 2 diabetes (non-insulin-dependent) for 10 years, presented to his physician's office with a nonhealing ulcer of 3 weeks' duration on his left foot. Screening studies done in the doctor's office revealed blood glucose of 356/fingerstick and urine Chemstix of 2%. Because of distance from medical provider and lack of local community services, he is admitted to the hospital.

Admitting Physician's Orders

Culture/sensitivity and Gram's stain of foot ulcer
Random blood glucose on admission and fingerstick BG qid
CBC, electrolytes, serum lipid profile, glycosylated Hb in AM
Chest x-ray and ECG in AM
DiaBeta 10 mg, PO bid
Glucophage 500 mg, PO daily to start—will increase gradually
Humulin N 10 U SC q AM and HS. Begin insulin instruction for
    postdischarge self-care if necessary
Dicloxacillin 500 mg PO q6h, start after culture obtained
Darvocet-N 100 mg PO q4h prn pain
Diet—2400 calories, 3 meals with 2 snacks
Up in chair ad lib with feet elevated
Foot cradle for bed
Irrigate lesion L foot with NS tid, then cover with wet to dry ster-
    ile dressing
Vital signs qid

Client Assessment Database

Name: R. S.   Informant: client
Reliability (Scale 1–4): 3
Age: 71   DOB: 5/3/38   Race: Caucasian   Gender: M
Adm. date: 6/28/2009   Time: 7 PM   From: home

Activity/Rest

Subjective (Reports)

Occupation: farmer
Usual activities/hobbies: reading, playing cards. "Don't have time to do much. Anyway, I'm too tired most of the time to do anything after the chores."

Limitations imposed by illness: "Have to watch what I order if I eat out."
Sleep: Hours: 6 to 8 hr/night   Naps: no   Aids: no
Insomnia: "Not unless I drink coffee after supper."
Usually feels rested when awakens at 4:30 AM

Objective (Exhibits)

Observed response to activity: limps, favors L foot when walking
Mental status: alert/active
Neuromuscular assessment: Muscle mass/tone: bilaterally equal/ firm Posture: erect
ROM: full Strength: equal 4 extremities/(favors L foot currently)

Circulation

Subjective (Reports)

History of slow healing: lesion L foot, 3 weeks' duration
Extremities: Numbness/tingling: "My feet feel cold and tingly like sharp pins poking the bottom of my feet when I walk the quarter mile to the mailbox."
Cough/character of sputum: occ./white
Change in frequency/amount of urine: yes/voiding more lately

Objective (Exhibits)

Peripheral pulses: radials 3+; popliteal, dorsalis, post-tibial/ pedal, all 1+
BP: R: Lying: 146/90   Sitting: 140/86   Standing: 138/90
   L: Lying: 142/88   Sitting: 138/88   Standing: 138/84
Pulse: Apical: 86   Radial: 86   Quality: strong
   Rhythm: regular
Chest auscultation: few wheezes clear with cough, no murmurs/ rubs
Jugular vein distention: 0
Extremities:

Temperature: feet cool bilaterally/legs warm
Color: Skin: legs pale
Capillary refill: slow both feet (approx. 4 sec)
Homans' sign: 0
Varicosities: few enlarged superficial veins both calves
Nails: toenails thickened, yellow, brittle
Distribution and quality of hair: coarse hair to midcalf; none on ankles/toes

Color:

General: ruddy face/arms
Mucous membranes/lips: pink
Nailbeds: pink
Conjunctiva and sclera: white

Ego Integrity

Subjective (Reports)

Report of stress factors: "Normal farmer's problems: weather, pests, bankers, etc."

Ways of handling stress: "I get busy with the chores and talk things over with my livestock. They listen pretty good."

Financial concerns: Medicare only and needs to hire someone to do chores while here

Relationship status: married

Cultural factors: rural/agrarian, eastern European descent, "American," no ethnic ties

Religion: Protestant/practicing

Lifestyle: middle class/self-sufficient farmer

Recent changes: no

Feelings: "I'm in control of most things, except the weather and this diabetes now."

Concerned re possible therapy change "from pills to shots."

Objective (Exhibits)

Emotional status: generally calm, appears frustrated at times

Observed physiological response(s): occasionally sighs deeply/frowns, fidgeting with coin, shoulders tense/shrugs shoulders, throws up hands

Elimination

Subjective (Reports)

Usual bowel pattern: almost every PM

Last BM: last night Character of stool: firm/brown
    Bleeding: 0   Hemorrhoids: 0   Constipation: occ.

Laxative used: hot prune juice on occ.

Urinary: no problems Character of urine: pale yellow

Objective (Exhibits)

Abdomen tender: no Soft/firm: soft Palpable mass: 0

Bowel sounds: active all 4 quads

Food/Fluid

Subjective (Reports)

Usual diet (type): 2400 calorie (occ. "cheats" with dessert; "My wife watches it pretty closely.")

No. of meals daily: 3/1 snack

Dietary pattern:

B: fruit juice/toast/ham/decaf coffee

L: meat/potatoes/veg/fruit/milk

D: $\frac{1}{2}$ meat sandwich/soup/fruit/decaf coffee

Snack: milk/crackers at HS. Usual beverage: skim milk, 2 to 3 cups decaf coffee, drinks "lots of water"—several quarts

Last meal/intake: Dinner: $\frac{1}{2}$ roast beef sandwich, vegetable soup, pear with cheese, decaf coffee

Loss of appetite: "Never, but lately I don't feel as hungry as usual."

Nausea/vomiting: 0   Food allergies: none

Heartburn/food intolerance: cabbage causes gas, coffee after supper causes heartburn

Mastication/swallowing problems: 0
   Dentures: partial upper plate—fits well

Usual weight: 175 lb Recent changes: has lost about 6 lb this month

Diuretic therapy: no

Objective (Exhibits)

Wt: 171 lb   Ht: 5 ft 10 in.   Build: stocky

Skin turgor: good/leathery Mucous membranes: moist

Condition of teeth/gums: good, no irritation/bleeding noted

Appearance of tongue: midline, pink

Mucous membranes: pink, intact

Breath sounds: few wheezes cleared with cough

Bowel sounds: active all 4 quads

Urine Chemstix: 2%   Fingerstick: 356 (Dr. office) 450 random BG on adm

Hygiene

Subjective (Reports)

Activities of daily living: independent in all areas

Preferred time of bath: PM

Objective (Exhibits)

General appearance: clean, shaven, short-cut hair; hands rough and dry; skin on feet dry, cracked, and scaly

Scalp and eyebrows: scaly white patches

No body odor

Neurosensory

Subjective (Reports)

Headache: "Occasionally behind my eyes when I worry too much."

Tingling/numbness: feet, 4 or 5 times/week (as noted)

Eyes: Vision loss, farsighted, "Seems a little blurry now." Examination: 2 yrs ago

Ears: Hearing loss R: "Some." L: no (has not been tested)

Nose: Epistaxis: 0   Sense of smell: "No problem."

Objective (Exhibits)

Mental status: alert, oriented to person, place, time, situation

Affect: concerned   Memory: Remote/recent: clear and intact

Speech: clear/coherent, appropriate
Pupil reaction: PERRLA/small
Glasses: reading   Hearing aid: no
Handgrip/release: strong/equal

Pain/Discomfort

Subjective (Reports)

Primary focus: Location: medial aspect, L heel
Intensity (0–10): 4 to 5   Quality: dull ache with occ. sharp
   stabbing sensation
Frequency/duration: "Seems like all the time."
   Radiation: no
Precipitating factors: shoes, walking
   How relieved: ASA, not helping
Other complaints: sometimes has back pain following chores/
   heavy lifting, relieved by ASA/liniment rubdown

Objective (Exhibits)

Facial grimacing: when lesion border palpated
Guarding affected area: pulls foot away
Narrowed focus: no
Emotional response: tense, irritated

Respiration

Subjective (Reports)

Dyspnea: 0   Cough: occ. morning cough, white sputum
Emphysema: 0   Bronchitis: 0   Asthma: 0   Tuberculosis: 0
Smoker: filters Pk/day: $\frac{1}{2}$ No. yrs: 50+
Use of respiratory aids: 0

Objective (Exhibits)

Respiratory rate: 22   Depth: good   Symmetry: equal, bilateral
Auscultation: few wheezes, clear with cough
Cyanosis: 0   Clubbing of fingers: 0
Sputum characteristics: none to observe
Mentation/restlessness: alert/oriented/relaxed

Safety

Subjective (Reports)

Allergies: 0   Blood transfusions: 0
Sexually transmitted disease: 0
Wears seat belt
Fractures/dislocations: L clavicle, 1960s, fell getting off tractor
Arthritis/unstable joints: "Some in my knees."
Back problems: occ. lower back pain
Vision impaired: requires glasses for reading

Hearing impaired: slightly (R), compensates by turning "good ear" toward speaker

Immunizations: current flu/pneumonia 3 yrs ago/tetanus maybe 8 yrs ago

Objective (Exhibits)

Temperature: 99.4°F (37.4°C) Tympanic

Skin integrity: impaired L foot   Scars: R inguinal, surgical

Rashes: 0   Bruises: 0   Lacerations: 0   Blisters: 0

Ulcerations: medial aspect L heel, 2.5-cm diameter, approx.
   3 mm deep, wound edges inflamed, draining small amount cream-color/pink-tinged matter, slight musty odor noted

Strength (general): equal all extremities   Muscle tone: firm

ROM: good   Gait: favors L foot   Paresthesia/paralysis:
   tingling, prickly sensation in feet after walking $\frac{1}{4}$ mile

Sexuality: Male

Subjective (Reports)

Sexually active: yes   Use of condoms: no (monogamous)

Recent changes in frequency/interest: "I've been too tired lately."

Penile discharge: 0   Prostate disorder: 0   Vasectomy: 0

Last proctoscopic examination: 2 yrs ago   Prostate examination: 1 yr ago

Practice self-examination: Breasts/testicles: no

Problems/complaints: "I don't have any problems, but you'd have to ask my wife if there are any complaints."

Objective (Exhibits)

Examination: Breasts: no masses   Testicles: deferred
   Prostate: deferred

Social Interactions

Subjective (Reports)

Marital status: married 45 yrs   Living with: wife

Report of problems: none

Extended family: 1 daughter lives in town (30 miles away); 1 daughter married/grandson, living out of state

Other: several couples, he and wife play cards/socialize with 2 to 3 times/mo, church fellowship weekly

Role: works farm alone; husband/father/grandfather

Report of problems related to illness/condition: none until now

Coping behaviors: "My wife and I have always talked things out. You know the 11th commandment is 'Thou shalt not go to bed angry.'"

Objective (Exhibits)

Speech: clear, intelligible

Verbal/nonverbal communication with family/SO(s): speaks quietly with wife, looking her in the eye; relaxed posture

Family interaction patterns: wife sitting at bedside, relaxed, both reading paper, making occasional comments to each other

Teaching/Learning

Subjective (Reports)

Dominant language: English   Second language: 0   Literate: yes

Education level: 2-yr college

Health and illness/beliefs/practices/customs: "I take care of the minor problems and see the doctor only when something's broken."

Presence of Advance Directives: yes—wife to bring in

Durable Medical Power of Attorney: wife

Familial risk factors/relationship:

    Diabetes: maternal uncle

    Tuberculosis: brother died, age 27

    Heart disease: father died, age 78, heart attack

    Strokes: mother died, age 81

    High BP: mother

Prescribed medications:

    Drug: DiaBeta Dose: 10 mg bid

    Schedule: 8 AM/6 PM, last dose 6 PM today

    Purpose: control diabetes

    Takes medications regularly? yes

    Home urine/glucose monitoring: "Only using TesTape, stopped some months ago when I ran out. It was always negative, anyway."

Nonprescription (OTC) drugs: occ. ASA

Use of alcohol (amount/frequency): socially, occ. beer

Tobacco: $\frac{1}{2}$ pk/day

Admitting diagnosis (physician): hyperglycemia with nonhealing lesion L foot

Reason for hospitalization (client): "Sore on foot and the doctor is concerned about my blood sugar, and says I'm supposed to learn this fingerstick test now."

History of current complaint: "Three weeks ago I got a blister on my foot from breaking in my new boots. It got sore so I lanced it but it isn't getting any better."

Client's expectations of this hospitalization: "Clear up this infection and control my diabetes."

Other relevant illness and/or previous hospitalizations/surgeries: 1960s, R inguinal hernia repair, tonsils age 5 or 6

Evidence of failure to improve: lesion L foot, 3 wk

Last physical examination: complete 1 yr ago, office follow-up 5 mo ago

Discharge Considerations (as of 6/28)

Anticipated discharge: 7/1/09 (3 days)

Resources: self, wife

Financial: "If this doesn't take too long to heal, we got some savings to cover things."

Community supports: diabetic support group (has not participated)

Anticipated lifestyle changes: become more involved in management of condition

Assistance needed: may require farm help for several days

Teaching: learn new medication regimen and wound care; review diet; encourage smoking cessation

Referral: Supplies: the Downtown Pharmacy or AARP

Equipment: Glucometer—AARP

Follow-up: primary care provider 1 wk after discharge to evaluate wound healing and potential need for additional changes in diabetic regimen

PLAN OF CARE FOR CLIENT WITH DIABETES MELLITUS

Client Diagnostic Statement:
impaired Skin Integrity related to pressure, altered metabolic state, circulatory impairment, and decreased sensation, as evidenced by draining wound L foot.

Outcome: Wound Healing: Secondary Intention (NOC) Indicators: Client Will:
Be free of purulent drainage within 48 hr (6/30 1900).
Display signs of healing with wound edges clean/pink within 60 hr (7/1 0700).

ACTIONS/ INTERVENTIONS	RATIONALE
Wound Care (NIC)	
Irrigate wound with room temperature sterile NS tid.	Cleans wound without harming delicate tissues.
Assess wound with each dressing change. Obtain wound tracing on adm and at discharge.	Provides information about effectiveness of therapy, and identifies additional needs.
Apply wet to dry sterile dressing.	Keeps wound clean/minimizes cross contamination.
Use paper tape.	Adhesive tape may be abrasive to fragile tissues.
Infection Control (NIC)	
Follow wound precautions.	Use of gloves and proper handling of contaminated dressings reduces likelihood of spread of infection.
Obtain sterile specimen of wound drainage on admission.	Culture/sensitivity identifies pathogens and therapy of choice.
Administer dicloxacillin 500 mg PO q6h, starting 10 PM.	Treatment of infection and prevention of complications. Food interferes with drug absorption, requiring scheduling around meals.
Observe for signs of hypersensitivity: pruritus, urticaria, rash.	Although no history of penicillin reaction, it may occur at any time.

Client Diagnostic Statement:
unstable blood Glucose Level related to lack of adherence to diabetes management and inadequate blood glucose monitoring as evidenced by fingerstick 450/adm.

Outcome: Blood Glucose Level (NOC)
Indicators: Client Will:

Demonstrate correction of metabolic state as evidenced by FBS less than 120 mg/dL within 36 hr (6/30 0700).

ACTIONS/ INTERVENTIONS	RATIONALE
Hyperglycemia Management (NIC)	
Perform fingerstick BG qid.	Bedside analysis of blood glucose levels is a more timely method for monitoring effectiveness of therapy and provides direction for alteration of medications.
Administer antidiabetic medications:	Treats underlying metabolic dysfunction, reducing hyperglycemia and promoting healing.
10 U Humulin N insulin SC q AM/HS after fingerstick BG;	Intermediate-acting preparation with onset of 2–4 hr, peak 6–12 hr, and duration 18–24 hr. Increases transport of glucose into cells and promotes the conversion of glucose to glycogen.
DiaBeta 10 mg PO bid;	Lowers blood glucose by stimulating the release of insulin from the pancreas and increasing the sensitivity to insulin at the receptor sites.
Glucophage 500 mg PO daily. Note onset of side effects.	Glucophage lowers serum glucose levels by decreasing hepatic glucose production and intestinal glucose absorption, and increasing sensitivity to insulin. By using in conjunction with DiaBeta, client may be able to discontinue insulin once target dosage is achieved (e.g., 2000 mg/day). Increase of 1 tablet per week is necessary to limit side effects of diarrhea, abdominal cramping, vomiting, possibly leading to

ACTIONS/ INTERVENTIONS	RATIONALE
	dehydration and prerenal azotemia.
Provide diet 2400 cals—3 meals/2 snacks.	Proper diet decreases glucose levels/insulin needs, prevents hyperglycemic episodes, can reduce serum cholesterol levels, and promote satiation.
Schedule consultation with dietitian to restructure meal plan and evaluate food choices.	Calories are unchanged on new orders but have been redistributed to 3 meals and 2 snacks. Dietary choices (e.g., increased vitamin C) may enhance healing.

Client Diagnostic Statement:
acute Pain related to physical agent (open wound L foot), as evidenced by verbal report of pain and guarding behavior.

Outcome: Pain Control (NOC) Indicators: Client Will:
Report pain is minimized/relieved within 1 hr of analgesic administration (ongoing).
Report absence or control of pain by discharge (7/1).

Outcome: Pain Disruptive Effects (NOC) Indicators: Client Will:
Ambulate normally, full weight bearing by discharge (7/1).

ACTIONS/ INTERVENTIONS	RATIONALE
Pain Management (NIC)	
Determine pain characteristics through client's description.	Establishes baseline for assessing improvement/ changes.
Place foot cradle on bed; encourage use of loose-fitting slipper when up.	Avoids direct pressure to area of injury, which could result in vasoconstriction/ increased pain.
Administer Darvocet-N 100 mg PO q4h as needed. Document effectiveness.	Provides relief of discomfort when unrelieved by other measures.

Client Diagnostic Statement:
ineffective peripheral tissue Perfusion related to decreased arterial flow evidenced by decreased pulses, pale/cool feet; thick, brittle nails; numbness/tingling of feet "when walks $\frac{1}{4}$ mile."

Outcome: Knowledge: Diabetes Management (NOC) Indicators: Client Will:

Verbalize understanding of relationship between chronic disease (diabetes mellitus) and circulatory changes within 48 hr (6/30 1900).

Demonstrate awareness of safety factors and proper foot care within 48 hr (6/30 1900).

Maintain adequate level of hydration to maximize perfusion, as evidenced by balanced intake/output, moist skin/mucous membranes, capillary refill less than 3 sec (ongoing).

ACTIONS/ INTERVENTIONS	RATIONALE
Circulatory Care: Arterial Insufficiency (NIC)	
Elevate feet when up in chair. Avoid long periods with feet in dependent position.	Minimizes interruption of blood flow, reduces venous pooling.
Assess for signs of dehydration.	Glycosuria may result in dehydration with consequent reduction of circulating volume and further impairment of peripheral circulation.
Monitor intake/output. Encourage oral fluids.	
Instruct client to avoid constricting clothing/socks and ill-fitting shoes.	Compromised circulation and decreased pain sensation may precipitate or aggravate tissue breakdown.
Reinforce safety precautions regarding use of heating pads, hot water bottles, or soaks.	Heat increases metabolic demands on compromised tissues. Vascular insufficiency alters pain sensation, increasing risk of injury.
Recommend cessation of smoking.	Vascular constriction associated with smoking and diabetes impairs peripheral circulation.
Discuss complications of disease that result from vascular changes: ulceration, gangrene, muscle or bony structure changes.	Although proper control of diabetes mellitus may not prevent complications, severity of effect may be minimized. Diabetic foot complications are the leading cause of nontraumatic lower extremity amputations.

ACTIONS/ INTERVENTIONS	RATIONALE
	Note: Skin dry, cracked, scaly; feet cool; pain when walking a distance suggest mild to moderate vascular disease (autonomic neuropathy) that can limit response to infection, impair wound healing, and increase risk of bony deformities.
Review proper foot care as outlined in teaching plan.	Altered perfusion of lower extremities may lead to serious or persistent complications at the cellular level.

Client Diagnostic Statement:

deficient Knowledge/Learning Need regarding diabetic condition related to misinterpretation of information and/or lack of recall as evidenced by inaccurate follow-through of instructions regarding home glucose monitoring and foot care, and failure to recognize signs/symptoms of hyperglycemia.

Outcome: Knowledge: Diabetes Management (NOC) Indicators: Client Will:

Perform procedure for home glucose monitoring correctly within 36 hr (6/30 0700).

Verbalize basic understanding of disease process and treatment within 38 hr (6/30 0900).

Explain reasons for actions within 38 hr (6/30 0900).

Perform insulin administration correctly within 60 hr (7/1 0700).

ACTIONS/ INTERVENTIONS	RATIONALE
Teaching: Disease Process (NIC)	
Determine client's level of knowledge, priorities of learning needs, desire/need for including wife in instruction.	Establishes baseline and direction for teaching/ planning. Involvement of wife, if desired, will provide additional resource for recall/understanding and may enhance client's follow through.
Provide teaching guide, "Understanding Your Diabetes," 6/29 AM. Show film "Living with Diabetes" 6/29 4 PM, when wife is visiting. Include in group	Provides different methods for accessing/reinforcing information and enhances opportunity for learning/ understanding.

ACTIONS/ INTERVENTIONS

RATIONALE

teaching session 6/30 AM. Review information and obtain feedback from client/wife.

Discuss factors related to/ altering diabetic control such as stress, illness, exercise.

Drug therapy/diet may need to be altered in response to both short-term and long-term stressors, changes in activity level.

Review signs/symptoms of hyperglycemia (e.g., fatigue, nausea, vomiting, polyuria, polydipsia). Discuss how to prevent and evaluate this situation and when to seek medical care. Have client identify appropriate interventions.

Recognition and understanding of these signs/symptoms and timely intervention will aid client in avoiding recurrences and preventing complications.

Review and provide information about necessity for routine examination of feet and proper foot care (e.g., daily inspection for injuries, pressure areas, corns, calluses; proper nail cutting; daily washing, application of good moisturizing lotion such as Eucerin, Keri, Nivea bid). Recommend wearing loose-fitting socks and properly fitting shoes (break new shoes in gradually) and avoiding going barefoot. If foot injury/skin break occurs, wash with soap/ dermal cleanser and water, cover with sterile dressing, inspect wound and change dressing daily; report redness, swelling, or presence of drainage.

Reduces risk of tissue injury; promotes understanding and prevention of stasis ulcer formation and wound-healing difficulties.

Teaching: Prescribed Medication (NIC)

Instruct regarding prescribed insulin therapy:

May be a temporary treatment of hyperglycemia with infection or may be permanent replacement of oral hypoglycemic agent.

ACTIONS/ INTERVENTIONS	RATIONALE
Humulin N Insulin, SC.	Intermediate-acting insulin generally lasts 18–24 hr, with peak effect 6–12 hr.
Keep vial in current use at room temperature (if used within 30 days).	Cold insulin is poorly absorbed.
Store extra vials in refrigerator.	Refrigeration prevents wide fluctuations in temperature, prolonging the drug shelf life.
Roll bottle and invert to mix, or shake gently, avoiding bubbles.	Vigorous shaking may create foam, which can interfere with accurate dose withdrawal and may damage the insulin molecule. *Note:* New research suggests that shaking the vial may be more effective in mixing suspension. Refer to Procedure Manual.
Choice of injection sites (e.g., across lower abdomen in Z pattern).	Provides for steady absorption of medication. Site is easily visualized and accessible by client, and Z pattern minimizes tissue damage.
Demonstrate, then observe client drawing insulin into syringe, reading syringe markings, and administering dose. Assess for accuracy.	May require several instruction sessions and practice before client/wife feel comfortable drawing up and injecting medication.
Instruct in signs/symptoms of insulin reaction or hypoglycemia: fatigue, nausea, headache, hunger, sweating, irritability, shakiness, anxiety, difficulty concentrating.	Knowing what to watch for and appropriate treatment such as $\frac{1}{2}$ cup of grape juice for immediate response and snack within $\frac{1}{2}$ hr (e.g., 1 slice bread with peanut butter or cheese, fruit and slice of cheese for sustained effect) may prevent or minimize complications.
Review "Sick Day Rules" (e.g., call the doctor if too sick to eat normally or stay active), take insulin as ordered. Keep record as noted in Sick Day Guide.	Understanding of necessary actions in the event of mild to severe illness promotes competent self-care and reduces risk of hyper/hypoglycemia.

ACTIONS/ INTERVENTIONS	RATIONALE
Instruct client/wife in fingerstick glucose monitoring to be done qid until stable, then bid, rotating times such as FBS and before dinner; before lunch and HS. Observe return demonstrations of the procedure.	Fingerstick monitoring provides accurate and timely information regarding diabetic status. Return demonstration verifies correct learning.
Recommend client maintain record/log of fingerstick testing, antidiabetic medication, and insulin dosage/site, unusual physiological response, dietary intake. Outline desired goals of FBS 80–110, premeal 80–130.	Provides accurate record for review by caregivers for assessment of therapy effectiveness/needs.
Discuss other healthcare issues, such as smoking habits, self-monitoring for cancer (breasts/testicles), and reporting changes in general well-being.	Encourages client involvement, awareness, and responsibility for own health; promotes wellness. *Note:* Smoking tends to increase client's resistance to insulin.

ANOTHER APPROACH TO PLANNING CLIENT CARE— MIND MAPPING

Mind mapping starts in the center of the page with a representation of the main concept—the client. (This helps keep in mind that the client is the focus of the plan, not the medical diagnosis or condition.) From that central thought, other main ideas that relate to the client are added. Different concepts can be grouped together by geometric shapes, color-coding, or by placement on the page. Connections and interconnections between groups of ideas are represented by the use of arrows or lines with defining phrases added that explain how the interconnected thoughts relate to one another. In this manner, many different pieces of information *about* the client can be connected directly *to* the client.

Whichever piece is chosen becomes the first layer of connections—clustered assessment data, nursing diagnoses, or outcomes. For example, a map could start with nursing diagnoses featured as the first "branches," each one being listed separately in some way on the map. Next, the signs and symptoms or data supporting the diagnoses could be added; or the plan could begin with the client outcomes to be achieved with connections then to nursing diagnoses. When the plan is completed, there should be a nursing diagnosis (supported by subjective and objective assessment data), nursing interventions, desired client outcomes, and any evaluation data, all connected in a manner that shows there is a relationship between them. It is critical to understand that there is no preset order for the pieces, because one cluster is not more or less important than another (or one is not "subsumed" under another). It is important, however, that those pieces within a branch be in the same order in each branch.

Figure 3.1 shows a Mind Map for Mr. R. S., the client with type 2 diabetes in our Client Situation at the beginning of this section of the chapter.

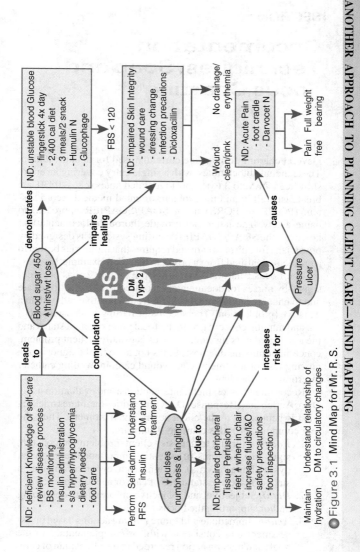

● Figure 3.1 Mind Map for Mr. R. S.

SECTION 4

Documentation Techniques: Soap and Focus Charting®

Several charting formats are currently used for documentation. These include block notes, with a single entry covering an entire shift (e.g., 7 AM to 3 PM); narrative timed notes (e.g., "0830, ate breakfast well"); and the problem-oriented medical record system (POMR or PORS) using SOAP/SOAPIER approach, to name a few. The latter can provide thorough documentation; however, the SOAP/SOAPIER charting system was designed by physicians for episodic care and requires that the entries be tied to a problem identified from a problem list. (See Example 1.)

The Focus Charting® system (see Example 2) has been designed by nurses for documentation of frequent or repetitive care and to encourage viewing the client from a positive rather than a negative (problem-only) perspective. Charting is focused on client and nursing concerns, with the focal point of client status and the associated nursing care. A Focus is usually a client problem, concern, or nursing diagnosis but is not a medical diagnosis or a nursing task or treatment (e.g., wound care, indwelling catheter insertion, tube feeding).

Recording of assessment, interventions, and evaluation using Data, Action, and Response (DAR) categories facilitates tracking what is happening to the client at any given moment. Thus, the four components of this charting system are:

1. *Focus:* Nursing diagnosis, client problem or concern, signs or symptoms of potential importance (e.g., fever, dysrhythmia, edema), a significant event or change in status, or specific standards of care or agency policy.
2. *Data:* Subjective and objective information describing and/or supporting the Focus.
3. *Action:* Immediate and future nursing actions based on assessment and consistent with, or complementary to the goals and nursing action recorded in the client plan of care.
4. *Response:* Describes the effects of interventions and whether the goal was met.

The following charting examples are based on the data within the client situation of Mr. R. S. in Chapter 3, Section 3, pages 46–53.

EXAMPLE 1 **SAMPLE SOAP/IER CHARTING FOR PROTOTYPE PLAN OF CARE**

| S = Subjective | O = Objective | A = Analysis | P = Plan |
| I = Implementation | E = Evaluation | R = Revision | |

Date	Time	Number/Problem*	Note
6/29/09	1900	No. 1 (impaired Skin Integrity)*	S: "That hurts" (when tissue surrounding wound palpated). O: Scant amount serous drainage on dressing. Wound borders pink. No odor present. A: Wound shows early signs of healing, free of infection. P: Continue skin care per plan of care.

To document more of the nursing process, some institutions have added the following: Implementation, Evaluation, and Revision (if plan was ineffective).

			I: NS irrig. as ordered. Applied sterile wet dressing with paper tape. E: Wound clean, no drainage present. R: None required. Signed: E. Moore, RN
6/29/09	2100	No. 3 (acute Pain)*	S: "Dull, throbbing pain in left foot." 4/10 States there is no radiation to other areas. O: Muscles tense. Moving about bed, appears uncomfortable. A: Persistent pain. P: Per plan of care. I: Foot cradle on bed. Darvocet-N given PO. Signed: M. Siskin, RN
	2200		E: Reports pain relieved 0/10. Appears relaxed. Signed: M. Siskin, RN

(table continues on page 66)

S = Subjective	O = Objective	A = Analysis	P = Plan
I = Implementation	E = Evaluation	R = Revision	

Date	Time	Number/Problem*	Note
6/30/09	1100	No. 5 (Learning Need, Diabetic Care)*	S: "My wife and I have some questions and concerns we wish to discuss." O: Copy of list of questions attached to teaching plan. A: R. S. and wife need review of information and practice for insulin administration. P: Attended group teaching session with wife and read "Understanding Your Diabetes." To meet with dietitian. I: R. S. demonstrated insulin administration techniques for wife to observe. Procedure handout sheet for future reference provided to couple. Scheduled meeting for them with dietitian at 1300 today to discuss remaining questions E: R. S. more confident in demonstration, performed activity correctly without hesitation or hand tremors. R. S. explained steps of procedure and reasons for actions to wife. Couple identified resources to contact if questions/problems arise. Signed: B. Briner, RN

*As noted on Plan of Care.

EXAMPLE 2 SAMPLE OF FOCUS CHARTING® FOR PROTOTYPE PLAN OF CARE

D = Data		A = Action	R = Response

Date	Time	Focus®	
6/29/09	1900	Skin integrity	D: Scant amount serous drainage on dressing, wound borders pink, no odor present, denies discomfort except with direct palpation of surrounding tissue. A: NS irrig. as ordered. Sterile wet dressing applied with paper tape. R: Wound clean—no drainage present. Signed: E. Moore, RN
6/29/09	2100	Pain L foot	D: Reports dull/throbbing ache L foot 4/10—no radiation. Muscles tense, restless in bed. A: Foot cradle on bed. Darvocet-N 100 mg given PO. Signed: M. Siskin, RN
	2200	Pain L foot	R: Reports pain relieved 0/10. Appears relaxed. Signed: M. Siskin, RN
6/30/09	1100	Learning Need, Diabetic Teaching	D: Attended group teaching session with wife. Both have read "Understanding Your Diabetes." A: Reviewed list of questions/concerns from R. S. and wife. (Copy attached to teaching plan.) R. S. demonstrated insulin administration technique for wife to observe.

(table continues on page 68)

D = Data	A = Action	R = Response

Date	Time	Focus®

Procedure handout sheet for future reference provided to couple.

Meeting scheduled with dietitian for 1300 today to discuss remaining questions.

R: R. S. more confident in demonstration, performed activity correctly without hesitation or hand tremors. He explained steps of procedure and reasons for actions to wife. Couple identified resources to contact if questions/problems arise.

The following is an example of documentation of a client need/concern that currently does not require identification as a client problem (nursing diagnosis) or inclusion in the plan of care and therefore is not easily documented in the SOAP format:

Date	Time	Focus®	
6/28/09	2120	Gastric distress	D: Awakened from light sleep by "indigestion/burning sensation." Places hand over epigastric area. Skin warm/dry, color pink, vital signs unchanged.
			A: Given Mylanta 30 mL PO. Head of bed elevated approximately 15 degrees.
			R: Reports pain relieved. Appears relaxed, resting quietly. Signed: E. Moore, RN

aFOCUS Charting®, Susan Lampe, RN, MS: Creative Nursing Management, Inc., 614 East Grant Street, Minneapolis, MN 55404.

CHAPTER 4

Nursing Diagnoses in Alphabetical Order

Activity Intolerance [specify level]

Taxonomy II: Activity/Rest—Class 4 Cardiovascular/
Pulmonary Responses (00092)
[Diagnostic Division: Activity/Rest]
Submitted 1982

Definition: Insufficient physiological or psychological
energy to endure or complete required or desired daily
activities

Related Factors

Generalized weakness
Sedentary lifestyle
Bedrest/immobility
Imbalance between oxygen supply and demand; [anemia]
Cognitive deficits/emotional status; secondary to underlying
    disease process/depression
Pain, vertigo, dysrhythmias, extreme stress

Defining Characteristics

Subjective
Verbal report of fatigue/weakness
Exertional discomfort/dyspnea
Verbalizes no desire and/or lack of interest in activity

Objective
Abnormal heart rate or blood pressure response to activity
Electrocardiographic changes reflecting arrhythmias or
    ischemia
Pallor, cyanosis

Information that appears in brackets has been added by the authors to clarify
and enhance the use of nursing diagnoses.

Functional Level Classification (Gordon, 2010):

Level I: Walk, regular pace, on level indefinitely; one flight or more but more short of breath than normally

Level II: Walk one city block [or] 500 ft on level; climb one flight slowly without stopping

Level III: Walk no more than 50 ft on level without stopping; unable to climb one flight of stairs without stopping

Level IV: Dyspnea and fatigue at rest

Desired Outcomes/Evaluation Criteria— Client Will:

- Identify negative factors affecting activity tolerance and eliminate or reduce their effects when possible.
- Use identified techniques to enhance activity tolerance.
- Participate willingly in necessary/desired activities.
- Report measurable increase in activity tolerance.
- Demonstrate a decrease in physiological signs of intolerance (e.g., pulse, respirations, and blood pressure remain within client's normal range).

Actions/Interventions

Nursing Priority No. 1.
To identify causative/precipitating factors:

- Note presence of factors contributing to fatigue (e.g., age, frail, acute or chronic illness, heart failure, hypothyroidism, cancer, and cancer therapies). **Fatigue affects both the client's actual and perceived ability to participate in activities.** (Refer to ND Fatigue.)
- Evaluate client's actual and perceived limitations, and severity of deficit in light of usual status. **Provides comparative baseline and information about needed education or interventions regarding quality of life.**
- Note client reports of weakness, fatigue, pain, difficulty accomplishing tasks, and/or insomnia. **Symptoms may be result of/or contribute to intolerance of activity.**
- Assess cardiopulmonary response to physical activity, including vital signs before, during, and after activity. Note accelerating fatigue.
- Ascertain ability to stand and move about, and degree of assistance necessary or use of equipment **to determine current**

Information that appears in brackets has been added by the authors to clarify and enhance the use of nursing diagnoses.

 Cultural　　Collaborative　　Community/Home Care

status and needs associated with participation in needed/ desired activities.

- Identify activity needs versus desires to evaluate appropriateness (e.g., is barely able to walk upstairs but would like to play tennis).
- Assess emotional and psychological factors affecting the current situation (e.g., stress and/or depression may be increasing the effects of an illness, or depression might be the result of forced inactivity).
- Note treatment-related factors, such as side effects and interactions of medications.

Nursing Priority No. 2.

To assist client to deal with contributing factors and manage activities within individual limits:

- Monitor vital and cognitive signs, watching for changes in blood pressure, heart and respiratory rate; note skin pallor and/ or cyanosis and presence of confusion.
- Adjust activities to prevent overexertion. Reduce intensity level or discontinue activities that cause undesired physiological changes.
- Provide and monitor response to supplemental oxygen, medications, and changes in treatment regimen.
- Increase exercise/activity levels gradually; teach methods to conserve energy, such as stopping to rest for 3 minutes during a 10-minute walk or sitting down to brush hair instead of standing.
- Plan care to carefully balance rest periods with activities to reduce fatigue.
- Provide positive atmosphere, while acknowledging difficulty of the situation for the client. Helps to minimize frustration and rechannel energy.
- Encourage expression of feelings contributing to, or resulting from condition.
- Involve client/SO(s) in planning of activities as much as possible.
- Assist with activities and provide/monitor client's use of assistive devices (e.g., crutches, walker, wheelchair, or oxygen tank) to protect client from injury.
- Promote comfort measures and provide for relief of pain to enhance ability to participate in activities. (Refer to NDs acute Pain; chronic Pain.)
- Provide referral to other disciplines, such as exercise physiologist, psychological counseling/therapy, occupational/

Information that appears in brackets has been added by the authors to clarify and enhance the use of nursing diagnoses.

physical therapists, and recreation/leisure specialists, as indicated, **to develop individually appropriate therapeutic regimens.**

Nursing Priority No. 3.
To promote wellness (Teaching/Discharge Considerations):

* Plan for maximal activity within the client's ability. **Promotes the idea of normalcy of progressive abilities in this area.**
* Review expectations of client/SO(s)/providers **to establish individual goals.** Explore conflicts and differences **to reach agreement for the most effective plan.**
* Instruct client/SO(s) in monitoring response to activity and in recognizing signs/symptoms that **indicate need to alter activity level.**
* Plan for progressive increase of activity level/participation in exercise training, as tolerated by client. **Both activity tolerance and health status may improve with progressive training.**
* Give client information that provides evidence of daily/weekly progress **to sustain motivation.**
* Assist client in learning and demonstrating appropriate safety measures **to prevent injuries.**
* Provide information about the effect of lifestyle and overall health factors on activity tolerance (e.g., nutrition, adequate fluid intake, smoking cessation, and mental health status).
* Encourage client to maintain positive attitude; suggest use of relaxation techniques, such as visualization or guided imagery, as appropriate, **to enhance sense of well-being.**
* Encourage participation in recreation, social activities, and hobbies appropriate for situation. (Refer to ND deficient Diversional Activity.)

Documentation Focus

Assessment/Reassessment
* Level of activity as noted in Functional Level Classification.
* Causative or precipitating factors.
* Client reports of difficulty or change.
* Vital signs before, during, and following activity.

Planning
* Plan of care and who is involved in planning.

Information that appears in brackets has been added by the authors to clarify and enhance the use of nursing diagnoses.

🌐 Cultural   🔄 Collaborative   🏠 Community/Home Care

Implementation/Evaluation
* Response to interventions, teaching, and actions performed.
* Implemented changes to plan of care based on assessment/reassessment findings.
* Teaching plan and understanding of material presented.
* Attainment or progress toward desired outcome(s).

Discharge Planning
* Referrals to other resources.
* Long-term needs and who is responsible for actions.

Sample Nursing Outcomes & Interventions Classifications (NOC/NIC) NIC

NOC—Activity Tolerance
NIC—Energy Management

---

risk for Activity Intolerance

Taxonomy II: Activity/Rest—Class 4 Cardiovascular/Pulmonary Response (00094)
[Diagnostic Division: Activity/Rest]
Submitted 1982

Definition: At risk of experiencing insufficient physiological or psychological energy to endure or complete required or desired daily activities

---

Risk Factors

History of previous intolerance
Presence of circulatory/respiratory problems; [dysrhythmias]
Deconditioned status; [aging]
Inexperience with the activity
Diagnosis of progressive disease state/debilitating condition, anemia
Verbalized reluctance/inability to perform expected activity

> **NOTE:** A risk diagnosis is not evidenced by signs and symptoms, as the problem has not occurred; rather, nursing interventions are directed at prevention.

Information that appears in brackets has been added by the authors to clarify and enhance the use of nursing diagnoses.

Desired Outcomes/Evaluation Criteria— Client Will:

- Verbalize understanding of potential loss of ability in relation to existing condition.
- Participate in conditioning/rehabilitation program to enhance ability to perform.
- Identify alternative ways to maintain desired activity level (e.g., if weather is bad, walking in a shopping mall).
- Identify conditions/symptoms that require medical reevaluation.

Actions/Interventions

Nursing Priority No. 1.

To assess factors affecting current situation:

- Note presence of medical diagnosis and/or therapeutic regimens (e.g., AIDS, chronic obstructive pulmonary disease [COPD], cancer, heart failure/other cardiac problems, anemia, multiple medications or treatment modalities, extensive surgical interventions, musculoskeletal trauma, neurological disorders, or renal failure) **that have potential for interfering with client's ability to perform at a desired level of activity.**
- Ask client/SO about usual level of energy **to identify potential problems and/or client's/SO's perception of client's energy and ability to perform needed/desired activities.**
- Identify factors, such as age, functional decline, client resistive to efforts, painful conditions, breathing problems, vision or hearing impairments, climate or weather, unsafe areas to exercise, and need for mobility assistance, **that could block/affect desired level of activity.**
- Determine current activity level and physical condition with observation, exercise tolerance testing, or use of functional level classification system (e.g., Gordon's), as appropriate. **Provides baseline for comparison and opportunity to track changes.**

Nursing Priority No. 2.

To develop alternative ways to remain active within the limits of the disabling condition/situation:

- Implement physical therapy/exercise program in conjunction with the client and other team members (e.g., physical and/or occupational therapist, exercise/rehabilitation physiologist). **Coordination of program enhances likelihood of success.**

Information that appears in brackets has been added by the authors to clarify and enhance the use of nursing diagnoses.

  Cultural Collaborative Community/Home Care

- Promote and implement conditioning program. Support inclusion in exercise and activity groups **to prevent/limit deterioration.**
- Instruct client in unfamiliar activities and in alternate ways of doing familiar activities **to conserve energy and promote safety.**

Nursing Priority No. 3.

To promote wellness (Teaching/Discharge Considerations):

- Discuss with client/SO the relationship of illness or debilitating condition and ability to perform desired activities. **Understanding these relationships can help with acceptance of limitations or reveal opportunity for changes of practical value.**
- Provide information regarding potential interfering factors with activity, such as smoking when one has respiratory problems or lack of motivation/interest in exercise, **which may be amenable to modification.**
- Assist client/SO(s) with planning for changes that may become necessary, such as use of supplemental oxygen **to improve client's ability to participate in desired activities.**
- Identify and discuss symptoms for which client needs to seek medical assistance/evaluation, **providing for timely intervention.**
- Refer to appropriate resources for assistance and/or equipment, as needed, **to sustain activity level.**

Documentation Focus

Assessment/Reassessment
- Identified or potential risk factors for individual.
- Current level of activity tolerance and blocks to activity.

Planning
- Treatment options, including physical therapy or exercise program, other assistive therapies and devices.
- Lifestyle changes that are planned, who is to be responsible for each action, and monitoring methods.

Implementation/Evaluation
- Responses to interventions, teaching, and actions performed.
- Attainment or progress toward desired outcome(s).
- Modification of plan of care.

Information that appears in brackets has been added by the authors to clarify and enhance the use of nursing diagnoses.

Discharge Planning
• Referrals for medical assistance/evaluation.

Sample Nursing Outcomes & Interventions Classifications (NOC/NIC) (NIC)

NOC—Endurance
NIC—Energy Management

ineffective Activity Planning

Taxonomy II: Perception/Cognition—Class 5 Cognition (00199)
[Diagnostic Division: Activity/Rest]
Submitted 2008

Definition: Inability to prepare for a set of actions fixed in time and under certain conditions

Related Factors

Unrealistic perception of events [or] personal competence
Lack of family/friend support
Compromised ability to process information
Defensive flight behavior when faced with proposed solution
Hedonism [motivated by pleasure and/or pain]

Defining Characteristics

Subjective
Verbalization of fear/worries toward a task to be undertaken
Excessive anxieties toward a task to be undertaken

Objective
Failure pattern of behavior
Lack of: plan; resources; sequential organization
Procrastination
Unmet goals for chosen activity

Desired Outcomes/Evaluation Criteria—Client Will: (Include Specific Time Frame)

• Acknowledge difficulty with follow-through of activity plan.
• Identify negative factors affecting ability to plan activities.

Information that appears in brackets has been added by the authors to clarify and enhance the use of nursing diagnoses.

  Cultural 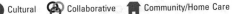 Collaborative 🏠 Community/Home Care

- Develop own plan for activity.
- Report lessened anxiety and fear toward planning.
- Be aware and make plan to deal with procrastination.

Actions/Interventions

Nursing Priority No. 1.
To identify causative/precipitating factors:

- Determine individual problems with planning and follow-through with activity plan. **Identifies individual difficulties (e.g., anxiety regarding what kind of activity to choose, lack of resources, lack of confidence in own ability).**
- Perform complete physical examination. **May have underlying problems such as allergies, hypertension, asthma, which contribute to fatigue and difficulty with undertaking task.**
- Review medication regimen **for possible side effects affecting client's desire to get involved in any activity.**
- Assess mental status, use Beck's Depression Inventory as indicated.
- Identify client's personal values and perception of self including strengths and weaknesses.
- Determine client's need to be in control; fear of dependency on others (although may need assistance from others), or belief he or she cannot do the task. **Indicative of external locus of control, where client sees others as having the control and ability.**
- Identify culture/religious issues **that may affect how individuals deal with issues of life, affect how they see their ability to make choices or manage own life.**
- Discuss awareness of procrastination, need for perfection, fear of failure. **Although client may not acknowledge it as a problem, this may be a factor in difficulty in planning for, choosing, and following through with activities that might be enjoyed.**
- Assess client's ability to process information. **May interfere with perception of the world and self.**
- Discuss possibility that client is motivated by pleasure to avoid pain (hedonism). **Individual may seek activities that bring pleasure to avoid painful experiences.**
- Note availability and use of resources.

Nursing Priority No. 2.
To assist client to recognize and deal with individual factors and begin to plan appropriate activities:

Information that appears in brackets has been added by the authors to clarify and enhance the use of nursing diagnoses.

- Encourage expression of feelings contributing/resulting from situation. Maintain a positive atmosphere without seeming overly cheerful.
- Discuss client's perception of self as worthless and not deserving of success and happiness. **Sometimes the underlying feelings are those of wanting to be perfect, and it is difficult to finish the task because of the fear that it will not be perfect (perfectionism).**
- Confront gently client's ambivalent, angry, or depressed feelings.
- Help client learn how to reframe negative thoughts about self into a positive view of what is happening.
- Involve client/SOs in planning an activity. **Having the support of family and nurse will help to promote success.**
- Direct client to break down desired activity in to specific steps. **Makes activity more manageable, and as each step is accomplished, individual feels more confident about ability to finish the task.**
- Encourage client to recognize procrastinating behaviors and make a decision to change. **Procrastination is a learned behavior and serves many purposes for the individual.**
- Accompany client to activity of own choosing, encouraging participation together if appropriate. **Support from caregiver may enable client to begin participating and gain confidence.**
- Assist client to develop skills of relaxation, imagery/visualization, and mindfulness. **Using these techniques can help the client learn to overcome stress and be able to manage life's difficulties more effectively.**
- Assist client to investigate the idea that seeking pleasure (hedonism) is interfering with motivation to accomplish goals. **Some philosophers believe that pleasure is the only good for a person and the individual does not see other aspects of life, interfering with accomplishments.**

Nursing Priority No. 3.
To promote wellness (Teaching/Discharge Criteria):

- Assist client to identify life goals and priorities.
- Review treatment goals and expectations of client and SOs. **Helps clarify what has been discussed and decisions that have been made; provides an opportunity to change goals as needed.**

Information that appears in brackets has been added by the authors to clarify and enhance the use of nursing diagnoses.

Cultural Collaborative 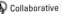 Community/Home Care

- Discuss progress in learning to relax and deal productively with anxieties and fears. **As client sees that progress is being made, feelings of worthwhileness will be enhanced and individual will be encouraged to continue working toward goals.**
- Identify community resources such as social services, senior center, or classes **to provide support and options for activities and change.**
- Refer for cognitive therapy as indicated. **This structured therapy can help the individual identify, evaluate, and modify any underlying assumptions and dysfunctional beliefs, and begin the process of change.**

Documentation Focus

Assessment/Reassessment
- Specific problems exhibited by client.
- Causative or precipitating factors.
- Client reports of difficulty making and following through with plans.

Planning
- Plan of care and who is involved in planning.
- Teaching plan.

Implementation/Evaluation
- Response to interventions, teaching, and actions performed.
- Attainment or progress toward desired outcome(s).

Discharge Planning
- Referrals to other resources.
- Long-term needs and who is responsible for actions.

Sample Nursing Outcomes & Interventions Classifications (NOC/NIC) NIC

NOC—Motivation
NIC—Self-Awareness Enhancement

Information that appears in brackets has been added by the authors to clarify and enhance the use of nursing diagnoses.

ineffective Airway Clearance

Taxonomy II: Safety/Protection—Class 2 Physical Injury
(00031)
[Diagnostic Division: Respiration]
Submitted 1980; Revised 1996, and Nursing Diagnosis
Extension and Classification (NDEC) 1998

Definition: Inability to clear secretions or obstructions
from the respiratory tract to maintain a clear airway

Related Factors

Environmental
Smoking; secondhand smoke; smoke inhalation

Obstructed Airway
Retained secretions; secretions in the bronchi; exudate in the
alveoli; excessive mucus; airway spasm; foreign body in airway; presence of artificial airway

Physiological
Chronic obstructive pulmonary disease [COPD]; asthma; aller-
gic airways; hyperplasia of the bronchial walls
Neuromuscular dysfunction
Infection

Defining Characteristics

Subjective
Dyspnea

Objective
Diminished/adventitious breath sounds [rales, crackles, rhonchi,
wheezes]
Cough ineffective/absent; excessive sputum
Changes in respiratory rate/rhythm
Difficulty vocalizing
Wide-eyed; restlessness
Orthopnea
Cyanosis

Information that appears in brackets has been added by the authors to clarify
and enhance the use of nursing diagnoses.

 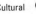 Cultural   Collaborative   Community/Home Care

Desired Outcomes/Evaluation Criteria— Client Will:

- Maintain airway patency.
- Expectorate/clear secretions readily.
- Demonstrate absence/reduction of congestion with breath sounds clear, respirations noiseless, improved oxygen exchange (e.g., absence of cyanosis, arterial blood gas [ABG]/ pulse oximetry results within client norms).
- Verbalize understanding of cause(s) and therapeutic management regimen.
- Demonstrate behaviors to improve or maintain clear airway.
- Identify potential complications and how to initiate appropriate preventive or corrective actions.

Actions/Interventions

Nursing Priority No. 1.
To maintain adequate, patent airway:

- Identify client populations at risk. **Persons with impaired ciliary function (e.g., cystic fibrosis); those with excessive or abnormal mucus production (e.g., asthma, emphysema, pneumonia, dehydration, mechanical ventilation); those with impaired cough function (e.g., neuromuscular diseases/conditions such as muscular dystrophy, Guillain-Barré); those with swallowing abnormalities (e.g., stroke, seizures, coma/sedation, head/neck cancer, facial burns, trauma, or surgery); immobility (e.g., spinal cord injury, developmental delay, fractures); infant/child feeding difficulties (e.g., congenital malformations, developmental delays, abdominal distention) are all at risk for problems with maintenance of open airways.**
- Monitor respirations and breath sounds, noting rate and sounds (e.g., tachypnea, stridor, crackles, wheezes) **indicative of respiratory distress and/or accumulation of secretions.**
- Evaluate client's cough/gag reflex and swallowing ability **to determine ability to protect own airway.**
- Position head appropriate for age and condition **to open or maintain open airway in at-rest or compromised individual.**
- Assist with appropriate testing (e.g., pulmonary function or sleep studies) **to identify causative/precipitating factors.**
- Suction naso/tracheal/oral prn **to clear airway when excessive or viscous secretions are blocking airway or client is unable to swallow or cough effectively.**

Information that appears in brackets has been added by the authors to clarify and enhance the use of nursing diagnoses.

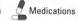

- Elevate head of bed and change position every 2 hours and prn **to take advantage of gravity decreasing pressure on the diaphragm and enhancing drainage of/ventilation to different lung segments.**
- Monitor infant/child for feeding intolerance, abdominal distention, and emotional stressors **that may compromise airway.**
- Insert oral airway (using correct size for adult or child) when needed, **to maintain anatomical position of tongue and natural airway, especially when tongue/laryngeal edema or thick secretions may block airway.**
- Assist with procedures (e.g., bronchoscopy, tracheostomy) **to clear/maintain open airway.**
- Keep environment allergen free (e.g., dust, feather pillows, smoke) according to individual situation.

Nursing Priority No. 2.

To mobilize secretions:

- Encourage deep-breathing and coughing exercises; splint chest/incision **to maximize effort.**
- Administer analgesics **to improve cough when pain is inhibiting effort. (Caution: Overmedication can depress respirations and cough effort.)**
- Give expectorants and bronchodilators as ordered.
- Increase fluid intake to at least 2000 mL/day within cardiac tolerance (may require IV in acutely ill, hospitalized client). Encourage/provide warm versus cold liquids as appropriate. Provide supplemental humidification, if needed (ultrasonic nebulizer, room humidifier). **Hydration can help liquefy viscous secretions and improve secretion clearance.** Monitor for signs/symptoms of congestive heart failure (crackles, edema, weight gain) when client is at risk.
- Perform/assist client with postural drainage and percussion as indicated if not contraindicated by condition, such as asthma.
- Assist with use of respiratory devices and treatments (e.g., intermittent positive-pressure breathing [IPPB]; incentive spirometer [IS]; positive expiratory pressure [PEP] mask; mechanical ventilation; oscillatory airway device [flutter]; assisted and directed cough techniques, etc.). **Various therapies/modalities may be required to acquire and maintain adequate airways, improve respiratory function and gas exchange.** (Refer to NDs ineffective Breathing Pattern; impaired Gas Exchange; impaired spontaneous Ventilation.)
- Support reduction/cessation of smoking **to improve lung function.**

Information that appears in brackets has been added by the authors to clarify and enhance the use of nursing diagnoses.

Cultural Collaborative Community/Home Care

- Position appropriately (e.g., head of bed elevated, side lying) and discourage use of oil-based products around nose **to prevent vomiting with aspiration into lungs.** (Refer to NDs risk for Aspiration; impaired Swallowing.)

Nursing Priority No. 3.
To assess changes, note complications:

- Auscultate breath sounds and assess air movement **to ascertain status and note progress.**
- Monitor vital signs, noting changes in blood pressure and heart rate.
- Observe for signs of respiratory distress (increased rate, restlessness/anxiety, use of accessory muscles for breathing).
- Evaluate changes in sleep pattern, noting insomnia or daytime somnolence.
- Document response to drug therapy and/or development of adverse side effects or interactions with antimicrobials, steroids, expectorants, bronchodilators.
- Observe for signs/symptoms of infection (e.g., increased dyspnea with onset of fever, change in sputum color, amount, or character) **to identify infectious process and promote timely intervention.**
- Obtain sputum specimen, preferably before antimicrobial therapy is initiated, **to verify appropriateness of therapy.**
- Monitor/document serial chest x-rays, ABGs, pulse oximetry readings.

Nursing Priority No. 4.
To promote wellness (Teaching/Discharge Considerations):

- Assess client's/SO's knowledge of contributing causes, treatment plan, specific medications, and therapeutic procedures. **Modalities to manage secretions and improve airflow vary according to client's diagnosis.**
- Provide information about the necessity of raising and expectorating secretions versus swallowing them, **to report changes in color and amount in the event that medical intervention may be needed to prevent or treat infection.**
- Demonstrate/assist client/SO in performing specific airway clearance techniques (e.g., forced expiratory breathing [also called huffing] or respiratory muscle strength training, chest percussion), as indicated.
- Review breathing exercises, effective coughing, and use of adjunct devices (e.g., IPPB or incentive spirometer) in preoperative teaching.

Information that appears in brackets has been added by the authors to clarify and enhance the use of nursing diagnoses.

- Encourage/provide opportunities for rest; limit activities to level of respiratory tolerance. **Prevents/reduces fatigue.**
- Refer to appropriate support groups (e.g., stop-smoking clinic, COPD exercise group, weight reduction).
- Determine that client has equipment and is informed in use of nocturnal continuous positive airway pressure (CPAP) **for treatment of obstructive sleep apnea, when indicated.** (Refer to NDs Insomnia; Sleep Deprivation.)

Documentation Focus

Assessment/Reassessment
- Related Factors for individual client.
- Breath sounds, presence and character of secretions, use of accessory muscles for breathing.
- Character of cough and sputum.
- Respiratory rate, pulse oximetry/O_2 saturation, vital signs.

Planning
- Plan of care and who is involved in planning.
- Teaching plan.

Implementation/Evaluation
- Client's response to interventions, teaching, and actions performed.
- Use of respiratory devices/airway adjuncts.
- Response to medications administered.
- Attainment or progress toward desired outcome(s).
- Modifications to plan of care.

Discharge Planning
- Long-term needs and who is responsible for actions to be taken.
- Specific referrals made.

Sample Nursing Outcomes & Interventions Classifications (NOC/NIC) NIC

NOC—Respiratory Status: Airway Patency
NIC—Airway Management

Information that appears in brackets has been added by the authors to clarify and enhance the use of nursing diagnoses.

latex Allergy Response

Taxonomy II: Safety/Protection—Class 5 Defensive
  Processes (00041)
[Diagnostic Division: Safety]
Submitted 1998; Revised 2006

Definition: A hypersensitive reaction to natural latex
rubber products

Related Factors

Hypersensitivity to natural latex rubber protein

Defining Characteristics

Subjective

*Life-threatening reactions occurring <1 hour after exposure to
  latex proteins:* Tightness in chest [feeling breathless]
Gastrointestinal characteristics: Abdominal pain; nausea
Orofacial characteristics: Itching of the eyes; nasal/facial/oral
  itching; nasal congestion
Generalized characteristics: Generalized discomfort; increasing complaint of total body warmth
*Type IV reactions occurring >1 hour after exposure to latex
  protein:* Discomfort reaction to additives such as thiurams
  and carbamates

Objective

*Life-threatening reactions occurring <1 hour after exposure to
  latex proteins:*
Contact urticaria progressing to generalized symptoms
Edema of the lips, tongue, uvula, throat
Dyspnea; wheezing; bronchospasm; respiratory arrest
Hypotension; syncope; cardiac arrest
Orofacial characteristics: Edema of sclera/eyelids; erythema/
  tearing of the eyes; nasal/facial erythema; rhinorrhea
Generalized characteristics: Flushing; generalized edema; restlessness
*Type IV reactions occurring >1 hour after exposure to latex
  protein:* Eczema; irritation; redness

Information that appears in brackets has been added by the authors to clarify
and enhance the use of nursing diagnoses.

Desired Outcomes/Evaluation Criteria—
Client Will:

- Be free of signs of hypersensitive response.
- Verbalize understanding of individual risks and responsibilities in avoiding exposure.
- Identify signs/symptoms requiring prompt intervention.

Actions/Interventions

Nursing Priority No. 1.
To assess contributing factors:

- Identify persons in high-risk categories such as those with history of certain food allergies (e.g., banana, avocado, chestnut, kiwi, papaya, peach, nectarine), prior allergies, asthma, and skin conditions (e.g., eczema and other dermatitis); those occupationally exposed to latex products (e.g., healthcare workers, police, firefighters, emergency medical technicians [EMTs], food handlers, hairdressers, cleaning staff, factory workers in plants that manufacture latex-containing products); those with neural tube defects (e.g., spina bifida); or those with congenital urological conditions requiring frequent surgeries and/or catheterizations (e.g., extrophy of the bladder). **The most severe reactions tend to occur with latex proteins contacting internal tissues during invasive procedures and when they touch mucous membranes of the mouth, vagina, urethra, or rectum.**
- Discuss history of recent exposure; for example, blowing up balloons or using powdered gloves (this might be an acute reaction to the powder); use of latex diaphragm/condoms (may affect either partner).
- Note positive skin-prick test (SPT) when client is skin-tested with latex extracts. **Sensitive, specific, and rapid test, and should be used with caution in persons with suspected sensitivity as it carries risk of anaphylaxis.**
- Perform challenge/patch test, if appropriate, **to identify specific allergens in client with known type IV hypersensitivity.**
- Note response to radioallergosorbent test (RAST) or enzyme-linked assays (ELISA) of latex-specific IgE. **This is the only safe test for the client with a history of life-threatening reaction.**

Information that appears in brackets has been added by the authors to clarify and enhance the use of nursing diagnoses.

    Cultural   Collaborative   Community/Home Care

Nursing Priority No. 2.

To take measures to reduce/limit allergic response/avoid exposure to allergens:

- Ascertain client's current symptoms, noting reports of rash, hives, itching, eye symptoms, edema, diarrhea, nausea, feeling of faintness.
- Determine time since exposure (e.g., immediate or delayed onset, such as 24–48 hours).
- Assess skin (usually hands but may be anywhere) for dry, crusty, hard bumps, scaling, lesions, and horizontal cracks. **May be irritant contact dermatitis (the least serious and most common type of hypersensitivity reaction) or allergic contact dermatitis (a delayed-onset and more severe form of skin/other tissue reaction).**
- Assist with treatment of dermatitis/type IV reaction (e.g., washing affected skin with mild soap and water, possible application of topical steroid ointment, avoidance of further exposure to latex).
- Monitor closely for signs of systemic reactions (e.g., difficulty breathing, wheezing, hypotension, tremors, chest pain, tachycardia, dysrhythmias). **Indicative of anaphylactic reaction and can lead to cardiac arrest.**
- Administer treatment, as appropriate, if severe/life-threatening reaction occurs, including antihistamines, epinephrine, IV fluids, corticosteroids, and oxygen/mechanical ventilation, if indicated.
- Ascertain that latex-safe environment (e.g., surgery/hospital room) and products are available according to recommended guidelines and standards, including equipment and supplies (e.g., powder-free, low-protein latex products and latex-free items: gloves, syringes, catheters, tubings, tape, thermometers, electrodes, oxygen cannulas, underpads, storage bags, diapers, feeding nipples), as appropriate.
- Educate all care providers in ways to prevent inadvertent exposure (e.g., post latex precaution signs in client's room, document allergy to latex in chart), and emergency treatment measures should they be needed.

Nursing Priority No. 3.

To promote wellness (Teaching/Learning):

- Instuct client/SO(s) to survey and routinely monitor environment for latex-containing products, and replace as needed.

Information that appears in brackets has been added by the authors to clarify and enhance the use of nursing diagnoses.

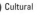 • Provide lists of products that can replace latex (e.g., rubber grip utensils/toys/hoses, rubber-containing pads, undergarments, carpets, shoe soles, computer mouse pad, erasers, rubber bands).

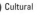 • Emphasize necessity of wearing medical ID bracelet and informing all new care providers of hypersensitivity **to reduce preventable exposures.**

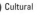 • Advise client to be aware of potential for related food allergies.

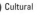 • Instruct client/family/SO about signs of reaction as well as how to implement emergency treatment. **Promotes awareness of problem and facilitates timely intervention.**

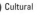 • Provide worksite review/recommendations to prevent exposure.

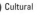 • Refer to resources (e.g., *Latex Allergy News*, National Institute for Occupational Safety and Health—NIOSH) **for further information and assistance.**

Documentation Focus

Assessment/Reassessment
• Assessment findings, pertinent history of contact with latex products, and frequency of exposure.
• Type and extent of symptomatology.

Planning
• Plan of care and interventions, and who is involved in planning.
• Teaching plan.

Implementation/Evaluation
• Response to interventions, teaching, and actions performed.
• Attainment or progress toward desired outcome(s).
• Modifications to plan of care.

Discharge Planning
• Discharge needs and referrals made, additional resources available.

Sample Nursing Outcomes & Interventions Classifications (NOC/NIC) [NIC]

NOC—Immune Hypersensitivity Control
NIC—Latex Precautions

Information that appears in brackets has been added by the authors to clarify and enhance the use of nursing diagnoses.

⊕ Cultural   🌐 Collaborative   🏠 Community/Home Care

risk for latex **Allergy Response**

Taxonomy II: Safety/Protection—Class 5 Defensive
Processes (00042)
[Diagnostic Division: Safety]
Submitted 1998; Revised 2006

Definition: Risk of hypersensitivity to natural latex rubber
products

Risk Factors

History of reactions to latex
Allergies to bananas, avocados, tropical fruits, kiwi, chestnuts,
poinsettia plants
History of allergies/asthma
Professions with daily exposure to latex
Multiple surgical procedures, especially from infancy

> **NOTE:** A risk diagnosis is not evidenced by signs and
> symptoms, as the problem has not occurred; rather,
> nursing interventions are directed at prevention.

Desired Outcomes/Evaluation Criteria— Client Will:

- Identify and correct potential risk factors in the environment.
- Demonstrate appropriate lifestyle changes to reduce risk of
  exposure.
- Identify resources to assist in promoting a safe environment.
- Recognize need for/seek assistance to limit response/compli-
  cations.

Actions/Interventions

Nursing Priority No. 1.

To assess causative/contributing factors:

- Identify persons in high-risk categories such as those with
  history of certain food allergies (e.g., banana, avocado, chestnut, kiwi, papaya, peach, nectarine), asthma, skin conditions
  (e.g., eczema); those occupationally exposed to latex products
  (e.g., healthcare workers, police, firefighters, EMTs, food handlers, hairdressers, cleaning staff, factory workers in plants
  that manufacture latex-containing products); those with neural

---

Information that appears in brackets has been added by the authors to clarify
and enhance the use of nursing diagnoses.

tube defects (e.g., spina bifida); or those with congenital urological conditions requiring frequent surgeries and/or catheterizations (e.g., extrophy of the bladder). **The most severe reactions tend to occur when latex proteins contact internal tissues during invasive procedures and when they touch mucous membranes of the mouth, vagina, urethra, or rectum.**

- Ascertain if client could be exposed through catheters, IV tubing, dental/other procedures in healthcare setting. **Although many healthcare facilities and providers use latex-safe equipment, latex is present in many medical supplies and/or in the healthcare environment, with possible risk to client and healthcare provider.**

Nursing Priority No. 2.
To assist in correcting factors that could lead to latex allergy:

- Discuss necessity of avoiding/limiting latex exposure if sensitivity is suspected.
- Recommend that client/family survey environment and remove any medical or household products containing latex.
- Create latex-safe environments (e.g., substitute nonlatex products, such as natural rubber gloves, PCV IV tubing, latex-free tape, thermometers, electrodes, oxygen cannulas) **to enhance client safety by reducing exposure.**
- Obtain lists of latex-free products and supplies for client/care provider if appropriate **in order to limit exposure.**
- Ascertain that facilities and/or employers have established policies and procedures to address safety and reduce risk to workers and clients.
- Promote good skin care when latex gloves may be preferred for barrier protection in specific disease conditions such as HIV or during surgery. Use powder-free gloves, wash hands immediately after glove removal; refrain from use of oil-based hand cream. **Reduces dermal and respiratory exposure to latex proteins that bind to the powder in gloves.**

Nursing Priority No. 3.
To promote wellness (Teaching/Discharge Considerations):

- Discuss ways to avoid exposure to latex products with client/SO/caregiver.
- Instruct client and care providers about potential for sensitivity reactions, how to recognize symptoms of latex allergy (e.g., skin rash; hives; flushing; itching; nasal, eye, or sinus symptoms; asthma; and [rarely] shock).

Information that appears in brackets has been added by the authors to clarify and enhance the use of nursing diagnoses.

Cultural   Collaborative   Community/Home Care

- Identify measures to take if reactions occur.
- Refer to allergist **for testing, as appropriate.** Perform challenge/patch test with gloves to skin. **Hives, itching, and reddened areas indicate sensitivity.**

Documentation Focus

Assessment/Reassessment
- Assessment findings, pertinent history of contact with latex products, and frequency of exposure.

Planning
- Plan of care, interventions, and who is involved in planning.
- Teaching plan.

Implementation/Evaluation
- Response to interventions, teaching, and actions performed.

Discharge Planning
- Discharge needs and referrals made.

Sample Nursing Outcomes & Interventions Classifications (NOC/NIC) NIC

NOC—Immune Hypersensitivity Control
NIC—Latex Precautions

Anxiety [specify level: mild, moderate, severe, panic]

Taxonomy II: Coping/Stress Tolerance—Class 2 Coping Responses (00146)
[Diagnostic Division: Ego Integrity]
Submitted 1973; Revised 1982, 1998 (by small group work 1996)

Definition: Vague uneasy feeling of discomfort or dread accompanied by an autonomic response (the source often nonspecific or unknown to the individual); a feeling of apprehension caused by anticipation of danger. It is an altering signal that warns of impending danger and enables the individual to take measures to deal with threat.

Information that appears in brackets has been added by the authors to clarify and enhance the use of nursing diagnoses.

Related Factors

Unconscious conflict about essential [beliefs,] goals, values of life

Situational/maturational crises

Stress

Familial association; heredity

Interpersonal transmission/contagion

Threat to self-concept [perceived or actual]; [unconscious conflict]

Threat of death [perceived or actual]

Threat to/change in: health status [progressive or debilitating disease, terminal illness]; interaction patterns; role function/status; environment [safety]; economic status

Unmet needs

Exposure to toxins; substance abuse

Positive or negative self-talk

Physiological factors, such as hyperthyroidism, pulmonary embolism, dysrhythmias, pheochromocytoma, drug therapy, including steroids

Defining Characteristics

Subjective

Behavioral
Expressed concerns due to change in life events; insomnia

Affective
Regretful; scared; rattled; distressed; apprehensive; fearful; feelings of inadequacy; uncertainty; jittery; worried; painful/persistent increased helplessness; [sense of impending doom]; [hopelessness]

Cognitive
Fear of unspecified consequences; awareness of physiological symptoms

Physiological
Shakiness

Sympathetic
Dry mouth; heart pounding; weakness; respiratory difficulties; anorexia; diarrhea

---

Information that appears in brackets has been added by the authors to clarify and enhance the use of nursing diagnoses.

 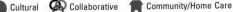 Cultural Collaborative Community/Home Care

Parasympathetic

Tingling in extremities; nausea; abdominal pain; diarrhea; urinary frequency/hesitancy; faintness; fatigue; sleep disturbance; [chest, back, neck pain]

Objective

Behavioral

Poor eye contact; glancing about; scanning; vigilance; extraneous movement [e.g., foot shuffling, hand/arm movements, rocking motion]; fidgeting; restlessness; diminished productivity; [crying/tearfulness]; [pacing/purposeless activity]; [immobility]

Affective

Increased wariness; focus on self; irritability; overexcited; anguish

Cognitive

Preoccupation; impaired attention; difficulty concentrating; forgetfulness; diminished ability to problem-solve; diminished ability to learn; rumination; tendency to blame others; blocking of thought; confusion; decreased perceptual field

Physiological

Voice quivering; trembling/hand tremors; increased tension; facial tension; increased perspiration

Sympathetic

Cardiovascular excitation; facial flushing; superficial vasoconstriction; increased pulse, respiration, blood pressure; pupil dilation; twitching; increased reflexes

Parasympathetic

Urinary urgency; decreased blood pressure/pulse

Desired Outcomes/Evaluation Criteria—Client Will:

- Appear relaxed and report anxiety is reduced to a manageable level.
- Verbalize awareness of feelings of anxiety.
- Identify healthy ways to deal with and express anxiety.
- Demonstrate problem-solving skills.
- Use resources/support systems effectively.

Information that appears in brackets has been added by the authors to clarify and enhance the use of nursing diagnoses.

Actions/Interventions

Nursing Priority No. 1.

To assess level of anxiety:

- Review familial and physiological factors (e.g., genetic depressive factors); psychiatric illness; active medical conditions (e.g., thyroid problems, metabolic imbalances, cardiopulmonary disease, anemia, or dysrhythmias); recent/ongoing stressors (e.g., family member illness or death, spousal conflict/abuse, or loss of job). **These factors can cause/exacerbate anxiety and anxiety disorders.**
- Determine current prescribed medications and recent drug history of prescribed or over-the-counter (OTC) medications (e.g., steroids, thyroid preparations, weight loss pills, or caffeine). **These medications can heighten feelings and sense of anxiety.**
- Identify client's perception of the threat represented by the situation.
- Monitor vital signs (e.g., rapid or irregular pulse, rapid breathing/hyperventilation, changes in blood pressure, diaphoresis, tremors, or restlessness) **to identify physical responses associated with both medical and emotional conditions.**
- Observe behaviors, **which can point to the client's level of anxiety:**

Mild

Alert; more aware of environment; attention focused on environment and immediate events

Restless; irritable; wakeful; reports of insomnia

Motivated to deal with existing problems in this state

Moderate

Perception narrower; concentration increased; able to ignore distractions in dealing with problem(s)

Voice quivers or changes pitch

Trembling; increased pulse/respirations

Severe

Range of perception is reduced; anxiety interferes with effective functioning

Preoccupied with feelings of discomfort, sense of impending doom

Increased pulse/respirations with reports of dizziness, tingling sensations, headache, and so forth

---

Information that appears in brackets has been added by the authors to clarify and enhance the use of nursing diagnoses.

 Cultural   Collaborative   Community/Home Care

Panic

Ability to concentrate is disrupted; behavior is disintegrated; client distorts the situation and does not have realistic perceptions of what is happening. Client may be experiencing terror or confusion or be unable to speak or move (paralyzed with fear).

- Note reports of insomnia or excessive sleeping, limited/avoidance of interactions with others, use of alcohol or other drugs of abuse, **which may be behavioral indicators of use of withdrawal to deal with problems.**
- Review results of diagnostic tests (e.g., drug screens, cardiac testing, complete blood count, and chemistry panel), **which may point to physiological sources of anxiety.**
- Be aware of defense mechanisms being used (e.g., denial or regression) **that interfere with ability to deal with problem.**
- Identify coping skills the individual is currently using, such as anger, daydreaming, forgetfulness, overeating, smoking, or lack of problem solving.
- Review coping skills used in past **to determine those that might be helpful in current circumstances.**

Nursing Priority No. 2.

To assist client to identify feelings and begin to deal with problems:

- Establish a therapeutic relationship, conveying empathy and unconditional positive regard. *Note:* Nurse needs to be aware of own feelings of anxiety or uneasiness, exercising care **to avoid the contagious effect or transmission of anxiety.**
- Be available to client for listening and talking.
- Encourage client to acknowledge and to express feelings: for example, crying (sadness), laughing (fear, denial), or swearing (fear, anger).
- Assist client to develop self-awareness of verbal and nonverbal behaviors.
- Clarify meaning of feelings and actions by providing feedback and checking meaning with the client.
- Acknowledge anxiety/fear. Do not deny or reassure client that everything will be all right.
- Provide accurate information about the situation. **Helps client identify what is reality based.**
- With a child, be truthful, avoid bribing, and provide physical contact (e.g., hugging or rocking) **to soothe fears and provide assurance.**

Information that appears in brackets has been added by the authors to clarify and enhance the use of nursing diagnoses.

ANXIETY [specify level: mild, moderate, severe, panic]

- Provide comfort measures (e.g., calm/quiet environment, soft music, warm bath, or back rub).
- Modify procedures as much as possible (e.g., substitute oral for intramuscular medications or combine blood draws/use fingerstick method) **to limit degree of stress and avoid over-whelming child or anxious adult.**
- Manage environmental factors, such as harsh lighting and high traffic flow, which may be confusing and stressful to older individuals.
- Accept client as is. **The client may need to be where he or she is at this point in time, such as in denial after receiving the diagnosis of a terminal illness.**
- Allow the behavior to belong to the client; do not respond personally. **The nurse may respond inappropriately, escalating the situation to a nontherapeutic interaction.**
- Assist client to use anxiety for coping with the situation, if helpful. **Moderate anxiety heightens awareness and permits the client to focus on dealing with problems.**

Panic

- Stay with client, maintaining a calm, confident manner.
- Speak in brief statements using simple words.
- Provide for nonthreatening, consistent environment/atmosphere. Minimize stimuli. Monitor visitors and interactions **to lessen effect of transmission of feelings.**
- Set limits on inappropriate behavior and help client to develop acceptable ways of dealing with anxiety.

> **NOTE:** Staff may need to provide safe controls and environment until client regains control.

- Gradually increase activities/involvement with others as anxiety is decreased.
- Use cognitive therapy **to focus on or correct faulty catastrophic interpretations of physical symptoms.**
- Administer medications (anti-anxiety agents/sedatives), as ordered.

Nursing Priority No. 3.
To promote wellness (Teaching/Discharge Considerations):

- Assist client to identify precipitating factors and new methods of coping with disabling anxiety.

Information that appears in brackets has been added by the authors to clarify and enhance the use of nursing diagnoses.

Cultural   Collaborative   Community/Home Care

- Review happenings, thoughts, and feelings preceding the anxiety attack.
- Identify actions and activities the client has previously used to cope successfully when feeling nervous/anxious.
- List helpful resources and people, including available "hotline" or crisis managers **to provide ongoing/timely support.**
- Encourage client to develop an exercise/activity program, **which may serve to reduce level of anxiety by relieving tension.**
- Assist in developing skills (e.g., awareness of negative thoughts, saying "Stop," and substituting a positive thought) **to eliminate negative self-talk. Mild phobias tend to respond well to behavioral therapy.**
- Review strategies, such as role playing, use of visualizations to practice anticipated events, prayer/meditation; **useful for being prepared for/dealing with anxiety-provoking situations.**
- Review medication regimen and possible interactions, especially with OTC drugs, other prescription drugs, and alcohol. Discuss appropriate drug substitutions, changes in dosage, or time of dose **to minimize side effects.**
- Refer to physician for drug management alteration of prescription regimen. **Drugs often causing symptoms of anxiety include aminophylline/theophylline, anticholinergics, dopamine, levodopa, salicylates, and steroids.**
- Refer to individual and/or group therapy, as appropriate, **to deal with chronic anxiety states.**

Documentation Focus

Assessment/Reassessment
- Level of anxiety and precipitating/aggravating factors.
- Description of feelings (expressed and displayed).
- Awareness and ability to recognize and express feelings.
- Related substance use, if present.

Planning
- Treatment plan and individual responsibility for specific activities.
- Teaching plan.

Implementation/Evaluation
- Client involvement and response to interventions, teaching, and actions performed.

Information that appears in brackets has been added by the authors to clarify and enhance the use of nursing diagnoses.

- Attainment or progress toward desired outcome(s).
- Modifications to plan of care.

Discharge Planning
- Referrals and follow-up plan.
- Specific referrals made.

Sample Nursing Outcomes & Interventions Classifications (NOC/NIC) NIC

NOC—Anxiety Self-Control
NIC—Anxiety Reduction

death Anxiety

Taxonomy II: Coping/Stress Tolerance—Class 2 Coping Response (00147)
[Diagnostic Division: Ego Integrity]
Submitted 1998; Revised 2006

Definition: Vague uneasy feeling of discomfort or dread generated by perceptions of a real or imagined threat to one's existence

Related Factors

Anticipating: pain; suffering; adverse consequences of general anesthesia; impact of death on others
Confronting reality of terminal disease; experiencing dying process; perceived proximity of death
Discussions on topic of death; observations related to death; near-death experience
Uncertainty of prognosis; nonacceptance of own mortality
Uncertainty about: the existence of a higher power; life after death; an encounter with a higher power

Defining Characteristics

Subjective
Fear of: developing a terminal illness; the process of dying; pain/suffering related to dying; loss of mental[/physical] abilities when dying; premature death; prolonged dying
Negative thoughts related to death and dying
Feeling powerlessness over dying

Information that appears in brackets has been added by the authors to clarify and enhance the use of nursing diagnoses.

Cultural   Collaborative   Community/Home Care

Worrying about the impact of one's own death on significant others

Concerns of overworking the caregiver; [about meeting one's creator or feeling doubtful about the existence of God or higher being]

Deep sadness

Desired Outcomes/Evaluation Criteria— Client Will:

* Identify and express feelings (e.g., sadness, guilt, fear) freely/effectively.
* Look toward/plan for the future one day at a time.
* Formulate a plan dealing with individual concerns and eventualities of dying as appropriate.

Actions/Interventions

Nursing Priority No. 1.

To assess causative/contributing factors:

* Determine how client sees self in usual lifestyle role functioning and perception and meaning of anticipated loss to him or her and SO(s).
* Ascertain current knowledge of situation **to identify misconceptions, lack of information, other pertinent issues.**
* Determine client's role in family constellation. Observe patterns of communication in family and response of family/SO to client's situation and concerns. **In addition to identifying areas of need/concern, also reveals strengths useful in addressing the concerns.**
* Assess impact of client reports of subjective experiences and past experience with death (or exposure to death); for example, witnessed violent death or as a child viewed body in casket, and so on.
* Identify cultural factors/expectations and impact on current situation and feelings.
* Note physical and mental condition, and complexity of therapeutic regimen.
* Determine ability to manage own self-care, end-of-life and other affairs, awareness/use of available resources.
* Observe behavior indicative of the level of anxiety present (mild to panic) **as it affects client's/SO's ability to process information and participate in activities.**
* Identify coping skills currently used and how effective they are. Be aware of defense mechanisms being used by the client.

Information that appears in brackets has been added by the authors to clarify and enhance the use of nursing diagnoses.

- Note use of alcohol or other drugs of abuse, reports of insomnia, excessive sleeping, avoidance of interactions with others, **which may be behavioral indicators of use of withdrawal to deal with problems.**
- 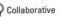 Note client's religious and spiritual orientation, involvement in religious activities, presence of conflicts regarding spiritual beliefs.
- Listen to client/SO reports/expressions of anger and concern, alienation from God, belief that impending death is a punishment for wrongdoing.
- Determine sense of futility; feelings of hopelessness, helplessness; lack of motivation to help self. **May indicate presence of depression and need for intervention.**
- Active-listen comments regarding sense of isolation.
- Listen for expressions of inability to find meaning in life or suicidal ideation.

Nursing Priority No. 2.
To assist client to deal with situation:
- Provide open and trusting relationship.
- Use therapeutic communication skills of Active-listening, silence, acknowledgment. Respect client's desire or request not to talk. Provide hope within parameters of the individual situation.
- Encourage expressions of feelings (anger, fear, sadness, etc.). Acknowledge anxiety/fear. Do not deny or reassure client that everything will be all right. Be honest when answering questions/providing information. **Enhances trust and therapeutic relationship.**
- Provide information about normalcy of feelings and individual grief reaction.
- Make time for nonjudgmental discussion of philosophic issues and questions about spiritual impact of illness/situation.
- Review life experiences of loss and previous use of coping skills, noting client's strengths and successes.
- Provide calm, peaceful setting and privacy as appropriate. **Promotes relaxation and ability to deal with situation.**
- Assist client to engage in spiritual growth activities, experience prayer/meditation and forgiveness to heal past hurts. Provide information that anger with God is a normal part of the grieving process. **Reduces feelings of guilt/conflict, allowing client to move forward toward resolution.**
- Refer to therapists, spiritual advisors, counselors **to facilitate grief work.**

Information that appears in brackets has been added by the authors to clarify and enhance the use of nursing diagnoses.

⊕ Cultural 🔬 Collaborative 🏠 Community/Home Care

• Refer to community agencies/resources **to assist client/SO for planning for eventualities (legal issues, funeral plans, etc.).**

Nursing Priority No. 3.

To promote independence:

• Support client's efforts to develop realistic steps to put plans into action.

• Direct client's thoughts beyond present state to enjoyment of each day and the future when appropriate.

• Provide opportunities for the client to make simple decisions. **Enhances sense of control.**

• Develop individual plan using client's locus of control **to assist client/family through the process.**

• Treat expressed decisions and desires with respect and convey to others as appropriate.

• Assist with completion of Advance Directives, cardiopulmonary resuscitation (CPR) instructions, and durable medical power of attorney.

Documentation Focus

Assessment/Reassessment
• Assessment findings, including client's fears and signs/symptoms being exhibited.
• Responses and actions of family/SO(s).
• Availability and use of resources.

Planning
• Plan of care and who is involved in planning.

Implementation/Evaluation
• Client's response to interventions, teaching, and actions performed.
• Attainment or progress toward desired outcome(s).
• Modifications to plan of care.

Discharge Planning
• Identified needs and who is responsible for actions to be taken.
• Specific referrals made.

Sample Nursing Outcomes & Interventions Classifications (NOC/NIC) NIC

NOC—Dignified Life Closure
NIC—Dying Care

Information that appears in brackets has been added by the authors to clarify and enhance the use of nursing diagnoses.

risk for **Aspiration**

Taxonomy II: Safety/Protection—Class 2 Physical Injury (00039)
[Diagnostic Division: Respiration]
Submitted 1988

Definition: At risk for entry of gastrointestinal secretions, oropharyngeal secretions, or [exogenous food] solids or fluids into tracheobronchial passages

Risk Factors

Reduced level of consciousness [sedation/anesthesia]

Depressed cough/gag reflexes

Impaired swallowing [inability of the epiglottis and true vocal cords to move to close off trachea]

Facial/oral/neck surgery or trauma; wired jaws; [congenital malformations]

Situation hindering elevation of upper body [weakness, paralysis]

Incompetent lower esophageal sphincter [hiatal hernia or other esophageal disease affecting stomach valve function]; delayed gastric emptying; decreased gastrointestinal motility; increased intragastric pressure; increased gastric residual

Presence of tracheostomy or endotracheal (ET) tube [inadequate or overinflation of tracheostomy/ET tube cuff]

[Presence of] gastrointestinal tubes; tube feedings; medication administration

NOTE: A risk diagnosis is not evidenced by signs and symptoms, as the problem has not occurred; rather, nursing interventions are directed at prevention.

Desired Outcomes/Evaluation Criteria— Client Will:

- Experience no aspiration as evidenced by noiseless respirations; clear breath sounds; clear, odorless secretions.
- Identify causative/risk factors.
- Demonstrate techniques to prevent and/or correct aspiration.

Information that appears in brackets has been added by the authors to clarify and enhance the use of nursing diagnoses.

🌐 Cultural 🔗 Collaborative 🏠 Community/Home Care

Nursing Priority No. 1.

To assess causative/contributing factors:

- Identify at-risk client according to condition or disease process, as listed in Risk Factors, **to determine when observation and/or interventions may be required.**
- Note client's level of consciousness, awareness of surroundings, and cognitive function, **as impairments in these areas increase client's risk of aspiration.**
- Determine presence of neuromuscular disorders, noting muscle groups involved, degree of impairment, and whether they are of an acute or progressive nature (e.g., stroke, Parkinson's disease, Guillain-Barré syndrome, or amyotrophic lateral sclerosis [ALS]).
- Assess client's ability to swallow and strength of gag/cough reflex and evaluate amount/consistency of secretions. **Helps to determine presence/effectiveness of protective mechanisms.**
- Observe for neck and facial edema. **Client with head/neck surgery, tracheal/bronchial injury (e.g., upper torso burns or inhalation/chemical injury) is at particular risk for airway obstruction and inability to handle secretions.**
- Note administration of enteral feedings **because of potential for regurgitation and/or displacement of tube.**
- Ascertain lifestyle habits; for example, use of alcohol, tobacco, and other CNS-suppressant drugs, **which can affect awareness and muscles of gag/swallow.**
- Assist with/review diagnostic studies (e.g., videofluoroscopy or fiberoptic endoscopy), **which may be done to assess for presence/degree of impairment.**

Nursing Priority No. 2.

To assist in correcting factors that can lead to aspiration:

- Monitor use of oxygen masks in clients at risk for vomiting. Refrain from using oxygen masks for comatose individuals.
- Keep wire cutters/scissors with client at all times when jaws are wired/banded **to facilitate clearing airway in emergency situations.**
- Maintain operational suction equipment at bedside/chairside.
- Suction (oral cavity, nose, and ET/tracheostomy tube), as needed, and avoid triggering gag mechanism when performing

---

Information that appears in brackets has been added by the authors to clarify and enhance the use of nursing diagnoses.

 Diagnostic Studies   ∞ Pediatric/Geriatric/Lifespan   Medications **103**

suction or mouth care **to clear secretions while reducing potential for aspiration of secretions.**

- Avoid keeping client supine/flat when on mechanical ventilation (especially when also receiving enteral feedings). **Supine positioning and enteral feedings have been shown to be independent risk factors for the development of aspiration pneumonia.**
- Assist with postural drainage **to mobilize thickened secretions that may interfere with swallowing.**
- Auscultate lung sounds frequently, especially in client who is coughing frequently or not coughing at all, or in client on ventilator being tube-fed, **to determine presence of secretions/silent aspiration.**
- Elevate client to highest or best possible position (e.g., sitting upright in chair) for eating and drinking and during tube feedings.
- Provide a rest period prior to feeding time. **The rested client may have less difficulty with swallowing.**
- Feed slowly, using small bites, instructing client to chew slowly and thoroughly.
- Vary placement of food in client's mouth according to type of deficit (e.g., place food in right side of mouth if facial weakness is present on left side).
- Provide soft foods that stick together/form a bolus (e.g., casseroles, puddings, or stews) **to aid swallowing effort.**
- Determine liquid viscosity best tolerated by client. Add thickening agent to liquids, as appropriate. **Some individuals may swallow thickened liquids better than thin liquids.**
- Offer very warm or very cold liquids. **Activates temperature receptors in the mouth that help to stimulate swallowing.**
- Avoid washing solids down with liquids.
- Ascertain that feeding tube (when used) is in correct position. Ask client about feeling of fullness and/or measure residuals (just prior to feeding and several hours after feeding), when appropriate, **to reduce risk of aspiration.**
- Determine best resting position for infant/child (e.g., with the head of bed elevated 30 degrees and infant propped on right side after feeding). **Upper airway patency is facilitated by upright position and turning to right side decreases likelihood of drainage into trachea.**
- Provide oral medications in elixir form or crush, if appropriate.
- Minimize use of sedatives/hypnotics whenever possible. **These agents can impair coughing and swallowing.**

Information that appears in brackets has been added by the authors to clarify and enhance the use of nursing diagnoses.

  Cultural 🄰 Collaborative 🏠 Community/Home Care

- Refer to physician/speech therapist for medical or surgical interventions and/or exercises **to strengthen muscles and learn techniques to enhance swallowing/reduce potential aspiration.**

Nursing Priority No. 3.

To promote wellness (Teaching/Discharge Considerations):

- Review with client/SO individual risk or potentiating factors.
- Provide information about the signs and effects of aspiration on the lungs. **Note: Severe coughing and cyanosis associated with eating or drinking or changes in vocal quality after swallowing indicates onset of respiratory symptoms associated with aspiration and requires immediate intervention.**
- Instruct in safety concerns regarding oral or tube feeing. (Refer to ND impaired Swallowing.)
- Train client how to self-suction or train family members in suction techniques (especially if client has constant or copious oral secretions) **to enhance safety/self-sufficiency.**
- Instruct individual/family member to avoid or limit activities after eating that increase intra-abdominal pressure (straining, strenuous exercise, or tight/constrictive clothing), **which may slow digestion/increase risk of regurgitation.**

Documentation Focus

Assessment/Reassessment

- Assessment findings, conditions that could lead to problems of aspiration.
- Verification of tube placement, observations of physical findings.

Planning

- Interventions to prevent aspiration or reduce risk factors and who is involved in the planning.
- Teaching plan.

Implementation/Evaluation

- Client's responses to interventions, teaching, and actions performed.
- Foods/fluids client handles with ease or difficulty.
- Amount and frequency of intake.
- Attainment or progress toward desired outcome(s).
- Modifications to plan of care.

Information that appears in brackets has been added by the authors to clarify and enhance the use of nursing diagnoses.

Discharge Planning
• Long-term needs and who is responsible for actions to be taken.

Sample Nursing Outcomes & Interventions Classifications (NOC/NIC) NIC

NOC—Aspiration Prevention
NIC—Aspiration Precautions

risk for impaired Attachment

Taxonomy II: Role Relationships—Class 2 Family Relationships (00058)
[Diagnostic Division: Social Interaction]
Submitted as risk for impaired parent/infant/child Attachment 1994

Definition: Disruption of the interactive process between parent/significant other and child/infant that fosters the development of a protective and nurturing reciprocal relationship

Risk Factors

Inability of parents to meet personal needs
Anxiety associated with the parent role; [parents who themselves experienced altered attachment]
Premature infant/ill child who is unable to effectively initiate parental contact due to altered behavioral organization; parental conflict resulting from altered behavioral organization
Separation; physical barriers; lack of privacy
Substance abuse
Difficult pregnancy and/or birth (actual or perceived)
Uncertainty of paternity; conception as a result of rape/sexual abuse

NOTE: A risk diagnosis is not evidenced by signs and symptoms, as the problem has not occurred; rather, nursing interventions are directed at prevention.

Desired Outcomes/Evaluation Criteria— Parent Will:

• Identify and prioritize family strengths and needs.
• Exhibit nurturant and protective behaviors toward child.

Information that appears in brackets has been added by the authors to clarify and enhance the use of nursing diagnoses.

- Identify and use resources to meet needs of family members.
- Demonstrate techniques to enhance behavioral organization of the infant/child.
- Engage in mutually satisfying interactions with child.

Actions/Interventions

Nursing Priority No. 1.
To identify causative/contributing factors:

- Interview parents, noting their perception of situation and individual concerns.
- Assess parent/child interactions.
- Ascertain availability and use of resources to include extended family, support groups, and financial resources.
- Evaluate parents' ability to provide protective environment and participate in reciprocal relationship.

Nursing Priority No. 2.
To enhance behavioral organization of child:

- ∞ Identify infant's strengths and vulnerabilities. **Each child is born with his or her own temperament that affects interactions with caregivers.**
- ∞ Educate parents regarding child growth and development, addressing parental perceptions. **Helps clarify realistic or unrealistic expectations.**
- ∞ Assist parents in modifying the environment **to provide appropriate stimulation.**
- Model caregiving techniques that best support behavioral organization.
- ∞ Respond consistently with nurturing to infant/child.

Nursing Priority No. 3.
To enhance best functioning of parents:

- Develop therapeutic nurse-client relationship. Provide a consistently warm, nurturing, and nonjudgmental environment.
- Assist parents in identifying and prioritizing family strengths and needs. **Promotes positive attitude by looking at what they already do well and using those skills to address needs.**
- Support and guide parents in process of assessing resources.
- ∞ Involve parents in activities with the child that they can accomplish successfully. **Promotes sense of confidence, thus enhancing self-concept.**

Information that appears in brackets has been added by the authors to clarify and enhance the use of nursing diagnoses.

- Recognize and provide positive feedback for nurturing and protective parenting behaviors. **Reinforces continuation of desired behaviors.**
- Minimize number of professionals on team with whom parents must have contact **to foster trust in relationships.**

Nursing Priority No. 4.
To support parent/child attachment during separation:
- Provide parents with telephone contact, as appropriate.
- Establish a routine time for daily phone calls/initiate calls, as indicated. **Provides sense of consistency and control; allows for planning of other activities.**
- Invite parents to use Ronald McDonald House or provide them with a listing of a variety of local accommodations and restaurants when child is hospitalized out of town.
- Arrange for parents to receive photos and progress reports from the child.
- Suggest parents provide a photo and/or audiotape of themselves for the child.
- Consider use of contract with parents **to clearly communicate expectations of both family and staff.**
- Suggest parents keep a journal of infant/child progress.
- Provide "homelike" environment for situations requiring supervision of visits.

Nursing Priority No. 5.
To promote wellness (Teaching/Discharge Considerations):
- Refer to individual counseling, family therapies, or addiction counseling/treatment, as indicated.
- Identify services for transportation, financial resources, housing, and so forth.
- Develop support systems appropriate to situation (e.g., extended family, friends, social worker).
- Explore community resources (e.g., church affiliations, volunteer groups, day/respite care).

Documentation Focus —————

Assessment/Reassessment
- Identified behaviors of both parents and child.
- Specific risk factors, individual perceptions and concerns.
- Interactions between parent and child.

Information that appears in brackets has been added by the authors to clarify and enhance the use of nursing diagnoses.

⊕ Cultural ⓐ Collaborative 🏠 Community/Home Care

Planning
- Plan of care and who is involved in planning.
- Teaching plan.

Implementation/Evaluation
- Parents'/child's responses to interventions, teaching, and actions performed.
- Attainment or progress toward desired outcomes.
- Modifications to plan of care.

Discharge Planning
- Long-term needs and who is responsible.
- Plan for home visits to support parents and to ensure infant/child safety and well-being.
- Specific referrals made.

Sample Nursing Outcomes & Interventions Classifications (NOC/NIC) NIC

NOC—Parent-Infant Attachment
NIC—Attachment Promotion

Autonomic Dysreflexia

Taxonomy II: Coping/Stress Tolerance—Class 3 Neurobehavioral Stress (00009)
[Diagnostic Division: Circulation]
Submitted 1988

Definition: Life-threatening, uninhibited sympathetic response of the nervous system to a noxious stimulus after a spinal cord injury [SCI] at T7 or above

Related Factors

Bladder/bowel distention; [catheter insertion, obstruction, irrigation; constipation]
Skin irritation
Deficient patient/caregiver knowledge
Sexual excitation; menstruation; pregnancy; labor and delivery
Environmental temperature extremes

Information that appears in brackets has been added by the authors to clarify and enhance the use of nursing diagnoses.

Defining Characteristics

Subjective

Headache (a diffuse pain in different portions of the head and not confined to any nerve distribution area)

Paresthesia; chilling; blurred vision; chest pain; metallic taste in mouth; nasal congestion

Objective

Paroxysmal hypertension [sudden periodic elevated blood pressure in which systolic pressure is greater than 140 mm Hg and diastolic pressure is greater than 90 mm Hg]

Bradycardia or tachycardia

Diaphoresis (above the injury), red splotches on skin (above the injury), pallor (below the injury)

Horner's syndrome [contraction of the pupil, partial ptosis of the eyelid, enophthalmos and sometimes loss of sweating over the affected side of the face]; conjunctival congestion

Pilomotor reflex [gooseflesh formation when skin is cooled]

Desired Outcomes/Evaluation Criteria— Client/Caregiver Will:

- Identify risk factors.
- Recognize signs/symptoms of syndrome.
- Demonstrate corrective techniques.
- Experience no episodes of dysreflexia or will seek medical intervention in a timely manner.

Actions/Interventions

Nursing Priority No. 1.

To assess precipitating risk factors:

- Monitor for bladder distention, presence of bladder spasms, stones, or infection. **The most common stimulus for autonomic dysreflexia (AD) is bladder irritation or overstretch associated with urinary retention or infection, blocked catheter, overfilled collection bag, or noncompliance with intermittent catheterization.**
- Assess for bowel distention, fecal impaction, problems with bowel management program. **Bowel irritation or overstretch is associated with constipation or impaction; digital stimulation, suppository or enema use during bowel program; hemorrhoids or fissures; and/or infection of**

Information that appears in brackets has been added by the authors to clarify and enhance the use of nursing diagnoses.

  🌐 Cultural   🔄 Collaborative   🏠 Community/Home Care

gastrointestinal tract, such as might occur with ulcers, appendicitis.
- Observe skin and tissue pressure areas, especially following prolonged sitting. **Skin and tissue irritants include direct pressure (e.g., object in chair or shoe, leg straps, abdominal support, orthotics), wounds (e.g., bruise, abrasion, laceration, pressure ulcer), ingrown toenail, tight clothing, sunburn or other burn.**
- Inquire about sexual activity and/or determine if reproductive issues are involved. **Overstimulation, vibration, sexual intercourse, ejaculation, scrotal compression, menstrual cramps, and/or pregnancy (especially labor and delivery) are known stimulants.**
- Inform client/care providers of additional precipitators during course of care. **Client is prone to numerous physical conditions or treatments (e.g., intolerance to temperature extremes; deep vein thrombosis [DVT]; kidney stones; fractures/other truama; surgical, dental, and diagnostic procedures), any of which can precipitate AD.**

Nursing Priority No. 2.
To provide for early detection and immediate intervention:
- Investigate associated complaints/symptoms (e.g., sudden severe headache, chest pains, blurred vision, facial flushing, nausea, metallic taste). **AD is a potentially life-threatening condition that requires immediate intervention.**
- Eliminate causative stimulus immediately when possible (e.g., perform immediate catheterization or restore urine flow if blocked; remove bowel impaction or stop digital stimulation; reduce skin pressure by changing position or removing restrictive clothing; protect from temperature extremes).
- Elevate head of bed as high as tolorated or place client in sitting position with legs dangling **to lower blood pressure.**
- Monitor vital signs frequently during acute episode. Continue to monitor blood pressure at intervals after symptoms subside **to evaluate effectiveness of interventions.**
- Administer medications as required **to block excessive autonomic nerve transmission, normalize heart rate, and reduce hypertension.**
- Adjust dosage of antihypertensive medications for children, the elderly, or pregnant women. **Assists in preventing seizures and maintaining blood pressure within desired range.**

Information that appears in brackets has been added by the authors to clarify and enhance the use of nursing diagnoses.

Nursing Priority No. 3.

To promote wellness (Teaching/Discharge Considerations):

• Discuss warning signs and how to avoid onset of syndrome with client/SO(s). **Knowledge can support adherence to preventive measures and promote prompt intervention when required. Note: If cause cannot be detected, or situation quickly resolved, contact physician immediately for further interventions to reduce risk of serious complications.**

• Instruct client/caregivers in preventive care (e.g., safe and timely bowel and bladder care; prevention of skin breakdown; care of existing skin breaks; prevention of infection).

• Instruct family member/caregiver in blood pressure monitoring and discuss plan for monitoring and treatment of high blood pressure during acute episodes.

• Review proper use/administration of medication if indicated. **Client may have medication(s) both for emergent situations and/or prevention of AD.**

• Assist client/family in identifying emergency referrals (e.g., physician, rehabilitation nurse, home-care supervisor). Place phone number(s) in prominent place.

• Recommend wearing medical alert bracelet/necklace and carrying information card reviewing client's typical signs/symptoms and usual methods of treatment. **Provides vital information to care providers in emergent situation.**

• Refer for advice or treatment of sexual and reproductive concerns as indicated.

• Refer to ND risk for Autonomic Dysreflexia.

Documentation Focus

Assessment/Reassessment

• Individual findings, noting previous episodes, precipitating factors, and individual signs/symptoms.

Planning

• Plan of care and who is involved in planning.
• Teaching plan.

Implementation/Evaluation

• Client's responses to interventions and actions performed, understanding of teaching.
• Attainment or progress toward desired outcome(s).
• Modifications to plan of care.

Information that appears in brackets has been added by the authors to clarify and enhance the use of nursing diagnoses.

Cultural   Collaborative   Community/Home Care

Discharge Planning

• Long-term needs and who is responsible for actions to be taken.

Sample Nursing Outcomes & Interventions Classifications (NOC/NIC) NIC

NOC—Neurological Status: Autonomic
NIC—Dysreflexia Management

risk for Autonomic Dysreflexia

Taxonomy II: Coping/Stress Tolerance—Class 3 Neuro-behavioral Stress (00010)
[Diagnostic Division: Circulation]
Nursing Diagnosis Extension and Classification (NDEC)
    Submission 1998/Revised 2000

Definition: At risk for life-threatening, uninhibited response of the sympathetic nervous system post-spinal shock, in an individual with a spinal cord injury [SCI] or lesion at T6 or above (has been demonstrated in patients with injuries at T7 and T8)

Risk Factors

An injury at T6 or above or a lesion at T6 or above and at least one of the following noxious stimuli:

Musculoskeletal—Integumentary Stimuli

Cutaneous stimulations (e.g., pressure ulcer, ingrown toenail, dressing, burns, rash); sunburns; wounds
Pressure over bony prominences/genitalia; range-of-motion exercises; spasms
Fractures; heterotrophic bone

Gastrointestinal Stimuli

Constipation; difficult passage of feces; fecal impaction; bowel distention; hemorrhoids
Digital stimulation; suppositories; enemas
GI system pathology; esophageal reflux; gastric ulcers; gallstones

Urological Stimuli

Bladder distention, spasm
Detrusor sphincter dyssynergia

Information that appears in brackets has been added by the authors to clarify and enhance the use of nursing diagnoses.

Diagnostic Studies   Pediatric/Geriatric/Lifespan   Medications **113**

Catheterization; instrumentation; surgery; calculi
Urinary tract infection; cystitis; urethritis; epididymitis

Regulatory Stimuli
Temperature fluctuations; extreme environmental temperatures

Situational Stimuli
Positioning; surgical procedure; [diagnostic procedures]
Constrictive clothing (e.g., straps, stockings, shoes)
Drug reactions (e.g., decongestants, sympathomimetics, vaso-
  constrictors, narcotic withdrawal)
Surgical or diagnostic procedures

Neurological Stimuli
Painful or irritating stimuli below the level of injury

Cardiac/Pulmonary Stimuli
Pulmonary emboli; deep vein thrombosis

Reproductive [and Sexuality] Stimuli
Sexual intercourse; ejaculation; [vibrator overstimulation; scro-
  tal compression]
Menstruation; pregnancy; labor and delivery; ovarian cyst

> **NOTE:** A risk diagnosis is not evidenced by signs and
> symptoms as the problem has not occurred; rather,
> nursing interventions are directed at prevention.

Desired Outcomes/Evaluation Criteria—
Client Will:

- Identify risk factors present.
- Demonstrate preventive or corrective techniques.
- Be free of episodes of dysreflexia.

Actions/Interventions

Nursing Priority No. 1.
To assess risk factors present:

- Monitor for potential precipitating factors, including urological
  (e.g., bladder distention, urinary tract infections, kidney stones);
  gastrointestinal (e.g., bowel overdistention, hemorrhoids,

Information that appears in brackets has been added by the authors to clarify
and enhance the use of nursing diagnoses.

  Cultural   Collaborative   Community/Home Care

digital stimulation); cutaneous (e.g., pressure ulcers, extreme external temperatures, dressing changes); reproductive (e.g., sexual activity, menstruation, pregnancy/delivery); and miscellaneous (e.g., pulmonary emboli, drug reaction, deep vein thrombosis).

Nursing Priority No. 2.
To prevent occurrence:

- Monitor vital signs, noting elevation in blood pressure, heart rate, and temperature, especially during times of physical stress, **to identify trends and intervene in a timely manner.**
- Instruct in appropriate interventions (e.g., regularly timed catheter and bowel care, appropriate padding for skin and tissues, proper positioning with frequent pressure-relief actions, checking frequently for tight clothes/leg straps, routine foot/toenail care, temperature control, sunburn/other burn prevention, compliance with preventive medications when used) **to prevent occurrence/limit severity.**
- Instruct all caregivers in safe bowel and bladder care, and immediate and long-term care for the prevention of skin stress/breakdown. **These problems are associated most frequently with AD.**
- Administer antihypertensive medications when at-risk client is placed on routine "maintenance dose," **as might occur when noxious stimuli cannot be removed (presence of chronic sacral pressure sore, fracture, or acute postoperative pain).**
- Refer to ND Autonomic Dysreflexia.

Nursing Priority No. 3.
To promote wellness (Teaching/Discharge Considerations):

- Discuss warning signs of AD with client/caregiver (i.e., sudden, severe pounding headache; flushed red face; increased blood pressure/acute hypertension; nasal congestion; anxiety; blurred vision; metallic taste in mouth; sweating and/or flushing above the level of SCI; goosebumps; bradycardia; cardiac irregularities). **AD can develop rapidly (in minutes), requiring quick intervention.**
- Review proper use and administration of medication if preventive medications are anticipated.
- Assist client/family in identifying emergency referrals (e.g., healthcare provider number in prominent place).

Information that appears in brackets has been added by the authors to clarify and enhance the use of nursing diagnoses.

Documentation Focus

Assessment/Reassessment
- Individual risk factors.
- Previous episodes, precipitating factors, and individual signs/symptoms.

Planning
- Plan of care and who is involved in planning.
- Teaching plan.

Implementation/Evaluation
- Client's responses to interventions and actions performed; understanding of teaching.
- Attainment or progress toward desired outcome(s).
- Modifications to plan of care.

Discharge Planning
- Long-term needs and who is responsible for actions to be taken.

Sample Nursing Outcomes & Interventions Classifications (NOC/NIC) NIC

NOC—Risk Control
NIC—Dysreflexia Management

---

risk-prone health Behavior

Taxonomy II: Coping/Stress Tolerance—Class 2 Coping Responses (00188)
[Diagnostic Division: Ego Integrity]
Submitted as impaired Adjustment 1986; Nursing Diagnosis Extension and Classification (NDEC) Revision 1998; Revised/Renamed 2006

Definition: Impaired ability to modify lifestyle/behaviors in a manner that improves health status

---

Related Factors

Inadequate comprehension; low self-efficacy
Multiple stressors
Smoking; excessive alcohol

Information that appears in brackets has been added by the authors to clarify and enhance the use of nursing diagnoses.

 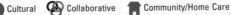 Cultural   Collaborative   Community/Home Care

Inadequate social support; low socioeconomic status
Negative attitude toward healthcare

Defining Characteristics

Subjective
Minimizes health status change
Failure to achieve optimal sense of control

Objective
Failure to take action that prevents health problems
Demonstrates nonacceptance of health status change

> **NOTE:** A risk diagnosis is not evidenced by signs and symptoms as the problem has not occurred; rather, nursing interventions are directed at prevention.

Desired Outcomes/Evaluation Criteria— Client Will:

* Demonstrate increasing interest/participation in self-care.
* Develop ability to assume responsibility for personal needs when possible.
* Identify stress situations leading to difficulties in adapting to change in health status and specific actions for dealing with them.
* Initiate lifestyle changes that will permit adaptation to current life situations.
* Identify and use appropriate support systems.

Actions/Interventions

Nursing Priority No. 1.
To assess degree of impaired function:

* Perform a physical and/or psychosocial assessment **to determine the extent of the limitation(s) of the current condition.**
* Listen to the client's perception of inability or reluctance to adapt to situations that are currently occurring.
* Survey (with the client) past and present significant support systems (e.g., family, church, groups, and organizations) **to identify helpful resources.**
* Explore the expressions of emotions signifying impaired adjustment by client/SO(s) (e.g., overwhelming anxiety, fear, anger, worry, passive and/or active denial).

Information that appears in brackets has been added by the authors to clarify and enhance the use of nursing diagnoses.

∞• Note child's interaction with parent/caregiver **Development of coping behaviors is limited at this age, and primary caregivers provide support for the child and serve as role models.**

∞• Determine whether child displays problems with school performance, withdraws from family or peers, or demonstrates aggressive behavior toward others/self.

Nursing Priority No. 2.

To identify the causative/contributing factors relating to the change in health behavior:

• Listen to client's perception of the factors leading to the present dilemma, noting onset, duration, presence or absence of physical complaints, and social withdrawal.

• Review previous life situations and role changes with client **to determine effects of prior experiences and coping skills used.**

• Note substance use/abuse (e.g., smoking, alcohol, prescription medications, street drugs) **that may be used as a coping mechanism, exacerbate health problem, or impair client's comprehension of situation.**

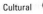• Determine lack of/inability to use available resources.

• Review available documentation and resources to determine actual life experiences (e.g., medical records, statements by SO[s], consultants' notes). **In situations of great stress, physical and/or emotional, the client may not accurately assess occurrences leading to the present situation.**

Nursing Priority No. 3.

To assist client in coping/dealing with impairment:

• Organize a team conference (including client and ancillary services) **to focus on contributing factors affecting adjustment and plan for management of the situation.**

• Acknowledge client's efforts to adjust: "Have done your best." **Lessens feelings of blame, guilt, or defensive response.**

∞• Share information with adolescent's peers with permission as indicated when illness/injury affects body image **Peers are primary support for this age group.**

• Explain disease process, causative factors, and prognosis, as appropriate, and promote questioning **to enhance understanding.**

• Provide an open environment encouraging communication **so that expression of feelings concerning impaired function can be dealt with realistically and openly.**

Information that appears in brackets has been added by the authors to clarify and enhance the use of nursing diagnoses.

⊕ Cultural ⊗ Collaborative 🏠 Community/Home Care

- Use therapeutic communication skills (Active-listening, acknowledgment, silence, I-statements).
- Discuss/evaluate resources that have been useful to the client in adapting to changes in other life situations (e.g., vocational rehabilitation, employment experiences, psychosocial support services).
- Develop a plan of action with client to meet immediate needs (e.g., physical safety and hygiene, emotional support of professionals and SO[s]) and assist in implementation of the plan. **Provides a starting point to deal with current situation for moving ahead with plan and for evaluation of progress.**
- Explore previously used coping skills and application to current situation. Refine or develop new strategies, as appropriate.
- Identify and problem-solve with the client frustration in daily health-related care. **Focusing on smaller factors of concern gives individual the ability to perceive impaired function from a less-threatening perspective, one-step-at-a-time concept.**
- Involve SO(s) in long-range planning for emotional, psychological, physical, and social needs.

Nursing Priority No. 4.
To promote wellness (Teaching/Discharge Considerations):

- Identify strengths the client perceives in current life situation. Keep focus on the present, **as unknowns of the future may be too overwhelming.**
- Refer to other resources in the long-range plan of care (e.g., occupational therapy, vocational rehabilitation, smoking cessation program, Alcoholics Anonymous) as indicated.
- Assist client/SO(s) to see appropriate alternatives and potential changes in locus of control.
- Assist SO(s) to learn methods for managing present needs. (Refer to NDs specific to client's deficits.)
- Pace and time learning sessions **to meet client's needs.** Provide feedback during and after learning experiences (e.g., self-catheterization, range-of-motion exercises, wound care, therapeutic communication) **to enhance retention, skill, and confidence.**

Documentation Focus

Assessment/Reassessment
- Reasons for, and degree of, impaired adaptation.
- Client's/SO's perception of the situation.
- Effect of behavior on health status/condition.

Information that appears in brackets has been added by the authors to clarify and enhance the use of nursing diagnoses.

Planning
- Plan for adjustments and interventions for achieving the plan and who is involved.
- Teaching plan.

Implementation/Evaluation
- Client responses to the interventions, teaching, and actions performed.
- Attainment or progress toward desired outcome(s).
- Modifications to plan of care.

Discharge Planning
- Resources that are available for the client and SO(s) and referrals that are made.

Sample Nursing Outcomes & Interventions Classifications (NOC/NIC) NIC

NOC—Acceptance: Health Status
NIC—Coping Enhancement

risk for Bleeding

Taxonomy II: Activity/Rest—Class 4: Cardiovascular/
Pulmonary Responses (00206)
[Diagnostic Division: Circulation]
Submitted 2008

Definition: At risk for a decrease in blood volume that may compromise health

Risk Factors

Aneurysm, trauma, history of falls

Gastrointestinal disorders (e.g. gastric ulcer disease, polyps, varices)

Impaired liver function (e.g. cirrhosis, hepatitis)

Pregnancy-related complications (e.g. placenta previa, molar pregnancy, abruption placenta); postpartum complications (e.g. uterine atony, retained placenta)

Inherent coagulopathies (e.g. thrombocytopenia, [hereditary hemorrhagic telangiectasia—HHT])

Treatment-related side effects (e.g., surgery, medications, administration of platelet-deficient blood products, chemotherapy); circumcision

---

Information that appears in brackets has been added by the authors to clarify and enhance the use of nursing diagnoses.

Cultural Collaborative Community/Home Care

Disseminated intravascular coagulopathy
Deficient knowledge

> **NOTE:** A risk diagnosis is not evidenced by signs and symptoms, as the problem has not occurred; rather, nursing interventions are directed at prevention.

Desired Outcomes/Evaluation Criteria— Client Will:

* Be free of signs of active bleeding such as hemoptysis, hematuria, or hematemesis; or excessive blood loss, as evidenced by stable vital signs, skin and mucous membranes free of pallor, usual mentation and urinary output.
* Display laboratory results for clotting times and factors within normal range for individual.
* Identify individual risks and engage in appropriate behaviors or lifestyle changes to prevent or reduce frequency of bleeding episodes.

Actions/Interventions

Nursing Priority No. 1.

* Assess client risk noting possible medical diagnoses or disease processes that may lead to bleeding as listed in risk factors.
* Note type of injury(ies) present when client presents with trauma. **The pattern and extent of injury may/may not be readily determined (e.g., unbroken skin can hide a significant injury with internal bleeding).**
* Determine presence of hereditary factors, obtain detailed history if a familial bleeding disorder is suspected such as HHT, hemophilia, other factor deficiencies; thrombocytopenia, and so on. **Hereditary bleeding or clotting disorders presdispose client to bleeding complications, necessitating specialized testing and/or referral to hematologist.**
* Note client's gender. **While bleeding disorders are common in both men and women, women are affected more owing to the increased risk of blood loss related to menstrual cycle and child delivery procedures.**
* Identify pregnancy-related factors such as overdistention of the uterus, lacerations of birth canal, or retained placenta.
* Evaluate client's medication regimen. **Use of medications, such as nonsteroidal anti-inflammatory drugs (NSAIDs),**

Information that appears in brackets has been added by the authors to clarify and enhance the use of nursing diagnoses.

anticoagulants, **corticosteroids, and certain herbals (gingko biloba), predispose client to bleeding.**

Nursing Priority No. 2.

- Monitor perineum and fundal height in postpartum client; and wounds, dressings or tubes in client with trauma, surgery, or other invasive procedures.
- Evaluate and mark boundaries of soft tissues in enclosed structures, such as a leg or abdomen, **to document expanding bruises or hematomas.**
- Assess vital signs, including blood pressure, pulse, and respirations. Measure blood pressure lying/sitting/standing as indicated to evaluate for orthostatic hypotension; monitor invasive hemodynamic parameters when present **to determine if intravascular fluid deficit exists.**
- Hematest all secretions and excretions for occult blood.
- Note client report of pain in specific areas, whether pain is increasing, diffuse, or localized. **Can help identify bleeding into tissues, organs, or body cavities.**
- Assess skin color and moisture, urinary output, level of consciousness or mentation. **Changes in these signs may be indicative of blood loss affecting systemic circulation or local organ function such as kidneys or brain.**
- Review laboratory data (e.g., complete blood count [CBC], platelet numbers and function; and other coagulation factors such as Factor I, Factor II, prothrombin time [PT], partial thromboplastin time [PTT], fibrinogen).
- Prepare client for, or assist with, diagnostic studies such as x-rays, computed tomography (CT) or magnetic resonance imaging (MRI) scans, ultrasound, **to determine presence of injuries or disorders that could cause internal bleeding.**

Nursing Priority No. 3.
To prevent bleeding/correct potential causes of excessive blood loss:

- Apply direct pressure and cold pack to bleeding site, insert nasal packing, or perform fundal massage as appropriate.
- Restrict activity, encourage bedrest or chair rest until bleeding abates.
- Maintain patency of vascular access **for fluid administration or blood replacement as indicated.**
- Assist with treatment of underlying conditions causing or contributing to blood loss such as medical treatment of systemic infections, or balloon tamponade of esophageal varices prior

risk for BLEEDING

Information that appears in brackets has been added by the authors to clarify and enhance the use of nursing diagnoses.

⊕ Cultural Collaborative Community/Home Care

to sclerotherapy; use of proton pump inhibitor medications or antibiotics for gastric ulcer; surgery for internal abdominal trauma, or retained placenta.

- Provide special intervention in at-risk client, such as individual with bone marrow suppression, chemotherapy, or uremia, **to prevent bleeding associated with tissue injury:**

  Monitor closely for overt bleeding.

  Observe for diffuse oozing from tubes, wounds, orifices with no observable clotting.

  Maintain pressure or pressure dressings as indicated for longer period of time **such as over arterial puncture site.**

  Hematest secretions and excretions for occult blood.

  Protect client from trauma such as falls, accidental or intentional blows, or lacerations.

  Use soft toothbrush or toothettes for oral care **to reduce risk of injury to oral mucosa.**

- Collaborate in evaluating need for replacing blood loss or specific components and be prepared for emergency interventions.

- Be prepared to administer hemostatic agents, which promote clotting and may stop bleeding by increasing coagulation factors; or medications to prevent bleeding such as proton pump inhibitors to reduce risk of gastrointestinal bleeding and need for replacement transfusion.

- Provide information to client/family about hereditary or familial problems that predispose to bleeding complications.

- Instruct at-risk client and family regarding:

  Specific signs of bleeding requiring healthcare provider notification, such as active bright bleeding anywhere, prolonged epistaxis or trauma in client with known factor bleeding tendencies, black tarry stools, weakness, vertigo, and syncope.

  Need to inform healthcare providers when taking aspirin and other anticoagulant-type agents (e.g., Coumadin, Plavix), especially when elective surgery or other invasive procedure is planned. **These agents will most likely be held for a period of time prior to elective procedures to reduce potential for excessive blood loss.**

  Importance of periodic review of client's medication regimen **to identify medications that might cause or exacerbate bleeding problems.**

  Necessity of regular medical and laboratory follow-up when on anticoagulants, such as Coumadin, **to determine needed dosage changes or client management issues requiring monitoring and/or modification.**

Information that appears in brackets has been added by the authors to clarify and enhance the use of nursing diagnoses.

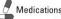

Dietary measures **to promote blood clotting, when indicated, such as foods rich in vitamin K.**

Need to avoid alcohol in diagnosed liver disorders or seek treatment for alcoholism in presence of alcoholic varices.

Techniques for postpartum client to check her own fundus and perform fundal massage as indicated; client to contact physician for postdischarge bleeding that is bright red or dark red with large clots. **May prevent blood loss complications, especially if client is discharged early from hospital.**

Documentation Focus

Assessment/Reassessment
- Individual factors that may potentiate blood loss—type of injuries, obstetrical complications, and so on.
- Baseline vital signs, mentation, urinary output, and subsequent assessments.
- Results of laboratory tests or diagnostic procedures.

Planning
- Plan of care and who is involved in the planning.
- Teaching plan.

Implementation/Evaluation
- Responses to interventions, teaching, and actions performed.
- Attainment or progress toward desired outcome(s).
- Modifications to plan of care.

Discharge Planning
- Long-term needs, identifying who is responsible for actions to be taken.
- Community resources or support for chronic problems.
- Specific referrals made.

Sample Nursing Outcomes & Interventions Classifications (NOC/NIC) NIC

NOC—Blood Loss Severity
NIC—Bleeding Precautions

Information that appears in brackets has been added by the authors to clarify and enhance the use of nursing diagnoses.

Cultural   Collaborative   Community/Home Care

disturbed Body Image

Taxonomy II: Perception/Cognition—Class 3 Body Image
(00118)
[Diagnostic Division: Ego Integrity]
Submitted 1973; Revised 1998 (by small group work
1996)

Definition: Confusion [and/or dissatisfaction] in mental
picture of one's physical self

Related Factors

Biophysical; illness; trauma; injury; surgery; [mutilation, pregnancy]
Illness treatment [change caused by biochemical agents (drugs),
dependence on machine]
Psychosocial
Cultural; spiritual
Cognitive; perceptual
Developmental changes [maturational changes]
Significance of body part or functioning with regard to age,
gender, developmental level, or basic human needs

Defining Characteristics

Subjective

Verbalization of feelings that reflect an altered view of one's
body (e.g., appearance, structure, function)
Verbalization of perceptions that reflect an altered view of one's
body in appearance
Verbalization of change in lifestyle
Fear of rejection/reaction by others
Focus on past strength, function, appearance
Negative feelings about body (e.g., feelings of helplessness,
hopelessness, or powerlessness); [depersonalization, grandiosity]
Preoccupation with change, loss
Refusal to verify actual change
Emphasis on remaining strengths; heightened achievement
Personalization of part/loss by name
Depersonalization of part/loss by impersonal pronouns

Objective

Behaviors of: acknowledgment of one's body; avoidance of
one's body; monitoring one's body

Information that appears in brackets has been added by the authors to clarify
and enhance the use of nursing diagnoses.

Nonverbal response to actual or perceived change in body (e.g., appearance, structure, function)

Missing body part

Actual change in structure or function

Not looking at/not touching body part

Trauma to nonfunctioning part

Change in ability to estimate spatial relationship of body to environment

Extension of body boundary to incorporate environmental objects

Intentional/unintentional hiding [or] overexposing of body part

Change in social involvement

Aggression; low frustration tolerance level

Desired Outcomes/Evaluation Criteria— Client Will:

- Verbalize understanding of body changes.
- Recognize and incorporate body image change into self-concept in accurate manner without negating self-esteem.
- Verbalize acceptance of self in situation (e.g., chronic progressive disease, amputee, decreased independence, weight as is, effects of therapeutic regimen).
- Verbalize relief of anxiety and adaptation to actual/altered body image.
- Seek information and actively pursue growth.
- Acknowledge self as an individual who has responsibility for self.
- Use adaptive devices/prosthesis appropriately.

Actions/Interventions

Nursing Priority No. 1.

To assess causative/contributing factors:

- Discuss pathophysiology present and/or situation affecting the individual and refer to additional NDs as appropriate. For example, when alteration in body image is related to neurological deficit (e.g., cerebrovascular accident—CVA), refer to ND unilateral Neglect; in the presence of severe, ongoing pain, refer to ND chronic Pain; or in loss of sexual desire/ability, refer to ND Sexual Dysfunction.
- Determine whether condition is permanent with no expectation for resolution. (May be associated with other NDs, such as Self-Esteem [specify] or risk for impaired parent/child

---

Information that appears in brackets has been added by the authors to clarify and enhance the use of nursing diagnoses.

Attachment, when child is affected.) **There is always something that can be done to enhance acceptance, and it is important to hold out the possibility of living a good life with the disability.**

- Assess mental and physical influence of illness or condition on the client's emotional state (e.g., diseases of the endocrine system, use of steroid therapy).
- Evaluate level of client's knowledge of and anxiety related to situation. Observe emotional changes, **which may indicate acceptance or nonacceptance of situation.**
- Recognize behavior indicative of overconcern with body and its processes.
- Have client describe self, noting what is positive and what is negative. Be aware of how client believes others see self.
∞• Discuss meaning of loss/change to client. **A small (seemingly trivial) loss may have a big impact (such as the use of a urinary catheter or enema for continence). A change in function (such as immobility in elderly) may be more difficult for some to deal with than a change in appearance. Or the change could be devastating, such as permanent facial scarring of child.**
∞• Use developmentally appropriate communication techniques for determining exact expression of body image in child (e.g., puppet play or constructive dialogue for toddler). **Developmental capacity must guide interaction to gain accurate information.**
• Note signs of grieving or indicators of severe or prolonged depression **to evaluate need for counseling and/or medications.**
• Determine ethnic background and cultural and religious perceptions or considerations. **May influence how individual deals with what has happened.**
- Identify social aspects of illness or condition (e.g., sexually transmitted diseases, sterility, chronic conditions).
- Observe interaction of client with SO(s). **Distortions in body image may be unconsciously reinforced by family members and/or secondary gain issues may interfere with progress.**

Nursing Priority No. 2.

To determine coping abilities and skills:

- Assess client's current level of adaptation and progress.
- Listen to client's comments and responses to the situation. **Different situations are upsetting to different people, depending on individual coping skills and past experiences.**

Information that appears in brackets has been added by the authors to clarify and enhance the use of nursing diagnoses.

- Note withdrawn behavior and the use of denial. **May be normal response to situation or may be indicative of mental illness (e.g., schizophrenia).** (Refer to ND ineffective Denial.)
- Note use of addictive substances, such as alcohol or other drugs, **which may reflect dysfunctional coping.**
- Identify previously used coping strategies and effectiveness.
- Determine individual/family/community resources available to client.

Nursing Priority No. 3.
To assist client and SO(s) to deal with/accept issues of self-concept related to body image:

- Establish therapeutic nurse-client relationship, conveying an attitude of caring and developing a sense of trust.
- Visit client frequently and acknowledge the individual as someone who is worthwhile. **Provides opportunities for listening to concerns and questions.**
- Assist in correcting underlying problems **to promote optimal healing and adaptation.**
- Provide assistance with self-care needs as necessary, while promoting individual abilities and independence.
- Work with client's self-concept, avoiding moral judgments regarding client's efforts or progress (e.g., "You should be progressing faster; You're weak or not trying hard enough"). **Positive reinforcement encourages client to continue efforts and strive for improvement.**
- Discuss concerns about fear of mutilation, prognosis, rejection when client is facing surgery or potentially poor outcome of procedure/illness, **to address realities and provide emotional support.**
- Acknowledge and accept feelings of dependency, grief, and hostility.
- Encourage verbalization of and role-play anticipated conflicts **to enhance handling of potential situations.**
- Encourage client and SO(s) to communicate feelings to each other.
- Assume all individuals are sensitive to changes in appearance but avoid stereotyping.
- Alert staff to monitor own facial expressions and other non-verbal behaviors **because they need to convey acceptance and not revulsion when the client's appearance is affected.**
- Encourage family members to treat client normally and not as an invalid.

Information that appears in brackets has been added by the authors to clarify and enhance the use of nursing diagnoses.

- Encourage client to look at/touch affected body part **to begin to incorporate changes into body image.**
- Allow client to use denial without participating (e.g., client may at first refuse to look at a colostomy; the nurse says "I am going to change your colostomy now" and proceeds with the task). **Provides individual time to adapt to situation.**
- Set limits on maladaptive behavior and assist client to identify positive behaviors **to aid in recovery.**
- Provide accurate information as desired/requested. Reinforce previously given information.
- Discuss the availability of prosthetics, reconstructive surgery, and physical/occupational therapy or other referrals as dictated by individual situation.
- Help client select and use clothing or makeup **to minimize body changes and enhance appearance.**
- Discuss reasons for infectious isolation and treatment procedures when used, and make time to sit down and talk/listen to client while in the room **to decrease sense of isolation/ loneliness.**

Nursing Priority No. 4.

To promote wellness (Teaching/Discharge Considerations):

- Begin counseling/other therapies (e.g., biofeedback, relaxation) as soon as possible **to provide early/ongoing sources of support.**
- Provide information at client's level of acceptance and in small segments **to allow easier assimilation.** Clarify misconceptions. Reinforce explanations given by other health team members.
- Include client in decision-making process and problem-solving activities.
- Assist client to incorporate therapeutic regimen into activities of daily living (ADLs) (e.g., including specific exercises, housework activities). **Promotes continuation of program.**
- Identify/plan for alterations to home and work environment/ activities **to accommodate individual needs and support independence.**
- Assist client in learning strategies for dealing with feelings and venting emotions.
- Offer positive reinforcement for efforts made (e.g., wearing makeup, using prosthetic device).
- Refer to appropriate support groups.

Information that appears in brackets has been added by the authors to clarify and enhance the use of nursing diagnoses.

Documentation Focus

Assessment/Reassessment
- Observations, presence of maladaptive behaviors, emotional changes, stage of grieving, level of independence.
- Physical wounds, dressings; use of life support–type machine (e.g., ventilator, dialysis machine).
- Meaning of loss or change to client.
- Support systems available (e.g., SOs, friends, groups).

Planning
- Plan of care and who is involved in planning.
- Teaching plan.

Implementation/Evaluation
- Client's response to interventions, teaching, and actions performed.
- Attainment or progress toward desired outcome(s).
- Modifications of plan of care.

Discharge Planning
- Long-term needs and who is responsible for actions.
- Specific referrals made (e.g., rehabilitation center, community resources).

Sample Nursing Outcomes & Interventions Classifications (NOC/NIC) NIC

NOC—Body Image
NIC—Body Image Enhancement

---

risk for imbalanced Body Temperature

Taxonomy II: Safety/Protection—Class 6 Thermoregulation (00005)
[Diagnostic Division: Safety]
Submitted 1986; Revised 2000

Definition: At risk for failure to maintain body temperature within normal range

---

Information that appears in brackets has been added by the authors to clarify and enhance the use of nursing diagnoses.

Risk Factors

Extremes of age, weight

Exposure to extremes of environmental temperature; inappropriate clothing for environmental temperature

Dehydration

Inactivity; vigorous activity

Medications causing vasoconstriction or vasodilation; sedation [use or overdose of certain drugs or exposure to anesthesia]

Illness or trauma affecting temperature regulation [e.g., infections, systemic or localized; neoplasms, tumors; collagen/vascular disease]; altered metabolic rate

> **NOTE:** A risk diagnosis is not evidenced by signs and symptoms as the problem has not occurred; rather, nursing interventions are directed at prevention.

Desired Outcomes/Evaluation Criteria—Client Will:

- Maintain body temperature within normal range.
- Verbalize understanding of individual risk factors and appropriate interventions.
- Demonstrate behaviors for monitoring and maintaining appropriate body temperature.

Actions/Interventions

Nursing Priority No. 1.
To identify causative/risk factors present:

- Determine if present illness/condition results from exposure to environmental factors, surgery, infection, trauma. **Helps in determining the scope of interventions that may be needed (e.g., simple addition of warm blankets after surgery, or hypothermia therapy following brain trauma).**
- Monitor laboratory values (e.g., tests indicative of infection, thyroid or other endocrine tests, drug screens) **to identify potential internal causes of temperature imbalances.**
- Note client's age (e.g., premature neonate, young child, or aging individual), **as it can directly impact ability to maintain/regulate body temperature and respond to changes in environment.**

Information that appears in brackets has been added by the authors to clarify and enhance the use of nursing diagnoses.

- Assess nutritional status **to determine metabolism effect on body temperature and to identify foods or nutrient deficits that affect metabolism.**

Nursing Priority No. 2.

To prevent occurrence of temperature alteration:

- Monitor and maintain comfortable ambient environment (e.g., provide heating/cooling measures such as space heaters/fans) as indicated.
- Supervise use of heating pads, electric blankets, ice bags, and hypothermia blankets, especially in clients who cannot self-protect.
- Dress client or discuss with client/caregiver(s) appropriate dressing (e.g., layering clothing, use of hat and gloves in cold weather, light loose clothing in warm weather, water-resistant outer gear).
- ∞ Cover infant's head with knit cap, place under adequate blankets. Place newborn infant under radiant warmer. **Heat loss in newborns/infants is greatest through head and by evaporation and convection.**
- ∞ Limit clothing or remove blanket from premature infant placed in incubator **to prevent overheating in climate-controlled environment.**
- ∞ Monitor core body temperature. **Tympanic temperature may be preferred, as it is the most accurate noninvasive method, except in infants, where skin electrode is preferred.**
- ⊛ Restore/maintain core temperature within client's normal range. **Client may require interventions to treat hypothermia or hyperthermia.** (Refer to NDs Hypothermia; Hyperthermia.)
- ⋔ Recommend lifestyle changes, such as cessation of smoking or substance use, normalization of body weight, nutritious meals, and regular exercise **to maximize metabolism to meet individual needs.**
- ⊛ Refer at-risk persons to appropriate community resources (e.g., home care, social services, foster adult care, housing agencies) **to provide assistance to meet individual needs.**

Nursing Priority No. 3.

To promote wellness (Teaching/Discharge Considerations):

- ⋔ Discuss potential problem/individual risk factors with client/SO(s).

Information that appears in brackets has been added by the authors to clarify and enhance the use of nursing diagnoses.

    Cultural   Collaborative   ⋔ Community/Home Care

∞ • Review age and gender issues, as appropriate. **Older or debilitated persons, babies, and young children typically feel more comfortable in higher ambient temperatures. Women notice feeling cooler quicker than men, which may be related to body size, or to differences in metabolism and the rate that blood flows to extremities to regulate body temperature.**

🏠 • Instruct in appropriate self-care measures (e.g., adding or removing clothing; adding or removing heat sources; reviewing medication regimen with physician to identify those which can affect thermoregulaton; evaluating home/shelter for ability to manage heat and cold; addressing nutritional and hydration status) **to protect from identified risk factors.**

🏠 • Review ways to prevent accidental temperature alterations, such as hypothermia resulting from overzealous cooling to reduce fever, or maintaining too warm an environment for client who has lost the ability to perspire.

Documentation Focus

Assessment/Reassessment
• Identified individual causative and risk factors.
• Record of core temperature, initially and prn.
• Results of diagnostic studies and laboratory tests.

Planning
• Plan of care and who is involved in planning.
• Teaching plan, including best ambient temperature, and ways to prevent hypothermia or hyperthermia.

Implementation/Evaluation
• Response to interventions, teaching, and actions performed.
• Attainment or progress toward desired outcome(s).
• Modifications to plan of care.

Discharge Planning
• Long-term needs and who is responsible for actions.
• Specific referrals made.

Sample Nursing Outcomes & Interventions Classifications (NOC/NIC) NIC

NOC—Thermoregulation
NIC—Temperature Regulation

Information that appears in brackets has been added by the authors to clarify and enhance the use of nursing diagnoses.

Bowel Incontinence

Taxonomy II: Elimination and Exchange—Class 2
  Gastrointestinal Function (00014)
[Diagnostic Division: Elimination]
Submitted 1975; Nursing Diagnosis Extension and
  Classification (NDEC) Revision 1998

Definition: Change in normal bowel habits characterized
by involuntary passage of stool

Related Factors

Toileting self-care deficit; environmental factors (e.g., inaccessible bathroom); impaired cognition; immobility
Dietary habits; medications; laxative abuse
Stress
Colorectal lesions; impaired reservoir capacity
Incomplete emptying of bowel; impaction; chronic diarrhea
General decline in muscle tone; abnormally high abdominal or intestinal pressure
Rectal sphincter abnormality; loss of rectal sphincter control; lower or upper motor nerve damage

Defining Characteristics

Subjective
Recognizes rectal fullness, but reports inability to expel formed stool
Urgency; inability to delay defecation
Self-report of inability to feel rectal fullness

Objective
Constant dribbling of soft stool
Fecal staining of clothing/bedding
Fecal odor
Red perianal skin
Inability to recognize/inattention to urge to defecate

Desired Outcomes/Evaluation Criteria—Client Will:

- Verbalize understanding of causative and controlling factors.
- Identify individually appropriate interventions.
- Participate in therapeutic regimen to control incontinence.

Information that appears in brackets has been added by the authors to clarify
and enhance the use of nursing diagnoses.

Cultural   Collaborative   Community/Home Care

- Establish/maintain as regular a pattern of bowel functioning as possible.

Actions/Interventions

Nursing Priority No. 1.
To assess causative/contributing factors:

- Identify pathophysiological factors present (e.g., multiple sclerosis [MS], acute or chronic cognitive and self-care impairments, spinal cord injury, stroke, ileus, ulcerative colitis).
- Determine historical aspects of incontinence with preceding/precipitating events. **The most common factors in incontinence include chronic constipation with leakage around impacted stool; severe diarrhea; decreased awareness of bowel fullness due to nerve or muscle damage (e.g., stroke, trauma, tumor, radiation); injury to anal muscles (e.g., due to childbirth, surgery, rectal prolapse); chronic laxative abuse; and emotional or psychological disorders.**
- Review medication regimen (e.g., sedatives/hypnotics, narcotics, muscle relaxants, antacids). **Many medications and their side effects or interactions can increase potential for bowel problems.**
- Review results of diagnostic studies (e.g., abdominal x-rays, colon endoscopy/other imaging, complete blood count, serum chemistries, stool for blood [guaiac]), as appropriate.
- Palpate abdomen **for distention, masses, tenderness.**

Nursing Priority No. 2.
To determine current pattern of elimination:

- Note stool characteristics (color, odor, consistency, amount, shape, and frequency). **Provides comparative baseline.**
- Encourage client or SO to record times at which incontinence occurs, **to note relationship to meals, activity, medications or client's behavior.**
- Auscultate abdomen **for presence, location, and characteristics of bowel sounds.**

Nursing Priority No. 3.
To promote control/management of incontinence:

- Assist in treatment of causative/contributing factors (e.g., as listed in the Related Factors and Defining Characteristics).
- Establish bowel program with predictable time for defecation efforts; use suppositories and/or digital stimulation when

---

Information that appears in brackets has been added by the authors to clarify and enhance the use of nursing diagnoses.

indicated. Maintain daily program initially. Progress to alternate days dependent on usual pattern or amount of stool.

- Take client to the bathroom, or place on commode or bedpan at specified intervals, taking into consideration individual needs and incontinence patterns **to maximize success of program.**
- Encourage and instruct client/caregiver in providing diet high in bulk/fiber and adequate fluids (minimum of 2000–2400 mL/day). Encourage warm fluids after meals.
- Identify and eliminate problem foods **to avoid diarrhea, constipation, and gas formation.**
- Give stool softeners/bulk formers as indicated.
- Provide pericare with frequent gentle cleansing and use of emollients **to avoid perineal excoriation.**
- Promote exercise program, as individually able, **to increase muscle tone/strength, including perineal muscles.**
- Provide incontinence aids/pads until control is obtained. Note: Incontinence pads should be changed frequently **to reduce incidence of skin rashes/breakdown.**
- Demonstrate techniques (e.g., contracting abdominal muscles, leaning forward on commode, manual compression) **to increase intra-abdominal pressure during defecation, and left to right abdominal massage to stimulate peristalsis.**
- Refer to ND Diarrhea if incontinence is due to uncontrolled diarrhea; ND Constipation if incontinence is due to impaction.

Nursing Priority No. 4.

To promote wellness (Teaching/Discharge Considerations):

- Review and encourage continuation of successful interventions as individually identified.
- Instruct in use of suppositories or stool softeners, if indicated, **to stimulate timed defecation.**
- Identify foods (e.g., daily bran muffins, prunes) that promote bowel regularity.
- Provide emotional support to client and SO(s), especially when condition is long-term or chronic. **Enhances coping with difficult situation.**
- Encourage scheduling of social activities within time frame of bowel program, as indicated (e.g., avoid a 4-hour excursion if bowel program requires toileting every 3 hours and facilities will not be available), **to maximize social functioning and success of bowel program.**

Information that appears in brackets has been added by the authors to clarify and enhance the use of nursing diagnoses.

🌐 Cultural   Collaborative   🏠 Community/Home Care

Assessment/Reassessment
• Current and previous pattern of elimination, physical findings, character of stool, actions tried.

Planning
• Plan of care and who is involved in planning.
• Teaching plan.

Implementation/Evaluation
• Client's/caregiver's responses to interventions, teaching, and actions performed.
• Changes in pattern of elimination, characteristics of stool.
• Attainment or progress toward desired outcome(s).
• Modifications to plan of care.

Discharge Planning
• Identified long-term needs, noting who is responsible for each action.
• Specific bowel program at time of discharge.

Sample Nursing Outcomes & Interventions Classifications (NOC/NIC) NIC

NOC—Bowel Continence
NIC—Bowel Incontinence Care

---

effective Breastfeeding*
[Learning Need]

Taxonomy II: Role Relationships—Class 3 Role Performance (00106)
[Diagnostic Division: Food/Fluid]
Submitted 1990

Definition: Mother-infant dyad/family exhibits adequate proficiency and satisfaction with breastfeeding process

---

*This ND is a challenge to address, as the Related Factors and Defining Characteristics are in fact the outcomes/evaluation criteria that would be desired. We believe that normal breastfeeding behaviors need to be learned and supported, with interventions directed at learning activities for enhancement.

Information that appears in brackets has been added by the authors to clarify and enhance the use of nursing diagnoses.

Related Factors

Basic breastfeeding knowledge
Normal breast structure
Normal infant oral structure
Infant gestational age greater than 34 weeks
Support sources [available]
Maternal confidence

Defining Characteristics

Subjective

Maternal verbalization of satisfaction with the breastfeeding process

Objective

Mother able to position infant at breast to promote a successful latch-on response
Infant content after feedings
Regular and sustained suckling/swallowing at the breast [e.g., 8–10 times/24 hr]
Appropriate infant weight patterns for age
Effective mother/infant communication patterns [infant cues, maternal interpretation and response]
Signs/symptoms of oxytocin release (let-down or milk ejection reflex)
Adequate infant elimination patterns for age [stools soft; more than 6 wet diapers/day of unconcentrated urine]
Eagerness of infant to nurse

Desired Outcomes/Evaluation Criteria— Client Will:

- Verbalize understanding of breastfeeding techniques.
- Demonstrate effective techniques for breastfeeding.
- Demonstrate family involvement and support.
- Attend classes, read appropriate materials, and access resources as necessary.

Actions/Interventions

Nursing Priority No. 1.

To assess individual learning needs:
- Assess mother's knowledge and previous experience with breastfeeding.

Information that appears in brackets has been added by the authors to clarify and enhance the use of nursing diagnoses.

  Cultural   Collaborative   Community/Home Care

- Identify cultural beliefs/practices regarding lactation, let-down techniques, maternal food preferences.
- Note incorrect myths/misunderstandings especially in teenage mothers, **who are more likely to have limited knowledge, as well as concerns about body image issues.**
- Monitor effectiveness of current breastfeeding efforts.
- Determine support systems available to mother/family. **Infant's father and maternal grandmother, in addition to caring healthcare providers, are important factors in whether breastfeeding is successful.**

Nursing Priority No. 2.
To promote effective breastfeeding behaviors:

- Initiate breastfeeding within first hour after birth.
- Demonstrate how to support and position infant.
- Observe mother's return demonstration.
- Encourage skin-to-skin contact.
- Keep infant with mother **for unrestricted breastfeeding duration and frequency.**
- Encourage mother to drink at least 2000 mL of fluid per day or 6 to 8 oz every hour.
- Provide information as needed about early infant feeding cues (e.g., rooting, lip smacking, sucking fingers/hand) versus late cue of crying. **Early recognition of infant hunger promotes timely/more rewarding feeding experience for infant and mother.**
- Discuss/demonstrate breastfeeding aids (e.g., infant sling, nursing footstool/pillows, breast pumps).
- Promote peer counseling for teen mothers. **Provides positive role model that teen can relate to and feel comfortable discussing concerns/feelings.**

Nursing Priority No. 3.
To enhance optimum wellness (Teaching/Discharge Considerations):

- Provide for follow-up contact or home visit 48 hours after discharge, as indicated or desired; repeat visits as necessary **to provide support and assist with problem solving.**
- Recommend monitoring number of infant's wet diapers. **(Some pediatric care providers suggest that six wet diapers in 24 hours indicate adequate hydration.)**
- Encourage mother/other family members to express feelings/concerns, and Active-listen **to determine nature of concerns.**

Information that appears in brackets has been added by the authors to clarify and enhance the use of nursing diagnoses.

• Educate father/SO about benefits of breastfeeding and how to manage common lactation challenges. **Enlisting support of father/SO is associated with higher ratio of successful breastfeeding at 6 months.**

• Review techniques for expression (breast pumping) and storage of breast milk **to help sustain breastfeeding activity.**

• Problem-solve return-to-work issues or periodic infant care requiring bottle/supplemental feeding.

• Recommend using expressed breast milk instead of formula or at least partial breastfeeding for as long as mother and child are satisfied.

• Explain changes in feeding needs/frequency. **Growth spurts require increased intake/more feedings by infant.**

• Review normal nursing behaviors of older breastfeeding infants/toddlers.

• Discuss importance of delaying introduction of solid foods until infant is at least 4 months, preferably 6 months old.

• Recommend avoidance of specific medications or substances (e.g., estrogen-containing contraceptives, bromocriptine, nicotine, alcohol) **that are known to decrease milk supply. Note: Small amounts of alcohol have not been shown to be detrimental.**

• Stress importance of client notifying healthcare providers, dentists, and pharmacists of breastfeeding status.

• Refer to support groups, such as La Leche League, as indicated.

• Refer to ND ineffective Breastfeeding for more specific information addressing challenges to breastfeeding, as appropriate.

Documentation Focus

Assessment/Reassessment
• Identified assessment factors (maternal and infant).
• Number of wet diapers daily and periodic weight.

Planning
• Plan of care, specific interventions, and who is involved in the planning.
• Teaching plan.

Implementation/Evaluation
• Mother's response to actions, teaching plan, and actions performed.
• Effectiveness of infant's efforts to feed.

Information that appears in brackets has been added by the authors to clarify and enhance the use of nursing diagnoses.

🌐 Cultural   🔵 Collaborative   🏠 Community/Home Care

- Attainment or progress toward desired outcome(s).
- Modifications to plan of care.

Discharge Planning
- Long-term needs, referrals, and who is responsible for follow-up actions.

Sample Nursing Outcomes & Interventions Classifications (NOC/NIC) NIC

NOC—Breastfeeding Maintenance
NIC—Lactation Counseling

---

ineffective **Breastfeeding**

Taxonomy II: Role Relationships—Class 3 Role Performance (00104)
[Diagnostic Division: Food/Fluid]
Submitted 1988

Definition: Dissatisfaction or difficulty a mother, infant, or child experiences with the breastfeeding process

---

Related Factors

Prematurity; infant anomaly; poor infant sucking reflex
Infant receiving [numerous or repeated] supplemental feedings with artificial nipple
Maternal anxiety, ambivalence
Knowledge deficit
Previous history of breastfeeding failure
Interruption in breastfeeding
Nonsupportive partner, family
Maternal breast anomaly; previous breast surgery

Defining Characteristics

Subjective
Unsatisfactory breastfeeding process
Persistence of sore nipples beyond the first week of breastfeeding
Insufficient emptying of each breast per feeding
Inadequate/perceived inadequate milk supply

Objective
Observable signs of inadequate infant intake [decrease in number of wet diapers, inappropriate weight loss/or inadequate gain]

Information that appears in brackets has been added by the authors to clarify and enhance the use of nursing diagnoses.

 Diagnostic Studies ∞ Pediatric/Geriatric/Lifespan 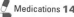 Medications **141**

Nonsustained/insufficient opportunity for suckling at the breast; infant inability [failure] to latch onto maternal breast correctly

Infant arching/crying at the breast; resistant latching on

Infant exhibiting fussiness/crying within the first hour after breastfeeding; unresponsive to other comfort measures

No observable signs of oxytocin release

Desired Outcomes/Evaluation Criteria— Client Will:

- Verbalize understanding of causative or contributing factors.
- Demonstrate techniques to enhance breastfeeding experience.
- Assume responsibility for effective breastfeeding.
- Achieve mutually satisfactory breastfeeding regimen with infant content after feedings and gaining weight appropriately.

Actions/Interventions

Nursing Priority No. 1.

To identify maternal causative or contributing factors:

- Assess client knowledge about breastfeeding and extent of instruction that has been given.
- Identify cultural expectations and conflicts about breastfeeding and beliefs or practices regarding lactation, let-down techniques, and maternal food preferences.
- Note incorrect myths/misunderstandings especially in teenage mothers, **who are more likely to have limited knowledge and more concerns about body image issues.**
- Encourage discussion of current and previous breastfeeding experience(s).
- Note previous unsatisfactory experience (including self or others) **because it may lead to negative expectations.**
- Perform physical assessment, noting appearance of breasts and nipples, marked asymmetry of breasts, obvious inverted or flat nipples, minimal or no breast enlargement during pregnancy.
- Determine whether lactation failure is primary **(i.e., maternal prolactin deficiency/serum prolactin levels, inadequate mammary gland tissue, breast surgery that has damaged the nipple, areola enervation [irremediable])** or secondary **(i.e., sore nipples, severe engorgement, plugged milk ducts, mastitis, inhibition of let-down reflex, maternal/infant separation with disruption of feedings [treatable]).** *Note: Overweight or obese women are 2.5 and 3.6 times less successful, respectively, in initiating breastfeeding than the general population.*

Information that appears in brackets has been added by the authors to clarify and enhance the use of nursing diagnoses.

  Cultural Collaborative Community/Home Care

- Note history of pregnancy, labor, and delivery (vaginal or cesarean section); other recent or current surgery; preexisting medical problems (e.g., diabetes, seizure disorder, cardiac diseases, or presence of disabilities); or adoptive mother.
- Identify maternal support systems; presence and response of SO(s), extended family, friends. **Infant's father and maternal grandmother (in addition to caring healthcare providers) are important factors that contribute to successful breastfeeding.**
- Ascertain mother's age, number of children at home, and need to return to work.
- Determine maternal feelings (e.g., fear/anxiety, ambivalence, depression).

Nursing Priority No. 2.

To assess infant causative/contributing factors:

- Determine suckling problems, as noted in Related Factors/ Defining Characteristics.
- Note prematurity and/or infant anomaly (e.g., cleft palate) **to determine special equipment/feeding needs.**
- Review feeding schedule **to note increased demand for feeding (at least eight times a day, taking both breasts at each feeding for more than 15 minutes on each side) or use of supplements with artificial nipple.**
- Evaluate observable signs of inadequate infant intake (e.g., baby latches onto mother's nipples with sustained suckling but minimal audible swallowing or gulping noted, infant arching and crying at the breasts with resistance to latching on, decreased urinary output and frequency of stools, inadequate weight gain).
- Determine whether baby is content after feeding, or exhibits fussiness and crying within the first hour after breastfeeding, **suggesting unsatisfactory breastfeeding process.**
- Note any correlation between maternal ingestion of certain foods and "colicky" response of infant.

Nursing Priority No. 3.

To assist mother to develop skills of adequate breastfeeding:

- Provide emotional support to mother. Use 1:1 instruction with each feeding during hospital stay, clinic, or home visit. Refer adoptive mothers choosing to breastfeed to a lactation consultant **to assist with induced lactation techniques.**
- Inform mother about early infant feeding cues (e.g., rooting, lip smacking, sucking fingers/hand) versus late cue of crying.

Information that appears in brackets has been added by the authors to clarify and enhance the use of nursing diagnoses.

Early recognition of infant hunger promotes timely/more rewarding feeding experience for infant and mother.

- Recommend avoidance or overuse of supplemental feedings and pacifiers (unless specifically indicated), **which can lessen infant's desire to breastfeed/increase risk of early weaning.** *Note:* Adoptive mothers may not develop a full breast milk supply, necessitating supplemental feedings.
- Restrict use of breast shields (i.e., only temporarily to help draw the nipple out), then place baby directly on nipple.
- Demonstrate use of piston-type electric breast pump with bilateral collection chamber when necessary **to maintain or increase milk supply.**
- Discuss/demonstrate breastfeeding aids (e.g., infant sling, nursing pillows or footstool).
- Recommend using a variety of nursing positions **to find the most comfortable for mother and infant. Positions particularly helpful for plus-sized women or those with large breasts include the "football" hold with infant's head to mother's breast and body curved around behind mother, or lying down to nurse.**
- Encourage frequent rest periods, sharing household/childcare duties **to limit fatigue and facilitate relaxation at feeding times.**
- Recommend abstinence/restriction of tobacco, caffeine, alcohol, drugs, excess sugar as appropriate **because they may affect milk production and let-down reflex or be passed on to the infant.**
- Promote early management of breastfeeding problems. For example:

    Engorgement: Heat and/or cool applications to the breasts, massage from chest wall down to nipple; use synthetic oxytocin nasal spray **to enhance let-down reflex;** soothe "fussy baby" before latching on the breast; properly position baby on breast/nipple; alternate the side baby starts nursing on; nurse round the clock and/or pump with piston-type electric breast pump with bilateral collection chambers at least 8 to 12 times a day.

    Sore nipples: Wear 100% cotton fabrics; do not use soap or alcohol/other drying agents on nipples; avoid use of nipple shields or nursing pads that contain plastic; cleanse and then air dry; use thin layers of lanolin (if mother/baby not sensitive to wool); expose to sunlight/sunlamps with extreme caution; administer mild pain reliever as appropriate; apply ice before nursing; soak with warm water before

---

Information that appears in brackets has been added by the authors to clarify and enhance the use of nursing diagnoses.

🌐 Cultural   🐾 Collaborative   🏠 Community/Home Care

attaching infant **to soften nipple and remove dried milk;** begin with least sore side or begin with hand expression **to establish let-down reflex;** properly position infant on breast/nipple; and use a variety of nursing positions.

Clogged ducts: Use larger bra or extender to avoid pressure on site; use moist or dry heat, gently massage from above plug down to nipple; nurse infant, hand express, or pump after massage; nurse more often on affected side.

Inhibited let-down: Use relaxation techniques before nursing (e.g., maintain quiet atmosphere, assume position of comfort, massage, apply heat to breasts, have beverage available); develop a routine for nursing, concentrate on infant; administer synthetic oxytocin nasal spray as appropriate.

Mastitis: Promote bedrest (with infant) for several days; administer antibiotics; provide warm, moist heat before and during nursing; empty breasts completely, continuing to nurse baby at least 8 to 12 times a day, or pumping breasts for 24 hours, then resuming breastfeeding as appropriate.

Nursing Priority No. 4.

To condition infant to breastfeed:

- Scent breast pad with breast milk and leave in bed with infant along with mother's photograph when separated from mother for medical purposes (e.g., prematurity).
- Increase skin-to-skin contact.
- Provide practice times at breast.
- Express small amounts of milk into baby's mouth.
- Have mother pump breast after feeding to enhance milk production.
- Use supplemental nutrition system cautiously when necessary.
- Identify special interventions for feeding in presence of cleft lip/palate.

Nursing Priority No. 5.

To promote wellness (Teaching/Discharge Considerations):

- Schedule follow-up visit with healthcare provider 48 hours after hospital discharge and 2 weeks after birth **for evaluation of milk intake/breastfeeding process.**
- Recommend monitoring number of infant's wet diapers. **(Some pediatric care providers suggest that six wet diapers in 24 hours indicate adequate hydration.)**
- Weigh infant at least every third day initially as indicated and record **to verify adequacy of nutritional intake.**

Information that appears in brackets has been added by the authors to clarify and enhance the use of nursing diagnoses.

- Educate father/SO about benefits of breastfeeding and how to manage common lactation challenges. **Enlisting support of father/SO is associated with higher ratio of successful breastfeeding at 6 months.**
- Promote peer counseling for teen mothers. **Provides positive role model that teen can relate to and feel comfortable discussing concerns/feelings.**
- Review mother's need for rest, relaxation, and time with other children as appropriate.
- Discuss importance of adequate nutrition and fluid intake, prenatal vitamins, or other vitamin/mineral supplements, such as vitamin C, as indicated.
- Address specific problems (e.g., suckling problems, prematurity facial anomalies).
- Inform mother that return of menses within first 3 months after infant's birth may indicate inadequate prolactin levels.
- Refer to support groups (e.g., La Leche League, parenting support groups, stress reduction, or other community resources, as indicated).
- Provide bibliotherapy/appropriate Web sites for further information.

Documentation Focus

Assessment/Reassessment
- Identified assessment factors, both maternal and infant (e.g., engorgement present, infant demonstrating adequate weight gain without supplementation).

Planning
- Plan of care, specific interventions, and who is involved in planning.
- Teaching plan.

Implementation/Evaluation
- Mother's/infant's responses to interventions, teaching, and actions performed.
- Changes in infant's weight.
- Attainment or progress toward desired outcome(s).
- Modifications to plan of care.

Discharge Planning
- Referrals that have been made and mother's choice of participation.

Information that appears in brackets has been added by the authors to clarify and enhance the use of nursing diagnoses.

 Cultural   Collaborative   Community/Home Care

Sample Nursing Outcomes & Interventions Classifications (NOC/NIC) NIC

NOC—Breastfeeding Establishment: Maternal [or] Infant
NIC—Breastfeeding Assistance

interrupted Breastfeeding

Taxonomy II: Role Relationships—Class 3 Role Performance (00105)
[Diagnostic Division: Food/Fluid]
Submitted 1992

Definition: Break in the continuity of the breastfeeding process as a result of inability or inadvisability to put baby to breast for feeding

Related Factors

Maternal/infant illness
Prematurity
Maternal employment
Contraindications to breastfeeding [e.g., drugs, true breast milk jaundice]
Need to abruptly wean infant

Defining Characteristics

Subjective

Infant receives no nourishment at the breast for some or all of feedings
Maternal desire to maintain breastfeeding for infant's/child's nutritional needs
Maternal desire to provide/eventually provide breast milk for infant's/child's nutritional needs
Lack of knowledge regarding expression/storage of breast milk

Objective
Separation of mother and infant

Desired Outcomes/Evaluation Criteria— Client Will:

• Identify and demonstrate techniques to sustain lactation until breastfeeding is reinitiated.

Information that appears in brackets has been added by the authors to clarify and enhance the use of nursing diagnoses.

Diagnostic Studies ∞ Pediatric/Geriatric/Lifespan   Medications **147**

- Achieve mutually satisfactory feeding regimen, with infant content after feedings and gaining weight appropriately.
- Achieve weaning and cessation of lactation if desired or necessary.

Actions/Interventions

Nursing Priority No. 1.

To identify causative/contributing factors:

- Assess client knowledge and perceptions about breastfeeding and extent of instruction that has been given.
- Note incorrect myths/misunderstandings especially in teenage mothers, **who are more likely to have limited knowledge and concerns about body image issues.**
- Ascertain cultural expectations/conflicts.
- Encourage discussion of current/previous breastfeeding experience(s).
- Determine maternal responsibilities, routines, and scheduled activities (e.g., caretaking of siblings, employment in/out of home, work/school schedules of family members, ability to visit hospitalized infant).
- Identify factors necessitating interruption, or occasionally cessation, of breastfeeding (e.g., maternal illness, drug use); desire or need to wean infant. **In general, infants with chronic diseases benefit from breastfeeding. Only a few maternal infections (e.g., HIV, active/untreated tuberculosis for initial 2 weeks of multidrug therapy, active herpes simplex of the breasts, development of chickenpox within 5 days prior to delivery or 2 days after delivery) are hazardous to breastfeeding infants. Also, use of antiretroviral medications/chemotherapy agents or maternal substance abuse usually requires weaning of infant. Exposure to radiation therapy requires interruption of breastfeeding for length of time radioactivity is known to be present in breast milk and is therefore dependent on agent used. (However, feedings with stored breast milk may be an option.)**
- Determine support systems available to mother/family. **Infant's father and maternal grandmother, in addition to caring healthcare providers, are important factors that contribute to successful breastfeeding.**

Nursing Priority No. 2.

To assist mother to maintain breastfeeding if desired:

- Provide information as needed regarding need/decision to interrupt breastfeeding.

Information that appears in brackets has been added by the authors to clarify and enhance the use of nursing diagnoses.

Cultural Collaborative Community/Home Care

- Promote peer counseling for teen mothers. **Provides positive role model that teen can relate to and feel comfortable with discussing concerns/feelings.**
- Educate father/SO about benefits of breastfeeding and how to manage common lactation challenges. **Enlisting support of father/SO is associated with higher ratio of successful breastfeeding at six months.**
- Discuss/demonstrate breastfeeding aids (e.g., infant sling, nursing footstool/pillows, manual and/or piston-type electric breast pumps).
- Suggest abstinence/restriction of tobacco, caffeine, alcohol, drugs, excess sugar, as appropriate when breastfeeding is reinitiated **because they may affect milk production/let-down reflex or be passed on to the infant.**
- Review techniques for expression and storage of breast milk **to help sustain breastfeeding activity.**
- Discuss proper techniques for expression of breast milk and use of expressed breast milk **to provide optimal nutrition and promote continuation of breastfeeding process.**
- Problem-solve return-to-work issues or periodic infant care requiring bottle/supplemental feeding.
- Provide privacy/calm surroundings when mother breastfeeds in hospital/work setting.
- Determine if a routine visiting schedule or advance warning can be provided **so that infant will be hungry/ready to feed.**
- Recommend using expressed breast milk instead of formula or at least partial breastfeeding for as long as mother and child are satisfied. **Prevents temporary interruption in breastfeeding, decreasing the risk of premature weaning.**
- Encourage mother to obtain adequate rest, maintain fluid and nutritional intake, and schedule breast pumping every 3 hours while awake as indicated **to sustain adequate milk production and breastfeeding process.**

Nursing Priority No. 3.

To assist mother in weaning process when desired:

- Provide emotional support to mother and accept decision regarding cessation of breastfeeding. **Feelings of sadness are common even if weaning is the mother's choice.**
- Discuss reducing frequency of daily feedings and breast pumping by one session every 2 to 3 days. **Preferred method of weaning, if circumstance permits, to reduce problems associated with engorgement.**

Information that appears in brackets has been added by the authors to clarify and enhance the use of nursing diagnoses.

- Encourage wearing a snug, well-fitting bra, but refrain from binding breasts **because of increased risk of clogged milk ducts and inflammation.**
- Recommend expressing some milk from breasts regularly each day over a period of 1 to 3 weeks, if necessary **to reduce discomfort associated with engorgement until milk production decreases.**
- Suggest holding infant differently during bottle feeding/interactions **to prevent infant rooting for breast and prevent stimulation of nipples.**
- Discuss use of ibuprofen/acetaminophen **for discomfort during weaning process.**
- Suggest use of ice packs to breast tissue (not nipples) for 15 to 20 minutes at least four times a day **to help reduce swelling during sudden weaning.**

Nursing Priority No. 4.
To promote successful infant feeding:

- Recommend/provide for infant sucking on a regular basis, especially if gavage feedings are part of the therapeutic regimen. **Reinforces that feeding time is pleasurable and enhances digestion.**
- Discuss proper use and choice of supplemental nutrition and alternate feeding method (e.g., bottle/syringe) if desired.
- Review safety precautions (e.g., proper flow of formula from nipple, frequency of burping, holding bottle instead of propping, formula preparation, and sterilization techniques).

Nursing Priority No. 5.
To promote wellness (Teaching/Discharge Considerations):

- Identify other means (other than breastfeeding) of nurturing and strengthening infant attachment (e.g., comforting, consoling, play activities).
- Explain anticipated changes in feeding needs/frequency. **Growth spurts require increased intake/more feedings by infant.**
- Refer to support groups (e.g., La Leche League, Lact-Aid), community resources (e.g., public health nurse, lactation specialist, Women, Infants, and Children [WIC] program).
- Promote use of bibliotherapy/appropriate Web sites for further information.

Information that appears in brackets has been added by the authors to clarify and enhance the use of nursing diagnoses.

      Cultural   Collaborative   Community/Home Care

Documentation Focus

Assessment/Reassessment
- Baseline findings maternal and infant factors.
- Reason for interruption or cessation of breastfeeding.
- Number of wet diapers daily, periodic weight.

Planning
- Method of feeding chosen.
- Plan of care and who is involved in planning.
- Teaching plan.

Implementation/Evaluation
- Maternal response to interventions, teaching, and actions performed.
- Infant's response to feeding and method.
- Whether infant appears satisfied or still seems to be hungry.
- Attainment or progress toward desired outcome(s).
- Modifications to plan of care.

Discharge Planning
- Plan for follow-up and who is responsible.
- Specific referrals made.

Sample Nursing Outcomes & Interventions Classifications (NOC/NIC) NIC

NOC—Breastfeeding Maintenance
NIC—Lactation Counseling

---

ineffective Breathing Pattern

Taxonomy II: Activity/Rest—Class 4 Cardiovascular/
  Pulmonary Responses (00032)
[Diagnostic Division: Respiration]
Submitted 1980; Revised 1996, and Nursing Diagnosis
  Extension and Classification (NDEC) 1998

Definition: Inspiration and/or expiration that does not
provide adequate ventilation

Related Factors

Neuromuscular dysfunction; spinal cord injury; neurological
  immaturity

Information that appears in brackets has been added by the authors to clarify
and enhance the use of nursing diagnoses.

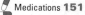

Musculoskeletal impairment; bony/chest wall deformity
Anxiety; [panic attacks]
Pain
Perception/cognitive impairment
Fatigue; [deconditioning]; respiratory muscle fatigue
Body position; obesity
Hyperventilation; hypoventilation syndrome [alteration of client's normal O_2:CO_2 ratio (e.g., lung diseases, pulmonary hypertension, airway obstruction, O_2 therapy in COPD)]

Defining Characteristics

Subjective
Feeling breathless

Objective
Dyspnea; orthopnea
Bradypnea; tachypnea
Alterations in depth of breathing
Timing ratio; prolonged expiration phases; pursed-lip breathing
Decreased minute ventilation, vital capacity
Decreased inspiratory/expiratory pressure
Use of accessory muscles to breathe; assumption of three-point position
Altered chest excursion; [paradoxical breathing patterns]
Nasal flaring; [grunting]
Increased anterior-posterior diameter

Desired Outcomes/Evaluation Criteria—Client Will:

• Establish a normal, effective respiratory pattern as evidenced by absence of cyanosis and other signs/symptoms of hypoxia, with ABGs within client's normal or acceptable range.
• Verbalize awareness of causative factors.
• Initiate needed lifestyle changes.
• Demonstrate appropriate coping behaviors.

Actions/Interventions

Nursing Priority No. 1.
To identify etiology/precipitating factors:
• Determine presence of factors/physical conditions as noted in Related Factors **that would cause breathing impairments.**

Information that appears in brackets has been added by the authors to clarify and enhance the use of nursing diagnoses.

⊕ Cultural   ⊗ Collaborative   🏠 Community/Home Care

- Auscultate chest **to evaluate presence/character of breath sounds and secretions.**
- Note rate and depth of respirations, type of breathing pattern (e.g., tachypnea, grunting, Cheyne-Stokes, other irregular patterns).
- Evaluate cough (e.g., tight or moist); presence of secretions, **indicating possible obstruction.**
- Assist with/review results of necessary testing (e.g., chest x-rays, lung volumes/flow studies, pulmonary function/sleep studies) **to diagnose presence/severity of lung diseases.**
- Review laboratory data; for example, ABGs **(determines degree of oxygenation, CO_2 retention);** drug screens; and pulmonary function studies **(determines vital capacity/tidal volume).**
- Note emotional responses (e.g., gasping, crying, reports of tingling fingers). **Anxiety may be causing or exacerbating acute or chronic hyperventilation.**
- Assess for concomitant pain/discomfort **that may restrict respiratory effort.**

Nursing Priority No. 2.

To provide for relief of causative factors:

- Administer oxygen at lowest concentration indicated and prescribed respiratory medications **for management of underlying pulmonary condition, respiratory distress, or cyanosis.**
- Suction airway, as needed, **to clear secretions.**
- Assist with bronchoscopy or chest tube insertion as indicated.
- Elevate head of bed and/or have client sit up in chair, as appropriate, **to promote physiological and psychological ease of maximal inspiration.**
- Encourage slower/deeper respirations, use of pursed-lip technique, and so on **to assist client in "taking control" of the situation.**
- Have client breathe into a paper bag, if appropriate, **to correct hyperventilation. (Research suggests this may not be effective and could actually stress the heart/respiratory system, potentially lowering O_2 saturation, especially if the hyperventilation is not simply anxiety based.)**
- Monitor pulse oximetry, as indicated, **to verify maintenance/ improvement in O_2 saturation.**
- Maintain calm attitude while dealing with client and SO(s) **to limit level of anxiety.**
- Assist client in the use of relaxation techniques.

Information that appears in brackets has been added by the authors to clarify and enhance the use of nursing diagnoses.

- Deal with fear/anxiety that may be present. (Refer to NDs Fear; Anxiety.)
- Encourage position of comfort. Reposition client frequently if immobility is a factor.
- Splint rib cage during deep-breathing exercises/cough, if indicated.
- Medicate with analgesics, as appropriate, **to promote deeper respiration and cough.** (Refer to NDs acute Pain; chronic Pain.)
- Encourage ambulation/exercise, as individually indicated.
- Avoid overeating/gas-forming foods **that may cause abdominal distention.**
- Provide/encourage use of adjuncts, such as incentive spirometer, **to facilitate deeper respiratory effort.**
- Supervise use of respirator/diaphragmatic stimulator, rocking bed, apnea monitor, and so forth **when neuromuscular impairment is present.**
- Ascertain that client possesses and properly operates continuous positive airway pressure (CPAP) machine **when obstructive sleep apnea is causing breathing problems.**
- Maintain emergency equipment in readily accessible location and include age/size appropriate ET/trach tubes (e.g., infant, child, adolescent, or adult) **when ventilatory support might be needed.**

Nursing Priority No. 3.
To promote wellness (Teaching/Discharge Considerations):

- Review etiology and possible coping behaviors.
- Stress importance of good posture and effective use of accessory muscles **to maximize respiratory effort.**
- Teach conscious control of respiratory rate, as appropriate.
- Assist client in breathing retraining (e.g., diaphragmatic, abdominal breathing, inspiratory resistive, and pursed-lip), as indicated.
- Recommend energy conservation techniques and pacing of activities.
- Refer for general exercise program (e.g., upper and lower extremity endurance and strength training), as indicated, **to maximize client's level of functioning.**
- Encourage adequate rest periods between activities **to limit fatigue.**
- Discuss relationship of smoking to respiratory function.
- Encourage client/SO(s) to develop a plan **for smoking cessation.** Provide appropriate referrals.

Information that appears in brackets has been added by the authors to clarify and enhance the use of nursing diagnoses.

  Cultural   Collaborative   Community/Home Care

- Review environmental factors (e.g., exposure to dust, high pollen counts, severe weather, perfumes, animal dander, household chemicals, fumes, secondhand smoke; insufficient home support for safe care) **that may require avoidance of triggers or modification of lifestyle or environment to limit impact on client's breathing.**
- Advise regular medical evaluation with primary care provider **to determine effectiveness of current therapeutic regimen and to promote general well-being.**
- Instruct in proper use and safety concerns for home oxygen therapy, as indicated.
- Make referral to support groups/contact with individuals who have encountered similar problems.

Documentation Focus

Assessment/Reassessment
- Relevant history of problem.
- Respiratory pattern, breath sounds, use of accessory muscles.
- Laboratory values.
- Use of respiratory aids or supports, ventilator settings, and so forth.

Planning
- Plan of care, specific interventions, and who is involved in the planning.
- Teaching plan.

Implementation/Evaluation
- Response to interventions, teaching, actions performed, and treatment regimen.
- Mastery of skills, level of independence.
- Attainment or progress toward desired outcome(s).
- Modifications to plan of care.

Discharge Planning
- Long-term needs, including appropriate referrals and action taken, available resources.
- Specific referrals provided.

Sample Nursing Outcomes & Interventions Classifications (NOC/NIC) NIC

NOC—Respiratory Status: Ventilation
NIC—Ventilation Assistances

Information that appears in brackets has been added by the authors to clarify and enhance the use of nursing diagnoses.

decreased **Cardiac Output**

Taxonomy II: Activity/Rest—Class 4 Cardiovascular/
  Pulmonary Responses (00029)
[Diagnostic Division: Circulation]
Submitted 1975; Revised 1996, 2000

Definition: Inadequate blood pumped by the heart to meet the metabolic demands of the body. [*Note:* In a hypermetabolic state, although cardiac output may be within normal range, it may still be inadequate to meet the needs of the body's tissues. Cardiac output and tissue perfusion are interrelated, although there are differences. When cardiac output is decreased, tissue perfusion problems will develop; however, tissue perfusion problems can exist without decreased cardiac output.]

Related Factors

Altered heart rate/rhythm; [conduction]
Altered stroke volume: altered preload [e.g., decreased venous return]; altered afterload [e.g., systemic vascular resistance]; altered contractility [e.g., ventricular-septal rupture, ventricular aneurysm, papillary muscle rupture, valvular disease]

Defining Characteristics

Subjective
Altered heart rate/rhythm: palpitations
Altered preload: fatigue
Altered afterload: [feeling breathless]
Altered contractility: orthopnea/paroxysmal nocturnal dyspnea [PND]
Behavioral/motional: anxiety

Objective
Altered heart rate/rhythm: [dys]arrhythmias; tachycardia; bradycardia; EKG [electrocardiogram—ECG] changes
Altered preload: Jugular vein distention (JVD); edema; weight gain; increased/decreased central venous pressure (CVP); increased/decreased pulmonary artery wedge pressure (PAWP); murmurs
Altered afterload: dyspnea; clammy skin; skin [and mucous membrane] color changes [cyanosis, pallor]; prolonged

---

Information that appears in brackets has been added by the authors to clarify and enhance the use of nursing diagnoses.

⊕ Cultural 🐾 Collaborative 🏠 Community/Home Care

capillary refill; decreased peripheral pulses; variations in blood pressure readings; increased/decreased systemic vascular resistance (SVR); increased/decreased pulmonary vascular resistance (PVR); oliguria; [anuria]

Altered contractility: crackles; cough; decreased cardiac output/cardiac index; decreased ejection fraction; decreased stroke volume index (SVI)/left ventricular stroke work index (LVSWI); S_3 or S_4 sounds [gallop rhythm]

Behavioral/emotional: restlessness

Desired Outcomes/Evaluation Criteria— Client Will:

- Display hemodynamic stability (e.g., blood pressure, cardiac output, renal perfusion/urinary output, peripheral pulses).
- Report/demonstrate decreased episodes of dyspnea, angina, and dysrhythmias.
- Demonstrate an increase in activity tolerance.
- Verbalize knowledge of the disease process, individual risk factors, and treatment plan.
- Participate in activities that reduce the workload of the heart (e.g., stress management or therapeutic medication regimen program, weight reduction, balanced activity/rest plan, proper use of supplemental oxygen, cessation of smoking).
- Identify signs of cardiac decompensation, alter activities, and seek help appropriately.

Actions/Interventions

Nursing Priority No. 1.
To identify causative/contributing factors:

- Review clients at risk as noted in Related Factors and Defining Characteristics, as well as individuals with conditions that stress the heart. **Persons with acute or chronic conditions (e.g., multiple trauma, renal failure, brainstem trauma, spinal cord injures at T8 or above, alcohol or other drug abuse/overdose, pregnant women in hypertensive state) may compromise circulation and place excessive demands on the heart.**
- Assess potential for/type of developing shock states: hematogenic, septicemic, cardiogenic, vasogenic, and psychogenic.
- Review laboratory data (e.g., cardiac markers, CBC, electrolytes, ABGs, blood urea nitrogen/creatinine (BUN/Cr), cardiac enzymes, and cultures, such as blood/wound/secretions).

Information that appears in brackets has been added by the authors to clarify and enhance the use of nursing diagnoses.

Nursing Priority No. 2.

To assess degree of debilitation:

- Evaluate client reports and evidence of extreme fatigue, intolerance for activity, sudden or progressive weight gain, swelling of extremities, and progressive shortness of breath **to assess for signs of poor ventricular function and/or impending cardiac failure.**
- Determine vital signs/hemodynamic parameters including cognitive status. Note vital sign response to activity or procedures and time required to return to baseline. **Provides baseline for comparison to follow trends and evaluate response to interventions.**
- Review signs of impending failure/shock, noting decreased cognition and unstable or subnormal low blood pressure/invasive hemodynamic parameters; tachypnea; labored respirations; changes in breath sounds (e.g., crackles, wheezing); distant or altered heart sounds (e.g., murmurs, dysrythmias); and reduced urinary output. **Early detection of changes in these parameters promotes timely intervention to limit degree of cardiac dysfunction.**
- Note presence of pulsus paradoxus, especially in the presence of distant heart sounds, **suggesting cardiac tamponade.**
- Review diagnostic studies (e.g., cardiac stress testing, ECG, scans, echocardiogram, heart catheterization, chest x-rays, electrolytes, CBC). **Helps determine underlying cause.**

Nursing Priority No. 3.

To minimize/correct causative factors, maximize cardiac output:

Acute Phase

- Keep client on bed or chair rest in position of comfort. (In congestive state, semi-Fowler's position is preferred.) May raise legs 20 to 30 degrees in shock situation. **Decreases oxygen consumption and risk of decompensation.**
- Administer high-flow oxygen via mask or ventilator, as indicated, **to increase oxygen available for cardiac function/tissue perfusion.**
- Monitor vital signs frequently **to note response to activities/interventions.**
- Perform periodic hemodynamic measurements, as indicated (e.g., arterial, CVP, pulmonary, and left atrial pressures and cardiac output).

Information that appears in brackets has been added by the authors to clarify and enhance the use of nursing diagnoses.

- Monitor cardiac rhythm continuously **to note effectiveness of medications and/or assistive devices, such as implanted pacemaker or defibrillator.**

 • Administer blood or fluid replacement, antibiotics, diuretics, inotropic drugs, antidysrhythmics, steroids, vasopressors, and/or dilators, as indicated. Evaluate response **to determine therapeutic, adverse, or toxic effects of therapy.**

- Restrict or administer fluids (IV/PO), as indicated. Provide adequate fluid/free water, depending on client needs.

- Assess urine ouput hourly or periodically; weigh daily, noting total fluid balance **to allow for timely alterations in therapeutic regimen.**

- Monitor rate of IV drugs closely, using infusion pumps, as appropriate, **to prevent bolus/overdose.**

- Decrease stimuli; provide quiet environment **to promote adequate rest.**

- Schedule activities and assessments **to maximize rest periods.**

- Assist with or perform self-care activities for client.

- Avoid the use of restraints whenever possible if client is confused. **May increase agitation and increase the cardiac workload.**

- Use sedation and analgesics, as indicated, with caution **to achieve desired effect without compromising hemodynamic readings.**

- Maintain patency of invasive intravascular monitoring and infusion lines. Tape connections **to prevent air embolus and/or exsanguination.**

- Maintain aseptic technique during invasive procedures. Provide site care, as indicated.

- Alter environment/bed linens and administer antipyretics or cooling measures, as indicated, **to maintain body temperature in near-normal range.**

- Instruct client to avoid/limit activities that may stimulate a Valsalva response (e.g., isometric exercises, rectal stimulation, bearing down during bowel movement, spasmodic coughing) **which can cause changes in cardiac pressures and/or impede blood flow.**

- Encourage client to breathe in/out during activities that increase risk for Valsalva effect; limit suctioning/stimulation of coughing reflex in intubated client; administer stool softeners when indicated.

- Provide psychological support. Maintain calm attitude, but admit concerns if questioned by the client. **Honesty can be**

Information that appears in brackets has been added by the authors to clarify and enhance the use of nursing diagnoses.

reassuring when so much activity and "worry" are apparent to the client.

- Provide information about testing procedures and client participation.
- Assist with special procedures, as indicated (e.g., invasive line placement, intra-aortic balloon pump (IABP) insertion, pericardiocentesis, cardioversion, pacemaker insertion).
- Explain dietary or fluid restrictions, as indicated.
- Refer to NDs risk for decreased cardiac tissue Perfusion; risk for Autonomic Dysreflexia.

Nursing Priority No. 4.
To promote venous return:

Postacute/Chronic Phase
- Provide for adequate rest, positioning client for maximum comfort.
- Administer analgesics, as appropriate, **to promote comfort/ rest.**
- Encourage relaxation techniques **to reduce anxiety and conserve energy.**
- Elevate legs when in sitting position; apply sequential compression devices (SCDs), if indicated, **to enhance venous return;** use tilt table or other circulatory support bed, as needed, **to prevent orthostatic hypotension.**
- Give skin care, provide sheepskin or special flotation mattress (e.g., air, water, gel, or foam) , and assist with frequent position changes **to avoid the development of pressure sores.**
- Elevate edematous extremities and avoid restrictive clothing. When support hose are used, be sure they are individually fitted and appropriately applied.
- Increase activity levels as permitted by individual condition/ physiological response.

Nursing Priority No. 5.
To maintain adequate nutrition and fluid balance:
- Provide for diet restrictions (e.g., low-sodium, bland, soft, low-calorie/fat diet, with frequent small feedings), as indicated.
- Note reports of anorexia or nausea and withhold oral intake, as indicated.
- Provide fluids and electrolytes, as indicated, **to minimize dehydration and dysrhythmias.**
- Monitor intake/output and calculate 24-hour fluid balance.

Information that appears in brackets has been added by the authors to clarify and enhance the use of nursing diagnoses.

Nursing Priority No. 6.

To promote wellness (Teaching/Discharge Considerations):

- Note individual risk factors present (e.g., smoking, stress, obesity), and specify interventions for reduction of identified factors.
- Review specifics of drug regimen, diet, exercise/activity plan. Emphasize necessity for long-term medical management of cardiac conditons.
- Discuss significant signs/symptoms that require prompt reporting to healthcare provider (e.g., muscle cramps, headaches, dizziness, skin rashes), **which may be signs of drug toxicity and/or electrolyte loss, especially potassium.**
- Review "danger" signs requiring immediate physician notification (e.g., unrelieved or increased chest pain, functional decline, dyspnea, edema), **which may indicate deteriorating cardiac function, heart failure.**
- Encourage changing positions slowly, dangling legs before standing **to reduce risk for orthostatic hypotension.**
- Give information about positive signs of improvement, such as decreased edema, improved vital signs/circulation, **to provide encouragement.**
- Teach home monitoring of weight, pulse, and/or blood pressure, as appropriate, **to detect change and allow for timely intervention.**
- Arrange time with dietitian **to determine/adjust individually appropriate diet plan.**
- Promote visits from family/SO(s) who provide positive social interaction.
- Encourage relaxing environment, using relaxation techniques, massage therapy, soothing music, quiet activities.
- Instruct in stress management techniques, as indicated, including appropriate exercise program.
- Identify resources for weight reduction, cessation of smoking, and so forth, **to provide support for change.**
- Refer to NDs Activity Intolerance; deficient Diversional Activity; ineffective Coping, compromised family Coping; Sexual Dysfunction; acute or chronic Pain; imbalanced Nutrition; deficient or excess Fluid Volume, as indicated.

Documentation Focus

Assessment/Reassessment

- Baseline and subsequent findings and individual hemodynamic parameters, heart and breath sounds, ECG pattern,

---

Information that appears in brackets has been added by the authors to clarify and enhance the use of nursing diagnoses.

presence/strength of peripheral pulses, skin/tissue status, renal output, and mentation.

Planning
- Plan of care and who is involved in planning.
- Teaching plan.

Implementation/Evaluation
- Client's responses to interventions, teaching, and actions performed.
- Status and disposition at discharge.
- Attainment or progress toward desired outcome(s).
- Modifications to plan of care.

Discharge Planning
- Discharge considerations and who will be responsible for carrying out individual actions.
- Long-term needs and available resources.
- Specific referrals made.

Sample Nursing Outcomes & Interventions Classifications (NOC/NIC) NIC

NOC—Cardiac Pump Effectiveness
NIC—Hemodynamic Regulations

Caregiver Role Strain

Taxonomy II: Role Relationships—Class 1 Caregiving Roles (00061)
[Diagnostic Division: Social Interaction]
Submitted 1992; Nursing Diagnosis Extension and Classification (NDEC) Revision 1998; 2000

Definition: Difficulty in performing caregiver role

Related Factors

Care Receiver Health Status
Illness severity/chronicity
Unpredictability of illness course; instability of care receiver's health
Increasing care needs; dependency
Problem behaviors; psychological or cognitive problems
Addiction; codependency

Information that appears in brackets has been added by the authors to clarify and enhance the use of nursing diagnoses.

⊕ Cultural   ✆ Collaborative   🏠 Community/Home Care

Caregiving Activities

Discharge of family member to home with significant care needs [e.g., premature birth/congenital defect, frail elder post stroke]

Unpredictability of care situation; 24-hour care responsibilities; amount/complexity of activities; years of caregiving

Ongoing changes in activities

Caregiver Health Status

Physical problems; psychological or cognitive problems

Inability to fulfill one's own or others' expectations; unrealistic expectations of self

Marginal coping patterns

Addiction; codependency

Socioeconomic

Competing role commitments

Alienation or isolation from others

Insufficient recreation

Caregiver-Care Receiver Relationship

Unrealistic expectations of caregiver by care receiver

History of poor relationship

Mental status of elder inhibits conversation

Presence of abuse or violence

Family Processes

History of marginal family coping or family dysfunction

Resources

Inadequate physical environment for providing care (e.g., housing, temperature, safety)

Inadequate equipment for providing care; inadequate transportation

Insufficient finances

Inexperience with caregiving; insufficient time, physical energy, emotional strength; lack of support

Lack of caregiver privacy

Deficient knowledge about or difficulty accessing community resources; inadequate community services (e.g., respite services, recreational resources)

Formal/informal assistance; formal/informal support

Caregiver is not developmentally ready for caregiver role

Information that appears in brackets has been added by the authors to clarify and enhance the use of nursing diagnoses.

NOTE: The presence of this problem may encompass other numerous problems/high-risk concerns, such as deficient Diversional Activity, Insomnia, Fatigue, Anxiety, ineffective Coping, compromised family Coping, disabled family Coping, decisional Conflict, ineffective Denial, Grieving, Hopelessness, Powerlessness, Spiritual Distress, ineffective Health Maintenance, impaired Home Maintenance, ineffective Sexuality Pattern, readiness for enhanced family Coping, interrupted Family Processes, Social Isolation. Careful attention to data gathering will identify and clarify the client's specific needs, which can then be coordinated under this single diagnostic label.

Defining Characteristics

Subjective

Caregiving Activities

Apprehension about: possible institutionalization of care receiver; the future regarding care receiver's health or caregiver's ability to provide care; care receiver's care if caregiver unable to provide care

Caregiver Health Status—Physical

GI upset; weight change
Headaches; fatigue; rash
Hypertension; cardiovascular disease; diabetes

Caregiver Health Status—Emotional

Feeling depressed; anger; stress; frustration; increased nervousness
Disturbed sleep
Lack of time to meet personal needs

Caregiver Health Status—Socioeconomic

Changes in leisure activities; refuses career advancement

Caregiver-Care Receiver Relationship

Difficulty watching care receiver go through the illness
Grief and uncertainty regarding changed relationship with care receiver

Family Processes—Caregiving Activities

Concerns about family members

Information that appears in brackets has been added by the authors to clarify and enhance the use of nursing diagnoses.

⊕ Cultural   ⊗ Collaborative   🏠 Community/Home Care

Objective

Caregiving Activities
Difficulty performing/completing required tasks
Preoccupation with care routine
Dysfunctional change in caregiving activities

Caregiver Health Status—Emotional
Impatience; increased emotional lability; somatization
Impaired individual coping

Caregiver Health Status—Socioeconomic
Low work productivity; withdraws from social life

Family Processes
Family conflict

Desired Outcomes/Evaluation Criteria— Client Will:

- Identify resources within self to deal with situation.
- Provide opportunity for care receiver to deal with situation in own way.
- Express more realistic understanding and expectations of the care receiver.
- Demonstrate behavior/lifestyle changes to cope with and/or resolve problematic factors.
- Report improved general well-being, ability to deal with situation.

Actions/Interventions

Nursing Priority No. 1.
To assess degree of impaired function:

- Inquire about and observe physical condition of care receiver and surroundings, as appropriate.
- Assess caregiver's current state of functioning (e.g., hours of sleep, nutritional intake, personal appearance, demeanor).
- Determine use of prescription/OTC drugs, alcohol to deal with situation.
- Identify safety issues concerning caregiver and receiver.
- Assess current actions of caregiver and how they are viewed by care receiver (e.g., caregiver may be trying to be helpful, but is not perceived as helpful; may be too protective or may

---

Information that appears in brackets has been added by the authors to clarify and enhance the use of nursing diagnoses.

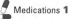

have unrealistic expectations of care receiver). **May lead to misunderstanding and conflict.**

* Note choice and frequency of social involvement and recreational activities.
* Determine use and effectiveness of resources and support systems.

Nursing Priority No. 2.

To identify the causative or contributing factors relating to the impairment:

* Note presence of high-risk situations (e.g., elderly client with total self-care dependence, or family with several small children with one child requiring extensive assistance due to physical condition/developmental delays). **May necessitate role reversal, resulting in added stress or place excessive demands on parenting skills.**
* Determine current knowledge of the situation, noting misconceptions, lack of information. **May interfere with caregiver/care receiver response to illness/condition.**
* Identify relationship of caregiver to care receiver (e.g., spouse/lover, parent/child, sibling, friend).
* Ascertain proximity of caregiver to care receiver. **Caregiver could be living in the home of care receiver (e.g., spouse or parent of disabled child), or be adult child stopping by to check on elderly parent each day, providing support, food preparation/shopping, assistance in emergencies. Either situation can be taxing.**
* Note care receiver's physical and mental condition, as well as the complexity of required therapeutic regimen. **Caregiving activities can be complex, requiring hands-on care, problem-solving skills, clinical judgment, and organizational and communication skills that can tax the caregiver.**
* Determine caregiver's level of involvement in/preparedness for the responsibilities of caring for the client, and anticipated length of care.
* Ascertain caregiver's physical and emotional health and developmental level, as well as additional responsibilities of caregiver (e.g., job, raising family). **Provides clues to potential stressors and possible supportive interventions.**
* Use assessment tool, such as Burden Interview, when appropriate, **to further determine caregiver's coping abilities.**
* Identify individual cultural factors and impact on caregiver. **Helps clarify expectations of caregiver/receiver, family, and community.**

Information that appears in brackets has been added by the authors to clarify and enhance the use of nursing diagnoses.

- Note codependency needs and enabling behaviors of caregiver.
- Determine availability/use of support systems and resources.
- Identify presence and degree of conflict between caregiver, care receiver, and family.
- Determine pre-illness and current behaviors that may be interfering with the care or recovery of the care receiver.

Nursing Priority No. 3.

To assist caregiver in identifying feelings and in beginning to deal with problems:

- Establish a therapeutic relationship, conveying empathy and unconditional positive regard. **A compassionate approach, blending the nurse's expertise in healthcare with the caregiver's firsthand knowledge of the care receiver can provide encouragement, especially in a long-term difficult situation.**
- Acknowledge difficulty of the situation for the caregiver/family. **Research shows that the two greatest predictors of caregiver strain are poor health and the feeling that there is no choice but to take on additional responsibilities.**
- Discuss caregiver's view of and concerns about situation.
- Encourage caregiver to acknowledge and express feelings. Discuss normalcy of the reactions without using false reassurance.
- Discuss caregiver's and family members' life goals, perceptions, and expectations of self **to clarify unrealistic thinking and identify potential areas of flexibility or compromise.**
- Discuss impact of and ability to handle role changes necessitated by situation.

Nursing Priority No. 4.

To enhance caregiver's ability to deal with current situation:

- Identify strengths of caregiver and care receiver.
- Discuss strategies to coordinate caregiving tasks and other responsibilities (e.g., employment, care of children/dependents, housekeeping activities).
- Facilitate family conference, as appropriate, **to share information and develop plan for involvement in care activities.**
- Identify classes and/or needed specialists (e.g., first aid/CPR classes, enterostomal/physical therapist).
- Determine need for, and sources of, additional resources (e.g., financial, legal, respite care, social, spiritual).
- Provide information and/or demonstrate techniques for dealing with acting out, violent, or disoriented behavior. **Enhances safety of caregiver and care receiver.**

Information that appears in brackets has been added by the authors to clarify and enhance the use of nursing diagnoses.

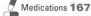

- Identify equipment needs or adaptive aids and resources **to enhance the independence and safety of the care receiver.**
- Provide contact person/case manager **to partner with care provider(s) in coordinating care, providing physical/social support, and assisting with problem solving, as needed/desired.**

Nursing Priority No. 5.

To promote wellness (Teaching/Discharge Considerations):

- Advocate for/assist caregiver to plan for and implement changes that may be necessary (e.g., home care providers, adult day care, placement in long-term care facility, hospice care).
- Support caregiver in setting practical goals for self (and care receiver) that are realistic for care receiver's condition/prognosis and caregiver's own abilities.
- Review signs of burnout (e.g., emotional/physical exaustion; changes in appetite and sleep; withdrawal from friends, family, life interests).
- Discuss/demonstrate stress management techniques (e.g., accepting own feelings/frustrations and limitations, talking with trusted friend, taking a break from situation) and importance of self-nurturing (e.g., eating and sleeping regularly; pursuing self-development interests, personal needs, hobbies, social activities, spiritual enrichment). **May provide care provider with options to look after self.**
- Encourage involvement in caregiver support group.
- Refer to classes/other therapies, as indicated.
- Identify available 12-step program, when indicated, to provide tools **to deal with enabling/codependent behaviors that impair level of function.**
- Refer to counseling or psychotherapy, as needed.
- Provide bibliotherapy of appropriate references **for self-paced learning** and encourage discussion of information.

Documentation Focus

Assessment/Reassessment

- Assessment findings, functional level or degree of impairment, caregiver's understanding and perception of situation.
- Identified risk factors.

Planning

- Plan of care and individual responsibility for specific activities.
- Needed resources, including type and source of assistive devices and durable equipment.
- Teaching plan.

Information that appears in brackets has been added by the authors to clarify and enhance the use of nursing diagnoses.

Implementation/Evaluation
- Caregiver/receiver response to interventions, teaching, and actions performed.
- Identification of inner resources, behavior and lifestyle changes to be made.
- Attainment or progress toward desired outcome(s).
- Modifications to plan of care.

Discharge Planning
- Plan for continuation and follow-through of needed changes.
- Referrals for assistance and reevaluation.

Sample Nursing Outcomes & Interventions Classifications (NOC/NIC) [NIC]

NOC—Caregiver Role Endurance
NIC—Caregiver Support

---

risk for **Caregiver Role Strain**

Taxonomy II: Role Relationships—Class 1 Caregiving Roles (00062)
[Diagnostic Division: Social Interaction]
Submitted 1992

Definition: Caregiver is vulnerable for felt difficulty in performing the family caregiver role

---

Risk Factors

Illness severity of the care receiver; psychological or cognitive problems in care receiver; addiction or codependency

Discharge of family member with significant home care needs; premature birth; congenital defect

Unpredictable illness course or instability in the care receiver's health

Duration of caregiving required; inexperience with caregiving; complexity/amount of caregiving tasks; caregiver's competing role commitments

Caregiver health impairment

Caregiver is female, spouse

Caregiver not developmentally ready for caregiver role [e.g., a young adult needing to provide care for middle-aged parent]; developmental delay or retardation of the care receiver or caregiver

---

Information that appears in brackets has been added by the authors to clarify and enhance the use of nursing diagnoses.

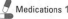

Presence of situational stressors that normally affect families (e.g., significant loss, disaster or crisis, economic vulnerability, major life events [e.g., birth, hospitalization, leaving home, returning home, marriage, divorce, change in employment, retirement, death])

Inadequate physical environment for providing care (e.g., housing, transportation, community services, equipment)

Family or caregiver isolation

Lack of respite or recreation for caregiver

Marginal family adaptation or dysfunction prior to the caregiving situation

Marginal caregiver coping patterns

Past history of poor relationship between caregiver and care receiver

Care receiver exhibits deviant, bizarre behavior

Presence of abuse or violence

> **NOTE:** A risk diagnosis is not evidenced by signs and symptoms, as the problem has not occurred; rather, nursing interventions are directed at prevention.

Desired Outcomes/Evaluation Criteria—Client Will:

- Identify individual risk factors and appropriate interventions.
- Demonstrate and initiate behaviors or lifestyle changes to prevent development of impaired function.
- Use available resources appropriately.
- Report satisfaction with current situation.

Actions/Interventions

Nursing Priority No. 1.

To assess factors affecting current situation:

∞• Note presence of high-risk situations (e.g., elderly client with total self-care dependence or several small children with one child requiring extensive assistance due to physical condition/developmental delays). **May necessitate role reversal, resulting in added stress or place excessive demands on parenting skills.**

- Identify relationship and proximity of caregiver to care receiver (e.g., spouse/lover, parent/child, friend).

Information that appears in brackets has been added by the authors to clarify and enhance the use of nursing diagnoses.

Cultural   Collaborative   Community/Home Care

- Note therapeutic regimen and physical and mental condition of care receiver **to ascertain potential areas of need (e.g., teaching, direct care support, respite)** .
- Determine caregiver's level of responsibility, involvement in, and anticipated length of caring role.
- Ascertain physical and emotional health and developmental level, as well as additional responsibilities of caregiver (e.g., job, school, raising family). **Provides clues to potential stressors and possible supportive interventions.**
- Use assessment tool, such as Burden Interview, when appropriate, **to further determine caregiver's abilities.**
- Identify strengths and weaknesses of caregiver and care receiver.
- Verify safety of caregiver/receiver.
- Discuss caregiver's and care receiver's views of and concerns about situation.
- Determine available supports and resources currently used.
- Note any codependency needs of caregiver.

Nursing Priority No. 2.
To enhance caregiver's ability to deal with current situation:

- Discuss strategies to coordinate care and other responsibilities (e.g., employment, care of children/dependents, housekeeping activities).
- Facilitate family conference, as appropriate, **to share information and develop plan for involvement in care activities.**
- Refer to classes and/or specialists (e.g., first aid/CPR classes, enterostomal/physical therapist) **for special training, as indicated.**
- Identify additional resources to include financial, legal, respite care.
- Identify equipment needs/resources, adaptive aids **to enhance the independence and safety of the care receiver.**
- Identify contact person or case manager as needed **to coordinate care, provide support, and assist with problem solving.**
- Provide information and/or demonstrate techniques for dealing with acting out, violent or disoriented behavior **to protect/prevent injury to caregiver and care receiver.**
- Assist caregiver to recognize codependent behaviors (i.e., doing things for others that others are able to do for themselves) and how these behaviors affect the situation.

Information that appears in brackets has been added by the authors to clarify and enhance the use of nursing diagnoses.

Nursing Priority No. 3.

To promote wellness (Teaching/Discharge Considerations):

🏠 • Stress importance of self-nurturing (e.g., pursuing self-development interests, personal needs, hobbies, and social activities) **to improve/maintain quality of life for caregiver.**

🔄 • Advocate for, and assist caregiver to plan and implement changes that may be necessary (e.g., home care providers, adult day care, eventual placement in long-term care facility, or hospice care).

🏠 • Review signs of burnout (e.g., emotional or physical exhaustion; changes in appetite and sleep; withdrawal from friends, family, life interests).

🏠 • Discuss and demonstrate stress management techniques and importance of self-nurturing (e.g., pursuing self-development interests, personal needs, hobbies, social activities, spiritual enrichment). **May provide care provider with options to protect self/promote well-being.**

🔄 • Encourage involvement in caregiver/other specific support group(s).

🏠 • Provide bibliotherapy of appropriate references and encourage discussion of information.

🔄 • Refer to classes/therapists as indicated.

🔄 • Identify available 12-step program, when indicated, **to provide tools to deal with codependent behaviors that impair level of function.**

🔄 • Refer to counseling or psychotherapy as needed.

Documentation Focus

Assessment/Reassessment
• Identified risk factors and caregiver perceptions of situation.
• Reactions of care receiver and family.
• Involvement of family members and others.

Planning
• Treatment plan and individual responsibility for specific activities.
• Teaching plan.

Implementation/Evaluation
• Caregiver/receiver response to interventions, teaching, and actions performed.
• Attainment or progress toward desired outcome(s).
• Modifications to plan of care.

Information that appears in brackets has been added by the authors to clarify and enhance the use of nursing diagnoses.

🌐 Cultural   🔄 Collaborative   🏠 Community/Home Care

Discharge Planning
- Long-term needs and who is responsible for actions to be taken.
- Specific referrals provided for assistance/evaluation.

Sample Nursing Outcomes & Interventions Classifications (NOC/NIC) NIC

NOC—Caregiver Stressors
NIC—Caregiver Support

---

readiness for enhanced **Childbearing Process**

Taxonomy II: Sexuality—Class 3 Reproduction (00208)
[Diagnostic Division: Safety]
Submitted 2008

Definition: A pattern of preparing for, maintaining, and strengthening a healthy pregnancy and childbirth process and care of newborn

---

Related Factors

To be developed

Defining Characteristics

During Pregnancy

Subjective

Reports: appropriate prenatal lifestyle (e.g., diet, elimination, sleep, bodily movement, exercise, personal hygiene), a realistic birth plan, appropriate physical preparations, availability of support systems

Reports managing unpleasant symptoms of pregnancy

Objective

Has regular prenatal health visits

Demonstrates respect for unborn baby; prepares necessary newborn care items

Seeks necessary knowledge (e.g., of labor and delivery, newborn care)

Information that appears in brackets has been added by the authors to clarify and enhance the use of nursing diagnoses.

During Labor and Delivery

Subjective
Reports lifestyle (e.g., diet, elimination, sleep, bodily movement, personal hygiene) that is appropriate for the stage of labor

Objective
Responds appropriately to onset of labor

Is proactive in labor and delivery; uses relaxation techniques appropriate for stage of labor; utilizes support systems appropriately

Demonstrates attachment behavior to the newborn baby

After Birth

Subjective
Reports appropriate postpartum lifestyle (e.g., diet, elimination, sleep, bodily movement, exercise, personal hygiene)

Objective
Demonstrates: attachment behavior to the baby, basic baby care techniques, appropriate baby feeding techniques

Provides safe environment for the baby

Utilizes support systems appropriately

Demonstrates appropriate breast care

Desired Outcomes/Evaluation Criteria—Client Will (Include Specific Time Frame)

- Demonstrate healthy pregnancy free of preventable complications.
- Engage in activities to prepare for birth process and care of newborn.
- Experience complication-free labor and childbirth.
- Verbalize understanding of care requirements to promote health of self and infant.

Actions/Interventions

Nursing Priority No. 1.
To determine individual needs:

Prenatal
- Evaluate current knowledge and cultural beliefs regarding normal physiological and psychological changes of pregnancy, as well as beliefs about activities, self-care, and so on.

Information that appears in brackets has been added by the authors to clarify and enhance the use of nursing diagnoses.

  Cultural Collaborative Community/Home Care

- Determine degree of motivation for learning. **Client may have difficulty learning unless the need for it is clear.**
- Identify who provides support/instruction within the clients culture (e.g., grandmother/other family member, cuerandero/ doula, other cultural healer). Work with support person(s) when possible, using interpreter as needed. **Helps ensure quality and continuity of care because support person(s) may be more successful than the healthcare provider in communicating information.**
- Determine client's commitments to work, family, community, and self; and roles/responsibilities within family unit, and use of supportive resources. **Helps in setting realistic priorities to assist client in making adjustments, such as changing work hours, shifting of household chores, curtailing some outside commitments.**
- Evaluate the client's/couple's response to pregnancy, individual and family stressors, and cultural implications of pregnancy/childbirth. **The ability to adapt positively depends on support systems, cultural beliefs, resources, and effective coping mechanisms developed in dealing with past stressors.**
- Determine client's/couple's perception of fetus as a separate entity and extent of preparations being made for this infant. **Activities such as choosing a name or nicknaming the baby in utero, and home preparations indicate completion of psychological tasks of pregnancy.** *Note:* **Cultural or familial beliefs may limit visible preparations out of concern that bad outcome might result.**
- Assess economic situation and financial needs to make necessary referrals.
- Determine usual pregravid weight and dietary patterns. **Research studies have found a positive correlation between pregravid maternal obesity and increased perinatal morbidity rates (e.g., hypertension and gestational diabetes) associated with preterm births and macrosomia.**

Labor and Delivery
- Ascertain clients understanding and expectations of the labor process.
- Review birth plan developed by client/partner. Note cultural expectations and preferences. **Verifies that choices made are amenable to the specific care setting, accommodate individual wishes, and reflect client/fetal status.**

Information that appears in brackets has been added by the authors to clarify and enhance the use of nursing diagnoses.

Postpartum/Newborn Care
- Determine plan for discharge after delivery and home care support/needs. **Early planning can facilitate discharge and help ensure that client/infant needs will be met.**
- Ascertain client's perception of labor and delivery, length of labor, and client's fatigue level. **There is a correlation between length of labor and the ability of some clients to assume responsibility for self-care/infant care tasks and activities.**
- Assess mother's strengths and needs, noting age, marital status/relationship, presence and reaction of siblings and other family members, available sources of support, and cultural background. **Identifies potential risk factors and sources of support, which influence the client's/couple's ability to assume role of parenthood. For example, an adolescent still formulating goals and an identity may have difficulty accepting the infant as a person. The single parent who lacks support systems may have difficulty assuming sole responsibility for parenting.**
- Appraise level of parent's understanding of infant's physiological needs and adaptation to extrauterine life associated with maintenance of body temperature, nutrition, respiratory needs, and bowel and bladder functioning.
- Evaluate nature of emotional and physical parenting that client/couple received during their childhood. **Parenting role is learned, and individuals use their own parents as role models. Those who experienced a negative upbringing or poor parenting may require additional support to meet the challenges of effective parenting.**
- Note father's/partner's response to birth and to parenting role. **Client's ability to adapt positively to parenting may be strongly influenced by the father's/partner's reaction.**
- Assess client's readiness and motivation for learning. Assist client/couple in identifying needs. **The postpartal period provides an opportunity to foster maternal growth, maturation, and competence.**

Nursing Priority No. 2.
To promote maximum participation in childbearing process:
Prenatal
- Maintain open attitude toward beliefs of client/couple. **Acceptance is important to developing and maintaining relationship and supporting independence.**
- Explain office visit routine, rationale for ongoing screening and close monitoring (e.g., urine testing, blood pressure

---

Information that appears in brackets has been added by the authors to clarify and enhance the use of nursing diagnoses.

 Cultural Collaborative Community/Home Care

monitoring, weight, fetal growth). Emphasize importance of keeping regular appointments. **Reinforces relationship between health assessment and positive outcome for mother and baby.**

- Suggest father and siblings attend prenatal office visits and listen to fetal heart tones (FHT) as appropriate. **Promotes a sense of involvement and helps make baby a reality for family members.**
- Provide information about need for additional laboratory studies, diagnostic tests or procedure(s). Review risks and potential side effects.
- Discuss any medications that may be needed to control or treat medical conditions. **Helpful in choosing treatment options because need must be weighed against possible harmful effects on the fetus.**
- Provide anticipatory guidance, including discussion of nutrition, regular moderate exercise, comfort measures, rest, employment, breast care, sexual activity, and health habits/lifestyle. **Information encourages acceptance of responsibility and promotes self-care:**
  - Review nutrition requirements and optimal prenatal weight gain to support maternal-fetal needs. **Inadequate prenatal weight gain and/or below normal prepregnancy weight increases the risk of intrauterine growth restriction (IUGR) in the fetus and delivery of a low-birth-weight (LBW) infant.**
  - Encourage moderate exercise such as walking, or non-weight-bearing activities (e.g., swimming, bicycling) in accordance with client's physical condition and cultural beliefs. **Tends to shorten labor, increases likelihood of a spontaneous vaginal delivery, and decreases need for oxytocin augmentation.**
  - Recommend a consistent sleep and rest schedule (e.g., 1- to 2-hour daytime nap and 8 hours of sleep each night) in a dark, comfortable room.
  - Identify anticipatory adaptations for SO/family necessitated by pregnancy. **Family members will need to be flexible in adjusting own roles and responsibilities in order to assist client to meet her needs related to the demands of pregnancy.**
  - Provide/reinforce information about potential teratogens, such as alcohol, nicotine, illicit drugs, STORCH group of viruses (**s**yphilis, **t**oxoplasmosis, **o**ther, **r**ubella, **c**ytomegalovirus [CMV], **h**erpes simplex), and HIV. **Helps client make informed decisions/choices about behaviors/**

Information that appears in brackets has been added by the authors to clarify and enhance the use of nursing diagnoses.

environment that can promote healthy offspring. *Note:* **Research supports the attribution of a wide range of negative effects in the neonate to alcohol, recreational drug use, and smoking.**

- Use various methods for learning, including pictures to discuss fetal development. **Visualization enhances reality of child and strengthens learning process.**

- Discuss signs of labor onset; how to distinguish between false and true labor, when to notify healthcare provider and to leave for hospital/birth center; and stages of labor/delivery. **Helps ensure timely arrival and enhances coping with labor/ delivery process.**

- Review signs/symptoms requiring evaluation by primary provider during prenatal period (e.g., excessive vomiting, fever, unresolved illness of any kind, decreased fetal movement). **Allows for timely intervention.**

Labor and Delivery

- Identify client's support person/coach and ascertain that the individual is providing support that client requires. **Coach may be client's husband or significant other or doula, and support can take the form of physical and emotional support for the mother, and aid in initiation of bonding with the neonate.**

- Demonstrate or review behaviors and techniques (e.g., breathing, focused imagery, music, other distractions; aromatherapy; abdominal effleurage, back or leg rubs, sacral pressure, repositioning, back rest; oral and perineal care, linen changes; shower/hot tub use) partner can use **to assist with pain control and relaxation.**

- Discuss available analgesics, usual responses and side effects (client and fetal), and duration of analgesic effect in light of current situation. **Allows client to make informed choice about means of pain control; can allay client's fears and anxieties about medication use.**

- Support client's decision about the use or nonuse of medication in a nonjudgmental manner. Continue encouragement for efforts and use of relaxation techniques. **Enhances client sense of control and may prevent or decrease need for medication.**

Postpartum/Newborn Care

- Initiate early breast- or oral feeding according to hospital protocol. **Initial feeding for breastfed infants usually occurs in the delivery room. Otherwise, 5 to 15 mL of sterile water may be offered in the nursery to assess effectiveness of sucking, swallowing, gag reflexes, and patency of esophagus.**

Information that appears in brackets has been added by the authors to clarify and enhance the use of nursing diagnoses.

⊕ Cultural 🐵 Collaborative 🏠 Community/Home Care

- Note frequency, amount, and length of feedings. Encourage demand feedings instead of scheduled feedings. Note frequency, amount, and appearance of regurgitation. **Hunger and length of time between feedings vary from feeding to feeding, and excessive regurgitation increases replacement needs.**
- Evaluate neonate and maternal satisfaction following feedings. **Provides opportunity to answer client questions, offer encouragement for efforts, identify needs, and problem-solve situations.**
- Demonstrate and supervise infant care activities related to feeding and holding; bathing, diapering, and clothing; care of circumcised male infant; and care of umbilical cord stump. Provide written/pictorial information for parents to refer to after discharge.
- Provide information about newborn interactional capabilities, states of consciousness, and means of stimulating cognitive development. **Helps parents recognize and respond to infant cues during interactional process; fosters optimal interaction, attachment behaviors, and cognitive development in infant.**
- Promote sleep and rest. **Reduces metabolic rate and allows nutrition and oxygen to be used for healing process rather than for energy needs.**
- Provide for unlimited participation for father and siblings. Ascertain whether siblings attended an orientation program. **Facilitates family development and ongoing process of acquaintance and attachment.**
- Monitor and document the client's/couple's interactions with infant. Note presence of bonding or acquaintance behaviors (e.g., making eye contact, using high-pitched voice and en face [face-to-face] position as culturally appropriate, calling infant by name, and holding infant closely).

Nursing Priority No. 3.
To enhance optimal well-being:

Prenatal
- Emphasize importance of maternal well-being. **Fetal well-being is directly related to maternal well-being, especially during the first trimester, when developing organ systems are most vulnerable to injury from environmental or hereditary factors.**
- Review physical changes to be expected during each trimester. **Prepares client/couple for managing common discomforts associated with pregnancy.**

Information that appears in brackets has been added by the authors to clarify and enhance the use of nursing diagnoses.

- Explain psychological reactions including ambivalence, introspection, stress reactions, and emotional lability as characteristic of pregnancy. **Helps client/couple understand mood swings and may provide opportunities for partner to offer support and affection at these times.**
- Provide necessary referrals (e.g., dietitian, social services, food stamps, or WIC food programs) as indicated. **Supplemental federally funded food program helps promote optimal maternal, fetal, and infant nutrition.**
- Review reportable danger signals of pregnancy, such as bleeding, cramping, acute abdominal pain, backache, edema, visual disturbance, headaches, and pelvic pressure. **Helps client distinguish normal from abnormal findings, thus assisting her in seeking timely, appropriate healthcare.**
- Encourage attendance at prenatal and childbirth classes. Provide information about father/sibling or grandparent participation in classes and delivery if client desires.
- Provide list of appropriate reading materials for client, couple, and siblings regarding adjusting to newborn. **Information helps individual realistically analyze changes in family structure, roles, and behaviors.**

Labor and Delivery
- Monitor labor progress, maternal and fetal well-being per protocol. Provide continuous intrapartal professional support/doula. **Fear of abandonment can intensify as labor progresses, and client may experience increased anxiety and/or loss of control when left unattended.**
- Reinforce use of positive coping mechanisms. **Enhances feelings of competence and fosters self-esteem.**

Postpartum/Newborn Care
- Provide information about self-care, including perineal care and hygiene; physiological changes, including normal progression of lochial discharge; needs for sleep and rest; importance of progressive postpartal exercise program; role changes.
- Review normal psychological changes and needs associated with the postpartal period. **Clients emotional state may be somewhat labile at this time and often is influenced by physical well-being.**
- Discuss sexuality needs and plans for contraception. Provide information about available methods, including advantages and disadvantages.
- Reinforce importance of postpartal examination by healthcare provider and interim follow-up as appropriate. **Follow-up visit is necessary to evaluate recovery of reproductive**

Information that appears in brackets has been added by the authors to clarify and enhance the use of nursing diagnoses.

🌐 Cultural Ⓐ Collaborative 🏠 Community/Home Care

organs, healing of episiotomy/laceration repair, general well-being, and adaptation to life changes.

- Provide oral and written information about infant care and development, feeding, and safety issues.
- Offer appropriate references reflecting cultural beliefs.
- Discuss physiology and benefits of breastfeeding, nipple and breast care, special dietary needs, factors that facilitate or interfere with successful breastfeeding, use of breast pump, and appropriate suppliers. **Helps ensure adequate milk supply, prevents nipple cracking and soreness, facilitates comfort, and establishes role of breastfeeding mother.**
- Refer client to support groups (e.g., La Leche League, Lact-Aid) or lactation consultant **to promote a successful breastfeeding outcome.**
- Identify available community resources as indicated (e.g., WIC program). **WIC and other federal programs support well-being through client education and enhanced nutritional intake for infant.**
- Discuss normal variations and characteristics of infant, such as caput succedaneum, cephalohematoma, pseudomenstruation, breast enlargement, physiological jaundice, and milia. **Helps parents recognize normal variations and may reduce anxiety.**
- Emphasize newborns need for follow-up evaluation by healthcare provider and timely immunizations.
- Identify manifestations of illness and infection and the times at which a healthcare provider should be contacted. Demonstrate proper technique for taking temperature, administering oral medications, or providing other care activities for infant as required. **Early recognition of illness and prompt use of healthcare facilitate treatment and positive outcome.**
- Refer client/couple to community postpartal parent groups. **Increases parent's knowledge of child rearing and child development, and provides supportive atmosphere while parents incorporate new roles.**

Documentation Focus

Assessment/Reassessment
- Assessment findings, general health, previous pregnancy experience.
- Cultural beliefs and expectations.
- Specific birth plan and individuals to be involved in delivery.
- Arrangements for postpartal recovery period.

Information that appears in brackets has been added by the authors to clarify and enhance the use of nursing diagnoses.

Planning
- Plan of care and who is involved in planning.
- Teaching plan.

Implementation/Evaluation
- Response to interventions, teaching, and actions performed.
- Attainment or progress toward desired outcome(s).
- Modifications to plan of care.

Discharge Planning
- Long-term needs and who is responsible for actions to be taken.
- Available resources, specific referrals made.

Sample Nursing Outcomes & Interventions Classifications (NOC/NIC) NIC

NOC—Childbirth Preparation
NIC—Knowledge: Pregnancy

---

impaired Comfort

Taxonomy II: Comfort—Class 1 Physical Comfort/Class 2 Environmental Comfort/Class 3 Social Comfort (00214)
[Diagnostic Division: Pain/Discomfort]
Submitted 2008

Definition: Perceived lack of ease, relief and transcendence in physical, psychospiritual, environmental and social dimensions

---

Related Factors

To be developed

Defining Characteristics

Subjective
Reports: distressing symptoms, lack of contentment/ease in situation, hunger, itching, being uncomfortable, cold, hot
Disturbed sleep pattern, inability to relax
Anxiety, fear
Illness-related symptoms, treatment-related side effects (e.g., medication, radiation)

Information that appears in brackets has been added by the authors to clarify and enhance the use of nursing diagnoses.

 Cultural Collaborative Community/Home Care

Insufficient resources (e.g., financial, social support)
Lack of privacy

Objective
Restlessness, irritability, moaning, crying
Lack of environmental control

Desired Outcomes/Evaluation Criteria—Client Will:

- Engage in behaviors or lifestyle changes to increase level of ease.
- Verbalize sense of comfort or contentment.
- Participate in desirable and realistic health-seeking behaviors.

Actions/Interventions

Nursing Priority No. 1.
To assess etiology/precipitating contributory factors:

- Determine the type of discomfort client is experiencing such as physical pain, feeling of discontent, lack of ease in social settings, or inability to rise above one's problems or pain (lack of transcendence).
- Note cultural/religious beliefs and values that impact perceptions and expectations of comfort.
- Ascertain locus of control. **Presence of external locus of control may hamper efforts to achieve sense of peace or contentment.**
- Discuss concerns with client and active-listen to identify underlying issues (e.g., physical and emotional stressors; or external factors such as environmental surroundings, social interactions) that could impact client's ability to control own well-being. **Helps to determine client's specific needs, ability to change own situation.**
- Establish context(s) in which lack of comfort is realized: physical—pertaining to bodily sensations; psychospiritual—pertaining to internal awareness of self and meaning in one's life, relationship to a higher order or being; environmental—pertaining to external surroundings, conditions, and influences; sociocultural—pertaining to interpersonal, family, and societal relationships.

Physical
- Determine how client is managing pain and pain components. **Lack of control may be related to other issues, or emotions such as fear, loneliness, anxiety, noxious stimuli, anger.**

Information that appears in brackets has been added by the authors to clarify and enhance the use of nursing diagnoses.

- Ascertain what has been tried or is required for comfort or rest (e.g., head of bed up/down, music on/off, white noise, rocking motion, certain person or thing).

Psychospiritual
- Determine how psychological and spiritual indicators overlap (e.g., meaningfulness, faith, identity, self-esteem) for client.
- Ascertain if client/SO desires support regarding spiritual enrichment, including prayer, meditation, or access to spiritual counselor of choice.

Environmental
- Determine that client's environment both respects privacy and provides natural lighting and readily accessible view to outdoors—**an aspect that can be manipulated to enhance comfort.**

Social
- Ascertain meaning of comfort in context of interpersonal, family, cultural values and societal relationships.
- Validate client/SO understanding of client's situation and ongoing methods of managing condition, as appropriate and/or desired by client. **Considers client/family needs in this area and/or shows appreciation for their desires.**

Nursing Priority No. 2.
To assist client to alleviate discomfort:
- Review knowledge base and note coping skills that have been used previously to change behavior/promote well-being. **Brings these to client's awareness and promotes use in current situation.**
- Acknowledge client's strengths in present situation and build on these in planning for future.

Physical
- Collaborate in treating or managing medical conditions involving oxygenation, elimination, mobility, cognitive abilities, electrolyte balance, thermoregulation, hydration, **to promote physical stability.**
- Work with client to prevent pain, nausea, itching, thirst/other physical discomforts.
- Review medications or treatment regimen **to determine possible changes or options to reduce side effects.**
- Suggest parent be present during procedures **to comfort child.**
- Provide age-appropriate comfort measures (e.g., back rub, change of position, cuddling, use of heat/cold) **to provide nonpharmacological pain management.**

Information that appears in brackets has been added by the authors to clarify and enhance the use of nursing diagnoses.

Cultural Collaborative Community/Home Care

∞• Discuss interventions/activities to promote ease, such as Therapeutic Touch (TT), massage, healing touch, biofeedback, self-hypnosis, guided imagery, breathing exercises; play therapy, and humor, **to promote ease and relaxation and to refocus attention.**

• Assist client to use and modify medication regimen **to make best use of pharmacological pain or symptom management.**

• Assist client/SO(s) to develop plan for activity and exercise within individual ability, emphasizing necessity of allowing sufficient time to finish activities.

• Maintain open and flexible visitation with client's desired persons.

• Encourage/plan care to allow individually adequate rest periods **to prevent fatigue.** Schedule activities for periods when client has the most energy **to maximize participation.**

• Discuss routines to promote restful sleep.

Psychospiritual

• Interact with client in therapeutic manner. **The nurse could be the most important comfort intervention for meeting client's needs. For example, assuring client that nausea can be treated successfully with both pharmacological and nonpharmacological methods may be more effective than simply administering antiemetic without reassurance and comforting presence.**

• Encourage verbalization of feelings and make time for listening/interacting.

• Identify ways (e.g., meditation, sharing oneself with others, being out in nature/garden, other spiritual activities) to achieve connectedness or harmony with self, others, nature, higher power.

• Establish realistic activity goals with client. **Enhances commitment to promoting optimal outcomes.**

• Involve client/SO(s) in schedule planning and decisions about timing and spacing of treatments **to promote relaxation/ reduce sense of boredom.**

• Encourage client to do whatever possible (e.g., self-care, sit up in chair, walk). **Enhances self-esteem and independence.**

∞• Use age-appropriate distraction with music, reading, chatting or texting with family and friends, watching TV or movies, playing video or computer games **to limit dwelling on and transcend unpleasant sensations and situations.**

• Encourage client to develop assertiveness skills, prioritizing goals/activities and to make use of beneficial coping behaviors. **Promotes sense of control and improves self-esteem.**

Information that appears in brackets has been added by the authors to clarify and enhance the use of nursing diagnoses.

- Identify opportunities for client to participate in experiences that enhance control and independence.

Environmental
- Provide quiet environment, calm activities.
- Provide for periodic changes in the personal surroundings when client is confined. Use the individual's input in creating the changes (e.g., seasonal bulletin boards, color changes, rearranging furniture, pictures). **Promotes client's sense of self-control and environmental comfort.**
- Suggest activities, such as bird feeders or baths for bird-watching, a garden in a window box/terrarium, or a fish bowl/aquarium, **to stimulate observation as well as involvement and participation in activity.**

Social
- Encourage age-appropriate diversional activities (e.g., TV/radio, computer games, playtime, socialization/outings with others).
- Avoid overstimulation/understimulation (cognitive and sensory).
- Make appropriate referrals to available support groups, hobby clubs, service organizations.

Nursing Priority No. 3.
To promote wellness (Teaching/Discharge Considerations):

- Provide information about conditions/health risk factors or concerns in desired format (e.g., pictures, TV programs, articles, handouts, audio/visual materials; classes, group discussions, Internet Web sites, and other databases) as appropriate. **Use of multiple modalities enhances acquisition/retention of information and gives client choices for accessing and applying information.**

Physical
- Promote overall health measures (e.g., nutrition, adequate fluid intake, elimination, appropriate vitamin and iron supplementation).
- Discuss potential complications and possible need for medical follow-up or alternative therapies. **Timely recognition and intervention can promote wellness.**
- Assist client/SO(s) to identify and acquire necessary equipment (e.g., lifts, commode chair, safety grab bars, personal hygiene supplies) to meet individual needs. Refer to appropriate suppliers.

Information that appears in brackets has been added by the authors to clarify and enhance the use of nursing diagnoses.

⊕ Cultural   Ⓐ Collaborative   🏠 Community/Home Care

Psychospiritual

- Collaborate with others when client expresses interest in lessons, counseling, coaching, and/or mentoring **to meet, enhance emotional and/or spiritual comfort.**
- Promote and encourage client's contributions toward meeting realistic goals.
- Encourage client take time to be introspective in the search for contentment/transcendence.

Environmental

- Create a compassionate, supportive, and therapeutic environment incorporating client's cultural and age or developmental factors.
- Correct environmental hazards that could influence safety or negatively affect comfort.
- Arrange for home visit or evaluation as needed.
- Discuss long-term plan for taking care of environmental needs.

Social

- Advocate for growth-promoting environment in conflict situations, and consider issues from client/family perspective.
- Identify resources or referrals (e.g., knowledge and skills, financial resources or assistance, personal or psychological support group, social activities).

Documentation Focus

Assessment/Reassessment
- Individual findings including client's description of current status/situation and factors impacting sense of comfort.
- Pertinent cultural and religious beliefs and values.
- Medication use and nonpharmacological measures.

Planning
- Plan of care, specific interventions, and who is involved in planning.
- Teaching plan.

Implementation/Evaluation
- Responses to interventions, teaching, and actions performed.
- Attainment or progress toward desired outcome(s).
- Modifications to plan of care.

Discharge Planning
- Long-term needs and who is responsible for actions to be taken.
- Specific referrals made.

Information that appears in brackets has been added by the authors to clarify and enhance the use of nursing diagnoses.

Sample Nursing Outcomes & Interventions Classifications (NOC/NIC) NIC

NOC—Comfort Level
NIC—Environmental Management: Comfort

readiness for enhanced Comfort

Taxonomy II: Comfort—Class 1 Physical Comfort/Class 2
  Environmental Comfort (00183)
[Diagnostic Division: Pain/Discomfort]
Submitted 2006

Definition: A pattern of ease, relief, and transcendence in physical, psychospiritual, environmental, and/or social dimensions that can be strengthened

Related Factors

To be developed

Defining Characteristics

Subjective
- Expresses desire to enhance comfort, feeling of contentment
- Expresses desire to enhance relaxation
- Expresses desire to enhance resolution of complaints

Objective
Appears relaxed, calm
Participating in comfort measures of choice

Desired Outcomes/Evaluation Criteria— Client Will:

- Verbalize sense of comfort or contentment.
- Demonstrate behaviors of optimal level of ease.
- Participate in desirable and realistic health-seeking behaviors.

Actions/Interventions

Nursing Priority No. 1.
To determine current level of comfort and motivation for change:

Information that appears in brackets has been added by the authors to clarify and enhance the use of nursing diagnoses.

 Cultural   Collaborative   Community/Home Care

- Determine the type of comfort client is experiencing: (1) relief (as from pain); (2) ease (a state of calm or contentment); or (3) transcendence (state in which one rises above one's problems or pain).
- Ascertain motivation or expectations for improvement.
- Establish context(s) in which comfort is realized: (1) physical (pertaining to bodily sensations); (2) psychospiritual (pertaining to internal awareness of self and meaning in one's life; relationship to a higher order or being); (3) environmental (pertaining to external surroundings, conditions, and influences); (4) sociocultural (pertaining to interpersonal, family, and societal relationships).

Physical
- Verify that client is managing pain and pain components effectively. **Success in this arena usually addresses other issues and emotions (e.g., fear, loneliness, anxiety, noxious stimuli, anger).**
- Ascertain what is used or required for comfort or rest (e.g., head of bed up or down, music on or off, white noise, rocking motion, certain person or thing).

Psychospiritual
- Determine how psychological and spiritual indicators overlap (e.g., meaningfulness, faith, identity, self-esteem) for client in enhancing comfort.
- Determine influence of cultural beliefs and values.
- Ascertain that client/SO has received desired support regarding spiritual enrichment, including prayer, meditation, access to spiritual counselor of choice.

Environmental
- Determine that client's environment respects privacy and provides natural lighting and readily accessible view to outdoors **(an aspect that can be manipulated to enhance comfort).**

Sociocultural
- Ascertain meaning of comfort in context of interpersonal, family, cultural values, spatial, and societal relationships.
- Validate client/SO understanding of client's diagnosis and prognosis and ongoing methods of managing condition, as appropriate and/or desired by client. **Considers client/family needs in this area and/or shows appreciation for their desires.**

Information that appears in brackets has been added by the authors to clarify and enhance the use of nursing diagnoses.

Nursing Priority No. 2.

To assist client in developing plan to improve comfort:

Physical

- Collaborate in treating and managing medical conditions involving oxygenation, elimination, mobility, cognitive abilities, electrolyte balance, thermoregulation, hydration, **to promote physical stability.**
- Work with client to prevent pain, nausea, itching, thirst or other physical discomforts.
- Suggest parent be present during procedures **to comfort child.**
- Provide age-appropriate comfort measures (e.g., back rub, change of position, cuddling, use of heat/cold) **to provide nonpharmacological pain management.**
- Review interventions and activities such as Therapeutic Touch (TT), biofeedback, self-hypnosis, guided imagery, breathing exercises, play therapy, and humor **to promote ease and relaxation and to refocus attention.**
- Assist client to use and modify medication regimen **to make best use of pharmacological pain management.**
- Assist client/SO(s) to develop plan for activity and exercise within individual ability, emphasizing necessity of allowing sufficient time to finish activities.
- Maintain open and flexible visitation with client's desired persons.
- Encourage adequate rest periods **to prevent fatigue.**
- Plan care to allow individually adequate rest periods. Schedule activities for periods when client has the most energy **to maximize participation.**
- Discuss routines to promote restful sleep.

Psychospiritual

- Interact with client in therapeutic manner. **The nurse could be the most important comfort intervention for meeting client's needs. For example, assuring client that nausea can be treated successfully with both pharmacological and nonpharmacological methods may be more effective than simply administering antiemetic without reassurance and comforting presence.**
- Encourage verbalization of feelings and make time for listening and interacting.
- Identify ways (e.g., meditation, sharing oneself with others, being out in nature/garden, other spiritual activities) **to**

Information that appears in brackets has been added by the authors to clarify and enhance the use of nursing diagnoses.

⊕ Cultural   ⊗ Collaborative   🏠 Community/Home Care

achieve connectedness or harmony with self, others, nature, higher power.

- Establish realistic activity goals with client. **Enhances commitment to promoting optimal outcomes.**
- Involve client/SO(s) in schedule planning and decisions about timing and spacing of treatments **to promote relaxation/ reduce sense of boredom.**
- Encourage client to do whatever possible (e.g., self-care, sit up in chair, walk). **Enhances self-esteem and independence.**
- Use age-appropriate distraction with music, chatting or texting with family and friends, watching TV, playing video or computer games, **to limit dwelling on or transcend unpleasant sensations and situations.**
- Encourage client to develop assertiveness skills, prioritizing goals/activities, and to make use of beneficial coping behaviors. **Promotes sense of control and improves self-esteem.**
- Offer or identify opportunities for client to participate in experiences that enhance control and independence.

Environmental

- Provide quiet environment, calm activities.
- Provide for periodic changes in the personal surroundings when client is confined. Use the individual's input in creating the changes (e.g., seasonal bulletin boards, color changes, rearranging furniture, pictures). **Enhances sense of comfort and control over environment.**
- Suggest activities, such as bird feeders or baths for bird-watching, a garden in a window box/terrarium, or a fish bowl/ aquarium, **to stimulate observation as well as involvement and participation in activity.**

Sociocultural

- Encourage age-appropriate diversional activities (e.g., TV/ radio, playtime/games, socialization/outings with others).
- Avoid cognitive or sensory overstimulation and understimulation.
- Make appropriate referrals to available support groups, hobby clubs, service organizations.

Nursing Priority No. 3.

To promote optimum wellness (Teaching/Discharge Considerations):

Information that appears in brackets has been added by the authors to clarify and enhance the use of nursing diagnoses.

Physical

- Promote overall health measures (e.g., nutrition, adequate fluid intake, elimination, appropriate vitamin/iron supplementation).
- Discuss potential complications and possible need for medical follow-up care or alternative therapies. **Timely recognition and intervention can promote wellness.**
- Assist client/SO(s) to identify and acquire necessary equipment (e.g., lifts, commode chair, safety grab bars, personal hygiene supplies) **to meet individual needs.**

Psychospiritual

- Collaborate with others when client expresses interest in lessons, counseling, coaching and/or mentoring **to meet/enhance emotional and/or spiritual comfort.**
- Encourage client's contributions toward meeting realistic goals.
- Encourage client to take time to be introspective in the search for contentment/transcendence.

Environmental

- Create a compassionate, supportive, and therapeutic environment incorporating client's cultural and age/developmental factors.
- Correct environmental hazards **that could influence safety/ negatively affect comfort.**
- Arrange for home visit/evaluation, as needed.
- Discuss long-term plan for taking care of environmental needs.

Sociocultural

- Advocate for growth-promoting environment in conflict situations, and consider issues from client/family perspective.
- Support client/SO access to resources (e.g., knowledge and skills; financial resources/assistance; personal/psychological support; social systems).

Documentation Focus ─────────────

Assessment/Reassessment

- Individual findings, including client's description of current status/situation.
- Motivation and expectations for change.
- Medication use/nonpharmacological measures.

Information that appears in brackets has been added by the authors to clarify and enhance the use of nursing diagnoses.

⊕ Cultural ⊛ Collaborative 🏠 Community/Home Care

Planning
- Plan of care, specific interventions, and who is involved in planning.
- Teaching plan.

Implementation/Evaluation
- Responses to interventions, teaching, and actions performed.
- Attainment or progress toward desired outcome(s).
- Modifications to plan of care.

Discharge Planning
- Long-term needs and who is responsible for actions to be taken.
- Specific referrals made.

Sample Nursing Outcomes & Interventions Classifications (NOC/NIC) NIC

NOC—Comfort Status
NIC—Self-Modification Assistance

---

impaired verbal Communication

Taxonomy II: Perception/Cognition—Class 5 Communication (00051)
[Diagnostic Division: Social Interaction]
Submitted 1983; Revised 1996, 1998

Definition: Decreased, delayed, or absent ability to receive, process, transmit, and/or use a system of symbols

---

Related Factors

Decrease in circulation to brain; brain tumor
Anatomical deficit (e.g., cleft palate, alteration of the neurovascular visual system, auditory system, or phonatory apparatus)
Difference related to developmental age
Physical barrier (tracheostomy, intubation)
Physiological conditions [e.g., dyspnea]; alteration of central nervous system (CNS); weakening of the musculoskeletal system
Psychological barriers (e.g., psychosis, lack of stimuli); emotional conditions [depression, panic, anger]; stress

---

Information that appears in brackets has been added by the authors to clarify and enhance the use of nursing diagnoses.

 Diagnostic Studies ∞ Pediatric/Geriatric/Lifespan 💊 Medications **193**

Environmental barriers
Cultural difference
Lack of information
Side effects of medication
Alteration in self-esteem or self-concept
Altered perceptions
Absence of SO(s)

Defining Characteristics

Subjective
Reports of difficulty expressing self

Objective
Inability to speak dominant language
Speaks/verbalizes with difficulty; stuttering; slurring
Does not/cannot speak; willful refusal to speak
Difficulty forming words or sentences (e.g., aphonia, dyslalia, dysarthria)
Difficulty expressing thoughts verbally (e.g., aphasia, dysphasia, apraxia, dyslexia)
Inappropriate verbalization [incessant, loose association of ideas; flight of ideas]
Difficulty in comprehending or maintaining usual communication pattern
Absence of eye contact/difficulty in selective attending; partial/total visual deficit
Inability or difficulty in use of facial or body expressions
Dyspnea
Disorientation to person, space, time
Inability to modulate speech
Message inappropriate to content
Use of nonverbal cues (e.g., pleading eyes, gestures, turning away)
Frustration, anger, hostility

Desired Outcomes/Evaluation Criteria— Client Will:

- Verbalize or indicate an understanding of the communication difficulty and plans for ways of handling.
- Establish method of communication in which needs can be expressed.

Information that appears in brackets has been added by the authors to clarify and enhance the use of nursing diagnoses.

🌐 Cultural   🔬 Collaborative   🏠 Community/Home Care

- Participate in therapeutic communication (e.g., using silence, acceptance, restating, reflecting, Active-listening, and I-messages).
- Demonstrate congruent verbal and nonverbal communication.
- Use resources appropriately.

Actions/Interventions

Nursing Priority No. 1.
To assess causative/contributing factors:

- Review history for neurological conditions **that could affect speech, such as stroke, tumor, MS, hearing or vision impairment.**
- Note results of neurological tests (e.g., electroencephalogram [EEG]; CT/MRI scans; and language/speech tests [e.g., Boston Diagnostic Aphasia Examination, the Action Naming Test]).
- Note whether aphasia is motor (expressive: loss of images for articulated speech), sensory (receptive: unable to understand words and does not recognize the defect), conduction (slow comprehension: uses words inappropriately but knows the error), and/or global (total loss of ability to comprehend and speak). Evaluate the degree of impairment.
- Evaluate mental status, note presence of psychiatric conditions (e.g., bipolar, schizoid/affective behavior). Assess psychological response to communication impairment, and willingness to find alternate means of communication.
- Note presence of ET tube/tracheostomy or other physical blocks to speech (e.g., cleft palate, jaws wired).
- Assess environmental factors that may affect ability to communicate (e.g., room noise level).
- Determine primary language spoken and cultural factors.
- Assess style of speech (as outlined in Defining Characteristics).
- Note level of anxiety present; presence of angry, hostile behavior; frustration.
- Interview parent to determine child's developmental level of speech and language comprehension.
- Note parental speech patterns and manner of communicating with child, including gestures.

Nursing Priority No. 2.
To assist client to establish a means of communication to express needs, wants, ideas, and questions:

- Ascertain that you have client's attention before communicating.

Information that appears in brackets has been added by the authors to clarify and enhance the use of nursing diagnoses.

- Determine ability to read and write. Evaluate musculoskeletal states, including manual dexterity (e.g., ability to hold a pen and write).
- Advise other healthcare providers of client's communication deficits (e.g., deafness, aphasia, presence of mechanical ventilation strategies) and needed means of communication (e.g., writing pad, signing, yes/no responses, gestures, picture board) **to minimize client's frustration and promote understanding (aphasia).**
- Obtain a translator, or provide written translation or picture chart **when writing is not possible or client speaks a different language than that spoken by healthcare provider.**
- Facilitate hearing and vision examinations **to obtain necessary aids.**
- Ascertain that hearing aid(s) are in place and batteries charged, and/or glasses are worn when needed **to facilitate and improve communication.** Assist client to learn to use and adjust to aids.
- Reduce environmental noise that can interfere with comprehension. Provide adequate lighting, especially if client is reading lips or attempting to write.
- Establish relationship with the client, listening carefully and attending to client's verbal/nonverbal expressions. **Conveys interest and concern.**
- Maintain eye contact, preferably at client's level. Be aware of cultural factors that may preclude eye contact (e.g., found in some American Indians, Indo-Chinese, Arabs, natives of Appalachia).
- Keep communication simple, speaking in short sentences, using appropriate words, and using all modes for accessing information: visual, auditory, and kinesthetic.
- Maintain a calm, unhurried manner. Provide sufficient time for client to respond. Downplay errors and avoid frequent corrections. **Individuals with expressive aphasia may talk more easily when they are rested and relaxed and when they are talking to one person at a time.**
- Determine meaning of words used by the client and congruency of communication and nonverbal messages.
- Validate meaning of nonverbal communication; do not make assumptions **because they may be wrong.** Be honest; if you do not understand, seek assistance from others.
- Individualize techniques using breathing for relaxation of the vocal cords, rote tasks (such as counting), and singing or

---

Information that appears in brackets has been added by the authors to clarify and enhance the use of nursing diagnoses.

Cultural Collaborative Community/Home Care

melodic intonation **to assist aphasic clients in relearning speech.**

- Anticipate needs and stay with client until effective communication is reestablished, and/or client feels safe/comfortable.
- Plan for alternative methods of communication (e.g., slate board, letter/picture board, hand/eye signals, typewriter/computer), incorporating information about type of disability present.
- Identify and use previous successful communication solutions used if situation is chronic or recurrent.
- Provide reality orientation by responding with simple, straightforward, honest statements.
- Provide environmental stimuli, as needed, **to maintain contact with reality,** or reduce stimuli **to lessen anxiety that may worsen problem.**
- Use confrontation skills, when appropriate, within an established nurse-client relationship **to clarify discrepancies between verbal and nonverbal cues.**

Nursing Priority No. 3.

To promote wellness (Teaching/Discharge Considerations):

- Review information about condition, prognosis, and treatment with client/SO(s).
- Reinforce that loss of speech does not imply loss of intelligence.
- Discuss individual methods of dealing with impairment.
- Recommend placing a tape recorder with a prerecorded emergency message near the telephone. Information to include: client's name, address, telephone number, and critical information (e.g., type of airway, person cannot speak), and a request for immediate emergency assistance.
- Use and assist client/SO(s) to learn therapeutic communication skills of acknowledgment, Active-listening, and I-messages. **Improves general communication skills.**
- Involve family/SO(s) in plan of care as much as possible. **Enhances participation and commitment to communication with loved one.**
- Refer to appropriate resources (e.g., speech/language therapist, support groups such as stroke club, individual/family, and/or psychiatric counseling).
- Refer to NDs ineffective Coping; disabled family Coping (as indicated); Anxiety; Fear.

Information that appears in brackets has been added by the authors to clarify and enhance the use of nursing diagnoses.

Documentation Focus

Assessment/Reassessment
- Assessment findings, pertinent history information (i.e., physical, psychological, cultural concerns).
- Meaning of nonverbal cues, level of anxiety client exhibits.

Planning
- Plan of care and interventions (e.g., type of alternative communication/translator).
- Teaching plan.

Implementation/Evaluation
- Response to interventions, teaching, and actions performed.
- Attainment or progress toward desired outcome(s).
- Modifications to plan of care.

Discharge Planning
- Discharge needs, referrals made; additional resources available.

Sample Nursing Outcomes & Interventions Classifications (NOC/NIC) NIC

NOC—Communication
NIC—Communication Enhancement: Speech Deficit

---

readiness for enhanced Communication

Taxonomy II: Perception/Cognition—Class 5 Communication (00161)
[Diagnostic Division: Teaching/Learning]
Submitted 2002

Definition: A pattern of exchanging information and ideas with others that is sufficient for meeting one's needs and life goals, and can be strengthened

---

Related Factors

To be developed

Information that appears in brackets has been added by the authors to clarify and enhance the use of nursing diagnoses.

🌐 Cultural   🔄 Collaborative   🏠 Community/Home Care

Defining Characteristics

Subjective
Expresses willingness to enhance communication
Expresses thoughts, feelings
Expresses satisfaction with ability to share information or ideas with others

Objective
Able to speak or write a language
Forms words, phrases, sentences
Uses and interprets nonverbal cues appropriately

Desired Outcomes/Evaluation Criteria— Client/SO/Caregiver Will:

- Verbalize or indicate an understanding of the communication process.
- Identify ways to improve communication.

Actions/Interventions

Nursing Priority No. 1.
To assess how client is managing communication/challenges:

- Ascertain circumstances that result in client's desire to improve communication. **Many factors are involved in communication, and identifying specific needs/expectations helps in developing realistic goals and determining likelihood of success.**
- Evaluate mental status. **Disorientation and psychotic conditions may be affecting speech and the communication of thoughts, needs, and desires.**
- Determine client's developmental level of speech and language comprehension. **Provides baseline information for developing plan for improvement.**
- Determine ability to read and write preferred language. **Evaluating grasp of language as well as musculoskeletal states, including manual dexterity (e.g., ability to hold a pen and write), provides information about nature of client's situation. Educational plan can address language skills. Neuromuscular deficits will require individual program in order to improve.**

Information that appears in brackets has been added by the authors to clarify and enhance the use of nursing diagnoses.

- Determine country of origin, dominant language, whether client is recent immigrant and what cultural, ethnic group client identifies as own. **Recent immigrant may identify with home country and its people, language, beliefs, and health-care practices, thus affecting language skills and ability to improve interactions in new country.**
- Ascertain if interpreter is needed/desired. **Law mandates that interpretation services be made available. A trained, professional interpreter who translates precisely and possesses a basic understanding of medical terminology and healthcare ethics is preferred to enhance client and provider satisfaction.**
- Determine comfort level in expression of feelings and concepts in nonproficient language. **Concern about language skills can impact perception of own ability to communicate.**
- Note any physical barriers to effective communication (e.g., talking tracheostomy, wired jaws) or physiological or neurological conditions (e.g., severe shortness of breath, neuromuscular weakness, stroke, brain trauma, hearing impairment, cleft palate, facial trauma). **Client may be dealing with speech/language comprehension difficulties or have voice production problems (pitch, loudness, or quality) that call attention to voice rather than what speaker is saying. These barriers may need to be addressed to enable client to improve communication skills.**
- Clarify meaning of words used by the client to describe important aspects of life and health/well-being (e.g., pain, sorrow, anxiety). **Words can easily be misinterpreted when sender and receiver have different ideas about their meanings. Restating what one has heard can clarify whether an expressed statement has been correctly understood or misinterpreted.**
- Determine presence of emotional lability (e.g., anger outbursts) and frequency of unstable behaviors. **Emotional and psychiatric issues can affect communication and interfere with understanding.**
- Evaluate congruency of verbal and nonverbal messages. **Communication is enhanced when verbal and nonverbal messages are congruent.**
- Evaluate need or desire for pictures or written communications and instructions as part of treatment plan. **Alternative methods of communication can help client feel understood and promote feelings of satisfaction with interaction.**

Information that appears in brackets has been added by the authors to clarify and enhance the use of nursing diagnoses.

Nursing Priority No. 2.

To improve client's ability to communicate thoughts, needs, and ideas:

* Maintain a calm, unhurried manner. Provide sufficient time for client to respond. **An atmosphere in which client is free to speak without fear of criticism provides the opportunity to explore all the issues involved in making decisions to improve communication skills.**

* Pay attention to speaker. Be an active listener. **The use of Active-listening communicates acceptance and respect for the client, establishing trust and promoting openness and honest expression. It communicates a belief that the client is a capable and competent person.**

* Sit down, maintain eye contact as culturally appropriate, preferably at client's level, and spend time with the client. **Conveys message that the nurse has time and interest in communicating.**

* Observe body language, eye movements, and behavioral cues. **May reveal unspoken concerns; for example, when pain is present, client may react with tears, grimacing, stiff posture, turning away, or angry outbursts.**

* Help client identify and learn to avoid use of nontherapeutic communication. **These barriers are recognized as detriments to open communication and learning to avoid them maximizes the effectiveness of communication between client and others.**

* Obtain interpreter with language or signing abilities, as needed. **May be needed to enhance understanding of words and language concepts or to ascertain that interpretation of communication is accurate.**

* Suggest use of pad and pencil, slate board, letter/picture board when interacting or attempting to interface in new situations. **When client has physical impairments that challenge verbal communication, alternate means can provide clear concepts that are understandable to both parties.**

* Obtain or provide access to voice-enabled computer, when indicated. **Use of these devices may be more helpful when communication challenges are long-standing and/or when client is used to working with them.**

* Respect client's cultural communication needs. **Different cultures can dictate beliefs of what is normal or abnormal (i.e., in some cultures, eye-to-eye contact is considered disrespectful, impolite, or an invasion of privacy; silence and**

Information that appears in brackets has been added by the authors to clarify and enhance the use of nursing diagnoses.

tone of voice have various meanings, and slang words can cause confusion).

- Encourage use of glasses, hearing aids, dentures, electronic speech devices, as needed. **These devices maximize sensory perception or speech formation, and can improve understanding and enhance speech patterns.**

- Reduce distractions and background noises (e.g., close the door, turn down the radio or TV). **A distracting environment can interfere with communication, limiting attention to tasks and making speech and communication more difficult. Reducing noise can help both parties hear clearly, thus improving understanding.**

- Associate words with objects—using repetition and redundancy—point to objects or demonstrate desired actions. **Speaker's own body language can be used to enhance client's understanding.**

- Use confrontation skills carefully, when appropriate, within an established nurse-client relationship. **Can be used to clarify discrepancies between verbal and nonverbal cues, enabling client to look at areas that may require change.**

Nursing Priority No. 3.

To promote optimum communication:

- Discuss with family/SO and other caregivers effective ways in which the client communicates. **Identifying positive aspects of current communication skills enables family members and other caregivers to learn and move forward in desire to enhance ways of interacting.**

- Encourage client/SO(s) to familiarize themselves with and use of new communication technologies. **Enhances family relationships and promotes self-esteem for all members as they are able to communicate regardless of the problems (e.g., progressive disorder) that could interfere with ability to interact.**

- Reinforce client/SO(s) learning and using therapeutic communication skills of acknowledgment, active-listening, and I-messages. **Improves general communication skills, emphasizes acceptance, and conveys respect, enabling family relationships to improve.**

- Refer to appropriate resources (e.g., speech therapist, language classes, individual/family and/or psychiatric counseling). **May be needed to help overcome challenges as family strives toward desired goal of enhanced communication.**

Information that appears in brackets has been added by the authors to clarify and enhance the use of nursing diagnoses.

  Cultural   Collaborative   Community/Home Care

Documentation Focus

Assessment/Reassessment
- Assessment findings, pertinent history information (i.e., physical, psychological, cultural concerns).
- Meaning of nonverbal cues, level of anxiety client exhibits.

Planning
- Plan of care and interventions (e.g., type of alternative communication, use of translator).
- Teaching plan.

Implementation/Evaluation
- Progress toward desired outcome(s).
- Modifications to plan of care.

Discharge Planning
- Discharge needs, referrals made, additional resources available.

Sample Nursing Outcomes & Interventions Classifications (NOC/NIC) `NIC`

NOC—Communication
NIC—Communication Enhancement [specify]

---

decisional **Conflict** [specify]

Taxonomy II: Life Principles—Class 3 Value/Belief/Action Congruence (00083)
[Diagnostic Division: Ego Integrity]
Submitted 1988; Revised 2006

Definition: Uncertainty about course of action to be taken when choice among competing actions involves risk, loss, or challenge to values and beliefs

---

Related Factors

Unclear personal values/beliefs; perceived threat to value system
Lack of experience or interference with decision making
Lack of relevant information; multiple or divergent sources of information

---

Information that appears in brackets has been added by the authors to clarify and enhance the use of nursing diagnoses.

Moral obligations require performing or not performing actions

Moral principles, rules, values support mutually inconsistent courses of action

Support system deficit

Age; developmental state

Family system; sociocultural factors

Cognitive, emotional, behavioral level of functioning

Defining Characteristics

Subjective

Verbalizes: uncertainty about choices; undesired consequences of alternative actions being considered

Verbalizes feeling of distress while attempting a decision

Questioning moral principles, rules, values or personal values and beliefs while attempting a decision

Objective

Vacillation between alternative choices; delayed decision making

Self-focusing

Physical signs of distress or tension (e.g., increased heart rate, increased muscle tension, restlessness)

Desired Outcomes/Evaluation Criteria— Client Will:

- Verbalize awareness of positive and negative aspects of choices and alternative actions.
- Acknowledge and ventilate feelings of anxiety and distress associated with choice, related to making difficult decision.
- Identify personal values and beliefs concerning issues.
- Make decision(s) and express satisfaction with choices.
- Meet psychological needs as evidenced by appropriate expression of feelings, identification of options, and use of resources.
- Display relaxed manner, calm demeanor, free of physical signs of distress.

Actions/Interventions

Nursing Priority No. 1.

To assess causative/contributing factors:

∞ • Determine usual ability to manage own affairs. Clarify who has legal right to intervene on behalf of a child, elder,

---

Information that appears in brackets has been added by the authors to clarify and enhance the use of nursing diagnoses.

 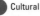 Cultural   Collaborative   Community/Home Care

impaired individual (e.g., parent/spouse, other relative, designee for durable medical power of attorney, or court appointed guardian/advocate). **Family disruption and conflicts can complicate decision process.**

* Note expressions of indecision, dependence on others, availability/involvement of support persons (e.g., client may have lack of/conflicting advice). Ascertain dependency of other(s) on client and/or issues of codependency.
* Active-listen/identify reason for indecisiveness. **Helps client to clarify problem and work toward a solution.**
* Determine effectiveness of current problem-solving techniques.
* Note presence/intensity of physical signs of anxiety (e.g., increased heart rate, muscle tension).
* Listen for expressions of client's inability to find meaning in life/reason for living, feelings of futility, or alienation from God and others around them. (Refer to ND Spiritual Distress, as indicated.)
* Review information client has about the healthcare decision. **Accurate and clearly understood information about situation will help the client make the best decision for self.**

Nursing Priority No. 2.

To assist client to develop/effectively use problem-solving skills:

* Promote safe and hopeful environment, as needed, while client regains inner control.
* Encourage verbalization of conflicts or concerns.
* Accept verbal expressions of anger or guilt, setting limits on maladaptive behavior **to promote client safety.**
* Clarify and prioritize individual goals, noting where the subject of the "conflict" falls on this scale. **Choices may have risky, uncertain outcomes; may reflect a need to make value judgments or may generate regret over having to reject positive choice and acccept negative consequences.**
* Identify strengths and presence of positive coping skills (e.g., use of relaxation technique, willingness to express feelings).
* Identify positive aspects of this experience and assist client to view it as a learning opportunity **to develop new and creative solutions.**

Information that appears in brackets has been added by the authors to clarify and enhance the use of nursing diagnoses.

 Diagnostic Studies ∞ Pediatric/Geriatric/Lifespan   Medications **205**

- Correct misperceptions client may have and provide factual information. **Provides for better decision making.**
- Provide opportunities for client to make simple decisions regarding self-care and other daily activities. Accept choice not to do so. Advance complexity of choices, as tolerated.
- Encourage child to make developmentally appropriate decisions concerning own care. **Fosters child's sense of self-worth, enhances ability to learn and exercise coping skills.**
- Discuss time considerations, setting time line for small steps and considering consequences related to not making/postponing specific decisions **to facilitate resolution of conflict.**
- Have client list some alternatives to present situation or decisions, using a brainstorming process. Include family in this activity as indicated (e.g., placement of parent in long-term care facility, use of intervention process with addicted member). (Refer to NDs interrupted Family Processes; dysfunctional Family Processes: alcoholism; compromised family Coping; moral Distress.)
- Practice use of problem-solving process with current situation/decision.
- Discuss or clarify cultural or spiritual concerns, accepting client's values in a nonjudgmental manner.

Nursing Priority No. 3.
To promote wellness (Teaching/Discharge Considerations):
- Promote opportunities for using conflict-resolution skills, identifying steps as client does each one.
- Provide positive feedback for efforts and progress noted. **Promotes continuation of efforts.**
- Encourage involvement of family/SO(s), as desired/available, **to provide support for the client.**
- Support client for decisions made, especially if consequences are unexpected, difficult to cope with.
- Encourage attendance at stress reduction, assertiveness classes.
- Refer to other resources, as necessary (e.g., clergy, psychiatric clinical nurse specialist/psychiatrist, family/marital therapist, addiction support groups).

Documentation Focus

Assessment/Reassessment
- Assessment findings, behavioral responses, degree of impairment in lifestyle functioning.

Information that appears in brackets has been added by the authors to clarify and enhance the use of nursing diagnoses.

- Individuals involved in the conflict.
- Personal values and beliefs.

Planning
- Plan of care, specific interventions, and who is involved in the planning process.
- Teaching plan.

Implementation/Evaluation
- Client's and involved individual's responses to interventions, teaching, and actions performed.
- Ability to express feelings, identify options; use of resources.
- Attainment or progress toward desired outcome(s).
- Modifications to plan of care.

Discharge Planning
- Long-term needs, referrals made, actions to be taken, and who is responsible for doing.
- Specific referrals made.

Sample Nursing Outcomes & Interventions Classifications (NOC/NIC) NIC

NOC—Decision Making
NIC—Decision-Making Support

---

parental role Conflict

Taxonomy II: Role Relationships—Class 1 Role Performance (00064)
[Diagnostic Division: Social Interaction]
Submitted 1988

Definition: Parent experience of role confusion and conflict in response to crisis

---

Related Factors

Separation from child due to chronic illness[/disability]
Intimidation with invasive modalities (e.g., intubation); restrictive modalities (e.g., isolation); specialized care centers
Home care of a child with special needs [e.g., apnea monitoring, postural drainage, parenteral nutrition]
Change in marital status; [conflicts of the role of the single parent]

Information that appears in brackets has been added by the authors to clarify and enhance the use of nursing diagnoses.

 Diagnostic Studies ∞ Pediatric/Geriatric/Lifespan 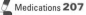 Medications **207**

Interruptions of family life due to home care regimen (e.g., treatments, caregivers, lack of respite)

Defining Characteristics

Subjective

Parent(s) express(es) concerns/feeling of inadequacy to provide for child's needs (e.g., physical and emotional)

Parent(s) express(es) concerns about changes in parental role; about family (e.g., functioning, communication, health)

Express(es) concern about perceived loss of control over decisions relating to their child

Verbalize(s) feelings of guilt, frustration; anxiety; fear

Verbalize(s) concern about role conflict of wanting to date while having responsibility of child care

Objective

Demonstrates disruption in caretaking routines

Reluctant to participate in usual caretaking activities, even with encouragement and support

Desired Outcomes/Evaluation Criteria— Parent(s) Will:

- Verbalize understanding of situation and expected parent's/child's role.
- Express feelings about child's illness or situation and effect on family life.
- Demonstrate appropriate behaviors in regard to parenting role.
- Assume caretaking activities as appropriate.
- Handle family disruptions effectively.

Actions/Interventions

Nursing Priority No. 1.

To assess causative/contributory factors:

- Assess individual situation and parent's perception of/concern about what is happening and expectations of self as caregiver.
- ∞ Note parental status, including age and maturity, stability of relationship, single parent, other responsibilities. (Increasing numbers of elderly individuals are providing full-time care

---

Information that appears in brackets has been added by the authors to clarify and enhance the use of nursing diagnoses.

   Cultural Collaborative Community/Home Care

for young grandchildren whose parents are unavailable or unable to provide care.)

- Ascertain parent's understanding of child's developmental stage and expectations for the future **to identify misconceptions and strengths.**
- Note coping skills currently being used by each individual as well as how problems have been dealt with in the past. **Provides basis for comparison and reference for client's coping abilities.**
- Determine use of substances (e.g., alcohol, other drugs, including prescription medications). **May interfere with individual's ability to cope and problem-solve.**
- Assess availability and use of resources, including extended family, support groups, and financial.
- Perform testing, such as Parent-Child Relationship Inventory (PCRI), for further evaluation as indicated.

Nursing Priority No. 2.
To assist parents to deal with current crisis:

- Encourage free verbal expression of feelings (including negative feelings of anger and hostility), setting limits on inappropriate behavior.
- Acknowledge difficulty of situation and normalcy of feeling overwhelmed and helpless. Encourage contact with parents who experienced similar situation with child and had positive outcome.
- Provide information, including technical information when appropriate, **to meet individual needs and correct misconceptions.**
- Promote parental involvement in decision making and care as much as possible/desired. **Enhances sense of control.**
- Encourage interaction/facilitate communication between parent(s) and children.
- Promote use of assertiveness, relaxation skills **to help individuals deal with situation/crisis.**
- Assist parent(s) to learn proper administration of medications and treatments, as indicated.
- Provide for, or encourage use of, respite care, parental time off **to enhance emotional well-being.**
- Help single parent distinguish between parent love and partner love. **Love is constant, but attention can be given to one or the other, as appropriate.**

Information that appears in brackets has been added by the authors to clarify and enhance the use of nursing diagnoses.

Nursing Priority No. 3.

To promote wellness (Teaching/Discharge Considerations):

 • Provide anticipatory guidance **to encourage making plans for future needs.**

 • Encourage parents to set realistic and mutually agreed-on goals.

 • Discuss attachment behaviors such as breastfeeding on cue, co-sleeping, and babywearing (carrying baby around on chest/back), and playing. **Dealing with ill child/home care pressures can strain the bond between parent and child. Activities such as these encourage secure relationships.**

 • Provide and identify learning opportunities specific to needs (e.g., parenting classes, healthcare equipment use/troubleshooting).

• Refer to community resources, as appropriate (e.g., visiting nurse, respite care, social services, psychiatric care or family therapy, well-baby clinics, special-needs support services).

• Refer to ND impaired Parenting for additional interventions.

Documentation Focus

Assessment/Reassessment

• Findings, including specifics of individual situation/parental concerns, perceptions, expectations.

Planning

• Plan of care and who is involved in the planning.
• Teaching plan.

Implementation/Evaluation

• Parent's responses to interventions, teaching, and actions performed.
• Attainment or progress toward desired outcome(s).
• Modifications to plan of care.

Discharge Planning

• Long-term needs and who is responsible for each action to be taken.
• Specific referrals made.

Sample Nursing Outcomes & Interventions Classifications (NOC/NIC) NIC

NOC—Parenting Performance
NIC—Parenting Promotion

Information that appears in brackets has been added by the authors to clarify and enhance the use of nursing diagnoses.

🌐 Cultural   🅐 Collaborative   🏠 Community/Home Care

acute Confusion

Taxonomy II: Perception/Cognition—Class 4 Cognition
(00128)
[Diagnostic Division: Neurosensory]
Submitted 1994; Revised 2006

Definition: Abrupt onset of reversible disturbances of
consciousness, attention, cognition, and perception that
develop over a short period of time

Related Factors

Alcohol abuse; drug abuse; [medication reaction/interaction;
anesthesia/surgery; metabolic imbalances]
Fluctuation in sleep-wake cycle
Over 60 years of age
Delirium [including febrile epilepticum (following or instead of
an epileptic attack), toxic and traumatic]
Dementia
Exacerbation of a chronic illness; hypoxemia
Severe pain

Defining Characteristics

Subjective
Hallucinations [visual or auditory]
Exaggerated emotional responses

Objective
Fluctuation in cognition or level of consciousness
Fluctuation in psychomotor activity [tremors, body movement]
Increased agitation or restlessness
Misperceptions [inappropriate responses]
Lack of motivation to initiate or follow-through with purposeful
behavior
Lack of motivation to initiate or follow-through with goal-
directed behavior

Desired Outcomes/Evaluation Criteria— Client Will:

- Regain and maintain usual reality orientation and level of consciousness.
- Verbalize understanding of causative factors when known.

Information that appears in brackets has been added by the authors to clarify
and enhance the use of nursing diagnoses.

- Initiate lifestyle or behavior changes to prevent or minimize recurrence of problem.

Actions/Interventions

Nursing Priority No. 1.

To assess causative/contributing factors:

- Identify factors present such as recent surgery, acute illness, trauma or fall, use of large numbers of medications (polypharmacy), intoxication, substance use or abuse, history of seizures or current seizure activity, episodes of fever, pain, presence of acute infection (especially urinary tract infection in elderly client), exposure to toxic substances, exposure to traumatic events, person with dementia experiencing sudden change in environment/unfamiliar surroundings or people. **Acute confusion is a symptom associated with numerous causes (e.g., hypoxia, abnormal metabolic conditions, ingestion of toxins or medications, electrolyte abnormalities, sepsis, nutritional deficiencies, endocrine disorders, central nervous system [CNS] infections or other neurological pathology, acute psychiatric disorders).**
- Investigate possibility of alcohol or other drug withdrawal.
- Evaluate vital signs **for indicators of poor tissue perfusion (i.e., hypotension, tachycardia, tachypnea), stress response (tachycardia, tachypnea).**
- Determine current medications/drug use—especially anti-anxiety agents, barbiturates, lithium, methyldopa, disulfiram, cocaine, alcohol, amphetamines, hallucinogens, opiates **(associated with high risk of confusion)**—and schedule of use, such as cimetidine + antacid or digoxin + diuretics **(combinations can increase risk of adverse reactions and interactions).**
- Assess diet and nutritional status **to identify possible deficiencies of essential nutrients and vitamins (e.g., thiamine) that could affect mental status.**
- Note presence of anxiety, agitation, fear.
- Evaluate for exacerbation of psychiatric conditions (e.g., mood or dissociative disorders, dementia).
- Monitor laboratory values (e.g., CBC, blood cultures, oxygen saturation, electrolytes, chemistries, ammonia levels, liver function studies, serum glucose, urinalysis, toxicology, and drug levels [including peak and trough, as appropriate]).
- Evaluate sleep and rest status, noting insomnia, sleep deprivation, or oversleeping. (Refer to NDs Insomnia; Sleep Deprivation, as appropriate.)

Information that appears in brackets has been added by the authors to clarify and enhance the use of nursing diagnoses.

Cultural   Collaborative   Community/Home Care

• Review results of medical diagnostic studies (e.g., brain scans, imaging studies, EEG, cardiopulmonary tests, lumbar puncture and cerebrospinal fluid [CSF] studies).

Nursing Priority No. 2.
To determine degree of impairment:

- Talk with SO(s) to determine historic baseline, observed changes, and onset or recurrence of changes **to understand and clarify current situation.**
- Evaluate mental status, noting extent of impairment in orientation, attention span, ability to follow directions, ability to send and receive communication, appropriateness of response.
- Note occurrence and timing of agitation, hallucinations, violent behaviors. **("Sundown syndrome" may occur, with client oriented during daylight hours but confused during nighttime.)**
- Determine threat to safety of client/others.

Nursing Priority No. 3.
To maximize level of function, prevent further deterioration:

- Assist with treatment of underlying problem (e.g., drug intoxication/substance abuse, infectious process, hypoxemia, biochemical imbalances, nutritional deficits, pain management).
- Monitor/adjust medication regimen and note response. Determine medications that can be changed or eliminated **when polypharmacy, side effects, or adverse reactions are determined to be associated with current condition.**
- Orient client to surroundings, staff, necessary activities, as needed. Present reality concisely and briefly. Avoid challenging illogical thinking—**defensive reactions may result.**
- Encourage family/SO(s) to participate in reorientation as well as providing ongoing input (e.g., current news and family happenings).
- Maintain calm environment and eliminate extraneous noise or other stimuli **to prevent overstimulation.** Provide normal levels of essential sensory and tactile stimulation—include personal items, pictures, and so forth.
- Encourage client to use vision or hearing aids when needed.
- Give simple directions. Allow sufficient time for client to respond, communicate, and make decisions.
- Provide for safety needs (e.g., supervision, seizure precautions, placing call bell within reach, positioning needed items within reach/clearing traffic paths, ambulating with devices).

Information that appears in brackets has been added by the authors to clarify and enhance the use of nursing diagnoses.

- Note behavior that may be indicative of potential for violence and take appropriate actions.
- Assist with treatment of alcohol or drug intoxication and/or withdrawal, as indicated.
- Administer psychotropics cautiously **to control restlessness, agitation, hallucinations.**
- Avoid or limit use of restraints—**may worsen situation, increase likelihood of untoward complications.**
- Provide undisturbed rest periods.
- Administer short-acting, nonbenzodiazepine sleeping medication (e.g., Benadryl) at bedtime.
- Refer to NDs impaired Memory; disturbed Thought Processes; impaired verbal Communication, for additional interventions.

Nursing Priority No. 4.

To promote wellness (Teaching/Discharge Considerations):

- Explain reason(s) for confusion, if known. **Although acute confusion usually subsides over time as client recovers from underlying cause and/or adjusts to situation, it can initially be frightening to client/SO. Therefore, information about the cause and appropriate treatment to improve condition may be helpful in managing sense of fear and powerlessness.**
- Discuss need for ongoing medical review of client's medications **to limit possibility of misuse and/or potential for dangerous side effects/interactions.**
- Assist in identifying ongoing treatment needs and emphasize necessity of periodic evaluation **to support early intervention.**
- Emphasize importance of keeping vision/hearing aids in good repair **to improve client's interpretation of environmental stimuli and communication.**
- Discuss situation with family and involve in planning **to meet identified needs.**
- Review ways to maximize sleep environment (e.g., prefered bedtime rituals, comfortable room temperature, bedding and pillows, elimination or reduction of extraneous noise or stimuli and interruptions.)
- Provide appropriate referrals (e.g., cognitive retraining, substance abuse treatment and support groups, medication monitoring program, Meals on Wheels, home health, and adult day care).

Information that appears in brackets has been added by the authors to clarify and enhance the use of nursing diagnoses.

    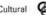 Cultural   Collaborative   Community/Home Care

Documentation Focus

Assessment/Reassessment
- Nature, duration, frequency of problem.
- Current and previous level of function, effect on independence and lifestyle (including safety concerns).

Planning
- Plan of care and who is involved in planning.
- Teaching plan.

Implementation/Evaluation
- Response to interventions and actions performed.
- Attainment or progress toward desired outcomes.
- Modifications to plan of care.

Discharge Planning
- Long-term needs and who is responsible for actions to be taken.
- Available resources and specific referrals.

Sample Nursing Outcomes & Interventions Classifications (NOC/NIC) NIC

NOC—Cognition
NIC—Delirium Management

---

chronic Confusion

Taxonomy II: Perception/Cognition—Class 4 Cognition (00129)
[Diagnostic Division: Neurosensory]
Submitted 1994

Definition: Irreversible, long-standing, and/or progressive deterioration of intellect and personality characterized by decreased ability to interpret environmental stimuli; decreased capacity for intellectual thought processes, manifested by disturbances of memory, orientation, and behavior

Related Factors

Alzheimer's disease [dementia of the Alzheimer's type]
Korsakoff's psychosis

Information that appears in brackets has been added by the authors to clarify and enhance the use of nursing diagnoses.

Multi-infarct dementia
Cerebral vascular attack
Head injury

Defining Characteristics

Objective
Clinical evidence of organic impairment
Altered interpretation
Altered response to stimuli
Progressive, long-standing cognitive impairment
No change in level of consciousness
Impaired socialization
Impaired short-term/long-term memory
Altered personality

Desired Outcome/Evaluation Criteria—Client Will:

• Remain safe and free from harm.

Family/SO Will:

• Verbalize understanding of disease process, prognosis, and client's needs.
• Identify and participate in interventions to deal effectively with situation.
• Provide for maximal independence while meeting safety needs of client.

Actions/Interventions

Nursing Priority No. 1.
To assess degree of impairment:

• Evaluate responses on diagnostic examinations (e.g., memory impairments, reality orientation, attention span, calculations). **A combination of tests (e.g., Confusion Assessment Method [CAM], Mini-Mental State Examination [MMSE], Alzheimer's Disease Assessment Scale [ADAS-cog], Brief Dementia Severity Rating Scale [BDSRS], Neuropsychiatric Inventory [NPI]) is often needed to complete an evaluation of the client's overall condition relating to a chronic/irreversible condition.**

Information that appears in brackets has been added by the authors to clarify and enhance the use of nursing diagnoses.

🌐 Cultural 🔵 Collaborative 🏠 Community/Home Care

- Test ability to receive and send effective communication. **Client may be nonverbal or require assistance with/ interpretation of verbalizations.**
- Talk with SO(s) regarding baseline behaviors, length of time since onset, and progression of problem, their perception of prognosis, and other pertinent information and concerns for client. **If the history reveals an insidious decline over months to years, and if abnormal perceptions, inattention, and memory problems are concurrent with confusion, a diagnosis of dementia is likely.**
- Ascertain interventions previously used or tried.
- Evaluate response to care providers and receptiveness to interventions **to determine areas of concern to be addressed.**
- Determine anxiety level in relation to situation and problem behaviors **that may be indicative of potential for violence.**

Nursing Priority No. 2.
To limit effects of deterioration/maximize level of function:

- Assist in treating conditions (e.g., infections, malnutrition, electrolyte imbalances, and adverse medication reactions) **that may contribute to/exacerbate confusion, discomfort, and agitation.**
- Provide calm environment, eliminate extraneous noise/stimuli **that may increase client's level of agitation/confusion.**
- Be open and honest in discussing client's disease, abilities, and prognosis.
- Use touch judiciously. Tell client what is being done before initiating contact **to reduce sense of surprise and negative reaction.**
- Avoid challenging illogical thinking **because defensive reactions may result.**
- Use positive statements; offer guided choices between two options. Simplify client's tasks and routines **to reduce agitation associated with multiple options or demands.**
- Be supportive when client is attempting to communicate, and be sensitive to increasing frustration, fears, and misperceived threats.
- Encourage family/SO(s) to provide ongoing orientation and input to include current news and family happenings.
- Maintain reality-oriented relationship and environment (e.g., clocks, calendars, personal items, seasonal decorations). Encourage participation in resocialization groups.
- Allow client to reminisce or exist in own reality, if not detrimental to well-being.

Information that appears in brackets has been added by the authors to clarify and enhance the use of nursing diagnoses.

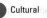

- Provide safety measures (e.g., close supervision, identification bracelet, medication lockup, lower temperature on hot water tank).
- Set limits on unsafe and/or inappropriate behavior, being alert to potential for violence.
- Avoid use of restraints as much as possible. Use vest (instead of wrist) restraints when required. **Although restraints may prevent falls, they can increase client's agitation and distress and are a safety risk.**
- Administer medications, as ordered (e.g., antidepressants, antipsychotics). Monitor for therapeutic action, as well as adverse reactions, side effects, and interactions. **Medications may be used judiciously to manage symptoms of psychosis, depression, or aggressive behavior.**
- Refer to NDs acute Confusion; impaired Memory; disturbed Thought Processes; impaired verbal Communication, for additional interventions.

Nursing Priority No. 3.
To assist SO(s) to develop coping strategies:
- Determine family resources, availability, and willingness to participate in meeting client's needs.
- Involve family/SO(s) in planning and care activities as needed/desired. Maintain frequent interactions with SO(s) **in order to relay information, change care strategies, obtain SO feedback, and offer support.**
- Discuss caregiver burden and signs of burnout, if appropriate.
- Provide educational materials, bibliographies, list of available local resources, help lines, Web sites, and so on, as desired, **to assist SO(s) in dealing and coping with long-term care issues.**
- Identify appropriate community resources (e.g., Alzheimer's Disease and Related Disorders Association [ARDA], stroke or brain injury support group, senior support groups, clergy, social services, respite care) **to provide client/SO with support and assist with problem solving.**
- Refer to ND risk for Caregiver Role Strain.

Nursing Priority No. 4.
To promote wellness (Teaching/Discharge Considerations):
- Discuss nature of client's condition (e.g., chronic stable, progressive, or degenerative), treatment concerns, and follow-up needed **to promote maintaining client at highest possible level of functioning.**

Information that appears in brackets has been added by the authors to clarify and enhance the use of nursing diagnoses.

Cultural Collaborative Community/Home Care

• Determine age-appropriate ongoing treatment and socialization needs and appropriate resources.

• Develop plan of care with family **to meet client's and SO's individual needs.**

• Provide appropriate referrals (e.g., Meals on Wheels, adult day care, home care agency, respite care).

Documentation Focus

Assessment/Reassessment
- Individual findings, including current level of function and rate of anticipated changes.
- Safety issues.

Planning
- Plan of care and who is involved in planning.

Implementation/Evaluation
- Response to interventions and actions performed.
- Attainment or progress toward desired outcomes.
- Modifications to plan of care.

Discharge Planning
- Long-term needs, referrals made and who is responsible for actions to be taken.
- Available resources, specific referrals made.

Sample Nursing Outcomes & Interventions Classifications (NOC/NIC) NIC

NOC—Cognitive Orientation
NIC—Dementia Management

---

risk for acute **Confusion**

Taxonomy II: Perception/Cognition—Class 4 Cognition (00173)
[Diagnostic Division: Neurosensory]
Submitted 2006

Definition: At risk for reversible disturbances of consciousness, attention, cognition, and perception that develop over a short period of time

---

Information that appears in brackets has been added by the authors to clarify and enhance the use of nursing diagnoses.

Risk Factors

Alcohol use; substance abuse
Infection; urinary retention
Pain
Fluctuation in sleep-wake cycle
Medication/drugs: anesthesia, anticholinergics, diphenhydramine, opioids, psychoactive drugs, multiple medications
Metabolic abnormalities: decreased hemoglobin, electrolyte imbalances, dehydration, increased BUN/Cr, azotemia, malnutrition
Decreased mobility; decreased restraints
History of stroke; impaired cognition; dementia; sensory deprivation
Over 50 years of age; male gender

> **NOTE:** A risk diagnosis is not evidenced by signs and symptoms, as the problem has not occurred; rather, nursing interventions are directed at prevention.

Desired Outcomes/Evaluation Criteria—Client Will:

- Verbalize understanding of individual cause and risk factor(s).
- Identify interventions to prevent or reduce risk of confusion.

Actions/Interventions

Nursing Priority No. 1.

To assess causative/contributing factors:

- Identify factors present such as recent trauma, fall; use of large numbers of medications or polypharmacy; substance use or abuse; history of seizures or current seizure activity; episodes of fever, pain; presence of acute infection; exposure to toxic substances; traumatic events in client's/SO's life; person with dementia experiencing sudden change in environment or unfamiliar surroundings or people. **Acute confusion is a symptom associated with numerous causes (e.g., hypoxia, abnormal metabolic conditions, ingestion of toxins or medications, electrolyte abnormalities, sepsis, nutritional deficiencies, endocrine disorders, CNS infections or other neurological pathology, acute psychiatric disorders).**
- Investigate possibility of alcohol or other drug withdrawal, exacerbation of psychiatric conditions (e.g., mood disorder, dissociative disorders, dementia).

Information that appears in brackets has been added by the authors to clarify and enhance the use of nursing diagnoses.

🌐 Cultural   🔄 Collaborative   🏠 Community/Home Care

- Determine client's functional level, including ability to provide self-care and move about at will. **Conditions and situations that limit client's mobility and independence (e.g., acute or chronic physical or psychiatric illnesses and their therapies, trauma or extensive immobility, confinement in unfamiliar surroundings, sensory deprivation) potentiate prospect of acute confusional state.**
- Ascertain life events (e.g., death of spouse/other family member, absence of known care provider, move from lifelong home, catastrophic natural disaster) **that can affect client's perceptions, attention, and concentration.**
- Assess diet and nutritional status **to identify possible deficiencies of essential nutrients and vitamins that could affect mental status.**
- Evaluate sleep and rest status, noting insomnia, sleep deprivation, or oversleeping. (Refer to NDs Insomnia; Sleep Deprivation, as appropriate.)

Nursing Priority No. 2.
To reduce/correct existing risk factors:

- Assist with treatment of underlying problem (e.g., drug intoxication/substance abuse, infectious processes, hypoxemia, biochemical imbalances, nutritional deficits, pain management).
- Monitor/adjust medication regimen and note response. **May identify medications that can be changed or eliminated in client who is prone to adverse or exaggerated responses (including confusion) to medications.**
- Administer medications, as appropriate (e.g., relieving pain in elderly client with hip fracture can improve cognitive responses).
- Orient client to surroundings, staff, necessary activities.
- Encourage family/SO(s) to participate in orientation by providing ongoing input (e.g., current news and family happenings).
- Maintain calm environment and eliminate extraneous noise or other stimuli **to prevent overstimulation.** Provide normal levels of essential sensory and tactile stimulation—include personal items, pictures, desired music, activities, contacts, and so on.
- Encourage client to use vision/hearing aids/other adaptive equipment, as needed, **to assist client in interpretation of environment and communication.**

Information that appears in brackets has been added by the authors to clarify and enhance the use of nursing diagnoses.

- Promote early ambulation activities **to enhance well-being and reduce effects of prolonged bedrest or inactivity.**
- Provide for safety needs (e.g., supervision; seizure precautions; placing needed items, such as a call bell, within reach; clearing traffic paths; ambulating with assistance; providing clear directions and instructions).

Nursing Priority No. 3.
To promote wellness (Teaching/Discharge Considerations):

- Assist with treatment of underlying medical conditions and/or management of risk factors **to reduce/limit complications.**
- Stress importance of ongoing monitoring of medication regimen **for potential adverse actions or reactions.**
- Provide undisturbed rest periods.
- Review ways to maximize sleep environment (e.g., preferred bedtime rituals, room temperature, bedding/pillows, elimination or reduction of extraneous noise/stimuli and interruptions).
- Provide appropriate referrals (e.g., medical or psychiatric specialists, medication monitoring program, nutritionist, substance abuse treatment, support groups, home health care, and adult day care).

Documentation Focus

Assessment/Reassessment
- Existing conditions, risk factors for individual.
- Current level of function, effect on independence and ability to meet own needs, including food and fluid intake, and medication use.

Planning
- Plan of care and who is involved in planning.
- Teaching plan.

Implementation/Evaluation
- Response to interventions and actions performed.
- Attainment or progress toward desired outcomes.
- Modifications to plan of care.

Discharge Planning
- Long-term needs and who is responsible for actions to be taken.
- Available resources and specific referrals.

Information that appears in brackets has been added by the authors to clarify and enhance the use of nursing diagnoses.

Cultural   Collaborative   Community/Home Care

Sample Nursing Outcomes & Interventions Classifications (NOC/NIC) NIC

NOC—Cognition
NIC—Reality Orientation

Constipation

Taxonomy II: Elimination and Exchange—Class 2
  Gastrointestinal Function (00011)
[Diagnostic Division: Elimination]
Submitted 1975; Nursing Diagnosis Extension and
  Classification (NDEC) Revision 1998

Definition: Decrease in normal frequency of defecation accompanied by difficult or incomplete passage of stool and/or passage of excessively hard, dry stool

Related Factors

Functional

Irregular defecation habits; inadequate toileting (e.g., timeliness, positioning for defecation, privacy)
Insufficient physical activity; abdominal muscle weakness
Recent environmental changes
Habitual denial or ignoring of urge to defecate

Psychological

Emotional stress; depression; mental confusion

Pharmacological

Antilipemic agents; laxative overdose; calcium carbonate; aluminum-containing antacids; NSAIDs; opiates; anticholinergics; diuretics; iron salts; phenothiazides; sedatives; sympathomimetics; bismuth salts; antidepressants; calcium channel blockers; anticonvulsants

Mechanical

Hemorrhoids; pregnancy; obesity
Rectal abscess, ulcer, or prolapse; rectal anal fissures or strictures; rectocele
Prostate enlargement; postsurgical obstruction
Neurological impairment; Hirschsprung's disease; tumors
Electrolyte imbalance

Information that appears in brackets has been added by the authors to clarify and enhance the use of nursing diagnoses.

Physiological

Poor eating habits; change in usual foods or eating patterns; insufficient fiber or fluid intake; dehydration

Inadequate dentition or oral hygiene

Decreased motility of gastrointestinal tract

Defining Characteristics

Subjective

Change in bowel pattern; unable to pass stool; decreased frequency, decreased volume of stool

Increased abdominal pressure; feeling of rectal fullness or pressure

Abdominal pain; pain with defecation; nausea; vomiting; headache; indigestion; generalized fatigue

Objective

Hard, formed stool

Straining with defecation

Hypoactive or hyperactive bowel sounds; borborygmi

Distended abdomen; abdominal tenderness with or without palpable muscle resistance; palpable abdominal or rectal mass

Percussed abdominal dullness

Presence of soft pastelike stool in rectum; oozing liquid stool; bright red blood with stool

Severe flatus; anorexia

Atypical presentations in older adults (e.g., change in mental status, urinary incontinence, unexplained falls, elevated body temperature)

Desired Outcomes/Evaluation Criteria— Client Will:

- Establish or regain normal pattern of bowel functioning.
- Verbalize understanding of etiology and appropriate interventions or solutions for individual situation.
- Demonstrate behaviors or lifestyle changes to prevent recurrence of problem.
- Participate in bowel program as indicated.

Actions/Interventions

Nursing Priority No. 1.

To identify causative/contributing factors:

- Review medical, surgical, and social history for conditions often associated with constipation (e.g., altered cognition;

Information that appears in brackets has been added by the authors to clarify and enhance the use of nursing diagnoses.

⊕ Cultural 🔗 Collaborative 🏠 Community/Home Care

metabolic, endocrine, or neurological disorders; surgery; bowel disorders [e.g., irritable bowel syndrome, intestinal obstructions or tumors]; pregnancy; advanced age; immobility).
- Review daily dietary regimen, noting if diet is deficient in fiber.
- Note general oral/dental health issues **that can impact dietary intake.**
- Determine fluid intake **to evaluate client's hydration status.**
 Evaluate client's medication/drug regimen (e.g., opioids, pain relievers, antidepressants, anticonvulsants, aluminum-containing antacids, chemotherapy, iron, contrast media, steroids) **that could cause/exacerbate constipation.**
- Note energy and activity levels and exercise pattern. **Sedentary lifestyle may affect elimination patterns.**
- Identify areas of stress (e.g., personal relationships, occupational factors, financial problems). **Individuals may fail to allow time for good bowel habits and/or suffer gastrointestinal effects from stress.**
- Determine access to bathroom, privacy, and ability to perform self-care activities.
- Investigate reports of pain with defecation. Inspect perianal area for hemorrhoids, fissures, skin breakdown, or other abnormal findings.
 Determine laxative/enema use. Note signs and reports of overuse of stimulant laxatives.
- Palpate abdomen **for presence of distention, masses.**
- Check rectum for presence of fecal impaction, as indicated.
- Assist with medical work-up (e.g., x-rays, abdominal imaging, proctosigmoidoscopy, colonic transit studies, stool sample tests) **for identification of other possible causative factors.**

Nursing Priority No. 2.
To determine usual pattern of elimination:
- Discuss usual elimination habits (e.g., normal urge time) and problems (e.g., client unable to eliminate unless in own home, passing hard stool after prolonged effort, anal pain).
- Identify elements that usually stimulate bowel activity (e.g., caffeine, walking, laxative use) and any interfering factors (e.g., taking opioid pain medications, unable to ambulate to bathroom, pelvic surgery).

Nursing Priority No. 3.
To assess current pattern of elimination:
- Note color, odor, consistency, amount, and frequency of stool. **Provides a baseline for comparison, promotes recognition of changes.**

Information that appears in brackets has been added by the authors to clarify and enhance the use of nursing diagnoses.

- Ascertain duration of current problem and client's degree of concern (e.g., long-standing condition that client has "lived with" may not cause undue concern, whereas an acute post-surgical occurrence of constipation can cause great distress). **Client's response may or may not reflect severity of condition.**
- Auscultate abdomen for presence, location, and characteristics of bowel sounds **reflecting bowel activity.**
- Note treatments client has tried to relieve current situation (e.g., laxatives, suppositories, enemas) and document failure or lack of effectiveness.

Nursing Priority No. 4.
To facilitate return to usual/acceptable pattern of elimination:

- Instruct in and encourage a diet of balanced fiber and bulk (e.g., fruits, vegetables, whole grains) and fiber supplements (e.g., wheat bran, psyllium) **to improve consistency of stool and facilitate passage through colon.** *Note:* Improvement in elimmination as a result of dietary changes takes time and is not a treatment for acute constipation.
- Promote adequate fluid intake, including high-fiber fruit juices; suggest drinking warm, stimulating fluids (e.g., coffee, hot water, tea) **to promote passage of soft stool.**
- Encourage activity and exercise within limits of individual ability **to stimulate contractions of the intestines.**
- Provide privacy and routinely scheduled time for defecation (bathroom or commode preferable to bedpan) **so client can respond to urge.**
- Encourage/support treatment of underlying medical causes where appropriate **to improve organ function, including the bowel.**
- Administer stool softeners, mild stimulants, or bulk-forming agents, as ordered or routinely, when appropriate (e.g., for client receiving opiates, decreased level of activity/immobility).
- Apply lubricant/anesthetic ointment to anus, if needed.
- Administer enemas; digitally remove impacted stool.
- Encourage sitz bath after stools **for soothing effect to rectal area.**
- Establish bowel program to include glycerin suppositories and digital stimulation, as appropriate, **when long-term or permanent bowel dysfunction is present.**
- Refer to primary care provider for medical therapies (e.g., added-emolient, saline, or hyperosmolar laxatives, enemas, or suppositories) **to best treat acute situation.**

Information that appears in brackets has been added by the authors to clarify and enhance the use of nursing diagnoses.

Cultural   Collaborative   Community/Home Care

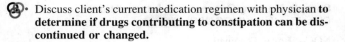

- Discuss client's current medication regimen with physician **to determine if drugs contributing to constipation can be discontinued or changed.**

Nursing Priority No. 5.
To promote wellness (Teaching/Discharge Considerations):

- Discuss client's particular physiology and acceptable variations in elimination.
- Provide information about relationship of diet, exercise, fluid, and appropriate use of laxatives, as indicated.
- Discuss rationale for and encourage continuation of successful interventions.
- Encourage client to maintain elimination diary, if appropriate, **to facilitate monitoring of long-term problem.**
- Identify specific actions to be taken if problem recurs **to promote timely intervention, enhancing client's independence.**

Documentation Focus

Assessment/Reassessment
- Usual and current bowel pattern, duration of the problem, and individual contributing factors, including diet and exercise/activity level.
- Characteristics of stool.
- Underlying dynamics.

Planning
- Plan of care, specific interventions, and changes in lifestyle that are necessary to correct individual situation, and who is involved in planning.
- Teaching plan.

Implementation/Evaluation
- Responses to interventions, teaching, and actions performed.
- Change in bowel pattern, character of stool.
- Attainment or progress toward desired outcomes.
- Modifications to plan of care.

Discharge Planning
- Individual long-term needs, noting who is responsible for actions to be taken.
- Recommendations for follow-up care.
- Specific referrals made.

Information that appears in brackets has been added by the authors to clarify and enhance the use of nursing diagnoses.

Sample Nursing Outcomes & Interventions Classifications (NOC/NIC) (NIC)

NOC—Bowel Elimination
NIC—Constipation/Impaction Management

perceived Constipation

Taxonomy II: Elimination and Exchange—Class 2
Gastrointestinal Function (00012)
[Diagnostic Division: Elimination]
Submitted 1988

Definition: Self-diagnosis of constipation and abuse of laxatives, enemas, and suppositories to ensure a daily bowel movement

Related Factors

Cultural or family health beliefs
Faulty appraisal [long-term expectations/habits]
Impaired thought processes

Defining Characteristics

Subjective
Expectation of a daily bowel movement
Expected passage of stool at same time every day
Overuse of laxatives, enemas, or suppositories

Desired Outcomes/Evaluation Criteria— Client Will:

- Verbalize understanding of physiology of bowel function.
- Identify acceptable interventions to promote adequate bowel function.
- Decrease reliance on laxatives or enemas.
- Establish individually appropriate pattern of elimination.

Actions/Interventions

Nursing Priority No. 1.
To identify factors affecting individual beliefs:

- Determine client's understanding of a "normal" bowel pattern and cultural expectations.

Information that appears in brackets has been added by the authors to clarify and enhance the use of nursing diagnoses.

Cultural   Collaborative   Community/Home Care

- Compare with client's current bowel functioning.
- Identify interventions used by client to correct perceived problem **to identify strengths and areas of concern to be addressed.**

Nursing Priority No. 2.
To promote wellness (Teaching/Discharge Considerations):

- Discuss physiology and acceptable variations in elimination.
- Identify detrimental effects of habitual laxative and/or enema use and discuss alternatives.
- Review relationship of diet, hydration, and exercise to bowel elimination.
- Provide support by Active-listening and discussing client's concerns/fears.
- Encourage use of stress-reduction activities and refocusing of attention while client works to establish individually appropriate pattern.
- Offer educational materials and resources for client/SO **to peruse at home to assist them in making informed decisions regarding constipation and management options.**
- Refer to ND Constipation.

Documentation Focus

Assessment/Reassessment
- Assessment findings, client's perceptions of the problem.
- Current bowel pattern, stool characteristics.

Planning
- Plan of care, specific interventions, and who is involved in the planning.
- Teaching plan.

Implementation/Evaluation
- Client's responses to interventions, teaching, and actions performed.
- Changes in bowel pattern, character of stool.
- Attainment or progress toward desired outcome(s).
- Modifications to plan of care.

Discharge Planning
- Referral for follow-up care.

Information that appears in brackets has been added by the authors to clarify and enhance the use of nursing diagnoses.

Diagnostic Studies ∞ Pediatric/Geriatric/Lifespan Medications **229**

perceived CONSTIPATION

Sample Nursing Outcomes & Interventions Classifications (NOC/NIC) `NIC`

NOC—Health Beliefs
NIC—Bowel Management

risk for **Constipation**

Taxonomy II: Elimination and Exchange—Class 2
  Gastrointestinal Function (00015)
[Diagnostic Division: Elimination]
Nursing Diagnosis Extension and Classification (NDEC)
  Submission 1998

Definition: At risk for a decrease in normal frequency of defecation accompanied by difficult or incomplete passage of stool and/or passage of excessively hard, dry stool

Risk Factors

Functional
Irregular defecation habits; inadequate toileting (e.g., timeliness, positioning for defecation, privacy)
Insufficient physical activity; abdominal muscle weakness
Recent environmental changes
Habitual denial or ignoring of urge to defecate

Psychological
Emotional stress; depression; mental confusion

Physiological
Change in usual foods or eating patterns; insufficient fiber/fluid intake, dehydration; poor eating habits
Inadequate dentition or oral hygiene
Decreased motility of gastrointestinal tract

Pharmacological
Phenothiazides; NSAIDs; sedatives; aluminum-containing antacids; laxative overuse; bismuth salts; iron salts; anticholinergics; antidepressants; anticonvulsants; antilipemic agents; calcium channel blockers; calcium carbonate; diuretics; sympathomimetics; opiates

---

Information that appears in brackets has been added by the authors to clarify and enhance the use of nursing diagnoses.

  Cultural 	Collaborative 	Community/Home Care

Mechanical
Hemorrhoids; pregnancy; obesity
Rectal abscess or ulcer; rectal anal stricture or fissures; rectal prolapse; rectocele
Prostate enlargement; postsurgical obstruction
Neurological impairment; Hirschsprung's disease; tumors
Electrolyte imbalance

> **NOTE:** A risk diagnosis is not evidenced by signs and symptoms, as the problem has not occurred; rather, nursing interventions are directed at prevention.

Desired Outcomes/Evaluation Criteria—Client Will:

- Maintain usual pattern of bowel functioning.
- Verbalize understanding of risk factors and appropriate interventions or solutions related to individual situation.
- Demonstrate behaviors or lifestyle changes to prevent developing problem.

Actions/Interventions

Nursing Priority No. 1.
To identify individual risk factors/needs:

- Review medical, surgical, and social history (e.g., altered cognition; metabolic, endocrine, or neurological disorders; certain medications; surgery; bowel disorders [e.g., irritable bowel syndrome, intestinal obstructions or tumors, hemorrhoids/rectal bleeding]; pregnancy; advanced age; weakness/debilitation; conditions associated with immobility; recent travel; stressors/changes in lifestyle; depression) **to identify conditions commonly associated with constipation.**
- Auscultate abdomen for presence, location, and characteristics of bowel sounds **reflecting bowel activity.**
- Discuss usual elimination pattern and use of laxatives.
- Ascertain client's beliefs and practices about bowel elimination, such as "must have a bowel movement every day or I need an enema."
- Evaluate current dietary and fluid intake and implications for effect on bowel function.
- Review medications (new and chronic use) **for impact on/effects of changes in bowel function.**

Information that appears in brackets has been added by the authors to clarify and enhance the use of nursing diagnoses.

Nursing Priority No. 2.

To facilitate normal bowel function:

* Instruct in/encourage balanced fiber and bulk in diet (e.g., fruits, vegetables, whole grains) and fiber supplements (e.g., wheat bran, psyllium) **to improve consistency of stool and facilitate passage through colon.**

* Promote adequate fluid intake, including water and high-fiber fruit juices; also suggest drinking warm fluids (e.g., coffee, hot water, tea) **to promote soft stool and stimulate bowel activity.**

* Encourage activity and exercise within limits of individual ability **to stimulate contractions of the intestines.**

* Provide privacy and routinely scheduled time for defecation (bathroom or commode preferable to bedpan) **so client can respond to urge.**

* Administer routine stool softeners, mild stimulants, or bulk-forming agents as needed, or routinely, as appropriate (e.g., for client taking pain medications, especially opiates, or who is inactive, immobile, or unconscious).

* Ascertain frequency, color, consistency, amount of stools. **Provides a baseline for comparison; promotes recognition of changes.**

Nursing Priority No. 3.

To promote wellness (Teaching/Discharge Considerations):

* Discuss physiology and acceptable variations in elimination. **May help reduce concerns/anxiety about situation.**

* Review individual risk factors, potential problems, and specific interventions.

* Educate client/SO about safe and risky practices for managing constipation. **Information can help client to make beneficial choices when need arises.**

* Encourage client to maintain elimination diary, if appropriate, **to help monitor bowel pattern.**

* Review appropriate use of medications. Discuss client's current medication regimen with physician **to determine if drugs contributing to constipation can be discontinued or changed.**

* Encourage/support treatment of underlying medical causes, where appropriate, **to improve organ function, including the bowel.**

* Refer to NDs Constipation; perceived Constipation.

Information that appears in brackets has been added by the authors to clarify and enhance the use of nursing diagnoses.

⊕ Cultural   ⊘ Collaborative   ♠ Community/Home Care

Documentation Focus

Assessment/Reassessment
- Current bowel pattern, characteristics of stool, medications and herbals used.
- Dietary intake.
- Exercise and activity level.

Planning
- Plan of care and who is involved in planning.
- Teaching plan.

Implementation/Evaluation
- Responses to interventions, teaching, and actions performed.
- Attainment or progress toward desired outcomes.
- Modifications to plan of care.

Discharge Planning
- Individual long-term needs, noting who is responsible for actions to be taken.
- Specific referrals made.

Sample Nursing Outcomes & Interventions Classifications (NOC/NIC) NIC

NOC—Bowel Elimination
NIC—Constipation/Impaction Management

Contamination

Taxonomy II: Safety/Protection—Class 4 Environmental Hazards (00181)
[Diagnostic Division: Safety]
Submitted 2006

Definition: Exposure to environmental contaminants in doses sufficient to cause adverse health effects

---

Related Factors

External
Chemical contamination of food or water; presence of atmospheric pollutants

---

Information that appears in brackets has been added by the authors to clarify and enhance the use of nursing diagnoses.

Inadequate municipal services (trash removal, sewage treatment facilities)

Geographical area (living in area where high levels of contaminants exist)

Playing in outdoor areas where environmental contaminants are used

Personal or household hygiene practices

Living in poverty (increases potential for multiple exposure, lack of access to healthcare, and poor diet)

Use of environmental contaminants in the home (e.g., pesticides, chemicals, environmental tobacco smoke)

Lack of breakdown of contaminants once indoors (breakdown is inhibited without sun and rain exposure)

Flooring surface (carpeted surfaces hold contaminant residue more readily than hard floor surfaces)

Flaking, peeling paint and plaster in presence of young children

Paint, lacquer, and so forth, in poorly ventilated areas or without effective protection

Inappropriate use or lack of protective clothing

Unprotected contact with heavy metals or chemicals (e.g., arsenic, chromium, lead)

Exposure to radiation (occupation in radiography, employment in or living near nuclear industries and electrical generating plants)

Exposure to disaster (natural or man-made); exposure to bioterrorism

Internal

Age (children less than age 5 years, older adults); gestational age during exposure; developmental characteristics of children

Female gender; pregnancy

Nutritional factors (e.g., obesity, vitamin and mineral deficiencies)

Preexisting disease states; smoking

Concomitant exposure; previous exposures

Defining Characteristics

Defining characteristics are dependent on the causative agent. Agents cause a variety of individual organ responses as well as systemic responses.

Subjective/Objective

Pesticides: (Major categories of pesticides: insecticides, herbicides, fungicides, antimicrobials, rodenticides; major

---

Information that appears in brackets has been added by the authors to clarify and enhance the use of nursing diagnoses.

🌐 Cultural 🔬 Collaborative 🏠 Community/Home Care

pesticides: organophosphates, carbamates, organochlorines, pyrethrum, arsenic, glycophosphates, bipyridyis, chlorophenoxy)

Dermatological, gastrointestinal, neurological, pulmonary, or renal effects of pesticide

Chemicals: (Major chemical agents: petroleum-based agents, anticholinesterases; Type I agents act on proximal tracheobronchial portion of the respiratory tract, Type II agents act on alveoli, Type III agents produce systemic effects)

Dermatological, gastrointestinal, immunological, neurological, pulmonary, or renal effects of chemical exposure

Biologicals: Dermatological, gastrointestinal, neurological, pulmonary,or renal effects of exposure to biologicals (toxins from living organisms—bacteria, viruses, fungi)

Pollution: (Major locations: air, water, soil; major agents: asbestos, radon, tobacco [smoke], heavy metal, lead, noise, exhaust)

Neurological or pulmonary effects of pollution exposure

Waste: (Categories of waste: trash, raw sewage, industrial waste)

Dermatological, gastrointestinal, hepatic,or pulmonary effects of waste exposure

Radiation: (Categories: Internal—ingestion of radioactive material [e.g., food/water contamination]; External—exposure through direct contact with radioactive material)

Immunological, genetic, neurological or oncological effects of radiation exposure

Desired Outcomes/Evaluation Criteria— Client Will:

- Be free of injury.
- Verbalize understanding of individual factors that contributed to injury and plans for correcting situation(s) where possible.
- Modify environment, as indicated, to enhance safety.

Client/Community Will:

- Identify hazards that lead to exposure or contamination.
- Correct environmental hazards, as identified.
- Demonstrate necessary actions to promote community safety.

Actions/Interventions

In reviewing this ND, it is apparent there is overlap with other diagnoses. We have chosen to present generalized interventions. Although there are commonalities to Contamination situations, we suggest that the reader refer to other primary

---

Information that appears in brackets has been added by the authors to clarify and enhance the use of nursing diagnoses.

 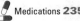

diagnoses as indicated, such as ineffective Airway Clearance, ineffective Breathing Pattern, impaired Gas Exchange, ineffective Home Maintenance, risk for Infection, risk for Injury, risk for Poisoning, impaired/risk for impaired Skin Integrity, Suffocation, ineffective tissue Perfusion [specify], Trauma.

Nursing Priority No. 1.

To evaluate degree/source of exposure:

- Ascertain: (1) type of contaminant(s) to which client has been exposed (e.g., chemical, biological, air pollutant), (2) manner of exposure (e.g., inhalation, ingestion, topical), (3) whether exposure was accidental or intentional, and (4) immediate/ delayed reactions. **Determines course of action to be taken by all emergency/other care providers. Note: Intentional exposure to hazardous materials requires notification of law enforcement for further investigation and possible prosecution.**

∞• Note age and gender: **Children less than 5 years of age are at greater risk for adverse effects from exposure to contaminants because: (1) smaller body size causes them to receive a more concentrated "dose" than adults; (2) they spend more time outside than most adults, increasing exposure to air and soil pollutants; (3) they spend more time on the floor, increasing exposure to toxins in carpets and low cupboards; (4) they consume more water and food per pound than adults, increasing their body weight to toxin ratio; and (5) fetus's/infant's and young children's developing organ systems can be disrupted. Older adults have a normal decline in function of immune, integumentary, cardiac, renal, hepatic, and pulmonary systems; an increase in adipose tissue mass; and a decline in lean body mass. Females, in general, have a greater proportion of body fat, increasing the chance of accumulating more lipid-soluble toxins than males.**

- Ascertain geographical location (e.g., home, work) where exposure occurred. **Individual and/or community intervention may be needed to correct problem.**

- Note socioeconomic status and availability and use of resources. **Living in poverty increases potential for multiple exposures, delayed/lack of access to healthcare, and poor general health, potentially increasing the severity of adverse effects of exposure.**

Information that appears in brackets has been added by the authors to clarify and enhance the use of nursing diagnoses.

⊕ Cultural   ∅ Collaborative   🏠 Community/Home Care

- Determine factors associated with particular contaminant:

  Pesticides: Determine if client has ingested contaminated foods (e.g., fruits, vegetables, commercially raised meats), or inhaled agent (e.g., aerosol bug sprays, in vicinity of crop spraying).

  Chemicals: Ascertain if client uses environmental contaminants in the home or at work (e.g., pesticides, chemicals, chlorine household cleaners), and fails to use/inappropriately uses protective clothing.

  Biologicals: Determine if client may have been exposed to biological agents (bacteria, viruses, fungi) or bacterial toxins (e.g., botulinum, ricin). **Exposure occurring as a result of an act of terrorism would be rare; however, individuals may be exposed to bacterial agents or toxins through contaminated or poorly prepared foods.**

  Pollution air/water: Determine if client has been exposed/is sensitive to atmospheric pollutants (e.g., radon, benzene [from gasoline], carbon monoxide, automobile emissions [numerous chemicals], chlorofluorocarbons [refrigerants, solvents], ozone or smog particles [acids, organic chemicals; particles in smoke; commercial plants, such as pulp and paper mills]).

  Investigate possibility of home-based exposure to air pollution—carbon monoxide (e.g., poor ventilation, especially in the winter months [poor heating systems, use of charcoal grill indoors, car left running in garage]; cigarette or cigar smoke indoors; ozone [spending a lot of time outdoors, such as playing children, adults participating in moderate to strenuous work or recreational activities]).

  Waste: Determine if client lives in area where trash or garbage accumulates, is exposed to raw sewage or industrial wastes that **can contaminate soil and water.**

  Radiation: Ascertain if client/household member experienced accidental exposure (e.g., occupation in radiography; living near, or working in, nuclear industries or electrical generation plants).

- Observe for signs and symptoms of infective agent and sepsis such as fatigue, malaise, headache, fever, chills, diaphoresis, skin rash, altered level of consciousness. **Initial symptoms of some diseases that mimic influenza may be misdiagnosed if healthcare providers do not maintain an index of suspicion.**

- Note presence and degree of chemical burns and initial treatment provided.

Information that appears in brackets has been added by the authors to clarify and enhance the use of nursing diagnoses.

 Diagnostic Studies   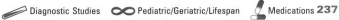 Pediatric/Geriatric/Lifespan   Medications **237**

- Obtain/assist with diagnostic studies, as indicated. **Provides information about type and degree of exposure/organ involvement or damage.**
- Identify psychological response (e.g., anger, shock, acute anxiety, confusion, denial) to accidental or mass exposure incident. **Although these are normal responses, they may recycle repeatedly and result in post-trauma syndrome if not dealt with adequately.**
- Alert proper authorities to presence of or exposure to contamination, as appropriate. **Depending on agent involved, there may be reporting requirements to local, state, or national agencies, such as the local health department and Centers for Disease Control and Prevention (CDC).**

Nursing Priority No. 2.
To assist in treating effects of exposure:

- Implement a coordinated decontamination plan (e.g., removal of clothing, showering with soap and water), when indicated, following consultation with medical toxicologist, hazardous materials team, and industrial hygiene and safety officer **to prevent further harm to client and to protect healthcare providers.**
- Insure availablity and use of personal protective equipment (PPE) (e.g., high-efficiency particulate air [HEPA] filter masks, special garments, and barrier materials including gloves/face shield) **to protect from exposure to biological, chemical, and radioactive hazards.**
- Provide for isolation or group/cohort individuals with same diagnosis or exposure, as resources require. **Limited resources may dictate open ward-like environment; however, the need to control the spread of infection still exists. Only plague, smallpox, and viral hemorrhagic fevers require more than standard infection-control precautions.**
- Provide/assist with therapeutic interventions, as individually appropriate. **Specific needs of the client and the level of care available at a given time/location determine response.**
- Refer pregnant client for individually appropriate diagnostic procedures or screenings. **Helps to determine effects of teratogenic exposure on fetus, allowing for informed choices/preparations.**
- Screen breast milk in lactating client following radiation exposure. **Depending on type and amount of exposure, breastfeeding may need to be briefly interrupted or, occasionally, terminated.**

Information that appears in brackets has been added by the authors to clarify and enhance the use of nursing diagnoses.

Cultural   Collaborative   Community/Home Care

- Cooperate with and refer to appropriate agencies (e.g., CDC; U.S. Army Medical Research Institute of Infectious Diseases [USAMRIID]; Federal Emergency Management Agency [FEMA]; U.S. Department of Health and Human Services [DHHS]; Office of Emergency Preparedness [OEP]; Environmental Protection Agency [EPA]) **to prepare for/manage mass casualty incidents.**

Nursing Priority No. 3.

To promote wellness (Teaching/Discharge Considerations):
Client/Caregiver

- Identify individual safety needs and injury/illness prevention in home, community, and work setting.
- Install carbon monoxide monitors and a radon detector in the home, as appropriate.
- Review individual nutritional needs, appropriate exercise program, and need for rest. **Essentials for well-being and recovery.**
- Repair, replace, or correct unsafe household items or situations (e.g., storage of solvents in soda bottles, flaking or peeling paint or plaster, filtering unsafe tap water).
- Emphasize importance of supervising infant/child or individuals with cognitive limitations.
- Encourage removal of or cleaning of carpeted floors, especially for small children and persons with respiratory conditions. **Carpets hold up to 100 times as much fine-particle material as a bare floor, and can contain metals and pesticides.**
- Identify commercial cleaning resources, if appropriate, **for safe cleaning of contaminated articles/surfaces.**
- Install dehumidifier in damp areas **to retard growth of molds.**
- Encourage timely replacement of air filters on furnace and/or air-conditioning unit. **Good ventilation cuts down on indoor air pollution from carpets, machines, paints, solvents, cleaning materials, and pesticides.**
- Discuss protective actions for specific "bad air" days (e.g., limiting or avoiding outdoor activities) **especially in sensitive groups (e.g., children who are active outdoors, adults involved in moderate or strenuous outdoor activities, persons with respiratory diseases).**
- Review effects of secondhand smoke and importance of refraining from smoking in home/car where others are likely to be exposed.

Information that appears in brackets has been added by the authors to clarify and enhance the use of nursing diagnoses.

🏠 • Recommend periodic inspection of well water and tap water **to identify possible contaminants.**

🏠 • Encourage client/caregiver to develop a personal/family disaster plan, to gather needed supplies to provide for self and family during a community emergency, and to learn how specific public health threats might affect client and actions **to reduce the risk to health and safety.**

🏠 • Instruct client to always refer to local authorities and health experts for specific up-to-date information for the community and to follow their advice.

🅐 • Refer to counselor/support groups **for ongoing assistance in dealing with traumatic incident/aftereffects of exposure.**

🏠 • Provide bibliotherapy including written resources and appropriate Web sites **for later review and self-paced learning.**

🅐 • Refer to smoking cessation program, as needed.

Community

🏠 • Promote community education programs in different modalities, languages, cultures, and educational levels geared to increasing awareness of safety measures and resources available to individuals/community.

🏠 • Review pertinent job-related health department and OSHA regulations.

🏠 • Refer to resources that provide information about air quality (e.g., pollen index, "bad air days").

🏠 • Encourage community members/groups to engage in problem-solving activities.

🏠 • Ascertain that there is a comprehensive disaster plan in place in the community to ensure an effective response to any emergency (e.g., flood, toxic spill, infectious disease outbreak, radiation release), including a chain of command, equipment, communication, training, decontamimation area(s), safety and security plans.

Documentation Focus

Assessment/Reassessment
• Details of specific exposure including location and circumstances.
• Client's/caregiver's understanding of individual risks and safety concerns.

Planning
• Plan of care and who is involved in planning.
• Teaching plan.

Information that appears in brackets has been added by the authors to clarify and enhance the use of nursing diagnoses.

Implementation/Evaluation

- Individual responses to interventions, teaching, and actions performed.
- Specific actions and changes that are made.
- Attainment or progress toward desired outcome(s).
- Modifications to plan of care.

Discharge Planning

- Long-range plans for discharge needs, lifestyle and community changes, and who is responsible for actions to be taken.
- Specific referrals made.

Sample Nursing Outcomes & Interventions Classifications (NOC/NIC) [NIC]

NOC—Community Disaster Readiness
NIC—Environmental Risk Protection

risk for Contamination

Taxonomy II: Safety/Protection—Class 4 Environmental Hazards (00180)
[Diagnostic Division: Safety]
Submitted 2006

Definition: Accentuated risk of exposure to environmental contaminants in doses sufficient to cause adverse health effects

Risk Factors

External

Chemical contamination of food/water; presence of atmospheric pollutants

Inadequate municipal services (trash removal, sewage treatment facilities)

Geographical area (living in area where high levels of contaminants exist)

Playing in outdoor areas where environmental contaminants are used

Personal/household hygiene practices

Living in poverty (increases potential for multiple exposure, lack of access to healthcare, and poor diet)

Use of environmental contaminants in the home (e.g., pesticides, chemicals, environmental tobacco smoke)

Information that appears in brackets has been added by the authors to clarify and enhance the use of nursing diagnoses.

Lack of breakdown of contaminants once indoors (breakdown is inhibited without sun and rain exposure)

Flooring surface (carpeted surfaces hold contaminant residue more readily than hard floor surfaces)

Flaking, peeling paint/plaster in presence of young children

Paint, lacquer, and so forth, in poorly ventilated areas or without effective protection

Inappropriate use or lack of protective clothing

Unprotected contact with heavy metals or chemicals (e.g., arsenic, chromium, lead)

Exposure to radiation (occupation in radiography, employment in/living near nuclear industries and electrical generating plants)

Exposure to disaster (natural or man-made); exposure to bioterrorism

Internal

Age (children less than age 5 years, older adults); gestational age during exposure; developmental characteristics of children

Female gender; pregnancy

Nutritional factors (e.g., obesity, vitamin and mineral deficiencies)

Preexisting disease states; smoking

Concomitant exposure; previous exposures

> **NOTE:** A risk diagnosis is not evidenced by signs and symptoms, as the problem has not occurred; rather, nursing interventions are directed at prevention.

Desired Outcomes/Evaluation Criteria— Client Will:

- Verbalize understanding of individual factors that contribute to possibility of injury and take steps to correct situation(s).
- Demonstrate behaviors or lifestyle changes to reduce risk factors and protect self from injury.
- Modify environment, as indicated, to enhance safety.
- Be free of injury.
- Support community activities for disaster preparedness.

Client/Community Will:

- Identify hazards that could lead to exposure or contamination.
- Correct environmental hazards, as identified.

Information that appears in brackets has been added by the authors to clarify and enhance the use of nursing diagnoses.

Cultural   Collaborative   Community/Home Care

- Demonstrate necessary actions to promote community safety and disaster preparedness.

Actions/Interventions

Nursing Priority No. 1.

To evaluate degree/source of risk inherent in the home/community/worksite:

- Ascertain type of contaminant(s) and exposure routes posing a potential hazard to client and/or community (e.g., air, soil, or water pollutants; food source, chemical, biological, radiation) as listed in Risk Factors. **Determines course of action to be taken by client, community, and care providers.**
- Note age and gender of client/community base (e.g., community health clinic serving primarily poor children or elderly; school near large industrial plant; family living in smog-prone area). **Young children, frail elderly, and females have been found to be at higher risk for effects of exposure to toxins.** (Refer to ND Contamination.)
- Ascertain client's geographical location at home or work (e.g., lives where crop spraying is routine; works in nuclear plant; contract worker/soldier in combat area). **Individual and/or community intervention may be needed to reduce risks of accidental/intentional exposures.**
- Note socioeconomic status, and availability and use of resources. **Living in poverty increases the potential for multiple exposures, delayed/lack of access to healthcare, and poor general health.**
- Determine client's/SO's understanding of potential risk and appropriate protective measures.

Nursing Priority No. 2.

To assist client to reduce or correct individual risk factors:

- Assist client to develop plan to address individual safety needs and injury/illness prevention in home, community, and work setting.
- Repair or replace unsafe household items and situations (e.g., flaking/peeling paint or plaster; filter for unsafe tap water).
- Review effects of secondhand smoke and importance of refraining from smoking in home/car **where others are likely to be exposed.**
- Encourage removal of/cleaning of carpeted floors, especially for small children and persons with respiratory conditions.

Information that appears in brackets has been added by the authors to clarify and enhance the use of nursing diagnoses.

Carpets hold up to 100 times as much fine-particle material as a bare floor and can contain metals and pesticides.

🏠 • Encourage timely cleaning and replacement of air filters on furnace and/or air-conditioning unit. **Good ventilation cuts down on indoor air pollution from carpets, machines, paints, solvents, cleaning materials, and pesticides.**

🏠 • Recommend periodic inspection of well water or tap water **to identify possible contaminants.**

🏠 • Encourage client to install carbon monoxide monitors and a radon detector in home, as appropriate.

🏠 • Recommend placing dehumidifier in damp areas **to retard growth of molds.**

🏠 • Review proper handling of household chemicals:

Read chemical labels. Know primary hazards (especially in commonly used household cleaning/gardening products).

Follow directions printed on product label (e.g., avoid use of certain chemicals on food preparation surfaces, refrain from spraying garden chemicals on windy days).

Choose least hazardous products for the job, preferably multiuse products **to reduce number of different chemicals used and stored.** Use products labeled "nontoxic" wherever possible.

Use form of chemical that most reduces risk of exposure (e.g., cream instead of liquid or aerosol).

Wear protective clothing, gloves, and safety glasses when using chemicals. Avoid mixing chemicals at all times, and use in well-ventilated areas.

Store chemicals in locked cabinets. Keep chemicals in original labeled containers and do not pour into other containers.

∞ Place safety stickers on chemicals **to warn children of harmful contents.**

🏠 • Review proper food handling, storage, and cooking techniques.

∞ • Stress importance of pregnant or lactating women following fish and wildlife consumption guidelines provided by state and U.S. territorial or Native American tribes. **Ingestion of noncommercial fish or wildlife can be a significant source of pollutants.**

Nursing Priority No. 3.

To promote wellness (Teaching/Discharge Considerations):
Home

🏠 • Discuss general safety concerns with client/SO.

Information that appears in brackets has been added by the authors to clarify and enhance the use of nursing diagnoses.

🌐 Cultural   ✆ Collaborative   🏠 Community/Home Care

- Stress importance of supervising infant, child or individuals with cognitive limitations.
- Stress importance of posting emergency and poison control numbers in a visible location.
- Encourage learning of CPR and first aid.
- Dissuss protective actions for specific "bad air days" (e.g., limiting or avoiding outdoor activities).
- Review pertinent job-related safety regulations. Stress necessity of wearing appropriate protective equipment.
- Encourage client/caregiver to develop a personal/family disaster plan, to gather needed supplies to provide for self and family during a community emergency, to learn how specific public health threats might affect client, and actions **to promote preparedness and reduce the risk to health and safety.**
- Provide information and refer to appropriate resources about potential toxic hazards and protective measures. Provide bibliotherapy including written resources and appropriate Web sites **for client review and self-paced learning.**
- Refer to smoking cessation program as needed.

Community

- Promote education programs **geared to increasing awareness of safety measures and resources available to individuals/community.**
- Review pertinent job-related health department and OSHA regulations **to safeguard the workplace and the community.**
- Ascertain that there is a comprehensive plan in place in the community to ensure an effective response to any emergency (e.g., flood, toxic spill, infectious disease outbreak, radiation release), including a chain of command, protective equipment, communication, training, decontamination area(s), safety and security plans).
- Refer to appropriate agencies (e.g., CDC; USAMRIID; FEMA; DHHS; OEP; EPA) **to prepare for and manage mass casualty incidents.**

Documentation Focus ──────────

Assessment/Reassessment
- Client's/caregiver's understanding of individual risks and safety concerns.

Information that appears in brackets has been added by the authors to clarify and enhance the use of nursing diagnoses.

Planning
- Plan of care and who is involved in planning.
- Teaching plan.

Implementation/Evaluation
- Individual responses to interventions, teaching, and actions performed.
- Specific actions and changes that are made.
- Attainment or progress toward desired outcome(s).
- Modifications to plan of care.

Discharge Planning
- Long-range plans, lifestyle and community changes, and who is responsible for actions to be taken.
- Specific referrals made.

Sample Nursing Outcomes & Interventions Classifications (NOC/NIC) NIC

NOC—Community Disaster Readiness
NIC—Environmental Risk Protection

compromised family Coping

Taxonomy II: Coping/Stress Tolerance—Class 2 Coping Responses (00074)
[Diagnostic Division: Social Interaction]
Submitted 1980; Revised 1996

Definition: Usually supportive primary person (family member or close friend [SO]) provides insufficient, ineffective, or compromised support, comfort, assistance, or encouragement that may be needed by the client to manage or master adaptive tasks related to his/her health challenge

Related Factors

Coexisting situations affecting the significant person
Developmental or situational crises the significant person may be facing
Prolonged disease [or disability progression] that exhausts the supportive capacity of SO(s)
Exhaustion of supportive capacity of significant people

Information that appears in brackets has been added by the authors to clarify and enhance the use of nursing diagnoses.

Inadequate or incorrect understanding of information by a primary person

Lack of reciprocal support; little support provided by client, in turn, for primary person; [unrealistic expectations of client/SO(s) or each other]

Temporary preoccupation by a significant person

Temporary family disorganization/role changes

Lack of mutual decision-making skills

Diverse coalitions of family members

Defining Characteristics

Subjective

Client expresses a complaint or concern about SO's response to health problem; SO expresses an inadequate knowledge base or understanding, which interferes with effective supportive behaviors

SO describes preoccupation with personal reaction (e.g., fear, anticipatory grief, guilt, anxiety) to client's need

Objective

SO attempts assistive or supportive behaviors with unsatisfactory results

SO displays protective behavior disproportionate to the client's abilities, or need for autonomy

SO enters into limited personal communication with client

SO withdraws from client

SO displays sudden outbursts of emotions or emotional lability, or interferes with necessary nursing or medical interventions

Desired Outcomes/Evaluation Criteria— Family Will:

• Identify and verbalize resources within themselves to deal with the situation.
• Interact appropriately with the client, providing support and assistance as indicated.
• Provide opportunity for client to deal with situation in own way.
• Verbalize knowledge and understanding of illness, disability, or disease.
• Express feelings honestly.
• Identify need for outside support and seek such.

Information that appears in brackets has been added by the authors to clarify and enhance the use of nursing diagnoses.

Actions/Interventions

Nursing Priority No. 1.

To assess causative/contributing factors:

- Identify underlying situation(s) that may contribute to the inability of family to provide needed assistance to the client. **Circumstances may have preceded the illness and now have a significant effect (e.g., client had a heart attack during sexual activity; mate is afraid any activity may cause repeat).**
- Note cultural factors related to family relationships that may be involved in problems of caring for member who is ill.
- Note the length of illness, such as cancer, MS, and/or other long-term situations that may exist.
- Assess information available to and understood by the family/SO(s).
- Discuss family perceptions of situation. **Expectations of client and family members may differ and/or be realistic.**
- Identify role of the client in family and how illness has changed the family organization.
- Note other factors besides the client's illness that are affecting abilities of family members **to provide needed support.**

Nursing Priority No. 2.

To assist family to reactivate/develop skills to deal with current situation:

- Listen to client's/SO's comments, remarks, and expression of concern(s). Note nonverbal behaviors and/or responses and congruency.
- Encourage family members to verbalize feelings openly and clearly.
- Discuss underlying reasons for behaviors with family **to help them understand and accept and deal with client behaviors.**
- Assist the family and client to understand "who owns the problem" and who is responsible for resolution. Avoid placing blame or guilt.
- Encourage client and family to develop problem-solving skills **to deal with the situation.**

Nursing Priority No. 3.

To promote wellness (Teaching/Discharge Considerations):

- Provide information for family/SO(s) about specific illness or condition.

Information that appears in brackets has been added by the authors to clarify and enhance the use of nursing diagnoses.

Cultural Collaborative Community/Home Care

• Involve client and family in planning care as often as possible. **Enhances commitment to plan.**

 • Promote assistance of family in providing client care, as appropriate. **Identifies ways of demonstrating support while maintaining client's independence (e.g., providing favorite foods, engaging in diversional activities).**

• Refer to appropriate resources for assistance, as indicated (e.g., counseling, psychotherapy, financial, spiritual).

• Refer to NDs Fear; Anxiety; death Anxiety; ineffective Coping; readiness for enhanced family Coping; disabled family Coping; Grieving, as appropriate.

Documentation Focus

Assessment/Reassessment
• Assessment findings, including current and past coping behaviors, emotional response to situation and stressors, support systems available.

Planning
• Plan of care, who is involved in planning, and areas of responsibility.
• Teaching plan.

Implementation/Evaluation
• Responses of family members/client to interventions, teaching, and actions performed.
• Attainment or progress toward desired outcome(s).
• Modifications to plan of care.

Discharge Planning
• Long-term plan and who is responsible for actions.
• Specific referrals made.

Sample Nursing Outcomes & Interventions Classifications (NOC/NIC) NIC

NOC—Family Coping
NIC—Family Involvement Promotion

Information that appears in brackets has been added by the authors to clarify and enhance the use of nursing diagnoses.

defensive Coping

Taxonomy II: Coping/Stress Tolerance—Class 2 Coping
Responses (00071)
[Diagnostic Division: Ego Integrity]
Submitted 1988; revised 2008

Definition: Repeated projection of falsely positive self-evaluation based on a self-protective pattern that defends against underlying perceived threats to positive self-regard

Related Factors

Conflict between self-perception and value system; uncertainty
Fear of failure, humiliation, or repercussions; low level of self-confidence
Low level of confidence in others; deficient support system
Unrealistic expectations of self
Lack of resilience

Defining Characteristics

Subjective
Denial of obvious problems or weaknesses
Projection of blame or responsibility
Hypersensitive to slight or criticism
Grandiosity
Rationalizes failures
Refuses or rejects assistance

Objective
Superior attitude toward others
Difficulty establishing or maintaining relationships [avoidance of intimacy]
Hostile laughter; ridicule of others [aggressive behavior]
Difficulty in perception of reality testing; reality distortion
Lack of participation or follow-through in treatment or therapy
Attention-seeking behavior

Desired Outcomes/Evaluation Criteria—Client Will:

- Verbalize understanding of own problems and stressors.
- Identify areas of concern or problems.

Information that appears in brackets has been added by the authors to clarify and enhance the use of nursing diagnoses.

  Cultural 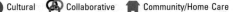 Collaborative 🏠 Community/Home Care

- Demonstrate acceptance of responsibility for own actions, successes, and failures.
- Participate in treatment program or therapy.
- Maintain involvement in relationships.

Actions/Interventions

- Refer to ND ineffective Coping for additional interventions.

Nursing Priority No. 1.
To determine degree of impairment:

- Assess ability to comprehend current situation, developmental level of functioning.
- Determine level of anxiety and effectiveness of current coping mechanisms.
- Perform or review results of testing such as Taylor Manifest Anxiety Scale (B-MAS) and Marlowe-Crowne Social Desirability Scale (LMC), as indicated, to identify coping styles.
- Determine coping mechanisms used (e.g., projection, avoidance, rationalization) and purpose of coping strategy (e.g., may mask low self-esteem) **to note how these behaviors affect current situation.**
- Observe interactions with others **to note difficulties and ability to establish satisfactory relationships.**
- Note availability of family/friends support for client in current situation. **SOs may not be supportive when person is denying problems or exhibiting unacceptable behaviors.**
- Note expressions of grandiosity in the face of contrary evidence (e.g., "I'm going to buy a new car" when the individual has no job or available finances).
- Assess physical condition. **Defensive coping style has been connected with a decline or alteration in physical well-being and illnesses, especially chronic health concerns (e.g., congestive heart failure [CHF], diabetes, chronic fatigue syndrome).**

Nursing Priority No. 2.
To assist client to deal with current situation:

- Develop therapeutic relationship to enable client **to test new behaviors in a safe environment.** Use positive, nonjudgmental approach and "I" language **to promote sense of self-esteem.**

Information that appears in brackets has been added by the authors to clarify and enhance the use of nursing diagnoses.

Diagnostic Studies ∞ Pediatric/Geriatric/Lifespan Medications **251**

- Assist client to identify and consider need to address problem differently.
- Use therapeutic communication skills such as active-listening to assist client to describe all aspects of the problem.
- Acknowledge individual strengths and incorporate awareness of personal assets and strengths in plan.
- Provide explanation of the rules of the treatment program, when indicated, and consequences of lack of cooperation.
- Set limits on manipulative behavior; be consistent in enforcing consequences when rules are broken and limits tested.
- Encourage control in all situations possible, include client in decisions and planning **to preserve autonomy.**
- Convey attitude of acceptance and respect (unconditional positive regard) **to avoid threatening client's self-concept, preserve existing self-esteem.**
- Encourage identification and expression of feelings.
- Provide healthy outlets for release of hostile feelings (e.g., punching bags, pounding boards). Involve client in outdoor recreation program or activities.
- Provide opportunities for client to interact with others in a positive manner, **promoting self-esteem.**
- Identify and discuss responses to situation, maladaptive coping skills. Suggest alternative responses to situation **to help client select more adaptive strategies for coping.**
- Use confrontation judiciously **to help client begin to identify defense mechanisms (e.g., denial/projection) that are hindering development of satisfying relationships.**
- Assist with treatments for physical illnesses, as appropriate.

Nursing Priority No. 3.
To promote wellness (Teaching/Discharge Considerations):

- Use cognitive-behavioral therapy. **Helps change negative thinking patterns when rigidly held beliefs are used by client to defend against low self-esteem.**
- Encourage client to learn relaxation techniques, use of guided imagery, and positive affirmation of self **in order to incorporate and practice new behaviors.**
- Promote involvement in activities or classes where client can practice new skills and develop new relationships.
- Refer to additional resources (e.g., substance rehabilitation, family/marital therapy), as indicated.

Information that appears in brackets has been added by the authors to clarify and enhance the use of nursing diagnoses.

    Cultural   Collaborative   Community/Home Care

Documentation Focus

Assessment/Reassessment
- Assessment findings, presenting behaviors.
- Client perception of the present situation and usual coping methods, degree of impairment.
- Health concerns.

Planning
- Plan of care and interventions and who is involved in development of the plan.
- Teaching plan.

Implementation/Evaluation
- Response to interventions, teaching, and actions performed.
- Attainment or progress toward desired outcome(s).
- Modifications to plan of care.

Discharge Planning
- Referrals and follow-up program.

Sample Nursing Outcomes & Interventions Classifications (NOC/NIC) NIC

NOC—Self-Esteem
NIC—Self-Awareness Enhancement

---

disabled family Coping

Taxonomy II: Coping/Stress Tolerance—Class 2 Coping Responses (00073)
[Diagnostic Division: Social Interaction]
Submitted 1980; Revised 1996, 2008

Definition: Behavior of significant person (family member or other primary person) that disables his or her capacities and the client's capacities to effectively address tasks essential to either person's adaptation to the health challenge

---

Related Factors

Significant person with chronically unexpressed feelings (e.g., guilt, anxiety, hostility, despair)

Information that appears in brackets has been added by the authors to clarify and enhance the use of nursing diagnoses.

disabled family COPING

Dissonant coping styles for dealing with adaptive tasks by the significant person and client/among significant people

Highly ambivalent family relationships

Arbitrary handling of family's resistance to treatment [that tends to solidify defensiveness as it fails to deal adequately with underlying anxiety]

High-risk family situations, such as single or adolescent parent, abusive relationship, substance abuse, acute or chronic disabilities, member with terminal illness

Defining Characteristics

Subjective
Expresses despair regarding family reactions or lack of involvement

Objective
Psychosomaticism

Intolerance; rejection; abandonment; desertion; agitation; aggression; hostility; depression

Carrying on usual routines without regard for client's needs; disregarding client's needs

Neglectful care of the client in regard to basic human needs or illness treatment

Neglectful relationships with other family members

Family behaviors that are detrimental to well-being

Distortion of reality regarding the client's health problem

Impaired restructuring of a meaningful life for self; impaired individualization; prolonged overconcern for client

Taking on illness signs of client

Client's development of dependence

Desired Outcomes/Evaluation Criteria— Family Will:

• Verbalize more realistic understanding and expectations of the client.
• Visit or contact client regularly.
• Participate positively in care of client, within limits of family's abilities and client's needs.
• Express feelings and expectations openly and honestly, as appropriate.

Information that appears in brackets has been added by the authors to clarify and enhance the use of nursing diagnoses.

Cultural   Collaborative   Community/Home Care

Actions/Interventions

Nursing Priority No. 1.
To assess causative/contributing factors:

- Ascertain pre-illness behaviors and interactions of the family. **Provides comparative baseline.**
- Identify current behaviors of the family members (e.g., withdrawal—not visiting, brief visits, and/or ignoring client when visiting; anger and hostility toward client and others; ways of touching between family members, expressions of guilt).
- Discuss family perceptions of situation. **Expectations of client and family members may/may not be realistic.**
- Note cultural factors related to family relationships that may be involved in problems of caring for member who is ill.
- Note other factors that may be stressful for the family (e.g., financial difficulties or lack of community support, as when illness occurs when out of town). **Provides opportunity for appropriate referrals.**
- Determine readiness of family members to be involved with care of the client.

Nursing Priority No. 2.
To provide assistance to enable family to deal with the current situation:

- Establish rapport with family members who are available. **Promotes therapeutic relationship and support for problem-solving solutions.**
- Acknowledge difficulty of the situation for the family. **Reduces blaming/feelings of guilt.**
- Active-listen to concerns; note both overconcern and lack of concern, which may interfere with ability to resolve situation.
- Allow free expression of feelings, including frustration, anger, hostility, and hopelessness. Place limits on acting-out/inappropriate behaviors **to minimize risk of violent behavior.**
- Give accurate information to SO(s) from the beginning.
- Act as liaison between family and healthcare providers **to provide explanations and clarification of treatment plan.**
- Provide brief, simple explanations about use and alarms when equipment (such as a ventilator) is involved. Identify appropriate professional(s) **for continued support/problem solving.**
- Provide time for private interaction between client/family.
- Include SO(s) in the plan of care; provide instruction **to assist them to learn necessary skills to help client.**

Information that appears in brackets has been added by the authors to clarify and enhance the use of nursing diagnoses.

- Accompany family when they visit, **to be available for questions, concerns, and support.**
- Assist SO(s) to initiate therapeutic communication with client.
- Refer client to protective services as necessitated by risk of physical harm. **Removing client from home enhances individual safety and may reduce stress on family to allow opportunity for therapeutic intervention.**

Nursing Priority No. 3.

To promote wellness (Teaching/Discharge Considerations):

- Assist family to identify coping skills being used and how these skills are/are not helping them deal with current situation.
- Answer family's questions patiently and honestly. Reinforce information provided by other healthcare providers.
- Reframe negative expressions into positive, whenever possible. **A positive frame contributes to supportive interactions and can lead to better outcomes.**
- Respect family needs for withdrawal and intervene judiciously. **Situation may be overwhelming and time away can be beneficial to continued participation.**
- Encourage family to deal with the situation in small increments rather than the whole picture at one time.
- Assist the family to identify familiar items that would be helpful to the client (e.g., a family picture on the wall), especially when hospitalized for long period of time, **to reinforce/ maintain orientation.**
- Refer family to appropriate resources, as needed (e.g., family therapy, financial counseling, spiritual advisor).
- Refer to ND Grieving, as appropriate.

Documentation Focus

Assessment/Reassessment

- Assessment findings, current and past behaviors, including family members who are directly involved and support systems available.
- Emotional response(s) to situation or stressors.
- Specific health or therapy challenges.

Planning

- Plan of care, specific interventions, and who is involved in planning.
- Teaching plan.

Information that appears in brackets has been added by the authors to clarify and enhance the use of nursing diagnoses.

⊕ Cultural ⓐ Collaborative 🏠 Community/Home Care

Implementation/Evaluation

- Responses of individuals to interventions, teaching, and actions performed.
- Attainment or progress toward desired outcome(s).
- Modifications to plan of care.

Discharge Planning

- Ongoing needs, resources, other follow-up recommendations, and who is responsible for actions.
- Specific referrals made.

Sample Nursing Outcomes & Interventions Classifications (NOC/NIC) NIC

NOC—Family Normalization
NIC—Family Therapy

---

ineffective Coping

Taxonomy II: Coping/Stress Tolerance—Class 2 Coping Responses (00069)
[Diagnostic Division: Ego Integrity]
Submitted 1978; Nursing Diagnosis Extension and Classification (NDEC) Revision 1998

Definition: Inability to form a valid appraisal of the stressors, inadequate choices of practiced responses, and/or inability to use available resources

---

Related Factors

Situational or maturational crises

High degree of threat

Inadequate opportunity to prepare for stressor; disturbance in pattern of appraisal of threat

Inadequate level of confidence in ability to cope; inadequate level of perception of control; uncertainty

Inadequate resources available; inadequate social support created by characteristics of relationships

Disturbance in pattern of tension release

Inability to conserve adaptive energies

Gender differences in coping strategies

Work overload, too many deadlines

Information that appears in brackets has been added by the authors to clarify and enhance the use of nursing diagnoses.

Impairment of nervous system; cognitive/sensory/perceptual impairment, memory loss

Severe, chronic pain

Defining Characteristics

Subjective
Verbalization of inability to cope or ask for help
Sleep disturbance; fatigue
Abuse of chemical agents
Reports of muscular or emotional tension; lack of appetite

Objective
Lack of goal-directed behavior or resolution of problem, including inability to attend to and difficulty with organizing information [lack of assertive behavior]

Use of forms of coping that impede adaptive behavior [including inappropriate use of defense mechanisms, verbal manipulation]

Inadequate problem solving

Inability to meet role expectations/basic needs [including skipping meals, little or no exercise, no time for self, no vacations]

Decreased use of social support

Poor concentration

Change in usual communication patterns

High illness rate [including high blood pressure, ulcers, irritable bowel, frequent headaches/neckaches]

Risk taking

Destructive behavior toward self [including overeating, excessive smoking/drinking, overuse of prescribed/OTC medications, illicit drug use]

Behavioral changes (e.g., impatience, frustration, irritability, discouragement)

Desired Outcomes/Evaluation Criteria—Client Will:

- Assess the current situation accurately.
- Identify ineffective coping behaviors and consequences.
- Verbalize awareness of own coping abilities.
- Verbalize feelings congruent with behavior.
- Meet psychological needs as evidenced by appropriate expression of feelings, identification of options, and use of resources.

Information that appears in brackets has been added by the authors to clarify and enhance the use of nursing diagnoses.

🌐 Cultural 🔬 Collaborative 🏠 Community/Home Care

Nursing Priority No. 1.

To determine degree of impairment:

- Determine individual stressors (e.g., family, social, work environment, life changes, or nursing or healthcare management).
- Evaluate ability to understand events, provide realistic appraisal of situation.
- Identify developmental level of functioning. **(People tend to regress to a lower developmental stage during illness or crisis.)**
- Assess current functional capacity and note how it is affecting the individual's coping ability.
- Determine alcohol intake, drug use, smoking habits, sleeping and eating patterns. **These mechanisms are often used when individual is not coping effectively with stressors.**
- Ascertain impact of illness on sexual needs and relationship.
- Assess level of anxiety and coping on an ongoing basis.
- Note speech and communication patterns. Be aware of negative/catastrophizing thinking.
- Observe and describe behavior in objective terms. Validate observations.

Nursing Priority No. 2.

To assess coping abilities and skills:

- Ascertain client's understanding of current situation and its impact on life and work.
- Active-listen and identify client's perceptions of what is happening.
- Evaluate client's decision-making ability.
- Determine previous methods of dealing with life problems **to identify successful techniques that can be used in current situation.**

Nursing Priority No. 3.

To assist client to deal with current situation:

- Call client by name. Ascertain how client prefers to be addressed. **Using client's name enhances sense of self and promotes individuality and self-esteem.**
- Encourage communication with staff/SO(s).
- Use reality orientation (e.g., clocks, calendars, bulletin boards) and make frequent references to time, place, as indicated. Place needed and familiar objects within sight for visual cues.

Information that appears in brackets has been added by the authors to clarify and enhance the use of nursing diagnoses.

- Provide for continuity of care with same personnel taking care of the client as often as possible.
- Explain disease process, procedures, and events in a simple, concise manner. Devote time for listening. **May help client to express emotions, grasp situation, and feel more in control.**
- Provide for a quiet environment and position equipment out of view as much as possible **when anxiety is increased by noisy surroundings or the sight of medical equipment.**
- Schedule activities so periods of rest alternate with nursing care. Increase activity slowly.
- Assist client in use of diversion, recreation, relaxation techniques.
- Emphasize positive body responses to medical conditions, but do not negate the seriousness of the situation (e.g., stable blood pressure during gastric bleed or improved body posture in depressed client).
- Encourage client to try new coping behaviors and gradually master situation.
- Confront client when behavior is inappropriate, pointing out difference between words and actions. **Provides external locus of control, enhancing safety.**
- Assist in dealing with change in concept of body image, as appropriate. (Refer to ND disturbed Body Image.)

Nursing Priority No. 4.
To provide for meeting psychological needs:

- Treat the client with courtesy and respect. Converse at client's level, providing meaningful conversation while performing care. **(Enhances therapeutic relationship.)**
- Help client learn how to substitute positive thoughts for negative ones (i.e., "I can do this; I am in charge of myself"). Take advantage of teachable moments.
- Allow client to react in own way without judgment by staff. Provide support and diversion, as indicated.
- Encourage verbalization of fears and anxieties and expression of feelings of denial, depression, and anger. Let the client know that these are normal reactions.
- Provide opportunity for expression of sexual concerns.
- Help client to set limits on acting-out behaviors and learn ways to express emotions in an acceptable manner. **(Promotes internal locus of control.)**

Nursing Priority No. 5.
To promote wellness (Teaching/Discharge Considerations):

Information that appears in brackets has been added by the authors to clarify and enhance the use of nursing diagnoses.

🌐 Cultural   Ⓐ Collaborative   🏠 Community/Home Care

- Give updated or additional information needed about events, cause (if known), and potential course of illness as soon as possible. **Knowledge helps reduce anxiety/fear, allows client to deal with reality.**
- Provide and encourage an atmosphere of realistic hope.
- Give information about purposes and side effects of medications/treatments.
- Stress importance of follow-up care.
- Encourage and support client in evaluating lifestyle, occupation, and leisure activities.
- Discuss ways to deal with identified stressors (e.g., family, social, work environment, or nursing or healthcare management).
- Provide for gradual implementation and continuation of necessary behavior/lifestyle changes. **Enhances commitment to plan.**
- Discuss or review anticipated procedures and client concerns, as well as postoperative expectations when surgery is recommended.
- Refer to outside resources and/or professional therapy, as indicated or ordered.
- Determine need/desire for religious representative/spiritual counselor and arrange for visit.
- Provide information, refer for consultation, as indicated, for sexual concerns. Provide privacy when client is not in own home.
- Refer to other NDs, as indicated (e.g., chronic Pain; Anxiety; impaired verbal Communication; risk for other-/self-directed Violence).

Documentation Focus

Assessment/Reassessment
- Baseline findings, specific stressors, degree of impairment, and client's perceptions of situation.
- Coping abilities and previous ways of dealing with life problems.

Planning
- Plan of care, specific interventions, and who is involved in planning.
- Teaching plan.

Implementation/Evaluation
- Client's responses to interventions, teaching, and actions performed.

Information that appears in brackets has been added by the authors to clarify and enhance the use of nursing diagnoses.

- Medication dose, time, and client's response.
- Attainment or progress toward desired outcome(s).
- Modifications to plan of care.

Discharge Planning
- Long-term needs and actions to be taken.
- Support systems available, specific referrals made, and who is responsible for actions to be taken.

Sample Nursing Outcomes & Interventions Classifications (NOC/NIC) NIC

NOC—Coping
NIC—Coping Enhancement

---

ineffective community Coping

Taxonomy II: Coping/Stress Tolerance—Class 2 Coping Responses (00077)
[Diagnostic Division: Social Interaction]
Submitted 1994; Nursing Diagnosis Extension and Classification (NDEC) Revision 1998

Definition: Pattern of community activities for adaptation and problem solving that is unsatisfactory for meeting the demands or needs of the community

---

Related Factors

Deficits in community social support services/resources
Inadequate resources for problem solving
Ineffective or nonexistent community systems (e.g., lack of emergency medical system, transportation system, or disaster planning systems)
Natural/man-made disasters

Defining Characteristics

Subjective
Community does not meet its own expectations
Expressed vulnerability; community powerlessness
Stressors perceived as excessive

Objective
Deficits of community participation
Excessive community conflicts

Information that appears in brackets has been added by the authors to clarify and enhance the use of nursing diagnoses.

High illness rates
Increased social problems (e.g., homicides, vandalism, arson, terrorism, robbery, infanticide, abuse, divorce, unemployment, poverty, militancy, mental illness)

Desired Outcomes/Evaluation Criteria— Community Will:

• Recognize negative and positive factors affecting community's ability to meet its own demands or needs.
• Identify alternatives to inappropriate activities for adaptation/problem solving.
• Report a measurable increase in necessary/desired activities to improve community functioning.

Actions/Interventions

Nursing Priority No. 1.
To identify causative or precipitating factors:

• Evaluate community activities **as related to meeting collective needs within the community itself and between the community and the larger society.**
• Note community reports of community functioning (e.g., transportation, financial needs, emergency response), including areas of weakness or conflict.
• Identify effects of Related Factors on community activities.
• Determine availability and use of resources.
• Identify unmet demands or needs of the community.

Nursing Priority No. 2.
To assist the community to reactivate/develop skills to deal with needs:

• Determine community strengths. **Provides a base upon which to build additional effective coping strategies.**
• Identify and prioritize community goals.
• Encourage community members to join groups and engage in problem-solving activities **to strengthen efforts and broaden base of support.**
• Develop a plan jointly with community **to deal with deficits in support to meet identified goals.**

Nursing Priority No. 3.
To promote wellness as related to community health:

Information that appears in brackets has been added by the authors to clarify and enhance the use of nursing diagnoses.

- Create plans managing interactions within the community itself and between the community and the larger society **to meet collective needs.**
- Assist the community to form partnerships within the community and between the community and the larger society. **Promotes long-term development of the community to deal with current and future problems.**
- Promote community involvement in developing a comprehensive disaster plan to ensure an effective response to any emergency (e.g., flood, tornado, toxic spill, infectious disease outbreak). (Refer to ND Contamination for additional interventions.)
- Provide channels for dissemination of information to the community as a whole (e.g., print media; radio/television reports and community bulletin boards; speakers' bureau; reports to committees, councils, advisory boards), keeping material on file and accessible to the public.
- Make information available in different modalities and geared to differing educational levels and cultural and ethnic populations of the community.
- Seek out and evaluate underserved populations, including the homeless.

Documentation Focus

Assessment/Reassessment
- Assessment findings, including perception of community members regarding problems.
- Availability and use of resources.

Planning
- Plan of care and who is involved in planning.
- Teaching plan.

Implementation/Evaluation
- Response of community entities to plan, interventions, and actions performed.
- Attainment or progress toward desired outcome(s).
- Modifications to plan of care.

Discharge Planning
- Long-term plans and who is responsible for actions to be taken.

Information that appears in brackets has been added by the authors to clarify and enhance the use of nursing diagnoses.

  Cultural Collaborative Community/Home Care

Sample Nursing Outcomes & Interventions Classifications (NOC/NIC) NIC

NOC—Community Competence
NIC—Community Health Development

readiness for enhanced Coping

Taxonomy II: Coping/Stress Tolerance—Class 2 Coping Responses (00158)
[Diagnostic Division: Ego Integrity]
Submitted 2002

Definition: A pattern of cognitive and behavioral efforts to manage demands that is sufficient for well-being and can be strengthened

Related Factors

To be developed

Defining Characteristics

Subjective
Defines stressors as manageable
Seeks social support or knowledge of new strategies
Acknowledges power
Aware of possible environmental changes

Objective
Uses a broad range of problem- or emotion-oriented strategies
Uses spiritual resources

Desired Outcomes/Evaluation Criteria— Client Will:

* Assess current situation accurately.
* Identify effective coping behaviors currently being used.
* Verbalize feelings congruent with behavior.
* Meet psychological needs as evidenced by appropriate expression of feelings, identification of options, and use of resources.

Information that appears in brackets has been added by the authors to clarify and enhance the use of nursing diagnoses.

 Diagnostic Studies ∞ Pediatric/Geriatric/Lifespan 💊 Medications **265**

Actions/Interventions

Nursing Priority No. 1.

To determine needs and desire for improvement:

* Evaluate ability to understand events, provide realistic appraisal of situation. **Provides information about client's perception, cognitive ability, and whether the client is aware of the facts of the situation. This is essential for planning care.**
* Determine stressors that are currently affecting client. **Accurate identification of situation that client is dealing with provides information for planning interventions to enhance coping abilities.**
* Ascertain motivation/expectations for change.
* Identify social supports available to client. **Available support systems, such as family and friends, can provide client with ability to handle current stressful events and often "talking it out" with an empathetic listener will help client move forward to enhance coping skills.**
* Review coping strategies client is aware of and currently using. **The desire to improve one's coping ability is based on an awareness of the current status of the stressful situation.**
* Determine alcohol intake, other drug use, smoking habits, sleeping and eating patterns. **Use of these substances impairs ability to deal with anxiety and affects ability to cope with life's stressors. Identification of impaired sleeping and eating patterns provides clues to need for change.**
* Assess level of anxiety and coping on an ongoing basis. **Provides information for baseline to develop plan of care to improve coping abilities.**
* Note speech and communication patterns. **Assesses ability to understand and provides information necessary to help client make progress in desire to enhance coping abilities.**
* Evaluate client's decision-making ability. **Understanding client's ability provides a starting point for developing plan and determining what information client needs to develop more effective coping skills.**

Nursing Priority No. 2.

To assist client to develop enhanced coping skills:

* Active-listen and clarify client's perceptions of current status. **Reflecting client's statements and thoughts can provide a**

Information that appears in brackets has been added by the authors to clarify and enhance the use of nursing diagnoses.

⊕ Cultural ⊗ Collaborative 🏠 Community/Home Care

forum for understanding perceptions in relation to reality for planning care and determining accuracy of interventions needed.

- Review previous methods of dealing with life problems. **Enables client to identify successful techniques used in the past, promoting feelings of confidence in own ability.**
- Discuss desire to improve ability to manage stressors of life. **Understanding client's desire to seek new information to enhance life will help client determine what is needed to learn new skills of coping.**
- Discuss understanding of concept of knowing what can and cannot be changed. **Acceptance of reality that some things cannot be changed allows client to focus energies on dealing with things that can be changed**.
- Help client develop problem-solving skills. **Learning the process for problem solving will promote successful resolution of potentially stressful situations that arise.**

Nursing Priority No. 3.
To promote optimum wellness:

- Discuss predisposing factors related to any individual's response to stress. **Understanding that genetic influences, past experiences, and existing conditions determine whether a person's response is adaptive or maladaptive will give client a base on which to continue to learn what is needed to improve life.**
- Encourage client to create a stress management program. **An individualized program of relaxation, meditation, involvement with caring for others/pets will enhance coping skills and strengthen client's ability to manage challenging situations.**
- Recommend involvement in activities of interest, such as exercise/sports, music, art. **Individuals must decide for themselves what coping strategies are adaptive for them. Most people find enjoyment and relaxation in these kinds of activities.**
- Discuss possibility of doing volunteer work in an area of the client's choosing. **Many people report satisfaction in helping others, and client may find pleasure in such involvement.**
- Refer to classes and/or reading material, as appropriate. **May be helpful to further learning and pursuing goal of enhanced coping ability.**

Information that appears in brackets has been added by the authors to clarify and enhance the use of nursing diagnoses.

Documentation Focus

Assessment/Reassessment
- Baseline information, client's perception of need to enhance abilities.
- Coping abilities and previous ways of dealing with life problems.
- Motivation and expectations for change.

Planning
- Plan of care, specific interventions, and who is involved in planning.
- Teaching plan.

Implementation/Evaluation
- Client's responses to interventions, teaching, and actions performed.
- Attainment or progress toward desired outcome(s).
- Modifications to plan of care.

Discharge Planning
- Long-term needs and actions to be taken.
- Support systems available, specific referrals made, and who is responsible for actions to be taken.

Sample Nursing Outcomes & Interventions Classifications (NOC/NIC) NIC

NOC—Coping
NIC—Coping Enhancement

---

readiness for enhanced community Coping

Taxonomy II: Coping/Stress Tolerance—Class 2 Coping Responses (00076)
[Diagnostic Division: Social Interaction]
Submitted 1994

Definition: Pattern of community activities for adaptation and problem solving that is satisfactory for meeting the demands or needs of the community but can be improved for management of current and future problems/stressors

---

Information that appears in brackets has been added by the authors to clarify and enhance the use of nursing diagnoses.

Cultural   Collaborative   Community/Home Care

Related Factors

Social supports available
Resources available for problem solving
Community has a sense of power to manage stressors

Defining Characteristics

One or more characteristics that indicate effective coping:

Subjective
Agreement that community is responsible for stress management

Objective
Active planning by community for predicted stressors
Active problem solving by community when faced with issues
Positive communication among community members
Positive communication between community, aggregates, and
larger community
Programs available for recreation and relaxation
Resources sufficient for managing stressors

Desired Outcomes/Evaluation Criteria—
Community Will:

- Identify positive and negative factors affecting management
  of current and future problems and stressors.
- Have an established plan in place to deal with identified problems and stressors.
- Describe management of challenges in characteristics that indicate effective coping.
- Report a measurable increase in ability to deal with problems
  and stressors.

Actions/Interventions

Nursing Priority No. 1.
To determine existence of and deficits or weaknesses in management of current and future problems/stressors:

- Review community plan for dealing with problems and stressors.
- Assess effects of Related Factors on management of problems/stressors.
- Determine community's strengths and weaknesses.

Information that appears in brackets has been added by the authors to clarify
and enhance the use of nursing diagnoses.

- Identify limitations in current pattern of community activities (such as transportation, water needs, roads) **that can be improved through adaptation and problem solving.**
- Evaluate community activities as related to management of problems and stressors within the community itself and between the community and the larger society.

Nursing Priority No. 2.

To assist the community in adaptation and problem solving for management of current and future needs/stressors:

- Define and discuss current needs and anticipated or projected concerns. **Agreement on scope/parameters of needs is essential for effective planning.**
- Prioritize goals **to facilitate accomplishment.**
- Identify available resources (e.g., persons, groups, financial, governmental, as well as other communities).
- Make a joint plan with the community to deal with adaptation and problem solving **for management of problems and stressors.**
- Seek out and involve underserved and at-risk groups within the community. **Supports communication and commitment of community as a whole.**

Nursing Priority No. 3.

To promote well-being of community:

- Assist the community to form partnerships within the community and between the community and the larger society **to promote long-term developmental growth of the community.**
- Support development of plans for maintaining these interactions.
- Establish mechanism for self-monitoring of community needs and evaluation of efforts. **Facilitates proactive rather than reactive responses by the community.**
- Use multiple formats, such as TV, radio, print media, billboards and computer bulletin boards, speakers' bureau, reports to community leaders/groups on file and accessible to the public, **to keep community informed regarding plans, needs, outcomes.**

Documentation Focus

Assessment/Reassessment

- Assessment findings and community's perception of situation.
- Identified areas of concern, community strengths and challenges.

Information that appears in brackets has been added by the authors to clarify and enhance the use of nursing diagnoses.

🌐 Cultural   🤝 Collaborative   🏠 Community/Home Care

Planning
- Plan of care and who is involved and responsible for each action.
- Teaching plan.

Implementation/Evaluation
- Response of community entities to the actions performed.
- Attainment or progress toward desired outcomes.
- Modifications to plan of care.

Discharge Planning
- Short- and long-term plans to deal with current, anticipated, and potential needs and who is responsible for follow-through.
- Specific referrals made, coalitions formed.

Sample Nursing Outcomes & Interventions Classifications (NOC/NIC) NIC

NOC—Community Competence
NIC—Program Development

---

readiness for enhanced family Coping

Taxonomy II: Coping/Stress Tolerance—Class 2 Coping Responses (00075)
[Diagnostic Division: Social Interaction]
Submitted 1980

Definition: Effective managing of adaptive tasks by family member involved with the client's health challenge, who now exhibits desire and readiness for enhanced health and growth in regard to self and in relation to the client

---

Related Factors

Needs sufficiently gratified to enable goals of self-actualization to surface
Adaptive tasks effectively addressed to enable goals of self-actualization to surface
Developmental stage, situational crises/supports

Information that appears in brackets has been added by the authors to clarify and enhance the use of nursing diagnoses.

Defining Characteristics

Subjective

Family member attempts to describe growth impact of crisis [on his or her own values, priorities, goals, or relationships]

Individual expresses interest in making contact with others who have experienced a similar situation

Objective

Family member moves in direction of health-promotion or en-riching lifestyle

Chooses experiences that optimize wellness

Desired Outcomes/Evaluation Criteria—Family Member Will:

- Express willingness to look at own role in the family's growth.
- Verbalize desire to undertake tasks leading to change.
- Report feelings of self-confidence and satisfaction with pro-gress being made.

Actions/Interventions

Nursing Priority No. 1.

To assess situation and adaptive skills being used by the family members:

- Determine individual situation and stage of growth family is experiencing or demonstrating. **Changes that are occurring may help family adapt, grow, and thrive when faced with these transitional events.**
- Ascertain motivation and expectations for change.
- Note expressions such as "Life has more meaning for me since this has occurred," **to identify changes in values.**
- Observe communication patterns of family. Listen to family's expressions of hope and planning and their effects on rela-tionships and life.
- Identify cultural/religious health beliefs and expectations. **For example, Navajo parents may define family as nuclear, extended, or a clan and it is important to identify who are the primary child-rearing persons.**

Nursing Priority No. 2.

To assist family member to develop/strengthen potential for growth:

Information that appears in brackets has been added by the authors to clarify and enhance the use of nursing diagnoses.

🌐 Cultural 🔄 Collaborative 🏠 Community/Home Care

- Provide time to talk with family **to discuss their view of the situation.**
- Establish a relationship with family/client **to foster trust and growth.**
- Provide a role model with which the family member may identify.
- Discuss importance of open communication and of not having secrets.
- Demonstrate techniques, such as Active-listening, I-messages, and problem solving, **to facilitate effective communication.**
- Establish social goals of achieving and maintaining harmony with oneself, family, and community.

Nursing Priority No. 3.
To promote wellness (Teaching/Discharge Considerations):

- Assist family member to support the client in meeting own needs within ability and/or constraints of the illness or situation.
- Provide experiences for the family **to help them learn ways of assisting or supporting client.**
- Identify other individuals or groups with similar conditions (e.g., Reach for Recovery, CanSurmount, Al-Anon, MS Society) and assist client/family member to make contact. **Provides ongoing support for sharing common experiences, problem solving, and learning new behaviors.**
- Assist family member to learn new, effective ways of dealing with feelings and reactions.
- Encourage family member to pursue personal interests, hobbies, and leisure activities **to promote individual well-being and strengthen coping abilities.**

Documentation Focus

Assessment/Reassessment
- Adaptive skills being used, stage of growth.
- Family communication patterns.
- Motivation and expectations for change.

Planning
- Plan of care, specific interventions, and who is involved in planning.
- Teaching plan.

Information that appears in brackets has been added by the authors to clarify and enhance the use of nursing diagnoses.

Implementation/Evaluation
- Client's/family's responses to interventions, teaching, and actions performed.
- Attainment or progress toward desired outcome(s).
- Modifications to plan of care.

Discharge Planning
- Identified needs/referrals for follow-up care, support systems.
- Specific referrals made.

Sample Nursing Outcomes & Interventions Classifications (NOC/NIC) NIC

NOC—Family Participation in Professional Care
NIC—Normalization Promotion

risk for sudden infant Death Syndrome

Taxonomy II: Safety/Protection—Class 2 Physical Injury (00156)
[Diagnostic Division: Safety]
Submitted 2002

Definition: Presence of risk factors for sudden death of an infant under 1 year of age

Sudden infant death syndrome (SIDS) is the sudden death of an infant under 1 year of age, which remains unexplained after a thorough case investigation, including performance of a complete autopsy, examination of the death scene, and review of the clinical history. SIDS is a subset of sudden unexpected death in infancy (SUDI), which is the sudden and unexpected death of an infant due to natural or unnatural causes.

Risk Factors

Modifiable
Delayed or lack of prenatal care
Infants placed to sleep in the prone or side-lying position
Soft underlayment (loose articles in the sleep environment)
Infant overheating or overwrapping
Prenatal or postnatal infant smoke exposure

Information that appears in brackets has been added by the authors to clarify and enhance the use of nursing diagnoses.

Cultural Collaborative Community/Home Care

Potentially Modifiable
Young maternal age
Low birth weight; prematurity

Nonmodifiable
Male gender
Ethnicity (e.g., African American or Native American)
Seasonality of SIDS deaths (higher in winter and fall months)
Infant age of 2 to 4 months

> **NOTE:** A risk diagnosis is not evidenced by signs and symptoms as the problem has not occurred; rather, nursing interventions are directed at prevention.

Desired Outcomes/Evaluation Criteria—Client Will:

* Verbalize understanding of modifiable factors.
* Make changes in environment to reduce risk of death occurring from other factors.
* Follow medically recommended prenatal and postnatal care.

Actions/Interventions

Nursing Priority No. 1.
To assess causative/contributing factors:

* Identify individual risk factors pertaining to situation. **Determines modifiable or potentially modifiable factors that can be addressed and treated. SIDS is the most common cause of unexplained death between 2 weeks and 1 year of age, with peak incidence occurring between the 2nd and 4th month of life.**
* Determine ethnicity, cultural background of family. **Although distribution is worldwide, African American infants are twice as likely to die of SIDS, and Native American infants are nearly three times more likely to die than other infants.**
* Note whether mother smoked during pregnancy or is currently smoking. **Smoking is known to negatively affect the fetus prenatally as well as after birth. Some reports indicate an increased risk of SIDS in babies of smoking mothers.**
* Assess extent of prenatal care and extent to which mother followed recommended care measures. **Prenatal care is important for all pregnancies to afford the optimal opportunity for all infants to have a healthy start to life.**

Information that appears in brackets has been added by the authors to clarify and enhance the use of nursing diagnoses.

• Note use of alcohol or other drugs/medications during and after pregnancy **that may have a negative impact on the developing fetus. Enables management to minimize any damaging effects.**

Nursing Priority No. 2.
To promote use of activities to minimize risk of SIDS:

• Recommend that infant be placed on his or her back to sleep, both at nighttime and naptime. **Research comfirms that fewer infants die of SIDS when they sleep on their backs and that a side-lying position is not to be used.**

• Advise all caregivers of the infant regarding the importance of maintaining correct sleep position. **Anyone who will have responsibility for the care of the child during sleep needs to be reminded of the importance of the back sleep position.**

• Encourage parents to schedule "tummy time" only while infant is awake. **This activity promotes strengthening of back and neck muscles while parents are close and baby is not sleeping.**

• Encourage early and medically recommended prenatal care and continue with well-baby checkups and immunizations after birth. Include information about signs of premature labor and actions to be taken to avoid problems if possible. **Prematurity presents many problems for the newborn, and keeping babies healthy prevents problems that could put the infant at risk for SIDS. Immunizing infants prevents many illnesses that can also be life threatening.**

• Encourage breastfeeding, if possible. Recommend sitting up in chair when nursing at night. **Breastfeeding has many advantages, immunological, nutritional, and psychosocial, promoting a healthy infant. Although this does not preclude the occurrence of SIDS, healthy babies are less prone to many illnesses/problems. The risk of the mother falling asleep while feeding infant in bed with resultant accidental suffocation has been shown to be of concern.**

• Discuss issues of bedsharing and the concerns regarding sudden and unexpected infant deaths from accidental entrapment under a sleeping adult or suffocation by becoming wedged in a couch or cushioned chair. **Bedsharing or putting infant to sleep in an unsafe situation results in dangerous sleep environments that place infants at substantial risk for SUDI or SIDS.**

• Note cultural beliefs about bedsharing. **Bedsharing is more common among breastfed infants and mothers who are**

Information that appears in brackets has been added by the authors to clarify and enhance the use of nursing diagnoses.

⊕ Cultural   ⊛ Collaborative   🏠 Community/Home Care

young, unmarried, low income, or from a minority group. **(Additional study is needed to better understand bedsharing practices and its associated risks and benefits.)**

Nursing Priority No. 3.

To promote wellness (Teaching/Discharge Considerations):

- Discuss known facts about SIDS with parents. **Corrects misconceptions and helps reduce level of anxiety.**
- Avoid overdressing or overheating infants during sleep. **Infants dressed in two or more layers of clothes as they slept had six times the risk of SIDS as those dressed in fewer layers.**
- Place the baby on a firm mattress in an approved crib. **Avoiding soft mattresses, sofas, cushions, waterbeds, and other soft surfaces, while not known to prevent SIDS, will minimize chance of suffocation/SUDI.**
- Remove fluffy and loose bedding from sleep area, making sure baby's head and face are not covered during sleep. **Minimizes possibility of suffocation.**
- Discuss the use of apnea monitors. **Apnea monitors are not recommended to prevent SIDS, but may be used to monitor other medical problems.**
- Recommend public health nurse or similar resource visit new mothers at least once or twice following discharge. **Researchers found that Native American infants whose mothers received such visits were 80% less likely to die from SIDS than those who were never visited.**
- Ascertain that day-care center/provider(s) are trained in observation and modifying risk factors (e.g., sleeping position) **to reduce risk of death while infant is in their care.**
- Refer parents to local SIDS programs/other resources for learning (e.g., National SIDS/Infant Death Resource Center and similar Web sites) and encourage consultation with healthcare provider if baby shows any signs of illness or behaviors that concern them. **Can provide information and support for risk reduction and correction of treatable problems.**

Documentation Focus

Assessment/Reassessment
- Baseline findings, degree of parental anxiety/concern.
- Individual risk factors.

Information that appears in brackets has been added by the authors to clarify and enhance the use of nursing diagnoses.

Planning
- Plan of care, interventions, and who is involved in planning.
- Teaching plan.

Implementation/Evaluation
- Parent's responses to interventions, teaching, and actions performed.
- Attainment or progress toward desired outcome(s).
- Modifications to plan of care.

Discharge Planning
- Long-term needs and actions to be taken.
- Support systems available, specific referrals made, and who is responsible for actions to be taken.

Sample Nursing Outcomes & Interventions Classifications (NOC/NIC) NIC

NOC—Risk Detection
NIC—Risk Identification

---

readiness for enhanced Decision Making

Taxonomy II: Life Principles—Class 3 Value/Belief/Action Congruence (00184)
[Diagnostic Division: Ego Integrity]
Submitted 2006

Definition: A pattern of choosing courses of action that is sufficient for meeting short- and long-term health-related goals and can be strengthened

---

Related Factors

To be developed

Defining Characteristics

Subjective
Expresses desire to enhance decision making, congruency of decisions with personal/sociocultural values and goals, use of reliable evidence for decisions, risk-benefit analysis of decisions, understanding of choices for decision making, understanding of the meaning of choices

---

Information that appears in brackets has been added by the authors to clarify and enhance the use of nursing diagnoses.

Desired Outcomes/Evaluation Criteria— Client Will:

- Explain possible choices for decision making.
- Identify risks and benefit of decisions.
- Express beliefs about the meaning of choices.
- Make decisions that are congruent with personal and socio-cultural values or goals.
- Use reliable evidence in making decisions.

Actions/Interventions

Nursing Priority No. 1.
To assess causative/contributing factors:

- Determine usual ability to manage own affairs. **Provides baseline for understanding client's decision-making process and measures growth.**
- Note expressions of decision, dependability, and availability of support persons.
- Active-listen and identify reason(s) client would like to improve decision-making abilities and expectations of change. **As client articulates/clarifies reasons for improvement, direction is provided for change.**
- Note presence of physical signs of excitement. **Enhances energy for quest for improvement and personal growth.**
- Discuss meaning of life and reasons for living, belief in God or higher power, and how these relate to current desire for improvement.

Nursing Priority No. 2.
To assist client to improve/effectively use problem-solving skills:

- Promote safe and hopeful environment. **Provides opportunity for client to discuss concerns/thoughts freely.**
- Provide opportunities for client to recognize own inner control in decision-making process. **Individuals with an internal locus of control believe they have some degree of control in outcomes and that their own actions/choices help determine what happens in their lives.**
- Encourage verbalization of ideas, concerns, particular decisions that need to be made.
- Clarify and prioritize individual's goals, noting possible conflicts or challenges that may be encountered.

Information that appears in brackets has been added by the authors to clarify and enhance the use of nursing diagnoses.

- Identify positive aspects of this experience, encouraging client to view it as a learning opportunity.
- Assist client in learning how to find factual information (e.g., use of the library, reliable Internet Web sites).
- Review the process of problem solving and how to do risk-benefit analysis of decisions.
- Encourage children to make age-appropriate decisions. **Learning problem solving at an early age will enhance sense of self-worth and ability to exercise coping skills.**
- Discuss and clarify spiritual beliefs, accepting client's values in a nonjudgmental manner.

Nursing Priority No. 3.
To promote optimum wellness:

- Identify opportunities for using conflict resolution skills, emphasizing each step as they are used.
- Provide positive feedback for efforts. **Enhances use of skills and learning efforts.**
- Encourage involvement of family/SO(s), as desired or appropriate, in decision-making process **to help all family members improve conflict-resolution skills**.
- Suggest participation in stress management or assertiveness classes, as appropriate.
- Refer to other resources, as necessary (e.g., clergy, psychiatric clinical nurse specialist or psychiatrist, family or marital therapist).

Documentation Focus ————————

Assessment/Reassessment
- Assessment findings, behavioral responses.
- Motivation and expectations for change.
- Individuals involved in improving conflict skills.
- Personal values and beliefs.

Planning
- Plan of care, intervention, and who is involved in the planning.
- Teaching plan.

Implementation/Evaluation
- Clients and involved individual's responses to interventions, teaching, and actions performed.
- Ability to express feelings, identify options, use resources.

Information that appears in brackets has been added by the authors to clarify and enhance the use of nursing diagnoses.

 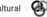

- Attainment or progress toward desired outcome(s).
- Modifications to plan of care.

Discharge Planning
- Long-term needs, noting who is responsible for actions to be taken.
- Specific referrals made.

Sample Nursing Outcomes & Interventions Classifications (NOC/NIC) NIC

NOC—Decision Making
NIC—Decision-Making Support

---

ineffective Denial

Taxonomy II: Coping/Stress Tolerance—Class 2 Coping Responses (00072)
[Diagnostic Division: Ego Integrity]
Submitted 1988; Revised 2006

Definition: Conscious or unconscious attempt to disavow the knowledge or meaning of an event to reduce anxiety/fear, but leading to the detriment of health

---

Related Factors

Anxiety; threat of inadequacy in dealing with strong emotions
Lack of control of life situation; fear of loss of autonomy
Overwhelming stress; lack of competency in using effective coping mechanisms
Threat of unpleasant reality
Fear of separation/death, loss of autonomy
Lack of emotional support from others

Defining Characteristics

Subjective
Minimizes symptoms; displaces source of symptoms to other organs
Unable to admit impact of disease on life pattern
Displaces fear of impact of the condition
Does not admit fear of death/invalidism

Information that appears in brackets has been added by the authors to clarify and enhance the use of nursing diagnoses.

Objective

Delays seeking or refuses healthcare attention to the detriment of health

Does not perceive personal relevance of symptoms

Unable to admit impact of disease on life pattern; does not perceive personal relevance of danger

Makes dismissive gestures or comments when speaking of distressing events

Displays inappropriate affect

Uses self-treatment

Desired Outcomes/Evaluation Criteria— Client Will:

- Acknowledge reality of situation or illness.
- Express realistic concern or feelings about symptoms/illness.
- Seek appropriate assistance for presenting problem.
- Display appropriate affect.

Actions/Interventions

Nursing Priority No. 1.

To assess causative/contributing factors:

- Identify situational crisis or problem and client's perception of the situation.
- Determine stage and degree of denial.
- Compare client's description of symptoms or conditions to reality of clinical picture.
- Note client's comments about impact of illness or problem on lifestyle.

Nursing Priority No. 2.

To assist client to deal appropriately with situation:

- Use therapeutic communication skills of Active-listening and I-messages **to develop trusting nurse-client relationship.**
- Provide safe, nonthreatening environment. **Encourages client to talk freely without fear of judgment.**
- Encourage expressions of feelings, accepting client's view of the situation without confrontation. Set limits on maladaptive behavior **to promote safety.**
- Present accurate information, as appropriate, without insisting that the client accept what has been presented. **Avoids confrontation, which may further entrench client in denial.**

Information that appears in brackets has been added by the authors to clarify and enhance the use of nursing diagnoses.

 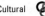

- Discuss client's behaviors in relation to illness (e.g., diabetes, hypertension, alcoholism) and point out the results of these behaviors.
- Encourage client to talk with SO(s)/friends. **May clarify concerns and reduce isolation and withdrawal.**
- Involve client in group sessions **so client can hear other views of reality and test own perceptions.**
- Avoid agreeing with inaccurate statements/perceptions **to prevent perpetuating false reality.**
- Provide positive feedback for constructive moves toward independence **to promote repetition of behavior.**

Nursing Priority No. 3.

To promote wellness (Teaching/Discharge Considerations):

- Provide written information about illness or situation **for client and family to refer to as they consider options.**
- Involve family members/SO(s) in long-range planning for meeting individual needs.
- Refer to appropriate community resources (e.g., Diabetes Association, MS Society, Alcoholics Anonymous) **to help client with long-term adjustment.**
- Refer to ND ineffective Coping.

Documentation Focus

Assessment/Reassessment

- Assessment findings, degree of personal vulnerability and denial.
- Impact of illness or problem on lifestyle.

Planning

- Plan of care and who is involved in the planning.
- Teaching plan.

Implementation/Evaluation

- Client's response to interventions, teaching, and actions performed.
- Use of resources.
- Attainment or progress toward desired outcome(s).
- Modifications to plan of care.

Discharge Planning

- Long-term needs and who is responsible for actions taken.
- Specific referrals made.

Information that appears in brackets has been added by the authors to clarify and enhance the use of nursing diagnoses.

Sample Nursing Outcomes & Interventions Classifications (NOC/NIC) ‹NIC›

NOC—Acceptance: Health Status
NIC—Anxiety Reduction

impaired **Dentition**

Taxonomy II: Safety/Protection—Class 2 Physical Injury (00048)
[Diagnostic Division: Food/Fluid]
Nursing Diagnosis Extension and Classification (NDEC) Submission 1998

Definition: Disruption in tooth development/eruption patterns or structural integrity of individual teeth

Related Factors

Dietary habits; nutritional deficits
Selected prescription medications; chronic use of tobacco, coffee, tea, red wine
Ineffective oral hygiene, sensitivity to heat/cold; chronic vomiting
Deficient knowledge regarding dental health; excessive intake of fluorides or use of abrasive cleaning agents
Barriers to self-care; lack of access or economic barriers to professional care
Genetic predisposition; bruxism
Traumatic injury; surgical intervention

Defining Characteristics

Subjective
Toothache

Objective
Halitosis
Tooth enamel discoloration; erosion of enamel; excessive plaque
Worn down and abraded teeth; crown or root caries; tooth fracture(s); loose teeth; missing teeth; absence of teeth
Premature loss of primary teeth; incomplete eruption for age (may be primary or permanent teeth)

Information that appears in brackets has been added by the authors to clarify and enhance the use of nursing diagnoses.

Excessive calculus

Malocclusion; tooth misalignment; asymmetrical facial expression

Desired Outcomes/Evaluation Criteria— Client Will:

* Display healthy gums, mucous membranes, and teeth in good repair.
* Report adequate nutritional and fluid intake.
* Verbalize and demonstrate effective dental hygiene skills.
* Follow through on referrals for appropriate dental care.

Action/Interventions

Nursing Priority No. 1.

To assess causative/contributing factors:

* Inspect oral cavity. Note presence or absence of teeth and/or dentures and ascertain significance of finding in terms of nutritional needs and aesthetics.
* Evaluate current status of dental hygiene and oral health **to determine need for instruction or coaching, assistive devices, and/or referral to dental care providers.**
* Document presence of factors affecting dentition (e.g., chronic use of tobacco, coffee, tea; bulimia/chronic vomiting; abscesses; tumors; braces; bruxism or chronic grinding of teeth) **to determine possible interventions and/or treatment needs.**
* Note current factors impacting dental health (e.g., presence of ET intubation, facial fractures, chemotherapy) **that require special mouth care.**
* Document (photo) facial injuries before treatment **to provide "pictorial baseline" for future comparison and evaluation.**

Nursing Priority No. 2.

To treat/manage dental care needs:

* Ascertain client's usual method of oral care **to provide continuity of care or to build on client's existing knowledge base and current practices in developing plan of care.**
* Assist with or provide oral care, as indicated:

  Tap water or saline rinses, diluted alcohol-free mouthwashes.
  Gentle gum massage and tongue brushing with soft toothbrush, using fluoride toothpaste to manage tartar buildup, if appropriate.

Information that appears in brackets has been added by the authors to clarify and enhance the use of nursing diagnoses.

Brushing and flossing **when client is unable to do self-care.**

Use of electric or battery-powered mouth care devices (e.g., toothbrush, plaque remover, waterpik), as indicated.

Denture care, when indicated (e.g., remove and clean after meals and at bedtime).

- Provide appropriate diet for optimal nutrition, limiting between-meal eating, sugary foods, and bedtime snacks, as **foods high in sugar or left on teeth at night are more likely to cause cavities.**
- Increase fluids, as needed, **to enhance hydration and general well-being of oral mucous membranes.**
- Reposition ET tubes and airway adjuncts routinely, carefully padding and protecting teeth or prosthetics. Suction with care, when indicated.
- Avoid thermal stimuli when teeth are sensitive. Recommend use of specific toothpastes **designed to reduce sensitivity of teeth.**
- Maintain good jaw and facial alignment when fractures are present.
- Administer antibiotics, as needed, **to treat oral/gum infections.**
- Recommend use of analgesics and topical analgesics, as needed, **when dental pain is present.**
- Administer antibiotic therapy prior to dental procedures in susceptible individuals (e.g., prosthetic heart valve clients) and/or ascertain that bleeding disorders or coagulation deficits are not present **to prevent excess bleeding.**
- Refer to appropriate care providers (e.g., dental hygienists, dentists, periodontists, oral surgeons).

Nursing Priority No. 3.

To promote wellness (Teaching/Discharge Considerations):

- Instruct client/caregiver in home-care interventions **to treat condition and/or prevent further complications.**
- Review resources that are needed for the client to perform adequate dental hygiene care (e.g., toothbrush/paste, clean water, dental floss, personal care assistant).
- Recommend that client (of any age) limit sugary and high-carbohydrate foods in diet and snacks **to reduce buildup of plaque and risk of cavities caused by acids associated with breakdown of sugar and starch.**
- Instruct older client and caregiver(s) concerning special needs and importance of regular dental care.
- Advise mother regarding age-appropriate concerns (e.g., refrain from letting baby fall asleep with milk or juice in bottle;

Information that appears in brackets has been added by the authors to clarify and enhance the use of nursing diagnoses.

⊕ Cultural   ⊗ Collaborative   ⌂ Community/Home Care

use water and pacifier during night; avoid sharing eating utensils among family members; teach children to brush teeth while young; provide child with safety devices such as helmet, face mask, or mouth guard to prevent facial injuries).

- Discuss with pregnant women special needs and regular dental care **to maintain maternal dental health and promote strong teeth and bones in fetal development.**
- Encourage cessation of tobacco, especially smokeless, and enrollment in smoking-cessation classes **to reduce incidence of gum disorders, oral cancer, and other health problems.**
- Discuss advisability of dental checkup and care prior to initiating chemotherapy or radiation treatments **to minimize oral and dental tissue damage.**
- Refer to resources to maintain dental hygiene (e.g., dental care providers, financial assistance programs).

Documentation Focus

Assessment/Reassessment
- Individual findings, including individual factors influencing dentition problems.
- Baseline photos, description of oral cavity and structures.

Planning
- Plan of care and who is involved in planning.
- Teaching plan.

Implementation/Evaluation
- Responses to interventions, teaching, and actions performed.
- Attainment or progress toward desired outcome(s).
- Modifications to plan of care.

Discharge Planning
- Individual long-term needs, noting who is responsible for actions to be taken.
- Specific referrals made.

Sample Nursing Outcomes & Interventions Classifications (NOC/NIC) NIC

NOC—Oral Hygiene
NIC—Oral Health Restoration

Information that appears in brackets has been added by the authors to clarify and enhance the use of nursing diagnoses.

risk for delayed Development

Taxonomy II: Growth/Development—Class 2 Development (00112)
[Diagnostic Division: Teaching/Learning]
Nursing Diagnosis Extension and Classification (NDEC) Submission 1998

Definition: At risk for delay of 25% or more in one or more of the areas of social or self-regulatory behavior, or cognitive, language, gross or fine motor skills

Risk Factors

Prenatal

Maternal age <15 or >35 years
Unplanned or unwanted pregnancy; lack of, late, or poor prenatal care
Inadequate nutrition; poverty
Illiteracy
Genetic or endocrine disorders; infections; substance abuse

Individual

Prematurity; congenital or genetic disorders
Vision or hearing impairment; frequent otitis media
Inadequate nutrition; failure to thrive
Chronic illness; chemotherapy; radiation therapy
Brain damage (e.g., hemorrhage in postnatal period, shaken baby, abuse, accident); seizures
Positive drug screening(s); substance abuse; lead poisoning
Foster or adopted child
Behavior disorders
Technology dependent
Natural disaster

Environmental
Poverty
Violence

Caregiver
Mental retardation; severe learning disability
Abuse
Mental illness

Information that appears in brackets has been added by the authors to clarify and enhance the use of nursing diagnoses.

Cultural   Collaborative   Community/Home Care

> **NOTE:** A risk diagnosis is not evidenced by signs and symptoms, as the problem has not occurred; rather, nursing interventions are directed at prevention.

Desired Outcomes/Evaluation Criteria— Client Will:

- Perform motor, social, self-regulatory behavior, cognitive and language skills appropriate for age within scope of present capabilities.

Caregiver Will:

- Verbalize understanding of age-appropriate development and expectations.
- Identify individual risk factors for developmental delay or deviation.
- Formulate plan(s) for prevention of developmental deviation.
- Initiate interventions and lifestyle changes promoting appropriate development.

Actions/Interventions

Nursing Priority No. 1.

To assess causative/contributing factors:

- Identify condition(s) that could contribute to developmental deviations; for example, genetic condition (e.g., Down syndrome, cerebral palsy) or complications of high-risk pregnancy (e.g., prematurity, extremes of maternal age, maternal substance abuse, brain injury or damage), chronic severe illness, infections, mental illness, poverty, shaken baby syndrome or child abuse, violence, failure to thrive, inadequate nutrition, and/or others as listed in Risk Factors.
- Collaborate in multidisciplinary evaluation to assess client's development in following areas: gross motor, fine motor, cognitive, social, emotional, adaptive, and communicative development **to determine area(s) of need/possible intervention.**
- Identify cultural beliefs, norms, and values **as they may impact parent/caregiver view of situation.**
- Ascertain nature of caregiver-required activities and abilities to perform needed activities.
- Note severity and pervasiveness of situation (e.g., potential for long-term stress leading to abuse or neglect versus situational disruption during period of crisis or transition).

Information that appears in brackets has been added by the authors to clarify and enhance the use of nursing diagnoses.

 Diagnostic Studies ∞ Pediatric/Geriatric/Lifespan Medications **289**

• Evaluate environment in which long-standing care will be provided **to determine ongoing services/other needs of child and care provider(s).**

Nursing Priority No. 2.

To assist in preventing and/or limiting developmental delays:

• Avoid blame when discussing contributing factors. **Blame engenders negative feelings and contributes nothing to solution of the situation.**

• Note chronological age and review expectations for "normal" development at this age **to help determine developmental expectations.**

• Review expected skills and activities using authoritative text (e.g., Gesell, Mussen-Congor) or assessment tools (e.g., Draw-a-Person, Denver Developmental Screening Test, Bender's Visual Motor Gestalt Test). **Provides guide for comparative measurement as child/individual progresses.**

• Consult professional resources (e.g., physical, occupational, rehabilitation, speech therapists; home health care agencies; social services; nutritionist; special-education teacher; family therapists; technological and adaptive equipment sources; vocational counselor) **to formulate plan and address specific individual needs and eligibility for intervention home- and/or community-based services.**

• Encourage setting of short-term realistic goals for achieving developmental potential. **Small incremental steps are often easier to deal with.**

• Identify equipment needs (e.g., adaptive/growth-stimulating computer programs, communication devices).

Nursing Priority No. 3.

To promote wellness (Teaching/Discharge Considerations):

• Provide information regarding normal development, as appropriate, including pertinent reference materials.

• Encourage attendance at appropriate educational programs (e.g., parenting classes, infant stimulation sessions, seminars on life stresses, aging process).

• Identify available community resources, as appropriate (e.g., early-intervention programs, seniors' activity/support groups, gifted and talented programs, sheltered workshop, crippled children's services, medical equipment/supplier). **Provides additional assistance to support family efforts in treatment program.**

Information that appears in brackets has been added by the authors to clarify and enhance the use of nursing diagnoses.

🌐 Cultural   🅐 Collaborative   🏠 Community/Home Care

Documentation Focus

Assessment/Reassessment
- Assessment findings, individual needs including developmental level and potential for improvement.
- Caregiver's understanding of situation and individual role.

Planning
- Plan of care and who is involved in the planning.
- Teaching plan.

Implementation/Evaluation
- Client's response to interventions, teaching, and actions performed.
- Caregiver response to teaching.
- Attainment or progress toward desired outcome(s).
- Modifications to plan of care.

Discharge Planning
- Identified long-range needs and who is responsible for actions to be taken.
- Specific referrals made, sources for assistive devices, educational tools.

Sample Nursing Outcomes & Interventions Classifications (NOC/NIC) NIC

NOC—Child Development: [specify age]
NIC—Developmental Enhancement: Child [or] Adolescent

Diarrhea

Taxonomy II: Elimination and Exchange—Class 2 Gastrointestinal Function (0013)
[Diagnostic Division: Elimination]
Submitted 1975; Nursing Diagnosis Extension and Classification (NDEC) Revision 1998

Definition: Passage of loose, unformed stools

Related Factors

Psychological
High stress levels; anxiety

Information that appears in brackets has been added by the authors to clarify and enhance the use of nursing diagnoses.

Diagnostic Studies   Pediatric/Geriatric/Lifespan   Medications **291**

Situational
Laxative or alcohol abuse; toxins; contaminants
Adverse effects of medications; radiation
Tube feedings
Travel

Physiological
Inflammation; irritation
Infectious processes; parasites
Malabsorption

Defining Characteristics

Subjective
Abdominal pain
Urgency, cramping

Objective
Hyperactive bowel sounds
At least three loose liquid stools per day

Desired Outcomes/Evaluation Criteria— Client Will:

- Reestablish and maintain normal pattern of bowel functioning.
- Verbalize understanding of causative factors and rationale for treatment regimen.
- Demonstrate appropriate behavior to assist with resolution of causative factors (e.g., proper food preparation or avoidance of irritating foods).

Actions/Interventions

Nursing Priority No. 1.
To assess causative factors/etiology:

- Ascertain onset and pattern of diarrhea, noting whether acute or chronic. **Acute diarrhea (caused by viral, bacterial, or parasitic infections [e.g., Norwalk, rotavirus; Salmonella, Shigella, Giardia; amebiasis, respectively]; bacterial food-borne toxins [e.g., *Staphylococcus aureus*, *Escherichia coli*]; medications [e.g., antibiotics, chemotherapy agents, cholchicine, laxatives]; and enteral tube feedings) lasts a few days up to a week. Chronic diarrhea (caused by irritable bowel syndrome, infectious diseases affecting colon [e.g., inflammatory bowel disease], colon cancer and**

Information that appears in brackets has been added by the authors to clarify and enhance the use of nursing diagnoses.

🌐 Cultural 🔬 Collaborative 🏠 Community/Home Care

treatments, severe constipation, malabsorption disorders, laxative abuse, certain endocrine disorders [e.g., hyperthyroidism, Addison's disease]) almost always lasts more than 3 weeks.

- Obtain history and observe stools for volume, frequency (e.g., more than normal number of stools per day), characteristics (e.g., slightly soft to watery stools), and precipitating factors (e.g., travel, recent antibiotic use, day care center attendance) related to occurrence of diarrhea.
- Note client's age. **Diarrhea in infant or young child and older or debilitated client can cause complications of dehydration and electrolyte imbalances.**
- Determine if incontinence is present. (Refer to ND Bowel Incontinence.)
- Note reports of abdominal or rectal pain associated with episodes.
- Auscultate abdomen **for presence, location, and characteristics of bowel sounds.**
- Observe for presence of associated factors, such as fever or chills, abdominal pain and cramping, bloody stools, emotional upset, physical exertion, and so forth.
- Evaluate diet history and note nutritional intake, fluid and electrolyte status.
- Determine recent exposure to different or foreign environments, change in drinking water or food intake, similar illness of others **that may help identify causative environmental factors.**
- Note history of recent gastrointestinal surgery; concurrent or chronic illnesses and treatment; food or drug allergies; lactose intolerance.
- Review results of laboratory testing (**e.g., parasites, cultures for bacteria, toxins, fat, blood) for acute diarrhea. Chronic diarrhea testing may include upper and lower gastrointestinal studies; stool examination for parasites; colonoscopy with biopsies, and so forth.**

Nursing Priority No. 2.
To eliminate causative factors:

- Restrict solid food intake, as indicated, **to allow for bowel rest and reduced intestinal workload.**
- Provide for changes in dietary intake **to avoid foods or substances that precipitate diarrhea.**
- Limit caffeine and high-fiber foods; avoid milk and fruits, as appropriate.

Information that appears in brackets has been added by the authors to clarify and enhance the use of nursing diagnoses.

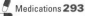

- Adjust strength or rate of enteral tube feedings; change formula, as indicated, **when diarrhea is associated with tube feedings.**
- Assess for and remove fecal impaction, especially in an elderly client **where impaction may be accompanied by diarrhea.** (Refer to NDs Constipation; Bowel Incontinence.)
- Recommend change in drug therapy, as appropriate (e.g., choice of antibiotic).
- Assist in treatment of underlying conditions (e.g., infections, malabsorption syndrome, cancer) and complications of diarrhea. **Therapies can include treatment of fever, pain, and infectious or toxic agents; rehydration; oral refeeding, and so forth.**
- Promote use of relaxation techniques (e.g., progressive relaxation exercise, visualization techniques) **to decrease stress and anxiety.**

Nursing Priority No. 3.
To maintain hydration/electrolyte balance:

- Assess for presence of postural hypotension, tachycardia, skin hydration/turgor, and condition of mucous membranes **indicating dehydration.**
- Weigh infant's diapers **to determine amount of output and fluid replacement needs.**
- Review laboratory studies for abnormalities.
- Administer antidiarrheal medications, as indicated, **to decrease gastrointestinal motility and minimize fluid losses.**
- Encourage oral intake of fluids containing electrolytes, such as juices, bouillon, or commercial preparations, as appropriate.
- Administer enteral and parenteral fluids, as indicated.

Nursing Priority No. 4.
To maintain skin integrity:

- Assist, as needed, with pericare after each bowel movement.
- Provide prompt diaper change and gentle cleansing, **because skin breakdown can occur quickly when diarrhea is present.**
- Apply lotion or ointment as skin barrier, as needed.
- Provide dry linen, as necessary.
- Expose perineum and buttocks to air; use heat lamp with caution, if needed to keep area dry.
- Refer to ND impaired Skin Integrity.

Information that appears in brackets has been added by the authors to clarify and enhance the use of nursing diagnoses.

Nursing Priority No. 5.

To promote return to normal bowel functioning:

- Increase oral fluid intake and return to normal diet, as tolerated.
- Encourage intake of nonirritating liquids.
- Discuss possible change in infant formula. **Diarrhea may be result of, or aggravated by, intolerance to specific formula.**
- Recommend products such as natural fiber, plain natural yogurt, Lactinex, **to restore normal bowel flora.**
- Administer medications, as ordered, **to treat infectious process, decrease motility, and/or absorb water.**
- Provide privacy during defecation and psychological support, as necessary.

Nursing Priority No. 6.

To promote wellness (Teaching/Discharge Considerations):

- Review causative factors and appropriate interventions **to prevent recurrence.**
- Discuss individual stress factors and coping behaviors.
- Review food preparation, emphasizing adequate cooking time and proper refrigeration or storage **to prevent bacterial growth and contamination.**
- Emphasize importance of hand hygiene **to prevent spread of infectious causes of diarrhea such as** *Clostridium difficile* (*C. difficile*) **or** *S. aureus*.
- Discuss possibility of dehydration and the importance of proper fluid replacement.
- Suggest use of incontinence pads **to protect bedding or furniture, depending on the severity of the problem.**

Documentation Focus

Assessment/Reassessment

- Assessment findings, including characteristics and pattern of elimination.
- Causative and aggravating factors.
- Methods used to treat problem.

Planning

- Plan of care and who is involved in planning.
- Teaching plan.

Implementation/Evaluation

- Client's response to treatment, teaching, and actions performed.

Information that appears in brackets has been added by the authors to clarify and enhance the use of nursing diagnoses.

- Attainment or progress toward desired outcome(s).
- Modifications to plan of care.

Discharge Planning
- Recommendations for follow-up care.

Sample Nursing Outcomes & Interventions Classifications (NOC/NIC) `NIC`

NOC—Bowel Elimination
NIC—Diarrhea Management

---

risk for compromised human Dignity

Taxonomy II: Self-Perception—Class 1 Self-Concept (00174)
[Diagnostic Division: Ego Integrity]
Submitted 2006

Definition: At risk for perceived loss of respect and honor

Risk Factors

Loss of control of body functions; exposure of the body
Perceived humiliation or invasion of privacy
Disclosure of confidential information; stigmatizing label; use of undefined medical terms
Perceived dehumanizing treatment/intrusion by clinicians
Inadequate participation in decision making
Cultural incongruity

Desired Outcomes/Evaluation Criteria— Client Will:

- Verbalize awareness of specific problem.
- Identify positive ways to deal with situation.
- Demonstrate problem-solving skills.
- Express sense of dignity in situation.

Actions/Interventions

Nursing Priority No. 1.
To evaluate source/degree of risk:
- Determine client's perceptions and specific factors that could lead to sense of loss of dignity. **Human dignity is a totality of the individual's uniqueness—mind, body, and spirit.**

Information that appears in brackets has been added by the authors to clarify and enhance the use of nursing diagnoses.

      Cultural   Collaborative   Community/Home Care

- Note labels or terms used by staff, friends/family that stigmatize the client. **Human dignity is threatened by insensitive, as well as inadequate, healthcare and lack of client participation in care decisions.**
- Ascertain cultural beliefs and values and degree of importance to client. **Some individuals cling to their basic culture, especially during times of stress, which may result in conflict with current circumstances.**
- Identify healthcare goals and expectations.
- Note availability of family/friends for support and encouragement.
- Ascertain response of family/SO(s) to client's situation.

Nursing Priority No. 2.

To assist client/caregiver to reduce or correct individual risk factors:

- Ask client by what name he or she would like to be called. **A person's name is important to his or her identity and recognizes one's individuality. Many older people prefer to be addressed in a formal manner (e.g., Mr. or Mrs.).**
- Active-listen feelings and be available for support and assistance, as desired, **so client's concerns can be addressed.**
- Provide for privacy when discussing sensitive or personal issues.
- Encourage family/SO(s) to treat client with respect and understanding, especially when the client is older and may be irritable and difficult to deal with. **Everyone should be treated with respect and dignity regardless of individual ability/frailty.**
- Use understandable terms when talking to client/family about the medical condition, procedures, and treatments. **Most laypeople do not understand medical terms and may be hesitant to ask what is meant.**
- Respect the client's needs and wishes for quiet, privacy, talking, or silence.
- Include client and family in decision making, especially regarding end-of-life issues. **Helps individuals feel respected and valued, and that they are participants in the care process.**
- Protect client's privacy when providing personal care or during procedures. Assure client is covered adequately when care is being given **to prevent unnecessary exposure/embarrassment.**
- Cleanse client immediately when vomiting, bleeding, or incontinence occurs. Speak in a gentle voice and assure client

---

Information that appears in brackets has been added by the authors to clarify and enhance the use of nursing diagnoses.

 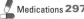

that these things cannot be helped and nurses are glad to take care of the problem.

• Involve facility/local ethics committee, as appropriate, **to facilitate mediation and resolution of issues.**

Nursing Priority No. 3.

To promote wellness (Teaching/Discharge Considerations):

• Discuss client's rights as an individual. **Hospitals and other care settings have a Patient's Bill of Rights, and a broader view of human dignity is stated in the U.S. Constitution.**
• Discuss and assist with planning for the future, taking into account client's desires and rights.
• Incorporate identified familial, religious, and cultural factors that have meaning for client.
• Refer to other resources (e.g., pastoral care, counseling, organized support groups, classes), as appropriate.

Documentation Focus

Assessment/Reassessment
• Assessment findings, including individual risk factors, client's perceptions, and concerns about involvement in care.
• Individual cultural and religious beliefs, values, healthcare goals.
• Responses and involvement of family/SO(s).

Planning
• Plan of care and who is involved in planning.
• Teaching plan.

Implementation/Evaluation
• Client's response to interventions, teaching, and actions performed.
• Attainment or progress toward desired outcome(s).
• Modifications to plan of care.

Discharge Planning
• Long-term needs and who is responsible for actions to be taken.
• Specific referrals made.

Sample Nursing Outcomes & Interventions Classifications (NOC/NIC) NIC

NOC—Client Satisfaction: Protection of Rights
NIC—Emotional Support

Information that appears in brackets has been added by the authors to clarify and enhance the use of nursing diagnoses.

Cultural   Collaborative   Community/Home Care

moral Distress

Taxonomy II: Life Principles—Class 3 Value/Belief/Action
   Congruence (00175)
[Diagnostic Division: Ego Integrity]
Submitted 2006

Definition: Response to the inability to carry out one's
chosen ethical/moral decision/action

Related Factors

Conflict among decision makers [e.g., family, healthcare providers, insurance payers]
Conflicting information guiding moral or ethical decision making; cultural conflicts
Treatment decisions; end-of-life decisions; loss of autonomy
Time constraints for decision making; physical distance of decision maker

Defining Characteristics

Objective
Expresses anguish (e.g., powerlessness, guilt, frustration, anxiety, self-doubt, fear) over difficulty of acting on one's
   moral choice

Desired Outcomes/Evaluation Criteria—
Client Will:

• Verbalize understanding of causes for conflict in own situation.
• Be aware of own moral values conflicting with desired/
   required course of action.
• Identify positive ways or actions necessary to deal with situation.
• Express sense of satisfaction with or acceptance of resolution.

Actions/Interventions

Nursing Priority No. 1.
To identify cause/situation in which moral distress is
   occurring:
• Determine client's perceptions and specific factors resulting
   in a sense of distress and all parties involved in situation.

Information that appears in brackets has been added by the authors to clarify
and enhance the use of nursing diagnoses.

Moral conflict centers around lessening the amount of harm suffered, with the involved individuals usually struggling with decisions about what "can be done" to prevent, improve, or cure a medical condition or what "ought to be done" in a specific situation, often within financial constraints or scarcity of resources.

- Note use of sarcasm, avoidance, apathy, crying, or reports of depression or loss of meaning. **Individuals may not understand their feelings of uneasiness/distress or know that the emotional basis for moral distress is anger.**

- Ascertain response of family/SO(s) to client's situation or healthcare choices.

- Identify healthcare goals and expectations. **New treatment options or technology can prolong life or postpone death based on the individual's personal viewpoint, increasing the possibility of conflict with others, including healthcare providers.**

- Ascertain cultural beliefs and values, and degree of importance to client. **Cultural diversity may lead to disparate views or expectations between clients, SO/family members, and healthcare providers. When tensions between conflicting values cannot be resolved, persons experience moral distress.**

- Note attitudes and expressions of dissatisfaction of caregivers/staff. **Client may feel pressure or disapproval if own views are not congruent with expectations of those perceived to be more knowledgeable or in "authority." Furthermore, healthcare providers may themselves feel moral distress in carrying out requested actions/interventions.**

- Determine degree of emotional and physical distress (e.g., fatigue, headaches, forgetfulness, anger, guilt, resentment) individual(s) are experiencing and impact on ability to function. **Moral distress can be very destructive, affecting one's ability to carry out daily tasks or care for self or others, and may lead to a crisis of faith.**

- Assess sleep habits of involved parties. **Evidence suggests that sleep deprivation can harm a person's physical health and emotional well-being, hindering the ability to integrate emotion and cognition to guide moral judgments.**

- Use a moral distress tool, such as the Moral Distress Assessment Questionnaire (MDAQ) **to help measure degree of involvement and identify possible actions to improve situation.**

Information that appears in brackets has been added by the authors to clarify and enhance the use of nursing diagnoses.

Cultural   Collaborative   Community/Home Care

• Note availability of family/friends for support and encouragement.

Nursing Priority No. 2.

To assist client/involved individuals to develop/effectively use problem-solving skills:

• Encourage involved individuals to recognize and name the experience resulting in moral sensitivity. **Brings concerns out in the open so they can be dealt with.**
• Use skills, such as Active-listening, I-messages, and problem solving to assist individual(s) **to clarify feelings of anxiety and conflict.**
• Make time available for support and provide information as desired **to help individuals understand the ethical dilemma that led to moral distress.**
• Provide for privacy when discussing sensitive or personal issues.
• Ascertain coping behaviors client has used successfully in the past that may be helpful in dealing with current situation.
• Provide time for nonjudgmental discussion of philosophic issues/questions about impact of conflict leading to moral questioning of current situation.
• Identify role models (e.g., other individuals who have experienced similar problems in their lives). **Sharing of experiences, identifying options can be helpful to deal with current situation.**
• Involve facility/local ethics committee or ethicist as appropriate **to educate, make recommendations, and facilitate mediation/resolution of issues.**

Nursing Priority No. 3.

To promote wellness (Teaching/Discharge Considerations):

• Engage all parties, as appropriate, in developing plan to address conflict. **Resolving one's moral distress requires making changes or compromises while preserving one's integrity and authenticity.**
• Incorporate identified familial, religious, and cultural factors that have meaning for client.
• Refer to appropriate resources for support and guidance (e.g., pastoral care, counseling, organized support groups, classes), as indicated.

Information that appears in brackets has been added by the authors to clarify and enhance the use of nursing diagnoses.

 Diagnostic Studies   ∞ Pediatric/Geriatric/Lifespan   Medications **301**

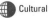 • Assist individuals to recognize that if they follow their moral decisions, they may clash with the legal system and refer to appropriate resource for legal opinion/options.

Documentation Focus

Assessment/Reassessment
- Individual findings, including nature of moral conflict, individuals involved in conflict.
- Physical and emotional responses to conflict.
- Individual cultural or religious beliefs and values, healthcare goals.
- Responses and involvement of family/SOs.

Planning
- Plan of care and who is involved in planning.
- Teaching plan.

Implementation/Evaluation
- Responses to interventions, teaching.
- Attainment or progress toward desired outcome(s).
- Modifications to plan of care.

Discharge Planning
- Long-term needs and who is responsible for actions to be taken.
- Available resources.
- Specific referrals made.

Sample Nursing Outcomes & Interventions Classifications (NOC/NIC) NIC

NOC—Decision Making
NIC—Decision-Making Support

---

risk for Disuse Syndrome

Taxonomy II: Activity/Rest—Class 2 Activity/Exercise (00040)
[Diagnostic Division: Activity/Rest]
Submitted 1988

Definition: At risk for deterioration of body systems as the result of prescribed or unavoidable musculoskeletal inactivity

---

Information that appears in brackets has been added by the authors to clarify and enhance the use of nursing diagnoses.

 Cultural   Collaborative   Community/Home Care

> **NOTE:** Complications from immobility can include pressure ulcer, constipation, stasis of pulmonary secretions, thrombosis, urinary tract infection and/or retention, decreased strength or endurance, orthostatic hypotension, decreased range of joint motion, disorientation, body image disturbance, and powerlessness.

Risk Factors

Severe pain; [chronic pain]
Paralysis; [other neuromuscular impairment]
Mechanical or prescribed immobilization
Altered level of consciousness
Chronic physical or mental illness

> **NOTE:** A risk diagnosis is not evidenced by signs and symptoms, as the problem has not occurred; rather, nursing interventions are directed at prevention.

Desired Outcomes/Evaluation Criteria—Client Will:

- Display intact skin and tissues or achieve timely wound healing.
- Maintain or reestablish effective elimination patterns.
- Be free of signs/symptoms of infectious processes.
- Demonstrate absence of pulmonary congestion with breath sounds clear.
- Demonstrate adequate peripheral perfusion with stable vital signs, skin warm and dry, palpable peripheral pulses.
- Maintain usual reality orientation.
- Maintain or regain optimal level of cognitive, neurosensory, and musculoskeletal functioning.
- Express sense of control over the present situation and potential outcome.
- Recognize and incorporate change into self-concept in accurate manner without negative self-esteem.

Actions/Interventions

Nursing Priority No. 1.

To evaluate probability of developing complications:

- Identify underlying conditions/pathology (e.g., cancer; trauma; fractures with casting; immobilization devices;

Information that appears in brackets has been added by the authors to clarify and enhance the use of nursing diagnoses.

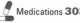 Diagnostic Studies ∞ Pediatric/Geriatric/Lifespan 🗲 Medications **303**

surgery; chronic disease conditions; malnutrition; neurological conditions [e.g., stroke/other brain injury, postpolio syndrome, MS, spinal cord injury]; chronic pain conditions; use of predisposing medications [e.g., steroids]) **that cause or exacerbate problems associated with inactivity and immobility.**

∞• Note specific and potential concerns including client's age, cognition, mobility and exercise status, and whether current condition is acute or short-term, or may be long-term or permanent. **Age-related physiological changes along with limitations imposed by illness or confinement predispose older adults to deconditioning and functional decline.**

• Assess and document client's ongoing functional status, including cognition, vision, and hearing; social support; psychological well-being; abilities in performance of ADLs **for comparative baseline; evaluate response to treatment and to identify preventive interventions or necessary services.**

• Evaluate client's risk for injury. **Risk is greater in client with cognitive difficulties, lack of safe or stimulating environment, inadequate or unsafe use of mobility aids, and/or sensory-perception problems.**

🏠• Ascertain availability and use of support systems.
• Evaluate client's/family's understanding and ability to manage care for long period.

Nursing Priority No. 2.
To identify individually appropriate preventive/corrective interventions:

🏠**Skin**
• Monitor skin over bony prominences.
• Reposition frequently as individually indicated **to relieve pressure.**
• Provide skin care daily and prn, drying well and using gentle massage and lotion **to stimulate circulation.**
• Use pressure-reducing devices (e.g., egg crate, gel, water, or air mattress or cushions).
• Review nutritional status and monitor nutritional intake.
• Provide or reinforce teaching regarding dietary needs, position changes, cleanliness.
• Refer to NDs impaired Skin Integrity; impaired Tissue Integrity.

Information that appears in brackets has been added by the authors to clarify and enhance the use of nursing diagnoses.

Elimination

- Encourage balanced diet, including fruits and vegetables high in fiber and with adequate fluids for optimal stool consistency and to facilitate passage through colon.
- Encourage intake of 8 oz of cranberry juice cocktail per day to reduce risk of urinary infections.
- Maximize mobility at earliest opportunity
- Evaluate need for stool softeners, bulk-forming laxatives.
- Implement consistent bowel management or bladder training programs, as indicated.
- Monitor urinary output and characteristics. Observe for signs of infection.
- Refer to NDs Constipation; Diarrhea; Bowel Incontinence; impaired Urinary Elimination; Urinary Retention.

Respiration

- Monitor breath sounds and characteristics of secretions for early detection of complications (e.g., pneumonia).
- Reposition, cough, deep-breathe on a regular schedule **to facilitate clearing of secretions/prevent atelectasis.**
- Suction, as indicated, **to clear airways.**
- Encourage use of incentive spirometry.
- Demonstrate techniques for, and assist with, postural drainage.
- Assist with, and instruct family and caregivers in, quad coughing techniques and diaphragmatic weight training **to maximize ventilation in presence of SCI.**
- Discourage smoking. Involve in smoking-cessation program, as indicated.
- Refer to NDs ineffective Airway Clearance; ineffective Breathing Pattern.

Vascular (Tissue Perfusion)

- Monitor cognition and mental status. **Changes can reflect state of cardiac health or cerebral oxygenation impairment, or can be indicative of mental or emotional state that could adversely affect safety and self-care.**
- Determine core and skin temperature. Investigate development of cyanosis, changes in mentation, **to identify changes in oxygenation status.**
- Routinely evaluate circulation and nerve function of affected body parts. Note changes in temperature, color, sensation, and movement.

Information that appears in brackets has been added by the authors to clarify and enhance the use of nursing diagnoses.

 Diagnostic Studies   Pediatric/Geriatric/Lifespan   Medications **305**

- Institute peripheral vascular support measures (e.g., elastic hose, Ace wraps, sequential compression devices [SCDs]) **to enhance venous return.**
- Encourage adequate fluid intake **to prevent dehydration and circulatory stasis.**
- Monitor blood pressure before, during, and after activity—sitting, standing, and lying—if possible, **to ascertain response to and tolerance of activity.**
- Assist with position changes as needed. Raise head gradually. Institute use of tilt table where appropriate. **Injury may occur as a result of orthostatic hypotension.**
- Maintain proper body position; avoid use of constricting garments/restraints **to prevent vascular congestion.**
- Provide range-of-motion exercises for bed or chair. Ambulate as quickly and often as possible, using mobility aids and frequent rest stops **to assist client in continuing activity and prevent circulatory problems related to inactivity.**
- Refer to physical therapy **for strengthening and restoration of optimal ROM and prevention of circulatory problems.**
- Refer to NDs ineffective peripheral tissue Perfusion; risk for Peripheral Neurovascular Dysfunction.

Musculoskeletal (Mobility/Range of Motion, Strength/Endurance)
- Perform range-of-motion exercises and involve client in active exercises with physical or occupational therapy (e.g., muscle strengthening).
- Maximize involvement in self-care.
- Pace activities as possible to increase strength and endurance.
- Apply functional positioning splints as appropriate.
- Evaluate role of pain in mobility problem.
- Implement pain management program as individually indicated.
- Monitor closely the use of restraints, if required, and immobilize client as little as possible. Remove restraints periodically and assist with ROM exercises.
- Refer to NDs Activity Intolerance; risk for Falls; impaired physical Mobility; acute or chronic Pain.

Sensory-Perception
- Orient client as necessary to time, place, person, and situation. Provide cues for orientation (e.g., clock, calendar).
- Provide appropriate level of environmental stimulation (e.g., music, TV/radio, personal possessions, visitors).

Information that appears in brackets has been added by the authors to clarify and enhance the use of nursing diagnoses.

⊕ Cultural ⓐ Collaborative ⌂ Community/Home Care

- Encourage participation in recreational and diversional activities and regular exercise program (as tolerated).
- Suggest use of sleep aids or presleep rituals to promote normal sleep or rest.
- Refer to NDs chronic Confusion; disturbed Sensory Perception; Insomnia; Social Isolation; deficient Diversional Activity.

Self-Esteem, Powerlessness
- Explain or review all care procedures.
- Provide for, and assist with, mutual goal setting involving SO(s). **Promotes sense of control and enhances commitment to goals.**
- Provide consistency in caregivers whenever possible.
- Ascertain that client can communicate needs adequately (e.g., call light, writing tablet, picture/letter board, interpreter).
- Encourage verbalization of feelings and questions.
- Refer to NDs Powerlessness; impaired verbal Communication; Self-Esteem [specify]; ineffective Role Performance.

Body Image
- Orient to body changes through verbal description, written information; encourage looking at and discussing changes **to promote acceptance.**
- Promote interactions with peers and normalization of activities within individual abilities.
- Refer to NDs disturbed Body Image; situational low Self-Esteem; Social Isolation; disturbed Personal Identity.

Nursing Priority No. 3.
To promote wellness (Teaching/Discharge Considerations):
- Promote self-care and SO-supported activities **to gain or maintain independence.**
- Provide or review information about individual needs and areas of concerns (e.g., client's mental status, living environment, nutritional needs) **to enhance safety and prevent or limit effects of disuse.**
- Encourage involvement in regular exercise program, including isometric or isotonic activities, active or assistive ROM, to limit consequences of disuse and maximize level of function.
- Review signs/symptoms requiring medical evaluation or follow-up to promote timely interventions.

Information that appears in brackets has been added by the authors to clarify and enhance the use of nursing diagnoses.

- Identify community support services (e.g., financial, counseling, home maintenance, respite care, transportation).
- Refer to appropriate rehabilitation/home-care resources.
- Note sources for assistive devices and necessary equipment.

Documentation Focus

Assessment/Reassessment
- Assessment findings, noting individual areas of concern, functional level, degree of independence, support systems and available resources.

Planning
- Plan of care and who is involved in planning.
- Teaching plan.

Implementation/Evaluation
- Client's response to interventions, teaching, and actions performed.
- Changes in level of functioning.
- Attainment or progress toward desired outcome(s).
- Modifications to plan of care.

Discharge Planning
- Long-term needs and who is responsible for actions to be taken.
- Specific referrals made, resources for specific equipment needs.

Sample Nursing Outcomes & Interventions Classifications (NOC/NIC) NIC

NOC—Immobility Consequences: Physiological
NIC—Exercise Promotion

---

deficient Diversional Activity

Taxonomy II: Activity/Rest—Class 2 Activity/Exercise (00097)
[Diagnostic Division: Activity/Rest]
Submitted 1980

Definition: Decreased stimulation from (or interest or engagement in) recreational or leisure activities [*Note:* Internal/external factors may or may not be beyond the individual's control.]

Information that appears in brackets has been added by the authors to clarify and enhance the use of nursing diagnoses.

Cultural · Collaborative · Community/Home Care

Related Factors

Environmental lack of diversional activity [e.g., long-term hos-
pitalization; frequent, lengthy treatments; home-bound]
Physical limitations; bedridden; fatigue; pain
Situational, developmental problem; lack of resources
Psychological condition, such as depression

Defining Characteristics

Subjective
Patient's statements regarding boredom (e.g., wish there were
something to do, to read)
Usual hobbies cannot be undertaken in hospital [home or other
care setting]
Changes in abilities/physical limitations

Objective
Flat affect; disinterest, inattentiveness
Restlessness; crying
Lethargy; withdrawal
Hostility
Overeating or lack of interest in eating; weight loss or gain

Desired Outcomes/Evaluation Criteria— Client Will:

* Recognize own psychological response (e.g., hopelessness
  and helplessness, anger, depression) and initiate appropriate
  coping actions.
* Engage in satisfying activities within personal limitations.

Actions/Interventions

Nursing Priority No. 1.
To assess precipitating/etiological factors:

* Assess client's physical, cognitive, emotional, and environmental status. **Validates reality of environmental deprivation when it exists, or considers potential for loss of desired
  diversional activities in order to plan for prevention or
  early interventions.**
* Note impact of disability or illness on lifestyle (e.g., young
  child with leukemia, elderly person with fractured hip, individual with severe depression). **Provides comparative baseline for assessments and interventions.**

Information that appears in brackets has been added by the authors to clarify
and enhance the use of nursing diagnoses.

∞ · Note age and developmental level, gender, cultural factors, and the importance of a given activity in client's life **in order to support client participation in something that promotes self-esteem and personal fulfillment.**
· Determine client's actual ability to participate and interest in available activities, noting attention span, physical limitations and tolerance, level of interest or desire, and safety needs. **Presence of acute illness, depression, problems of mobility, protective isolation, or sensory deprivation may interfere with desired activity.**

Nursing Priority No. 2.
To motivate and stimulate client involvement in solutions:

· Institute and continue appropriate actions to deal with concomitant conditions such as anxiety, depression, grief, dementia, physical injury, isolation and immobility, malnutrition, acute or chronic pain. **These interfere with the individual's ability to engage in meaningful diversional activities.**
· Acknowledge reality of situation and feelings of the client **to establish therapeutic relationship and support hopeful emotions.**
· Review history of lifelong activities and hobbies client has enjoyed. Discuss reasons client is not doing these activities now and determine whether client can and would like to resume these activites.
· Encourage mix of desired activities and stimuli (e.g., music, news, educational presentations—TV/tapes, movies, computer or Internet access, books and other reading materials, visitors, games, arts and crafts, sensory enrichment [e.g., massage, aromatherapy], grooming and beauty care, cooking, social outings, gardening, discussion groups, as appropriate). **Activities need to be personally meaningful and not physically or emotionally overwhelming for client to derive the most benefit.**
· Participate in decisions about timing and spacing of lengthy treatments **to promote relaxation and reduce sense of boredom.**
· Encourage client to assist in scheduling required and optional activity choices (e.g., if client's favorite TV show occurs at bathtime, reschedule bath for a later time), **enhancing client's sense of control.**
· Refrain from making changes in schedule without discussing with client. **It is important for staff to be responsible in making and following through on commitments to client.**

Information that appears in brackets has been added by the authors to clarify and enhance the use of nursing diagnoses.

• Provide change of scenery (indoors and outdoors where possible) to **provide positive sensory stimulation, reduce sense of boredom, improve sense of normalcy and control.**

• Identify requirements for mobility (wheelchair, walker, van, volunteers, etc.).

• Provide for periodic changes in the personal environment when the client is confined. Use the individual's input in creating the changes (e.g., seasonal bulletin boards, color changes, rearranging furniture, pictures).

• Suggest activities, such as bird feeders or baths for bird watching, a garden in a window box or terrarium, or a fish bowl or aquarium **to stimulate observation as well as involvement and participation in activity, such as identification of birds, choice of seeds, and so forth.**

• Accept hostile expressions while limiting aggressive acting-out behavior. **Permission to express feelings of anger, hopelessness allows for beginning resolution. However, destructive behavior is counterproductive to self-esteem and problem solving.**

• Involve recreational, occupational, play, music, and/or movement therapist as appropriate **to help identify enjoyable activities for client; to procure assistive devices and/or modify activities for individual situation.**

Nursing Priority No. 3.

To promote wellness (Teaching/Discharge Considerations):

• Explore options for useful activities using the person's strengths and abilities.

• Make appropriate referrals to available support groups, hobby clubs, service organizations.

• Refer to NDs Powerlessness; Social Isolation.

Documentation Focus

Assessment/Reassessment

• Specific assessment findings, including blocks to desired activities.

• Individual choices for activities.

Planning

• Plan of care, specific interventions, and who is involved in planning.

Information that appears in brackets has been added by the authors to clarify and enhance the use of nursing diagnoses.

Implementation/Evaluation
- Client's responses to interventions, teaching, and actions performed.
- Attainment or progress toward desired outcome(s).
- Modifications to plan of care.

Discharge Planning
- Long-term needs and who is responsible for actions to be taken.
- Referrals and community resources.

Sample Nursing Outcomes & Interventions Classifications (NOC/NIC) NIC

NOC—Leisure Participation
NIC—Recreation Therapy

risk for Electrolyte Imbalance

Taxonomy II: Nutrition—Class 5 Hydration (00195)
[Diagnostic Division: Food/Fluid]]
Submitted 2008

Definition: For change in serum electrolyte levels that may compromse health

Risk Factors

Fluid imbalance (e.g., dehydration, water intoxication); diarrhea; vomiting
Endocrine dysfunction
Renal dysfunction
Impaired regulatory mechanisms (e.g., diabetes insipidus, syndrome of inappropriate secretion of antidiuretic hormone)
Treatment-related side effects (e.g., medications, drains)

NOTE: A risk diagnosis is not evidenced by signs and symptoms, as the problem has not occurred; rather, nursing interventions are directed at prevention.

Desired Outcomes/Evaluation Criteria— Client Will:

- Display laboratory results within normal range for individual.
- Be free of complications resulting from electrolyte imbalance.

Information that appears in brackets has been added by the authors to clarify and enhance the use of nursing diagnoses.

Cultural   Collaborative   Community/Home Care

- Identify individual risks and engage in appropriate behaviors or lifestyle changes to prevent or reduce frequency of electrolyte imbalances.

Actions/Interventions

Nursing Priority No. 1.

To assess causative/contributing factors:

- Identify client with current or newly diagnosed condition commonly associated with electrolyte imbalances, such as inability to eat or drink, febrile illness, active bleeding or other fluid loss, including vomiting, diarrhea, gastrointestinal drainage, burns.
- Assess specific client risk, noting chronic disease processes that may lead to electrolyte imbalances, including kidney disease, metabolic or endocrine disorders, chronic alcoholism, cancer or cancer treatments, conditions causing hemolysis such as massive trauma, multiple blood transfusions; sickle cell disease.
- Note client's age and developmental level, which may increase risk for electrolyte imbalance. **This risk group can include the very young or elderly, or individuals unable to meet their own needs or monitor their health status, including clients who are unconcious for unknown cause or period of time, trauma victim, and so on. Note: Elderly clients are more prone to electrolyte imbalances related to fluid imbalances, use of multiple medications including diuretics, heart and blood pressure medications, lack of appetite or interest in eating or drinking, lack of appropriate dietary and/or medication supervision at home, and so on.**
- Review client's medications **for those associated with electrolyte imbalance, such as diurectics, laxatives, corticosteroids, barbiturates, and some antibiotics.**

Nursing Priority No. 2.

To identify potential electrolyte deficit:

- Assess mental status, noting client/caregiver report of change—altered attention span, recall of recent events, other cognitive functions. **Can be associated with electrolyte imbalance; for example, it is the most common problem of hypernatremia.**
- Monitor heart rate and rhythm by palapation and asculatation. **Tachycardia, bradycardia, and other dysrhythmias are**

Information that appears in brackets has been added by the authors to clarify and enhance the use of nursing diagnoses.

balances.*Weak pulse and thready pulse can be associated with hypokalemia.*

- Ascultate breath sounds, assess rate and depth of respirations and ease of respiratory effort, observe color of nailbeds and mucous membranes, and note pulse oximetry or blood gas measurement, as indicated. **Certain electrolyte imbalances, such as hypokalemia, can cause or exacerbate respiratory insufficiency.**
- Review electrocardiogram (ECG). **Because the ECG reflects electrophysiological, anatomical, metabolic, and hemodynamic alterations, it is routinely used for the diagnosis of electrolyte and metabolic disturbances, as well as myocardial ischemia, cardiac dysrhythmias, structural changes of the myocardium, and drug effects.**
- Assess gastrointestinal symptoms, noting presence, absence, and character of bowel sounds; presence of acute or chronic diarrhea; persistent vomiting, high nasogastric tube output. **Any disturbance of the gastrointestional functioning carries with it the potential for electrolyte imbalances.**
- Review client's food intake. Note presence of anorexia, vomiting, or recent fad or unusual diet; look for chronic malnutrition.
- Evaluate motor strength and function, noting steadiness of gait, handgrip strength, and reactivity of refluxes, **which can provide clues to electrolyte imbalance.**
- Assess fluid intake and output. **Many factors, such as inability to drink, large diuresis or chronic kidney failure, trauma, and surgery, affect individual's fluid balance, disrupting electrolyte transport, function, and excretion.**
- Review laboratory results for abnormal findings. **Electrolytes include sodium, potassium, calcium, chloride, bicarbonate (carbon dioxide) and magnesium. These chemicals are essential in many bodily functions including fluid balance, movement of fluid within and between body compartments, nerve conduction, muscle contraction—including the heart; blood clotting and pH balance.**
- Assess for specific imbalances:

  - Sodium (Na^+) **Dominant extracellular cation and cannot freely cross the cell membrane.**

  - Review laboratory results—normal range in adults is 135 to 145 mEq/L. **Elevated sodium (hypernatremia) can**

Information that appears in brackets has been added by the authors to clarify and enhance the use of nursing diagnoses.

⊕ Cultural 🔄 Collaborative 🏠 Community/Home Care

occur if client has an overall deficit of total body water owing to inadequate fluid intake or water loss, and can be associated with low potassium, metabolic acidosis, and hypoglycemia.

- Monitor for physical or mental disorders impacting fluid intake. **Impaired thirst sensation, inability to express thirst or obtain needed fluids may lead to hypernatremia.**
- Note presence of medical conditions that may impact sodium level. **Hyponatremia may be associated with disorders such as congestive heart failure, liver and kidney failure, pneumonia, metabolic acidosis, intestinal conditions resulting in prolonged gastrointestinal suction. Hypernatremia can result from simple conditions such as febrile illness causing fluid loss and/or restricted fluid intake, or complicated conditions such as kidney and endocrine diseases affecting sodium intake or excretion.**
- Note presence of cognitive dysfunction such as confusion, restlessness, abnormal speech (**which may be cause or effect of sodium imbalance**).
- Assess for orthostatic blood pressure changes, tachycardia, low urine output; or other clinical findings, such as generalized weakness, swollen tongue, weight loss, seizures. **Signs suggesting hypernatremia.**
- Assess for nausea, abdominal cramping, lethargy, orthostatic blood pressure changes—if fluid volume is also depleted; confusion, decreased level of consciousness, or headache. **Signs and symptoms suggestive of hyponatremia, which can lead to seizures and coma if untreated.**
- Review drug regimen. **Drugs such as anabolic steroids, angiotensin, cisplatin, and mannitol may increase sodium level. Diuretics, laxatives, theophylline, and trimeterine can decrease sodium level.**
- <u>Potassium (K+)</u> **Most abundant intracellular cation, obtained through diet, excreted via kidneys.**
- Review laboratory results—normal range in adults is 3.5 to 5.0 mEq/L.
- Note current medical conditions that may impact potassium level. **Metabolic acidosis, burn or crush injuries, massive hemolysis, diabetes, kidney disease/renal failure, cancer, and sickle cell trait are associated with hyperkalemia, fasting, diarrhea or nasogastric suctioning, alkalosis,**

Information that appears in brackets has been added by the authors to clarify and enhance the use of nursing diagnoses.

administration of IV potassium boluses, or transfusions of whole blood or packed cells increases the risk of hypokalemia.

- Identify conditions or situations **that potentiate risk for hyperkalemia, including ingestion of unusual diet with high-potassium, low-sodium foods, or use of potassium supplements, including OTC herbals or salt substitutes.**
- Monitor ECG, as indicated. **Abnormal potassium levels, both low and high, are associated with changes in the ECG.**
- Evaluate reports of abdominal cramping, fatigue, hyperactive bowel motility, muscle twitching, and cramps, followed by muscle weakness. Note presence of depressed reflexes, ascending flaccid paralysis of legs and arms. **Signs/ symptoms suggesting hyperkalemia.**
- Note presence of anorexia, abdominal distention, diminished bowel sounds, postural hypotension, muscle weakness, flaccid paralysis. **May be manifestations of hypokalemia.**
- Review drug regimen. **Use of potassium-sparing diuretics, other medications, such as NSAIDs, angiotensin-converting enzyme (ACE) inhibitors, certain antibiotics such as pentamidine may increase potassium level. Medications such as albuterol, terbutaline, or some diuretics may decrease potassium level.**
- Calcium (Ca^{2+}) **Most abundant cation in the body, participates in almost all vital processes, working with sodium to regulate depolarization and the generation of action potentials.**
- Review laboratory results—normal range for adults is 8.5 to 10.5 mg/dL.
- Note presence of medical conditions impacting calcium level. **Acidosis, Addison's disease, cancers (e.g., bone, lymphoma, leukemias), hyperparathyroidism, lung disease (e.g., TB, histoplasmosis), thyrotoxicosis, polycythemia may lead to increased calcium level. Chronic diarrhea, intestinal disorders such as Crohn's disease; pancreatitis, alcoholism, renal failure or renal tubular disease; recent orthopedic surgery or bone healing, history of thyroid surgery or irradiation of upper middle chest and neck; and psychosis may result in decreased calcium levels.**

Information that appears in brackets has been added by the authors to clarify and enhance the use of nursing diagnoses.

⊕ Cultural 🌐 Collaborative 🏠 Community/Home Care

- Monitor for excessive urination (polyuria), constipation, lethargy, muscle weakness, anorexia, headache, coma, **which can be associated with hypercalcemia.**
- Monitor for cardiac dysrhythmias, hypotension, and heart failure; muscle cramps, facial spasms—postive Chvostek's sign; numbness and tingling sensations, muscle twitching—postive Trousseau's sign; seizures or tetany, **which suggest hypocalcemia.**
- Review drug regimen. **Drugs such as anabolic steroids, some antacids, lithium, oral contraceptives, vitamins A and D, amoxapine, can increase calcium levels. Drugs such as albuterol, anticonvulsants, glucocorticoids, insulin, phosphates, trazadone, laxative overuse, or long-term anticonvulsant therapy can decrease calcium levels.**
- Magnesium (Mg^{2+}) **Second most abundant intracellular cation after potassium, magnesium controls absorption or function of sodium, potassium, calcium, and phosphorus.**

- Review laboratory results—normal range in adults is 1.5 to 2.0 mEq/L.
- Note presence of medical condition impacting magnesium level. **Diabetic acidosis, multiple myeloma, renal insufficiency, eclampsia, asthma, GI hypomotility; adrenal insufficiency, extensive soft tissue injury, severe burns, shock, sepsis, cardiac arrest are associated with hypermagnesemia. Conditions resulting in decreased intake— starvation, alcoholism, parenteral feeding; excess gastrointestinal losses—diarrhea, vomiting, nasogastric suction, malabsorption; renal losses—inherited renal tubular defects among others; or miscellaneous causes including calcium abnormalities, chronic metabolic acidosis, diabetic ketoacidosis can lead to hypomagnesemia.**
- Note GI and renal function. **Main controlling factors of magnesium are GI absorption and renal excretion. Low levels of magnesium, potassium, calcium, and phosphorus may be manifest at the same time if absorption is impaired. High levels of magnesium, calcium, phosphate, and potassium often occur together in setting of kidney disease.**

Information that appears in brackets has been added by the authors to clarify and enhance the use of nursing diagnoses.

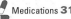

- Monitor for nausea, vomiting, weakness, vasodilaton, **which suggests mild to moderate elevation of magnesium level (>3.5–5.0 mEq/L).**
- Monitor ECG, as indicated. **Presence of heart blocks, especially if accompanied by ventilatory failure and stupor, suggest severe hypermagnesemia (>10.0 mEq/L). Hypomagenesemia can lead to potentially fatal ventricular dysrthythmias, coronary artery vasospasm, and sudden death.**
- Review drug regimen. **Drugs such as aspirin and progesterone may increase magnesium level; albuterol, digoxin, diuretics, oral contraceptives, aminoglycosides, proton-pump inhibitors, immunosuppressants, cisplatin, and cyclosporines are some of the medications that may decrease magnesium levels.**

Nursing Priority No. 3.
To prevent imbalances:

- Collaborate in treatment of underlying conditions **to prevent or limit effects of electrolyte imbalances caused by disease or organ dysfunction.**
- Provide or recommend balanced nutrition, using best route for feeding. Monitor intake, weight and bowel function. **Obtaining and utilizing electrolytes and other minerals depends on client regularly receiving them in a readily available form, including food and supplements via ingestion, enteral or parenteral routes.**
- Measure and report all fluid losses, including emesis, diarrhea, wound or fistula drainage. **Loss of fluids rich in electrolytes can lead to imbalances.**
- Maintain fluid balance **to prevent dehydration and shifts of electrolytes.**
- Use pump or controller device when administering intravenous electrolyte solutions **to provide medication at desired rate and prevent untoward effects of excessive or too rapid delivery.**

Nursing Priority No. 4.
To promote wellness (Teaching/Discharge Considerations):

- Discuss ongoing concerns for client with chronic health problems, such as kidney disease, diabetes, cancer; individuals taking multiple medications, and/or client deciding to take

---

Information that appears in brackets has been added by the authors to clarify and enhance the use of nursing diagnoses.

   ⊕ Cultural   🐢 Collaborative   🏠 Community/Home Care

medications or drugs differently than prescribed. **Early intervention can help prevent serious complications.**

- Consult with dietician or nutritionist for specific teaching needs. **Learning how to incorporate foods that increase electrolyte intake, or identifying food or condiment alternatives increases client's self-sufficiency and likelihood of success.**
- Teach client/caregiver to take, or administer, drugs as prescribed—especially diuretics, antihypertensives, and cardiac drugs **to reduce potential of complications associated with medication-induced electrolyte imbalances.**
- Instruct client/caregiver in reportable symptoms. **For example, sudden change in mentation or behavior 2 days after starting a new diuretic could indicate hyponatremia; or elderly person taking digitalis (for atrial fibrillation) and a diuretic may be hypokalemic.**
- Provide information regarding calcium supplements, as indicated. **It is popular wisdom to instruct people, women in particular, to take calcium for prevention of osteoporosis. However, calcium absorption cannot take place without vitamins D and K and magnesium. Client taking calcium may need additional information or resources.**
- Review client's medications at each visit and discuss with primary care provider **for possible change in dosage or drug choice.**

Documentation Focus

Assessment/Reassessment
- Identified or potential risk factors for individual.
- Assessment findings, including vital signs, mentation, muscle strength and reflexes, presence of fatigue, respiratory distress.
- Results of laboratory tests and diagnostic studies.

Planning
- Plan of care, specific interventions, and who is involved in the planning.
- Teaching plan.

Implementation/Evaluation
- Client's responses to treatment, teaching, and actions performed.

Information that appears in brackets has been added by the authors to clarify and enhance the use of nursing diagnoses.

- Attainment or progress toward desired outcome(s).
- Modifications to plan of care.

Discharge Planning
- Long-term needs, identifying who is responsible for actions to be taken.
- Specific referrals made.

Sample Nursing Outcomes & Interventions Classifications (NOC/NIC) `NIC`

NOC—Electrolyte & Acid Base Balance
NIC—Electrolyte Management

---

disturbed Energy Field

Taxonomy II: Activity/Rest—Class 3 Energy Balance (00050)
[Diagnostic Division: Ego Integrity]
Submitted 1994, Revised 2004

Definition: Disruption of the flow of energy [aura] surrounding a person's being that results in a disharmony of the body, mind, and/or spirit

---

Related Factors

Slowing or blocking of energy flows secondary to:
Pathophysological factors—Illness, pregnancy, injury
Treatment-related factors—Immobility, labor and delivery, perioperative experience, chemotherapy
Situational factors—Pain, fear, anxiety, grieving
Maturational factors—Age-related developmental difficulties or crisis

Defining Characteristics

Objective
Perception of changes in patterns of energy flow, such as:
Movement (wave, spike, tingling, dense, flowing)
Sounds (tone, words)
Temperature change (warmth, coolness)

Information that appears in brackets has been added by the authors to clarify and enhance the use of nursing diagnoses.

Cultural Collaborative Community/Home Care

Visual changes (image, color)
Disruption of the field (deficient, hole, spike, bulge, obstruction, congestion, diminished flow in energy field)

Desired Outcomes/Evaluation Criteria— Client Will:

- Acknowledge feelings of anxiety and distress.
- Verbalize sense of relaxation and well-being.
- Display reduction in severity or frequency of symptoms.

Actions/Interventions

Nursing Priority No. 1.

To determine causative/contributing factors:

- Review current situation and concerns of client. Provide opportunity for client to talk about condition, past history, emotional state, or other relevant information. Note body gestures, tone of voice, words chosen to express feelings or issues.
- Determine client's motivation or desire for treatment. **Although attitude can affect success of therapy, Therapeutic Touch is often successful even when the client is skeptical. Recent studies reported that TT produced positive outcomes by decreasing levels of anxiety and pain perception and improving sense of well-being/quality of life; TT may also be beneficial in reducing behavioral symptoms of dementia (e.g., manual manipulation/restlessness, vocalization, pacing).**
- Note use of medications, other drug use (e.g., alcohol). **TT may be helpful in reducing anxiety level in individuals undergoing alcohol withdrawal.**
- Perform/review results of testing, as indicated, such as the State-Trait Anxiety Inventory (STAI) or the Affect Balance Scale, **to provide measures of the client's anxiety.**

Nursing Priority No. 2.

To evaluate energy field:

- Develop therapeutic nurse-client relationship, initially accepting role of healer/guide as client desires.
- Place client in sitting or supine position with legs and arms uncrossed. Place pillows or other supports to enhance comfort and relaxation.
- Center self physically and psychologically **to quiet mind and turn attention to the healing intent.**

Information that appears in brackets has been added by the authors to clarify and enhance the use of nursing diagnoses.

• Move hands slowly over the client at level of 2 to 6 inches above skin to assess state of energy field and flow of energy within the system.

• Identify areas of imbalance or obstruction in the field (i.e., areas of asymmetry; feelings of heat or cold, tingling, congestion, or pressure).

Nursing Priority No. 3.

To provide therapeutic intervention:

• Explain the process of TT and answer questions, as indicated, **to prevent unrealistic expectations. Fundamental focus of TT is on healing and wholeness, not curing signs/ symptoms of disease.**

• Discuss findings of evaluation with client.

• Assist client with exercises to promote "centering" and increase potential to self-heal, enhance comfort, reduce anxiety.

• Perform unruffling process, keeping hands 2 to 6 inches from client's body **to dissipate impediments to free flow of energy within the system and between nurse and client.**

• Focus on areas of disturbance identified, holding hands over or on skin, and/or place one hand in back of body with other hand in front. **Allows client's body to pull or repattern energy as needed.** At the same time, concentrate on the intent to help the client heal.

• Shorten duration of treatment to 2 to 3 minutes, as appropriate. **Children, elderly individuals, those with head injuries, and others who are severely debilitated are generally more sensitive to overloading energy fields.**

• Make coaching suggestions (e.g., pleasant images or other visualizations, deep breathing) in a soft voice **for enhancing feelings of relaxation.**

• Use hands-on massage/apply pressure to acupressure points, as appropriate, during process.

• Note changes in energy sensations as session progresses. Stop when the energy field is symmetric and there is a change to feelings of peaceful calm.

• Hold client's feet for a few minutes at end of session **to assist in "grounding" the body energy.**

• Provide client time following procedure **for a period of peaceful rest.**

Nursing Priority No. 4.

To promote wellness (Teaching/Discharge Considerations):

• Allow period of client dependency, as appropriate, **for client to strengthen own inner resources.**

Information that appears in brackets has been added by the authors to clarify and enhance the use of nursing diagnoses.

- Encourage ongoing practice of the therapeutic process.
- Instruct in use of stress-reduction activities (e.g., centering/ meditation, relaxation exercises) **to promote mind-body-spirit harmony.**
- Discuss importance of integrating techniques into daily activity plan **for sustaining/enhancing sense of well-being.**
- Have client practice each step and demonstrate the complete TT process following the session as client displays readiness to assume responsibilities for self-healing.
- Promote attendance at a support group, **where members can help each other practice and learn the techniques of TT.**
- Reinforce that TT is a complementary intervention and stress importance of seeking timely evaluation and continuing other prescribed treatment modalities, as appropriate.
- Refer to other resources, as identified (e.g., psychotherapy, clergy, medical treatment of disease processes, hospice), **for the individual to address total well-being and facilitate peaceful death.**

Documentation Focus

Assessment/Reassessment
- Assessment findings, including characteristics and differences in the energy field.
- Client's perception of problem or need for treatment.

Planning
- Plan of care and who is involved in planning.
- Teaching plan.

Implementation/Evaluation
- Changes in energy field.
- Client's response to interventions, teaching, and actions performed.
- Attainment or progress toward desired outcomes.
- Modifications to plan of care.

Discharge Planning
- Long-term needs and who is responsible for actions to be taken.
- Specific referrals made.

Information that appears in brackets has been added by the authors to clarify and enhance the use of nursing diagnoses.

Sample Nursing Outcomes & Interventions Classifications (NOC/NIC) (NIC)

NOC—Personal Well-Being
NIC—Therapeutic Touch

impaired Environmental Interpretation Syndrome

Taxonomy II: Perception/Cognition—Class 2 Orientation (00127)
[Diagnostic Division: Safety]
Submitted 1994

Definition: Consistent lack of orientation to person, place, time, or circumstances over more than 3 to 6 months, necessitating a protective environment

Related Factors

Dementia [Alzheimer's disease, multi-infarct dementia, Pick's disease, AIDS dementia]
Huntington's disease
Depression

Defining Characteristics

Objective
Consistent disorientation
Chronic confusional states
Inability to follow simple directions
Inability to reason or concentrate; slow in responding to questions
Loss of occupation, social functioning

Desired Outcomes/Evaluation Criteria— Client Will:

• Be free of harm.

Caregiver Will:

• Identify individual client safety concerns/needs.
• Modify activities and environment to provide for safety.

Information that appears in brackets has been added by the authors to clarify and enhance the use of nursing diagnoses.

⊕ Cultural   ✺ Collaborative   🏠 Community/Home Care

Actions/Interventions

Nursing Priority No. 1.

To assess causative/precipitating factors:

Refer to NDs acute Confusion; chronic Confusion; impaired Memory; [disturbed Thought Processes] for additional relevant assessment and interventions.

- Determine presence of medical conditions and/or behaviors leading to client's current situation **to identify potentially useful interventions and therapies.**
- **Note presence, or reports of, client's misinterpretation of environmental information** (e.g., sensory, cognitive, or social cues).
- **Discuss history and progression of condition, length of time since onset, future expectations, and incidents of injury or accidents.**
- Review client's behavioral changes with SO(s) **to note differences in viewpoint, as well as to identify additional impairments (e.g., decreased agility, reduced range of motion of joints, loss of balance, decline in visual acuity, failure to eat, loss of interest in personal grooming, and forgetfulness resulting in unsafe actions).**
- Identify actual and/or potential environmental dangers and client's level of awareness (if any) of threat.
- Test ability to receive and send effective communication. **Client may be nonverbal or require assistance with/ interpretation of verbalizations.**
- Review client/SO(s) usual habits for activities, such as sleeping, eating, self-care, **to include in plan of care.**
- Determine anxiety level in relation to situation. Note behavior **that may be indicative of potential for violence.**
- Evaluate responses on diagnostic examinations (e.g., memory impairments, reality orientation, attention span, calculations). **A combination of tests (e.g., Confusion Assessment Method [CAM], Mini-Mental State Examination [MMSE], Alzheimer's Disease Assessment Scale [ADAS-cog], Brief Dementia Severity Rating Scale [BDSRS], and Neuropsychiatric Inventory [NPI]) is often needed to determine client's overall condition relating to chronic/ irreversible condition.**

Nursing Priority No. 2.

To promote safe environment:

- Collaborate in management of treatable conditions (e.g., infections, malnutrition, electrolyte imbalances, and adverse

---

Information that appears in brackets has been added by the authors to clarify and enhance the use of nursing diagnoses.

Diagnostic Studies   ∞ Pediatric/Geriatric/Lifespan   Medications **325**

medication reactions) **that may contribute to or exacerbate confusion.**

- Provide calm environment; eliminate extraneous noise/stimuli **that may increase client's level of agitation/confusion.**
- Keep communications simple. Use concrete terms and words that client can recognize. (Refer to ND impaired verbal Communication for additional interventions.)
- Use family/other interpreter, as needed, to comprehend client's communications.
- Provide and promote use of glasses, hearing aids, and adequate lighting **to optimize sensory input.**
- Use touch judiciously. Tell client what is being done before touching **to reduce sense of surprise or negative reaction.**
- Maintain reality-oriented environment (e.g., clocks, calendars, personal items, seasonal decorations, social events).
- Explain environmental cues to client (ongoing) **to protect safety and attempt to diminish fears.**
- Provide consistent caregivers and family-centered care as much as possible **for consistency and to decrease confusion.**
- Incorporate previous/usual patterns for activities (e.g., sleeping, eating, hygiene, desired clothing, leisure/play, or rituals) to the extent possible **to keep environment predictable and prevent client from feeling overwhelmed.**
- Limit number of visitors client interacts with at one time, if needed, **to prevent overstimulation.**
- Implement complementary therapies, as indicated and desired (e.g., music or movement therapy, massage, Therapeutic Touch, aromatherapy, bright-light treatment). **May help client relax, refocus attention, and stimulate memories.**
- Set limits on unsafe and/or inappropriate behavior, being alert to potential for violence.
- Provide for safety and protection against hazards, such as locking doors to unprotected areas and stairwells, prohibiting or supervising smoking, and monitoring ADLs (e.g., choice of clothing in relation to environment and season).
- Use identity tags in clothes and belongings, bracelet/necklace **to provide identification if client wanders away or becomes lost.**
- Avoid use of restraints as much as possible. Use vest (instead of wrist) restraints, when required. **Although restraints can prevent falls, they can increase client's agitation and distress.**
- Administer medications, as ordered (e.g., antidepressants, antipsychotics). Monitor for expected and/or adverse reactions

---

Information that appears in brackets has been added by the authors to clarify and enhance the use of nursing diagnoses.

🌐 Cultural 🤝 Collaborative 🏠 Community/Home Care

and side effects and interactions. **May be used to manage symptoms of psychosis, depression, or aggressive behavior.**

Nursing Priority No. 3.

To assist caregiver to deal with situation:

- Determine family dynamics, cultural values, resources, and availability and willingness to participate in meeting client's needs.
- Involve family/SO(s) in planning and care activities, as needed/desired. Maintain frequent interactions with SO(s) **in order to relay information, change care strategies, obtain feedback, and offer support.**
- Evaluate SO's attention to own needs, including health status, grieving process, and respite. **Caregivers often feel guilty when taking time for themselves. Without adequate support and respite, the caregiver cannot meet the needs of the client.**
- Discuss caregiver burden, if appropriate. (Refer to NDs Caregiver Role Strain; risk for Caregiver Role Strain for additional interventions.)
- Provide educational materials and list of available resources (help lines, Web sites, etc.) as desired, **to assist SO(s) in coping with long-term care issues.**
- Identify appropriate community resources (e.g., Alzheimer's Disease and Related Disorders Association [ARDA], stroke or brain injury support group, senior support groups, clergy, social services, or respite care) **to provide client/SO with support and assist with problem solving.**

Nursing Priority No. 4.

To promote wellness (Teaching/Discharge Considerations):

- Provide specific information about disease process/prognosis and client's particular needs. **Individuals with conditions requiring ongoing monitoring of their environment usually need more social and behavioral support than medical management, although medical concerns will occur occasionally.**
- Review age-appropriate ongoing treatment and social needs and appropriate resources for client and family.
- Develop plan of care with family **to meet client's and SO's individual needs.**
- Reinforce that caregiver cannot physically watch client at all times.

Information that appears in brackets has been added by the authors to clarify and enhance the use of nursing diagnoses.

• Perform home assessment, if indicated, to identify safety issues, such as securing medications and poisonous substances and locking exterior doors, **to prevent client from wandering off while SO is engaged in other household activities,** or removing matches and smoking material and knobs from the stove **to prevent client from starting fires or turning on stove burner and leaving it unattended.**

• Refer to appropriate outside resources, such as adult day care, homemaker services, or support groups. **Provides assistance and promotes problem solving.**

Documentation Focus

Assessment/Reassessment
* Assessment findings, including degree of impairment.
* Involvement and availability of family members to provide care.

Planning
* Plan of care and who is involved in planning.
* Teaching plan.

Implementation/Evaluation
* Response to treatment plan, interventions, and actions performed.
* Attainment or progress toward desired outcomes.
* Modifications to plan of care.

Discharge Planning
* Long-term needs, who is responsible for actions to be taken.
* Specific referrals made.

Sample Nursing Outcomes & Interventions Classifications (NOC/NIC) NIC

NOC—Cognition
NIC—Surveillance: Safety

Information that appears in brackets has been added by the authors to clarify and enhance the use of nursing diagnoses.

⊕ Cultural   ⊛ Collaborative   🏠 Community/Home Care

adult Failure to Thrive

Taxonomy II: Growth/Development—Class 1 Growth
(00101)
[Diagnostic Division: Food/Fluid]
Submitted 1998

Definition: Progressive functional deterioration of a
physical and cognitive nature. The individual's ability
to live with multisystem diseases, cope with ensuing
problems, and manage his/her care are remarkably
diminished.

Related Factors

Depression
Major disease or degenerative condition
Aging process

Defining Characteristics

Subjective
Expresses loss of interest in pleasurable outlets
Altered mood state
Verbalizes desire for death

Objective
Inadequate nutritional intake; consumption of minimal to no
food at most meals (i.e., consumes less than 75% of normal
requirements); anorexia
Unintentional weight loss (e.g., 5% in 1 month, 10% in 6
months)
Physical decline (e.g., fatigue, dehydration, incontinence of
bowel and bladder)
Cognitive decline: problems with responding to environmental
stimuli; demonstrated difficulty in reasoning, decision making, judgment, memory, concentration; decreased perception
Apathy
Decreased participation in activities of daily living; self-care
deficit; neglect of home environment/financial responsibilities
Decreased social skills; social withdrawal
Frequent exacerbations of chronic health problems

Information that appears in brackets has been added by the authors to clarify
and enhance the use of nursing diagnoses.

Desired Outcomes/Evaluation Criteria— Client Will:

- Acknowledge presence of factors affecting well-being.
- Identify corrective or adaptive measures for individual situation.
- Demonstrate behaviors and lifestyle changes necessary to enhance functional status.

Actions/Interventions

Refer to NDs Activity Intolerance, risk-prone health Behaviors, chronic Confusion, ineffective Coping, impaired Dentition, risk for Falls, complicated Grieving, risk for Loneliness, imbalanced Nutrition: less than body requirements, Relocation Stress Syndrome, chronic low Self-Esteem, Self-Care Deficit (specify), risk for Spiritual Distress, impaired Swallowing, as appropriate, for additional relevant interventions.

Nursing Priority No. 1.

To identify causative/contributing factors:

- Assess client's/SO's perception of factors leading to present condition, noting onset, duration, presence/absence of physical complaints, social withdrawal, **to provide comparative baseline.**
- Review with client previous and current life situations, including role changes and losses (e.g., death of loved ones; change in living arrangements, finances, independence), **to identify stressors affecting current situation.**
- Identify cultural beliefs and expectations regarding condition or situation, presence of conflicts.
- Determine presence of malnutrition and factors contributing to failure to eat (e.g., chronic nausea, loss of appetite, no access to food or cooking, poorly fitting dentures, no one with whom to share meals, depression, financial problems).
- Determine client's medical, cognitive, emotional, and perceptual status and effect on self-care ability.
- Evaluate level of adaptive behavior, knowledge, and skills about health maintenance, environment, and safety.
- Ascertain safety and effectiveness of home environment, persons providing care, and potential for or presence of neglect, abusive situations.

Nursing Priority No. 2.

To assess degree of impairment:

- Collaborate in comprehensive assessment (e.g., physical, nutritional, self-care, and psychosocial) status **to determine the**

Information that appears in brackets has been added by the authors to clarify and enhance the use of nursing diagnoses.

extent of limitations affecting ability to thrive and potential for positive intervention.

- Obtain current weight **to provide comparative baseline and evaluate response to interventions.**
- Active-listen to client's/caregiver's perception of problem(s).
- Discuss individual concerns about feelings of loss/loneliness and relationship between these feelings and current decline in well-being. Note desire and willingness to change situation. **Motivation can impede—or facilitate—achieving desired outcomes.**
- Survey past and present availability/use of support systems.

Nursing Priority No. 3.

To assist client to achieve/maintain general well-being:

- Assist with treatment of underlying medical and psychiatric conditions **that could positively influence current situation (e.g., resolution of infection, addressing depression).**
- Coordinate session with client/SO(s) and nutritionist **to identify specific dietary needs and creative ways to stimulate intake (e.g., offering client's favorite foods, family-style meals, participation in social events such as ice cream social, happy hour).**
- Develop plan of action with client/caregiver **to meet immediate needs for nutrition, safety, and self-care and facilitate implementation of actions.**
- Explore strengths/successful coping behaviors the individual has used previously. **Incorporating these into problem solving builds on past successes.** Refine/develop new strategies as appropriate.
- Assist client to develop goals for dealing with life or illness situation. Involve SO/family in long-range planning. **Promotes commitment to goals and plan, maximizing outcomes.**

Nursing Priority No. 4.

To promote wellness (Teaching/Discharge Considerations):

- Assist client/SO(s) to identify useful community resources (e.g., support groups, Meals on Wheels, social worker, home care or assistive care, placement services). **Enhances coping, assists with problem solving, and may reduce risks to client and caregiver.**
- Encourge client to talk about positive aspects of life and to keep as physically active as possible **to reduce effects of dispiritedness (e.g., "feeling low," sense of being unimportant, disconnected).**

Information that appears in brackets has been added by the authors to clarify and enhance the use of nursing diagnoses.

- Introduce concept of mindfulness (living in the moment). **Promotes feeling of capability and belief that this moment can be dealt with.**
- Offer opportunities to discuss life goals and support client/SO in setting and attaining new goals for this time of life to **enhance hopefulness for future.**
- Promote socialization within individual limitations. **Provides additional stimulation, reduces sense of isolation.**
- Assist client/SO/family to understand that failure to thrive commonly occurs near the end of life, and cannot always be reversed.
- Help client explore reasons for living, or begin to deal with end-of-life issues and provide support for grieving. **Enhances hope and sense of control.**
- Refer to pastoral care, counseling or psychotherapy **for grief work.**
- Discuss appropriateness of, and refer to, palliative services or hospice care as indicated.

Documentation Focus

Assessment/Reassessment
- Individual findings, including current weight, dietary pattern, perceptions of self, food and eating.
- Perception of losses and life changes.
- Ability to perform activities of daily living and participate in care, meet own needs.
- Motivation for change, support, and feedback from SO(s).

Planning
- Plan of care, specific interventions, and who is involved in planning.
- Teaching plan.

Implementation/Evaluation
- Responses to interventions and actions performed, general well-being, weekly weight.
- Attainment or progress toward desired outcome(s).
- Modifications to plan of care.

Discharge Planning
- Long-term needs and who is responsible for actions to be taken.
- Community resources and support groups.
- Specific referrals made.

Information that appears in brackets has been added by the authors to clarify and enhance the use of nursing diagnoses.

⊕ Cultural Collaborative Community/Home Care

Sample Nursing Outcomes & Interventions Classifications (NOC/NIC) [NIC]

NOC—Will to Live
NIC—Mood Management

risk for Falls

Taxonomy II: Safety/Protection—Class 2 Physical Injury (00155)
[Diagnostic Division: Safety]
Submitted 2000

Definition: Increased susceptibility to falling that may cause physical harm

Risk Factors

Adults
History of falls
Wheelchair use; use of assistive devices (e.g., walker, cane)
Age 65 or over; lives alone
Lower limb prosthesis

Physiological
Presence of acute illness; postoperative conditions
Visual or hearing difficulties
Arthritis
Orthostatic hypotension; faintness when turning or extending neck
Sleeplessness
Anemias; vascular disease
Neoplasms (i.e., fatigue/limited mobility)
Urgency; incontinence; diarrhea
Postprandial blood sugar changes
Impaired physical mobility; foot problems; decreased lower extremity strength
Impaired balance; difficulty with gait; proprioceptive deficits [e.g., unilateral neglect]
Neuropathy

Cognitive
Diminished mental status [e.g., confusion, delirium, dementia, impaired reality testing]

Information that appears in brackets has been added by the authors to clarify and enhance the use of nursing diagnoses.

 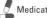

Medications
Antihypertensive agents; angiotensin-converting enzyme
(ACE) inhibitors; diuretics; tricyclic antidepressants; anti-
anxiety agents; hypnotics; tranquilizers; narcotics/opiates
Alcohol use

Environment
Restraints
Weather conditions (e.g., wet floors, ice)
Cluttered environment; throw rugs; no antislip material in bath/
shower
Unfamiliar or dimly lit room

Children
<2 years of age; male gender when <1 year of age
Lack of gate on stairs, window guards, auto restraints
Unattended infant on elevated surface (e.g., bed/changing ta-
ble); bed located near window
Lack of parental supervision

> **NOTE:** A risk diagnosis is not evidenced by signs and
> symptoms, as the problem has not occurred; rather,
> nursing interventions are directed at prevention.

Desired Outcomes/Evaluation Criteria— Client/Caregivers Will:

- Verbalize understanding of individual risk factors that con-
tribute to possibility of falls.
- Demonstrate behaviors, lifestyle changes to reduce risk fac-
tors and protect self from injury.
- Modify environment as indicated to enhance safety.
- Be free of injury.

Actions/Interventions

Nursing Priority No. 1.
To evaluate source/degree of risk:
- Observe individual's general health status, **noticing factors
that might affect safety, such as chronic or debilitating
conditions, use of multiple medications, recent trauma.**
- ∞ Note factors associated with age, gender, and developmental
level. **Infants, young children (e.g., climbing on objects),**

Information that appears in brackets has been added by the authors to clarify
and enhance the use of nursing diagnoses.

⊕ Cultural ⓐ Collaborative 🏠 Community/Home Care

young adults (e.g., sports activities), and elderly are at greatest risk because of developmental issues and impaired or lack of ability to self-protect.

- Assess muscle strength, gross and fine motor coordination. Review history of past or current physical injuries (e.g., musculoskeletal injuries; orthopedic surgery) **altering coordination, gait, and balance.**

- Review history of prior falls associated with immobility, weakness, prolonged bedrest, sedentary lifestyle (changes in body due to disuse); unsafe environment **to predict current risk for falls.**

- Evaluate use, misuse, or failure to use assistive aids, when indicated. **Client may have assistive device, but is at high risk for falls while adjusting to altered body state and use of unfamiliar device; or might refuse to use devices for various reasons (e.g., waiting for help; perception of weakness).**

- Evaluate client's cognitive status (e.g., brain injury, neurological disorders; depression). **Affects ability to perceive own limitations or recognize danger.**

- Assess mood, coping abilities, personality styles. **Individual's temperament, typical behavior, stressors, and level of self-esteem can affect attitude toward safety issues, resulting in carelessness or increased risk-taking without consideration of consequences.**

- Ascertain client's/SO's level of knowledge about and attendance to safety needs. **May reveal lack of understanding, insufficient resources, or simple disregard for personal safety (e.g., "I can't watch him every minute; we can't hire a home assistant; it's not manly . . .").**

- Consider environmental hazards in the care setting and/or home/other environment. **Identifying needs or deficits provides opportunities for intervention and/or instruction (e.g., concerning clearing of hazards, intensifying client supervision, obtaining safety equipment, referring for vision evaluation).**

- Review results of various fall risk assessment tools (e.g., Functional Ambulation Profile [FAP]; the Johns Hopkins Hospital Fall Risk Assessment Tool; Tinetti Balance and Gait Assessment [not a comprehensive listing]).

- Note socioeconomic status and availability and use of resources in other circumstances. **Can affect current coping abilities.**

Information that appears in brackets has been added by the authors to clarify and enhance the use of nursing diagnoses.

Nursing Priority No. 2.

To assist client/caregiver to reduce or correct individual risk factors:

- Assist in treatments and provide information regarding client's disease/condition(s) **that may result in increased risk of falls.**
- Discuss consequences of previously determined risk factors (e.g., falls caused by failure to make provisions for previously identified impairments or safety needs) **for follow-up instruction or interventions.**
- Review medication regimen and how it affects client. Instruct in monitoring of effects and side effects. **Use of certain medications (e.g., narcotics/opiates, psychotropics, antihypertensives, diuretics) can contribute to weakness, confusion, balance and gait disturbances).**
- Stress importance of monitoring conditions and risks that may contribute to occurrence of falls (e.g., client fatigue; acute illness; depression; objects that block traffic patterns in home; insufficient lighting; unfamiliar surroundings; client attempting tasks that are too difficult for present level of functioning; unable to contact someone when help is needed).
- Practice client safety. **Demonstrates behaviors for client/caregiver(s) to emulate.**
- Determine caregiver's expectations of children, cognitively impaired, and/or elderly family members and compare with actual abilities. **Reality of client's abilities and needs may be different than perception or desires of caregivers.**
- Discuss need for and sources of supervision (e.g., babysitters, before- and after-school programs, elderly day care, personal companions).
- Perform home visit when appropriate. Determine that home safety issues are addressed, including supervision, access to emergency assistance, and client's ability to manage self-care in the home. **May be needed to adequately determine client's needs and available resources.**
- Refer to rehabilitation team, physical or occupational therapist, as appropriate, **to improve client's balance, strength, or mobility; to improve or relearn ambulation; to identify and obtain appropriate assistive devices for mobility, environmental safety, or home modification.**

Nursing Priority No. 3.

To promote wellness (Teaching/Discharge Considerations):

- Refer to other resources as indicated. **Client/caregivers may need financial assistance, home modifications, referrals for**

Information that appears in brackets has been added by the authors to clarify and enhance the use of nursing diagnoses.

   Cultural Collaborative Community/Home Care

counseling, home care, sources for safety equipment, or placement in extended-care facility.

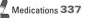• Provide educational resources (e.g., home safety checklist; equipment directions for proper use, appropriate Web sites) **for later review and reinforcement of learning.**

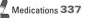• Promote community awareness about the problems of design of buildings, equipment, transportation, and workplace accidents that contribute to falls.

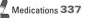• Connect client/family with community resources, neighbors, friends **to assist elderly or handicapped individuals in providing such things as structural maintenance and clearing of snow, gravel, or ice from walks and steps.**

Documentation Focus

Assessment/Reassessment
* Individual risk factors noting current physical findings (e.g., signs of injury—bruises, cuts; anemia, fatigue; use of alcohol, drugs, and prescription medications).
* Client's/caregiver's understanding of individual risks and safety concerns.

Planning
* Plan of care and who is involved in planning.
* Teaching plan.

Implementation/Evaluation
* Individual responses to interventions, teaching, and actions performed.
* Specific actions and changes that are made.
* Attainment or progress toward desired outcomes.
* Modifications to plan of care.

Discharge Planning
* Long-term plans for discharge needs, lifestyle, home setting and community changes, and who is responsible for actions to be taken.
* Specific referrals made.

Sample Nursing Outcomes & Interventions Classifications (NOC/NIC) NIC

NOC—Fall Prevention Behavior
NIC—Fall Prevention

Information that appears in brackets has been added by the authors to clarify and enhance the use of nursing diagnoses.

dysfunctional Family Processes

Taxonomy II: Role Relationships—Class 2 Family
  Relationships (00063)
[Diagnostic Division: Social Interaction]
Submitted as dysfunction Family Processes: Alcoholism
  1994; name change 2008

Definition: Psychosocial, spiritual, and physiological
functions of the family unit are chronically disorganized,
which leads to conflict, denial of problems, resistance to
change, ineffective problem solving, and a series of self-
perpetuating crises

Related Factors

Abuse of alcohol, [addictive substances]
Family history of alcoholism/resistance to treatment
Inadequate coping skills; addictive personality; lack of prob-
  lem-solving skills
Biochemical influences; genetic predisposition

Defining Characteristics

Subjective

Feelings
Anxiety, tension, distress; decreased self-esteem; worthless-
  ness; lingering resentment
Anger; suppressed rage; frustration; shame; embarrassment;
  hurt; unhappiness; guilt
Emotional isolation; loneliness; powerlessness; insecurity;
  hopelessness; rejection
Responsibility for alcoholic's behavior; vulnerability; mistrust
Depression; hostility; fear; confusion; dissatisfaction; loss
Being different from other people; misunderstood
Emotional control by others; being unloved; lack of identity
Abandonment; confused love and pity; moodiness; failure

Roles and Relationships
Family denial; deterioration in family relationships; disturbed
  family dynamics; ineffective spouse communication; marital
  problems; intimacy dysfunction
Altered role function; disrupted family roles; inconsistent parenting; low perception of parental support; chronic family
  problems

Information that appears in brackets has been added by the authors to clarify
and enhance the use of nursing diagnoses.

🌐 Cultural ♨ Collaborative 🏠 Community/Home Care

Lack of skills necessary for relationships; lack of cohesiveness; disrupted family rituals

Pattern of rejection; economic problems; neglected obligations

Objective

Feelings
Repressed emotions

Roles and Relationships
Closed communication systems

Triangulating family relationships; reduced ability of family members to relate to each other for mutual growth and maturation

Family does not demonstrate respect for individuality/autonomy of its members

Behavioral
Alcohol abuse; substance abuse other than alcohol; nicotine addiction

Enabling maintenance of alcohol drinking pattern, [substance use]; inadequate understanding of, or deficient knowledge about, alcoholism, [substance abuse]

Family special occasions are alcohol centered

Rationalization; denial of problems; refusal to get help; inability to accept or receive help appropriately

Inappropriate expression of anger; blaming; criticizing; verbal abuse of children, spouse, or parent

Lying; broken promises; lack of reliability; manipulation; dependency

Inability to express or accept wide range of feelings; difficulty with intimate relationships; diminished physical contact

Harsh self-judgment; difficulty having fun; self-blaming; isolation; unresolved grief; seeking approval or affirmation

Impaired communication; controlling, contradictory, or paradoxical communication; power struggles

Ineffective problem-solving skills; lack of dealing with conflict; orientation toward tension relief rather than achievement of goals; agitation; escalating conflict; chaos

Disturbances in concentration; disturbances in academic performance in children; failure to accomplish developmental tasks; difficulty with life cycle transitions

Inability to meet emotional, security, or spiritual needs of its members

---

Information that appears in brackets has been added by the authors to clarify and enhance the use of nursing diagnoses.

Inability to adapt to change; immaturity; stress-related physical illnesses; inability to accept health; inability to deal constructively with traumatic experiences

Desired Outcomes/Evaluation Criteria— Family Will:

- Verbalize understanding of dynamics of codependence.
- Participate in individual/family treatment programs.
- Identify ineffective coping behaviors and consequences of choices and actions.
- Demonstrate and plan for necessary lifestyle changes.
- Take action to change self-destructive behaviors and alter behaviors that contribute to client's drinking or substance use.
- Demonstrate improvement in parenting skills.

Actions/Interventions

Nursing Priority No. 1.

To assess contributing factors/underlying problem(s):

- Assess current level of functioning of family members.
- Ascertain family's understanding of current situation; note results of previous involvement in treatment.
- Review family history, explore roles of family members and circumstances involving substance use.
- Determine history of accidents or violent behaviors within family and safety issues.
- Discuss current and past methods of coping. **May be able to identify methods that would be useful in the current situation.**
- Determine extent and understanding of enabling behaviors being evidenced by family members.
- Identify sabotage behaviors of family members. **Issues of secondary gain (conscious or unconscious) may impede recovery.**
- Note presence and extent of behaviors of family, client, and self that might be "too helpful," such as frequent requests for help, excuses for not following through on agreed-on behaviors, feelings of anger or irritation with others. **Enabling behaviors can complicate acceptance and resolution of problem.**

Information that appears in brackets has been added by the authors to clarify and enhance the use of nursing diagnoses.

   Cultural   Collaborative   Community/Home Care

Nursing Priority No. 2.
To assist family to change destructive behaviors:

- Mutually agree on behaviors and responsibilities for nurse and client. **Maximizes understanding of what is expected of each individual.**
- Confront and examine denial and sabotage behaviors used by family members. **Helps individuals recognize and move beyond blocks to recovery.**
- Discuss use of anger, rationalization, and/or projection and ways in which these interfere with problem resolution.
- Encourage family to deal with anger **to prevent escalation to violence.** Problem-solve concerns.
- Determine family strengths, areas for growth, individual/family successes.
- Remain nonjudgmental in approach to family members and to member who uses alcohol/drugs.
- Provide information regarding effects of addiction on mood/personality of the involved person. **Helps family members understand and cope with negative behaviors without being judgmental or reacting angrily.**
- Distinguish between destructive aspects of enabling behavior and genuine motivation to aid the user.
- Identify use of manipulative behaviors and discuss ways to avoid or prevent these situations. **Manipulation has the goal of controlling others; when family members accept self-responsibility and commit to stop using it, new healthy behaviors will ensue.**

Nursing Priority No. 3.
To promote wellness (Teaching/Discharge Considerations):

- Provide factual information to client/family about the effects of addictive behaviors on the family and what to expect after discharge.
- Provide information about enabling behavior, addictive disease characteristics for both user and nonuser who is codependent.
- Discuss importance of restructuring life activities, work/leisure relationships. **Previous lifestyle/relationships supported substance use, requiring change to prevent relapse.**
- Encourage family to refocus celebrations excluding alcohol use **to reduce risk of relapse.**
- Provide support for family members; encourage participation in group work. **Involvement in a group provides**

Information that appears in brackets has been added by the authors to clarify and enhance the use of nursing diagnoses.

information about how others are dealing with problems, provides role models, and gives individual an opportunity to practice new healthy skills.

- Encourage involvement with, and refer to, self-help groups (e.g., Al-Anon, AlaTeen, Narcotics Anonymous, family therapy groups) **to provide ongoing support and assist with problem solving.**
- Provide bibliotherapy as appropriate.
- In addition, refer to NDs interrupted Family Processes; compromised/disabled family Coping, as appropriate.

Documentation Focus

Assessment/Reassessment
- Assessment findings, including history of substance(s) that have been used and family risk factors and safety concerns.
- Family composition and involvement.
- Results of prior treatment involvement.

Planning
- Plan of care and who is involved in planning.
- Teaching plan.

Implementation/Evaluation
- Responses of family members to treatment, teaching, and actions performed.
- Attainment or progress toward desired outcome(s).
- Modifications to plan of care.

Discharge Planning
- Long-term needs, who is responsible for actions to be taken.
- Specific referrals made.

Sample Nursing Outcomes & Interventions Classifications (NOC/NIC) NIC

NOC—Family Support During Treatment
NIC—Substance Use Treatment

Information that appears in brackets has been added by the authors to clarify and enhance the use of nursing diagnoses.

Cultural   Collaborative   Community/Home Care

interrupted Family Processes

Taxonomy II: Role Relationships—Class 2 Family
  Relationships (00060)
[Diagnostic Division: Social Interactions]
Submitted 1982; Nursing Diagnosis Extension and
  Classification (NDEC) Revision 1998

Definition: Change in family relationships and/or
functioning

Related Factors

Situational transition or crises [e.g., economic, change in roles,
  illness, trauma, disabling, or expensive treatments]
Developmental transition or crises [e.g., loss or gain of a family
  member, adolescence, leaving home for college]
Shift in health status of a family member
Family roles shift; power shift of family members
Modification in family finances or status
Interaction with community

Defining Characteristics

Subjective

Changes in: power alliances; satisfaction with family; expressions of conflict within family; effectiveness in completing
  assigned tasks; stress-reduction behaviors; expressions of
  conflict with or isolation from community resources; somatic
  complaints
Family expresses confusion about what to do; verbalizes they
  are having difficulty responding to change

Objective

Changes in: assigned tasks; participation in problem solving or
  decision making; communication patterns; mutual support;
  availability for emotional support or effective responsiveness; patterns; rituals; intimacy

Desired Outcomes/Evaluation Criteria—
Family Will:

• Express feelings freely and appropriately.
• Demonstrate individual involvement in problem-solving processes directed at appropriate solutions for the situation or
  crisis.

Information that appears in brackets has been added by the authors to clarify
and enhance the use of nursing diagnoses.

Diagnostic Studies   Pediatric/Geriatric/Lifespan   Medications **343**

- Direct energies in a purposeful manner to plan for resolution of the crisis.
- Verbalize understanding of condition, treatment regimen, and prognosis.
- Encourage and allow effected member to handle situation in own way, progressing toward independence.

Actions/Interventions

Nursing Priority No. 1.
To assess individual situation for causative/contributing factors:

- Determine pathophysiology, illness/trauma, developmental crisis present.
- Identify family developmental stage (e.g., marriage, birth of a child, children leaving home). **Provides baseline for establishing plan of care.**
- Note components of family: parent(s), children, male/female, extended family available.
- Observe patterns of communication in family. Are feelings expressed? Freely? Who talks to whom? Who makes decisions? For whom? Who visits? When? What is the interaction between family members? **Identifies weakness/areas of concern to be addressed as well as strengths that can be used for resolution of problem.**
- Assess boundaries of family members. Do members share family identity and have little sense of individuality? Do they seem emotionally distant, not connected with one another? **Answers to these questions help identify specific problems needing to be addressed.**
- Ascertain role expectations of family members. Who is the ill member (e.g., nurturer, provider)? How does the illness affect the roles of others?
- Identify "family rules." For example, how adult concerns (finances, illness, etc.) are kept from the children.
- Determine effectiveness of parenting skills and parents' expectations.
- Note energy direction. Are efforts at resolution/problem solving purposeful or scattered?
- Listen for expressions of despair or helplessness (e.g., "I don't know what to do") **to note degree of distress and inability to handle what is happening.**
- Note cultural and/or religious factors **that may affect perceptions/expectations of family members.**

Information that appears in brackets has been added by the authors to clarify and enhance the use of nursing diagnoses.

Cultural Collaborative Community/Home Care

- Assess availability and use of support systems outside of the family.

Nursing Priority No. 2.

To assist family to deal with situation/crisis:

- Deal with family members in warm, caring, respectful way.
- Acknowledge difficulties and realities of the situation. **Reinforces that some degree of conflict is to be expected and can be used to promote growth.**
- Encourage expressions of anger. Avoid taking comments personally as the client is usually only angry at the situation over which he or she has little or no control. **Maintains boundaries between nurse and family.**
- Stress importance of continuous, open dialogue between family members **to facilitate ongoing problem solving.**
- Provide information, as necessary, in verbal and written formats. Reinforce as necessary.
- Assist family to identify and encourage their use of previously successful coping behaviors.
- Recommend contact by family members on a regular, frequent basis.
- Arrange for and encourage family participation in multidisciplinary team conference or group therapy, as appropriate.
- Involve family in social support and community activities of their interest and choice.

Nursing Priority No. 3.

To promote wellness (Teaching/Discharge Considerations):

- Encourage use of stress-management techniques (e.g., appropriate expression of feelings, relaxation exercises).
- Provide educational materials and information **to assist family members in resolution of current crisis.**
- Refer to classes (e.g., parent effectiveness, specific disease/disability support groups, self-help groups, clergy, psychological counseling, family therapy), as indicated.
- Assist family to identify situations that may lead to fear or anxiety. (Refer to NDs Fear; Anxiety.)
- Involve family in planning for future and mutual goal setting. **Promotes commitment to goals/continuation of plan.**
- Identify community agencies (e.g., Meals on Wheels, visiting nurse, trauma support group, American Cancer Society, Veterans Administration) for both immediate and long-term support.

Information that appears in brackets has been added by the authors to clarify and enhance the use of nursing diagnoses.

Documentation Focus

Assessment/Reassessment
- Assessment findings, including family composition, developmental stage of family, and role expectations.
- Family communication patterns.

Planning
- Plan of care, specific interventions, and who is involved in planning.
- Teaching plan.

Implementation/Evaluation
- Each individual's response to interventions, teaching, and actions performed.
- Attainment or progress toward desired outcome(s).
- Modifications to plan of care.

Discharge Planning
- Long-term needs, noting who is responsible for actions to be taken.
- Specific referrals made.

Sample Nursing Outcomes & Interventions Classifications (NOC/NIC) NIC

NOC—Family Functioning
NIC—Family Process Maintenance

readiness for enhanced Family Processes

Taxonomy II: Role Relationships—Class 2 Family Relationships (00159)
[Diagnostic Division: Social Interaction]
Submitted 2002

Definition: A pattern of family functioning that is sufficient to support the well-being of family members and can be strengthened

Defining Characteristics

Subjective
Expresses willingness to enhance family dynamics
Communication is adequate

Information that appears in brackets has been added by the authors to clarify and enhance the use of nursing diagnoses.

Cultural   Collaborative   Community/Home Care

Relationships are generally positive; interdependent with community; family tasks are accomplished

Energy level of family supports activities of daily living

Family adapts to change

Objective

Family functioning meets needs of family members

Activities support the safety, growth of family members

Family roles are appropriate, flexible for developmental stages

Family resilience is evident

Respect for family members is evident

Boundaries of family members are maintained

Balance exists between autonomy and cohesiveness

Desired Outcomes/Evaluation Criteria— Client Will:

- Express feelings freely and appropriately.
- Verbalize understanding of desire for enhanced family dynamics.
- Demonstrate individual involvement in problem solving to improve family communications.
- Acknowledge awareness of and respect for boundaries of family members.

Actions/Interventions

Nursing Priority No. 1.

To determine status of family:

- Determine family composition: parent(s), children, male/female, extended family. **Many family forms exist in society today, such as biological, nuclear, single-parent, step-family, communal, and same-sex couple or family. A better way to determine a family may be to determine the attribute of affection, strong emotional ties, a sense of belonging, and durability of membership.**
- Identify participating members of family and how they define family. **Establishes members of family who need to be directly involved/taken into consideration when developing plan of care to improve family functioning.**
- ∞ Note stage of family development (e.g., single, young adult, newly married, family with young children, family with adolescents, grown children, later in life).

Information that appears in brackets has been added by the authors to clarify and enhance the use of nursing diagnoses.

- Ascertain motivation and expectations for change.
- Observe patterns of communication in the family. Are feelings expressed? Freely? Who talks to whom? Who makes decisions? For whom? Who visits? When? What is the interaction between family members? **Identifies possible weaknesses to be addressed, as well as strengths that can be used for improving family communication.**
- Assess boundaries of family members. Do members share family identity and have little sense of individuality? Do they seem emotionally connected with one another? **Individuals need to respect one another and boundaries need to be clear so family members are free to be responsible for themselves.**
- Identify "family rules" that are accepted in the family. **Families interact in certain ways over time and develop patterns of behavior that are accepted as the way "we behave" in this family. "Functional family" rules are constructive and promote the needs of all family members.**
- Note energy direction. **Efforts at problem solving and resolution of different opinions may be purposeful or may be scattered and ineffective.**
- Determine cultural and/or religious factors influencing family interactions. **Expectations related to socioeconomic beliefs may be different in various cultures. For instance, traditional views of marriage and family life may be strongly influenced by Roman Catholicism in Italian-American and Latino-American families. In some cultures, the father is considered the authority figure and the mother is the homemaker. These beliefs may change with stressors or circumstances (e.g., financial, loss or gain of a family member, personal growth).**
- Note health of married individuals. **Recent reports have determined that marriage increases life expectancy by as much as 5 years.**

Nursing Priority No. 2.

To assist the family to improve interactions:

- Establish nurse-family relationship. **Promotes a warm, caring atmosphere in which family members can share thoughts, ideas, and feelings openly and nonjudgmentally.**
- Acknowledge realities, and possible difficulties, of individual situation. **Reinforces that some degree of conflict is to be**

Information that appears in brackets has been added by the authors to clarify and enhance the use of nursing diagnoses.

Cultural Collaborative Community/Home Care

expected in family interactions that can be used to promote growth.

- Stress importance of continuous, open dialogue between family members. **Facilitates ongoing expression of open, honest feelings and opinions and effective problem solving.**

- Assist family to identify and encourage use of previously successful coping behaviors. **Promotes recognition of previous successes and confidence in own abilities to learn and improve family interactions.**

- Acknowledge differences among family members with open dialogue about how these differences have occurred. **Conveys an acceptance of these differences among individuals and helps to look at how they can be used to strengthen the family.**

- Identify effective parenting skills already being used and additional ways of handling difficult behaviors. **Allows individual family members to realize that some of what has been done already has been helpful and encourages them to learn new skills to manage family interactions in a more effective manner.**

Nursing Priority No. 3.
To promote optimum well-being:

 • Discuss and encourage use and participation in stress-management techniques. **Relaxation exercises, visualization, and similar skills can be useful for promoting reduction of anxiety and ability to manage stress that occurs in their lives.**

• Encourage participation in learning role-reversal activities. **Helps individuals to gain insight and understanding of other person's feelings and perspective/point of view.**

• Involve family members in setting goals and planning for the future. **When individuals are involved in the decision making, they are more committed to carrying out a plan to enhance family interactions as life goes on.**

• Provide educational materials and information. **Enhances learning to assist in developing positive relationships among family members.**

• Assist family members to identify situations that may create problems and lead to stress/anxiety. **Thinking ahead can help individuals anticipate helpful actions to handle/prevent conflict and untoward consequences.**

Information that appears in brackets has been added by the authors to clarify and enhance the use of nursing diagnoses.

• Refer to classes/support groups, as appropriate. **Family effectiveness, self-help, psychology, and religious affiliations can provide role models and new information to enhance family interactions.**

Documentation Focus

Assessment/Reassessment
• Assessment findings, including family composition, developmental stage of family, and role expectations.
• Cultural or religious values and beliefs regarding family and family functioning.
• Family communication patterns.
• Motivation and expectations for change.

Planning
• Plan of care, specific interventions, and who is involved in planning.
• Educational plan.

Implementation/Evaluation
• Each individual's response to interventions, teaching, and actions performed.
• Attainment or progress toward desired outcome(s).
• Modifications to lifestyle.
• Changes in treatment plan.

Discharge Planning
• Long-term needs, noting who is responsible for actions to be taken.
• Specific referrals made.

Sample Nursing Outcomes & Interventions Classifications (NOC/NIC) NIC

NOC—Family Social Climate
NIC—Family Support

Information that appears in brackets has been added by the authors to clarify
and enhance the use of nursing diagnoses.

Cultural Collaborative Community/Home Care

Fatigue

Taxonomy II: Activity/Rest—Class 3 Energy Balance
(00093)
[Diagnostic Division: Activity/Rest]
Submitted 1988; Nursing Diagnosis Extension and
Classification (NDEC) Revision 1998

Definition: An overwhelming sustained sense of exhaustion and decreased capacity for physical and mental
work at usual level

Related Factors

Psychological
Stress; anxiety; boring lifestyle; depression

Environmental
Noise; lights; humidity; temperature

Situational
Occupation; negative life events

Physiological
Increased physical exertion; sleep deprivation
Pregnancy; disease states; malnutrition; anemia
Poor physical condition
Altered body chemistry (e.g., medications, drug withdrawal,
chemotherapy)

Defining Characteristics

Subjective
Verbalization of an unremitting or overwhelming lack of energy; inability to maintain usual routines or level of physical
activity
Perceived need for additional energy to accomplish routine
tasks; increase in rest requirements
Tired; inability to restore energy even after sleep
Feelings of guilt for not keeping up with responsibilities
Compromised libido
Increase in physical complaints

Information that appears in brackets has been added by the authors to clarify
and enhance the use of nursing diagnoses.

Objective

Lethargic; listless; drowsy; lack of energy
Compromised concentration
Disinterest in surroundings; introspection
Decreased performance [accident prone]

Desired Outcomes/Evaluation Criteria— Client Will:

- Report improved sense of energy.
- Identify basis of fatigue and individual areas of control.
- Perform activities of daily living and participate in desired activities at level of ability.
- Participate in recommended treatment program.

Actions/Interventions

Nursing Priority No. 1.

To assess causative/contributing factors:

- Identify presence of physical and/or psychological conditions (e.g., pregnancy; infectious processes; blood loss, anemia; connective tissue disorders [e.g., MS, lupus]; trauma, chronic pain syndromes [e.g., arthritis]; cardiopulmonary disorders; cancer and cancer treatments; hepatitis; AIDS; major depressive disorder; anxiety states; substance use or abuse).
- Note age, gender, and developmental stage. **Although some studies show a prevalence of fatigue in adolescent girls, the condition may be present in any person at any age.**
- Review medication regimen/use. **Certain medications, including prescription (especially beta-adrenergic blockers, chemotherapy), OTC drugs, herbal supplements, and combinations of drugs and/or substances, are known to cause and/or exacerbate fatigue.**
- Ascertain client's belief about what is causing the fatigue.
- Assess vital signs **to evaluate fluid status and cardiopulmonary response to activity.**
- Determine presence/degree of sleep disturbances. **Fatigue can be a consequence of, and/or exacerbated by, sleep deprivation.**
- Note recent lifestyle changes, including conflicts (e.g., expanded responsibilities, demands of others, job-related conflicts); maturational issues (e.g., adolescent with eating disorder); and developmental issues (e.g., new parenthood, loss of spouse/SO).

Information that appears in brackets has been added by the authors to clarify and enhance the use of nursing diagnoses.

⊕ Cultural Ⓐ Collaborative 🏠 Community/Home Care

- Assess psychological and personality factors that may affect reports of fatigue level.
- Evaluate aspect of "learned helplessness" that may be manifested by giving up. **Can perpetuate a cycle of fatigue, impaired functioning, and increased anxiety and fatigue.**

Nursing Priority No. 2.

To determine degree of fatigue/impact on life:

- Obtain client/SO descriptions of fatigue (i.e., lacking energy or strength, tiredness, weakness lasting over length of time). Note presence of additional concerns (e.g., irritability, lack of concentration, difficulty making decisions, problems with leisure, relationship difficulties) **to assist in evaluating impact on client's life.**
- Ask client to rate fatigue (1–10 scale) and its effects on ability to participate in desired activities.
- Discuss lifestyle changes or limitations imposed by fatigue state.
- Interview parent/caregiver regarding specific changes observed in child or elder client. **These individuals may not be able to verbalize feelings or relate meaningful information.**
- Note daily energy patterns (i.e., peaks and valleys). **Helpful in determining pattern/timing of activity.**
- Measure physiological response to activity (e.g., changes in blood pressure or heart and respiratory rate).
- Evaluate need for individual assistance or assistive devices.
- Review availability and current use of support systems and resources.
- Perform, or review results of, testing, such as the Multidimensional Assessment of Fatigue (MAF); Piper Fatigue Scale; Global Fatigue Index, as appropriate. **Can help determine manifestation, intensity, duration, and emotional meaning of fatigue.**

Nursing Priority No. 3.

To assist client to cope with fatigue and manage within individual limits of ability:

- Accept reality of client reports of fatigue, and do not underestimate effect on client's quality of life. **For example, clients with MS are prone to more frequent and severe fatigue following minimal energy expenditure and require a longer recovery period than is usual; postpolio clients**

Information that appears in brackets has been added by the authors to clarify and enhance the use of nursing diagnoses.

often display a cumulative effect if they fail to pace themselves and rest when early signs of fatigue develop.

- Establish realistic activity goals with client and encourage forward movement. **Enhances commitment to promoting optimal outcomes.**
- Plan interventions to allow individually adequate rest periods. Schedule activities for periods when client has the most energy **to maximize participation.**
- Involve client/SO(s) in schedule planning.
- Encourage client to do whatever possible (e.g., self-care, sit up in chair, go for walk, interact with family, play game). Increase activity level, as tolerated.
- Instruct in methods to conserve energy:

  Sit instead of stand during daily care and other activities.
  Carry several small loads instead of one large load.
  Combine and simplify activities.
  Take frequent, short breaks during activities.
  Delegate tasks.
  Ask for and accept assistance.
  Say "No" or "Later."
  Plan steps of activity before beginning so that all needed materials are at hand.

- Encourage use of assistive devices (e.g., wheeled walker, handicap parking spot, elevator, backpack for carrying objects), as needed, **to extend active time/conserve energy for other tasks.**
- Assist with self-care needs; keep bed in low position and travelways clear of furniture; assist with ambulation, as indicated.
- Avoid or limit exposure to temperature and humidity extremes, **which can negatively impact energy level.**
- Provide diversional activities. Avoid both over- and understimulation (cognitive and sensory). **Participating in pleasurable activities can refocus energy and diminish feelings of unhappiness, sluggishness, and worthlessness that can accompany fatigue.**
- Discuss routines to promote restful sleep. (Refer to ND Insomnia)
- Encourage nutritionally dense, easy to prepare and consume foods and avoidance of caffeine and high-sugar foods and beverages **to promote energy.**
- Instruct in/implement stress-management skills of visualization, relaxation, and biofeedback, when appropriate.
- Refer to comprehensive rehabilitation program, physical and occupational therapy for programmed daily exercises and

---

Information that appears in brackets has been added by the authors to clarify and enhance the use of nursing diagnoses.

activities **to improve stamina, strength, and muscle tone and to enhance sense of well-being.**

Nursing Priority No. 4.

To promote wellness (Teaching/Discharge Considerations):

- Discuss therapy regimen relating to individual causative factors (e.g., physical and/or psychological illnesses) and help client/SO(s) to understand relationship of fatigue to illness.
- Assist client/SO(s) to develop plan for activity and exercise within individual ability. Stress necessity of allowing sufficient time to finish activities.
- Instruct client in ways to monitor responses to activity and significant signs/symptoms **that indicate the need to alter activity level.**
- Promote overall health measures (e.g., nutrition, adequate fluid intake, appropriate vitamin and iron supplementation).
- Provide supplemental oxygen, as indicated. **Presence of anemia and hypoxemia reduces oxygen available for cellular uptake and contributes to fatigue.**
- Encourage client to develop assertiveness skills, to prioritize goals and activities, to learn to delegate duties or tasks, or to say "No." Discuss burnout syndrome, when appropriate, and actions client can take to change individual situation.
- Assist client to identify appropriate coping behaviors. **Promotes sense of control and improves self-esteem.**
- Identify support groups and community resources.
- Refer to counseling or psychotherapy, as indicated.
- Identify resources to assist with routine needs (e.g., Meals on Wheels, homemaker or housekeeper services, yard care).

Documentation Focus

Assessment/Reassessment

- Manifestations of fatigue and other assessment findings.
- Degree of impairment and effect on lifestyle.
- Expectations of client/SO(s) relative to individual abilities and specific condition.

Planning

- Plan of care, specific interventions, and who is involved in the planning.
- Teaching plan.

Information that appears in brackets has been added by the authors to clarify and enhance the use of nursing diagnoses.

Implementation/Evaluation

- Client's response to interventions, teaching, and actions performed.
- Attainment or progress toward desired outcome(s).
- Modifications to plan of care.

Discharge Planning

- Discharge needs/plan, actions to be taken, and who is responsible.
- Specific referrals made.

Sample Nursing Outcomes & Interventions Classifications (NOC/NIC) NIC

NOC—Endurance
NIC—Energy Management

> ### Fear [specify focus]
>
> Taxonomy II: Coping/Stress Tolerance—Class 2 Coping Responses (00148)
> [Diagnostic Division: Ego Integrity]
> Submitted 1980; Revised 2000
>
> **Definition:** Response to perceived threat [real or imagined] that is consciously recognized as a danger

Related Factors

Innate origin (e.g., sudden noise, height, pain, loss of physical support); innate releasers (neurotransmitters); phobic stimulus

Learned response (e.g., conditioning, modeling from or identification with others)

Unfamiliarity with environmental experience(s)

Separation from support system in potentially stressful situation (e.g., hospitalization, hospital procedures[/treatments])

Language barrier; sensory impairment

Defining Characteristics

Subjective

Report of apprehension; excitement; being scared; alarm; panic; terror; dread; decreased self-assurance; increased tension; jitteriness

---

Information that appears in brackets has been added by the authors to clarify and enhance the use of nursing diagnoses.

Cultural Collaborative Community/Home Care

Cognitive
Identifies object of fear; stimulus believed to be a threat

Physiological
Anorexia; nausea; fatigue; dry mouth; [palpitations]

Objective

Cognitive
Diminished productivity, learning ability, or problem solving

Behaviors
Increased alertness; avoidance behaviors; attack behaviors; impulsiveness; narrowed focus on the source of the fear

Physiological
Increased pulse; vomiting; diarrhea; muscle tightness; increased respiratory rate; dyspnea; increased systolic blood pressure; pallor; increased perspiration; pupil dilation

Desired Outcomes/Evaluation Criteria— Client Will:

- Acknowledge and discuss fears, recognizing healthy versus unhealthy fears.
- Verbalize accurate knowledge of and sense of safety related to current situation.
- Demonstrate understanding through use of effective coping behaviors (e.g., problem solving) and resources.
- Display appropriate range of feelings and lessened fear.

Actions/Interventions

Nursing Priority No. 1.
To assess degree of fear and reality of threat perceived by the client:

- Ascertain client's/SO's perception of what is occurring and how this affects life. **Fear is a defensive mechanism in protecting oneself but, if left unchecked, can become disabling to the client's life.**
- ∞ Determine client's age and developmental level. **Helps in understanding usual or typical fears experienced by individuals (e.g., toddler often has different fears than adolescent or older person suffering with dementia).**
- Note degree of incapacitation (e.g., "frozen with fear," inability to engage in necessary activities).
- Compare verbal and nonverbal responses **to note congruencies or misperceptions of situation.**

Information that appears in brackets has been added by the authors to clarify and enhance the use of nursing diagnoses.

- Be alert to signs of denial or depression.
- Identify sensory deficits that may be present, such as vision or hearing impairment. **Affects sensory reception and interpretation of environment.**
- Note degree of concentration, focus of attention.
- Investigate client's reports of subjective experiences, which could be indicative of delusions/hallucinations, **to help determine client's interpretation of surroundings and/or stimuli.**
- Be alert to and evaluate potential for violence.
- Measure vital signs and physiological responses to situation.
- Assess family dynamics. Refer to other NDs, such as interrupted Family Processes; readiness for enhanced family Coping; compromised or disabled family Coping; Anxiety.

Nursing Priority No. 2.
To assist client/SO(s) in dealing with fear/situation:

- Stay with the client or make arrangements to have someone else be there. **Providing client with usual or desired support persons can diminish feelings of fear.**
- Discuss client's perceptions and fearful feelings. Listen and Active-listen to client's concerns. **Promotes atmosphere of caring and permits explanation or correction of misperceptions.**
- Provide information in verbal and written form. Speak in simple sentences and concrete terms. **Facilitates understanding and retention of information.**
- Acknowledge normalcy of fear, pain, despair, and give "permission" to express feelings appropriately and freely. **Promotes attitude of caring, opens door for discussion about feelings and/or addressing reality of situation.**
- Provide opportunity for questions and answer honestly. **Enhances sense of trust and nurse-client relationship.**
- ∞• Provide presence and physical contact (e.g., hugging, refocusing attention, rocking a child), as appropriate, when painful procedures are anticipated **to soothe fears and provide assurance.**
- ∞• Modify procedures, if possible (e.g., substitute oral for intramuscular medications, combine blood draws or use finger-stick method), **to limit degree of stress, avoid overwhelming a fearful individual.**
- ∞• Manage environmental factors, such as loud noises, harsh lighting, changing person's location without knowledge of family/SO(s), strangers in care area, unfamiliar people, high

---

Information that appears in brackets has been added by the authors to clarify and enhance the use of nursing diagnoses.

traffic flow, **which can cause or exacerbate stress, especially to very young or to older individuals.**
* Present objective information, when available, and allow client to use it freely. Avoid arguing about client's perceptions of the situation. **Limits conflicts when fear response may impair rational thinking.**
* Promote client control, where possible, and help client identify and accept those things over which control is not possible. **Strengthens internal locus of control.**
* Encourage contact with a peer who has successfully dealt with a similarly fearful situation. **Provides a role model, and client is more likely to believe others who have had similar experience(s).**

Nursing Priority No. 3.
To assist client in learning to use own responses for problem solving:
* Acknowledge usefulness of fear for taking care of self.
* Identify client's responsibility for the solutions while reinforcing that the nurse will be available for help if desired or needed. **Enhances sense of control.**
* Determine internal and external resources for assistance (e.g., awareness and use of effective coping skills in the past; SOs who are available for support).
* Explain procedures within level of client's ability to understand and handle. (Be aware of how much information client wants **to prevent confusion or information overload.**)
* Explain relationship between disease and symptoms, if appropriate.
* Review use of antianxiety medications and reinforce use as prescribed.

Nursing Priority No. 4.
To promote wellness (Teaching/Discharge Considerations):
* Support planning for dealing with reality. **Assists in identifying areas in which control can be exercised and those in which control is not possible, thus enabling client to handle fearful situations/feelings.**
* Instruct in use of relaxation or visualization and guided imagery skills.
* Encourage regular physical activity within limits of ability. Refer to physical therapist to develop exercise program to meet individual needs. **Provides a healthy outlet for energy generated by fearful feelings and promotes relaxation.**

Information that appears in brackets has been added by the authors to clarify and enhance the use of nursing diagnoses.

- Provide for and deal with sensory deficits in appropriate manner (e.g., speak clearly and distinctly, use touch carefully, as indicated by situation).
- Refer to support groups, community agencies and organizations, as indicated. **Provides ongoing assistance for individual needs.**

Documentation Focus

Assessment/Reassessment
- Assessment findings, noting individual factors contributing to current situation, source of fear.
- Manifestations of fear.

Planning
- Plan of care and who is involved in the planning.
- Teaching plan.

Implementation/Evaluation
- Client's responses to treatment plan, interventions, and actions performed.
- Attainment or progress toward desired outcome(s).
- Modifications to plan of care.

Discharge Planning
- Long-term needs and who is responsible for actions to be taken.
- Specific referrals made.

Sample Nursing Outcomes & Interventions Classifications (NOC/NIC) NIC

NOC—Fear Self-Control
NIC—Anxiety Reduction

---

ineffective infant Feeding Pattern

Taxonomy II: Nutrition—Class 1 Ingestion (00107)
[Diagnostic Division: Food/Fluid]
Submitted 1992; Revised 2006

Definition: Impaired ability of an infant to suck or coordinate the suck/swallow response resulting in inadequate oral nutrition for metabolic needs

---

Information that appears in brackets has been added by the authors to clarify and enhance the use of nursing diagnoses.

  Cultural   Collaborative   Community/Home Care

Related Factors

Prematurity
Neurological impairment or delay
Oral hypersensitivity
Prolonged NPO
Anatomic abnormality

Defining Characteristics

Subjective
[Caregiver reports infant's inability to achieve an effective
suck]

Objective
Inability to initiate or sustain an effective suck
Inability to coordinate sucking, swallowing, and breathing

Desired Outcomes/Evaluation Criteria— Client Will:

* Display adequate output as measured by sufficient number of
wet diapers daily.
* Demonstrate appropriate weight gain.
* Be free of aspiration.

Actions/Interventions

Nursing Priority No. 1.
To identify contributing factors/degree of impaired function:

* Assess infant's suck, swallow, and gag reflexes. **Provides
comparative baseline and is useful in determining appropriate feeding method.**
* Note developmental age, structural abnormalities (e.g., cleft
lip/palate), mechanical barriers (e.g., ET tube, ventilator).
* Determine level of consciousness, neurological impairment,
seizure activity, presence of pain.
* Observe parent/infant interactions **to determine level of
bonding and comfort that could impact stress level during
feeding activity.**
* Note type and scheduling of medications **that could cause
sedative effect and impair feeding activity.**
* Compare birth and current weight and length measurements
to note progress.

Information that appears in brackets has been added by the authors to clarify
and enhance the use of nursing diagnoses.

 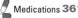

- Assess signs of stress when feeding (e.g., tachypnea, cyanosis, fatigue or lethargy).
- Note presence of behaviors indicating continued hunger after feeding.

Nursing Priority No. 2.

To promote adequate infant intake:

• Determine appropriate method for feeding (e.g., special nipple or feeding device, gavage or enteral tube feeding) and choice of breast milk or formula to meet infant needs.
- Review early infant feeding cues (e.g., rooting, lip smacking, sucking fingers or hand) versus late cue of crying. **Early recognition of infant hunger promotes timely/more rewarding feeding experience for infant and mother.**
- Demonstrate techniques and procedures for feeding. Note proper positioning of infant, "latching-on" techniques, rate of delivery of feeding, frequency of burping. (Refer to ND ineffective Breastfeeding, as appropriate.)
- Limit duration of feeding to maximum of 30 minutes based on infant's response (e.g., signs of fatigue) **to balance energy expenditure with nutrient intake.**
- Monitor caregiver's efforts. Provide feedback and assistance, as indicated. **Enhances learning, encourages continuation of efforts.**
- Refer nursing mother to lactation specialist for assistance and support in dealing with unresolved issues (e.g., teaching infant to suck).
- Emphasize importance of calm, relaxed environment during feeding **to reduce detrimental stimuli and enhance mother's and infant's focus on feeding activity.**
- Adjust frequency and amount of feeding according to infant's response. **Prevents stress associated with under- or overfeeding.**
- Advance diet, adding solids or thickening agent, as appropriate for age and infant needs.
- Alternate feeding techniques (e.g., nipple and gavage) according to infant's ability and level of fatigue.
- Alter medication/feeding schedules, as indicated, **to minimize sedative effects and have infant in alert state.**

Nursing Priority No. 3.

To promote wellness (Teaching/Discharge Considerations):

Information that appears in brackets has been added by the authors to clarify and enhance the use of nursing diagnoses.

⊕ Cultural ⊛ Collaborative 🏠 Community/Home Care

• Instruct caregiver in techniques to prevent or alleviate aspiration.

 • Discuss anticipated growth and development goals for infant, corresponding caloric needs.

 • Suggest monitoring infant's weight and nutrient intake periodically.

• Recommend participation in classes, as indicated (e.g., first aid, infant CPR).

• Refer to support groups (e.g., La Leche League, parenting support groups, stress reduction, or other community resources, as indicated).

 • Provide bibliotherapy and appropriate Web sites for further information.

Documentation Focus

Assessment/Reassessment
• Type and route of feeding, interferences to feeding and reactions.
• Infant's measurements.

Planning
• Plan of care, specific interventions, and who is involved in planning.
• Teaching plan.

Implementation/Evaluation
• Infant's response to interventions (e.g., amount of intake, weight gain, response to feeding) and actions performed.
• Caregiver's involvement in infant care, participation in activities, response to teaching.
• Attainment of or progress toward desired outcome(s).
• Modifications to plan of care.

Discharge Planning
• Long-term needs, referrals made, and who is responsible for follow-up actions.

Sample Nursing Outcomes & Interventions Classifications (NOC/NIC) NIC

NOC—Swallowing Status: Oral Phase
NIC—Nutrition Therapy

Information that appears in brackets has been added by the authors to clarify and enhance the use of nursing diagnoses.

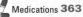

readiness for enhanced **Fluid Balance**

Taxonomy II: Nutrition—Class 5 Hydration (00160)
[Diagnostic Division: Food/Fluid]
Submitted 2002

Definition: A pattern of equilibrium between fluid volume and chemical composition of body fluids that is sufficient for meeting physical needs and can be strengthened

Related Factors

To be developed

Defining Characteristics

Subjective
Expresses willingness to enhance fluid balance
No excessive thirst

Objective
Stable weight; no evidence of edema
Moist mucous membranes
Intake adequate for daily needs
Straw-colored urine; specific gravity within normal limits; urine output appropriate for intake
Good tissue turgor; [no signs of] dehydration

Desired Outcomes/Evaluation Criteria—Client Will:

- Maintain fluid volume at a functional level as indicated by adequate urinary output, stable vital signs, moist mucous membranes, good skin turgor.
- Demonstrate behaviors to monitor fluid balance.
- Be free of thirst.
- Be free of evidence of fluid overload (e.g., absence of edema and adventitious lung sounds).

Actions/Interventions

Nursing Priority No. 1.
To determine potential for fluid imbalance and ways that client is managing:

Information that appears in brackets has been added by the authors to clarify and enhance the use of nursing diagnoses.

🌐 Cultural   🔘 Collaborative   🏠 Community/Home Care

- Note presence of factors with potential for fluid imbalance: (1) diagnoses or disease processes (e.g., hyperglycemia, ulcerative colitis, COPD, burns, cirrhosis of the liver, vomiting, diarrhea, hemorrhage), or situations (e.g., diuretic therapy, hot or humid climate, prolonged exercise, getting overheated or feverish, diuretic effect of caffeine and alcohol) that may lead to deficits; or (2) conditions or situations potentiating fluid excess (e.g., renal failure, cardiac failure, stroke, cerebral lesions, renal or adrenal insufficiency, psychogenic polydipsia, acute stress, surgical procedures, use of anesthesia, excessive or rapid infusion of IV fluids). **Body fluid balance is regulated by intake (food and fluid), output (kidney, gastrointestinal [GI] tract, skin, and lungs), and regulatory hormonal mechanisms. Balance is maintained within a relatively narrow margin and can be easily disrupted by multiple factors.**
- Determine potential effects of age and developmental stage. **Elderly individuals have less body water than younger adults, decreased thirst response, and reduced effectiveness of compensatory mechanisms (e.g., kidneys are less efficient in conserving sodium and water). Infants and children have a relatively higher percentage of total body water and metabolic rate and are often less able than adults to control their fluid intake.**
- Evaluate environmental factors that could impact fluid balance. **Persons with impaired mobility, diminished vision, or confined to bed cannot as easily meet their own needs and may be reluctant to ask for assistance. Persons whose work environment is restrictive or outside may also have greater challenges in meeting fluid needs.**
- Assess vital signs (e.g., temperature, blood pressure, heart rate), skin and mucous membrane moisture, and urine output. Weigh, as indicated. **Predictors of fluid balance that should be in client's usual range in a healthy state.**

Nursing Priority No. 2.
To prevent occurrence of imbalance:
- Monitor I&O (e.g., frequency of voids or diaper changes), as appropriate, being aware of insensible losses (e.g., diaphoresis in hot environment, use of oxygen, permanent tracheostomy), and "hidden sources" of intake (e.g., foods high in water content) **to ensure accurate picture of fluid status.**
- Weigh client and compare with recent weight history. **Provides baseline for future monitoring.**

Information that appears in brackets has been added by the authors to clarify and enhance the use of nursing diagnoses.

- Establish and review with client individual fluid needs and replacement schedule. **Active participation in planning for own needs enhances likelihood of adhering to plan.**
- Encourage regular oral intake (e.g., fluids between meals, additional fluids during hot weather or when exercising) **to maximize intake and maintain fluid balance.**
- Distribute fluids over 24-hour period in presence of fluid restriction. **Prevents peaks/valleys in fluid level and associated thirst.**
- Administer or discuss judicious use of medications, as indicated (e.g., antiemetics, antidiarrheals, antipyretics, diuretics). **Medications may be indicated to prevent fluid imbalance if individual becomes sick.**

Nursing Priority No. 3.
To promote optimum wellness:

- Discuss client's individual conditions and factors that could cause occurrence of fluid imbalance, as individually appropriate (such as prevention of hyperglycemic episodes) **so that client/SO can take corrective action.**
- Identify and instruct in ways to meet specific fluid needs (e.g., client could carry water bottle when going to sports events or measure specific 24-hour fluid portions if restrictions apply) **to manage fluid intake over time.**
- Recommend restriction of caffeine, alcohol, as indicated. **Prevents untoward diuretic effect and possible dehydration.**
- Instruct client/SO(s) in how to measure and record I&O, if needed for home management. **Provides means of monitoring status and adjusting therapy to meet changing needs.**
- Establish regular schedule for weighing **to help monitor changes in fluid status.**
- Identify actions (if any) client may take to correct imbalance. **Encourages responsibility for self-care.**
- Review any dietary needs or restrictions and safe substitutes for salt, as appropriate. **Helps prevent fluid retention/edema formation.**
- Review or instruct in medication regimen and administration, and discuss potential for interactions/side effects that could disrupt fluid balance.
- Instruct in signs and symptoms indicating need for immediate/further evaluation and follow-up care **to prevent complications and/or allow for early intervention.**

Information that appears in brackets has been added by the authors to clarify and enhance the use of nursing diagnoses.

Cultural Collaborative Community/Home Care

Documentation Focus

Assessment/Reassessment
- Individual findings, including factors affecting ability to manage (regulate) body fluids.
- I&O, fluid balance, changes in weight, and vital signs.

Planning
- Plan of care and who is involved in the planning.
- Teaching plan.

Implementation/Evaluation
- Client's responses to treatment, teaching, and actions performed.
- Attainment or progress toward desired outcome(s).
- Modifications to plan of care.

Discharge Planning
- Long-term needs, noting who is responsible for actions to be taken.
- Specific referrals made.

Sample Nursing Outcomes & Interventions Classifications (NOC/NIC) [NIC]

NOC—Fluid Balance
NIC—Fluid Monitoring

[deficient hyper/hypotonic Fluid Volume]

[Diagnostic Division: Food/Fluid]

Definition: [Decreased intravascular, interstitial, and/or intracellular fluid. This refers to dehydration with changes in sodium.]

NOTE: NANDA has restricted Fluid Volume, deficient, to address only isotonic dehydration. For client needs related to dehydration associated with alterations in sodium, the authors have provided this second diagnostic category.

Information that appears in brackets has been added by the authors to clarify and enhance the use of nursing diagnoses.

Related Factors

Hypertonic dehydration: uncontrolled diabetes mellitus/insipidus, hyperosmolar nonketotic diabetic coma (HHNC), increased intake of hypertonic fluids/IV therapy, inability to respond to thirst reflex, inadequate free water supplementation (high-osmolarity enteral feeding formulas), renal insufficiency or failure

Hypotonic dehydration: chronic illness, malnutrition, excessive use of hypotonic IV solutions (e.g., D5W), renal insufficiency

Defining Characteristics

Subjective
Reports of fatigue, nervousness, exhaustion
Thirst

Objective
Increased urine output, dilute urine (initially) and/or decreased output/oliguria
Weight loss
Decreased venous filling; [hypotension (postural)]
Increased pulse rate; decreased pulse volume and pressure
Decreased skin turgor; [dry skin/mucous membranes]
Increased body temperature
Change in mental status (e.g., confusion)
Hemoconcentration; altered serum sodium

Desired Outcomes/Evaluation Criteria— Client Will:

- Maintain fluid volume at a functional level, as evidenced by individually adequate urinary output, stable vital signs, moist mucous membranes, good skin turgor.
- Verbalize understanding of causative factors and purpose of individual therapeutic interventions and medications.
- Demonstrate behaviors to monitor and correct deficit, as indicated, when condition is chronic.

Actions/Interventions

Nursing Priority No. 1.
To assess causative/precipitating factors:

- Note possible conditions or processes that may lead to deficits: (1) fluid loss (e.g., diarrhea, vomiting, excessive

---

Information that appears in brackets has been added by the authors to clarify and enhance the use of nursing diagnoses.

🌐 Cultural 🐢 Collaborative 🏠 Community/Home Care

sweating; heat stroke; diabetic ketoacidosis; burns, other draining wounds; GI obstruction; salt-wasting diuretics; rapid breathing or mechanical ventilation; surgical drains); (2) limited intake (e.g., sore throat or mouth; client dependent on others for eating or drinking; NPO status); (3) fluid shifts (e.g., ascites, effusions, burns, sepsis); and (4) environmental factors (e.g., isolation, restraints, malfunctioning air conditioning, exposure to extreme heat).

 • Determine effects of age. **Very young and extremely elderly individuals are quickly affected by fluid volume deficit, and are least able to express need. For example, elderly people often have a decreased thirst reflex and/or may not be aware of water needs. Infants/young children and other nonverbal persons cannot describe thirst.**

• Evaluate nutritional status, noting current intake, weight changes, problems with oral intake, use of supplements/tube feedings. Measure subcutaneous fat and muscle mass.

Nursing Priority No. 2.

To evaluate degree of fluid deficit:

• Assess vital signs, including temperature (often elevated), pulse (may be elevated), and respirations. Note strength of peripheral pulses.

• Measure blood pressure (may be low) with the client lying, sitting, and standing, when possible, and monitor invasive hemodynamic parameters, as indicated (e.g., CVP, PAP/PCWP).

• Note presence of physical signs (e.g., dry mucous membranes, poor skin turgor, delayed capillary refill).

• Note change in usual mentation, behavior, or functional abilities (e.g., confusion, falling, loss of ability to carry out usual activities, lethargy, dizziness). **These signs indicate sufficient dehydration to cause poor cerebral perfusion and/or electrolyte imbalance.**

• Observe urinary output, color, and measure amount and specific gravity. Measure or estimate other fluid losses (e.g., gastric, respiratory, wound losses) **to more accurately determine replacement needs.**

• Review laboratory data (e.g., Hb/Hct; electrolytes [sodium, potassium, chloride, bicarbonate]; BUN; creatinine; total protein/albumin).

Nursing Priority No. 3.

To correct/replace fluid losses to reverse pathophysiological mechanisms:

Information that appears in brackets has been added by the authors to clarify and enhance the use of nursing diagnoses.

(A) • Assist with treatment of underlying conditions causing or contributing to dehydration and electrolyte imbalances.

(A) • Administer fluids and electrolytes, as indicated. **Fluids used for replacement depend on (1) the type of dehydration present (e.g., hypertonic or hypotonic) and (2) the degree of deficit determined by age, weight, and type of condition causing the deficit.**

• Establish 24-hour replacement needs and routes to be used (e.g., IV, PO, enteral feedings). **Steady rehydration over time prevents peaks and valleys in fluid level.**

• Note client preferences, and provide beverages and foods with high fluid content.

• Limit intake of alcohol and caffeinated beverages, **which tend to exert a diuretic effect.**

• Provide nutritious diet via appropriate route; give adequate free water with enteral feedings.

(A) • Maintain accurate intake and output (I&O), calculate 24-hour fluid balance, and weigh daily.

Nursing Priority No. 4.

To promote comfort and safety:

• Bathe less frequently, using mild cleanser or soap, and provide optimal skin care with suitable emollients **to maintain skin integrity and prevent excessive dryness.**

• Provide frequent oral and eye care **to prevent injury from dryness.**

• Change position frequently **to reduce pressure on fragile, dehydrated skin and tissues.**

• Provide for safety measures when client is confused.

(A) • Replace electrolytes, as ordered.

💊 • Administer or discontinue medications, as indicated, **when disease process or medications are contributing to dehydration.**

Nursing Priority No. 5.

To promote wellness (Teaching/Discharge Considerations):

🏠 • Discuss factors related to occurrence of deficit, as individually appropriate. **Early identification of risk factors can decrease occurrence and severity of complications associated with hypovolemia.**

🏠 • Identify and instruct in ways to meet specific nutritional needs.

🏠 • Instruct client/SO(s) in how to measure and record I&O, monitor fluid status.

Information that appears in brackets has been added by the authors to clarify and enhance the use of nursing diagnoses.

🌐 Cultural   (A) Collaborative   🏠 Community/Home Care

• Identify actions (if any) client may take to correct deficiencies.
• Review or instruct in medication regimen, administration, and interactions and side effects.
• Instruct in signs and symptoms indicating need for immediate or further evaluation and follow-up care.

Documentation Focus

Assessment/Reassessment
• Individual findings, including factors affecting ability to manage (regulate) body fluids and degree of deficit.
• I&O, fluid balance, changes in weight, urine specific gravity, and vital signs.
• Results of diagnostic testing and laboratory studies.

Planning
• Plan of care and who is involved in the planning.
• Teaching plan.

Implementation/Evaluation
• Client's responses to treatment, teaching, and actions performed.
• Attainment or progress toward desired outcome(s).
• Modifications to plan of care.

Discharge Planning
• Long-term needs, noting who is responsible for actions to be taken.
• Specific referrals made.

Sample Nursing Outcomes & Interventions Classifications (NOC/NIC) NIC

NOC—Fluid Balance
NIC—Fluid/Electrolyte Management

[deficient hyper/hypotonic FLUID VOLUME]

Information that appears in brackets has been added by the authors to clarify and enhance the use of nursing diagnoses.

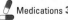

deficient Fluid Volume [isotonic]

NOTE: This diagnosis has been structured to address isotonic dehydration (hypovolemia) excluding states in which changes in sodium occur. For client needs related to dehydration associated with alterations in sodium, refer to [deficient Fluid Volume: hyper/hypotonic].

Taxonomy II: Nutrition—Class 5 Hydration (00027)
[Diagnostic Division: Food/Fluid]
Submitted 1978; Revised 1996

Definition: Decreased intravascular, interstitial, and/or intracellular fluid. This refers to dehydration, water loss alone without change in sodium.

Related Factors

Active fluid volume loss [e.g., hemorrhage, gastric intubation, acute or prolonged diarrhea, wounds, abdominal cancer; burns, fistulas, ascites (third spacing), use of hyperosmotic radiopaque contrast agents]

Failure of regulatory mechanisms [e.g., fever, thermoregulatory response, renal tubule damage]

Defining Characteristics

Subjective
Thirst
Weakness

Objective
Decreased urine output; increased urine concentration
Decreased venous filling; decreased pulse volume or pressure
Sudden weight loss (except in third spacing)
Decreased blood pressure; increased pulse rate, body temperature
Decreased skin or tongue turgor; dry skin and mucous membranes
Change in mental state
Elevated hematocrit (Hct)

Desired Outcomes/Evaluation Criteria— Client Will:

• Maintain fluid volume at a functional level as evidenced by individually adequate urinary output with normal specific

Information that appears in brackets has been added by the authors to clarify and enhance the use of nursing diagnoses.

⊕ Cultural ⊛ Collaborative ⌂ Community/Home Care

gravity, stable vital signs, moist mucous membranes, good skin turgor and prompt capillary refill, resolution of edema (e.g., ascites).
- Verbalize understanding of causative factors and purpose of individual therapeutic interventions and medications.
- Demonstrate behaviors to monitor and correct deficit, as indicated.

Actions/Interventions

Nursing Priority No. 1.
To assess causative/precipitating factors:
- Note possible diagnoses that may create a fluid volume deficit (e.g., diarrhea, ulcerative colitis, burns, cirrhosis of the liver, abdominal cancer) and other factors (e.g., bleeding or drainage from wounds and fistulas or suction devices, hemorrhage, water deprivation, fluid restrictions, vomiting, dialysis, decreased level of consciousness, prolonged exercise, increased metabolic rate secondary to fever, hot or humid climate, overuse of diuretics, caffeine or alcohol).
- Determine effects of age. **Elderly individuals are at higher risk because of decreasing response and effectiveness of compensatory mechanisms (e.g., kidneys are less efficient in conserving sodium and water). Infants and children have a relatively high percentage of total body water, are sensitive to loss, and are less able to control their fluid intake.**

Nursing Priority No. 2.
To evaluate degree of fluid deficit:
- Estimate traumatic or procedural fluid losses and note possible routes of insensible fluid losses.
- Assess vital signs, noting low blood pressure—severe hypotension, rapid heart beat, and thready peripheral pulses. **These changes in vital signs are associated with fluid volume loss and/or hypovolemia.**
- Note complaints and physical signs associated with dehydration (e.g., scanty, concentrated urine; lack of tears when crying [infant, child]; dry, sticky mucous membranes; lack of sweating; delayed capillary refill; poor skin turgor; confusion; sleepiness; lethargy; muscle weakness; dizziness or lightheadedness; headache).
- Compare usual and current weight.
- Measure abdominal girth when ascites or third spacing of fluid occurs. Assess for peripheral edema formation.

Information that appears in brackets has been added by the authors to clarify and enhance the use of nursing diagnoses.

• Review laboratory data (e.g., hemoglobin [Hb]/Hct, electrolytes, total protein or albumin, BUN/Cr).

Nursing Priority No. 3.

To correct/replace losses to reverse pathophysiological mechanisms:

- Stop blood loss (e.g., gastric lavage with room temperature or cool saline solution, drug administration) and prepare for surgical intervention.
- Establish 24-hour fluid replacement needs and routes to be used. **Prevents peaks and valleys in fluid level.**
- Note client preferences regarding fluids and foods with high fluid content.
- Keep fluids within client's reach and encourage frequent intake, as appropriate.
- Administer IV fluids, as indicated. Replace blood products, administer plasma expanders, as ordered.
- Control humidity and ambient air temperature, as appropriate, especially when major burns are present; or increase or decrease in presence of fever. Reduce bedding and clothes; provide tepid sponge bath. Assist with hypothermia, when ordered, **to reduce high fever and elevated metabolic rate.** (Refer to ND Hyperthermia.)
- Maintain accurate I&O and weigh daily. Monitor urine specific gravity.
- Monitor vital signs (lying/sitting/standing) and invasive hemodynamic parameters, as indicated (e.g., CVP, pulmonary artery pressure/pulmonary capillary wedge pressure [PAP/PCWP]).

Nursing Priority No. 4.

To promote comfort and safety:

- Change position frequently **to reduce pressure on fragile skin and tissues.**
- Bathe every other day, provide optimal skin care with emollients.
- Provide frequent oral as well as eye care **to prevent injury from dryness.**
- Change dressings frequently, use adjunct appliances as indicated, for draining wounds **to protect skin and monitor losses.**
- Provide for safety measures when client is confused.
- Administer medications (**e.g., antiemetics or antidiarrheals to limit gastric or intestinal losses; antipyretics to reduce fever**).
- Refer to ND Diarrhea.

Information that appears in brackets has been added by the authors to clarify and enhance the use of nursing diagnoses.

🌐 Cultural   🅐 Collaborative   🏠 Community/Home Care

Nursing Priority No. 5.

To promote wellness (Teaching/Discharge Considerations):

• Discuss factors related to occurrence and ways client/SO(s) can prevent dehydration, as indicated.

• Assist client/SO(s) to learn to measure own I&O.

• Recommend restriction of caffeine, alcohol, as indicated **to reduce effects of diuresis.**

• Review medications, and interactions and side effects.

• Note signs/symptoms indicating need for emergent or further evaluation and follow-up care.

Documentation Focus

Assessment/Reassessment

• Assessment findings, including degree of deficit and current sources of fluid intake.
• I&O, fluid balance, changes in weight, presence of edema, urine specific gravity, and vital signs.
• Results of diagnostic studies.

Planning

• Plan of care and who is involved in planning.
• Teaching plan.

Implementation/Evaluation

• Client's responses to interventions, teaching, and actions performed.
• Attainment or progress toward desired outcome(s).
• Modifications to plan of care.

Discharge Planning

• Long-term needs, plan for correction, and who is responsible for actions to be taken.
• Specific referrals made.

Sample Nursing Outcomes & Interventions Classifications (NOC/NIC) NIC

NOC—Hydration
NIC—Hypovolemia Management

Information that appears in brackets has been added by the authors to clarify and enhance the use of nursing diagnoses.

excess Fluid Volume

Taxonomy II: Nutrition—Class 5 Hydration (00026)
[Diagnostic Division: Food/Fluid]
Submitted 1982; Revised 1996

Definition: Increased isotonic fluid retention

Related Factors

Compromised regulatory mechanism [e.g., syndrome of inappropriate antidiuretic hormone (SIADH) or decreased plasma proteins as found in conditions such as malnutrition, draining fistulas, burns, organ failure]

Excess fluid intake

Excess sodium intake

Drug therapies, such as chlorpropamide, tolbutamide, vincristine, triptylines, carbamazepine

Defining Characteristics

Subjective
Orthopnea [difficulty breathing]
Anxiety

Objective
Edema; anasarca; weight gain over short period of time

Intake exceeds output; oliguria

Adventitious breath sounds [rales or crackles]; changes in respiratory pattern; dyspnea

Increased CVP; jugular vein distention; positive hepatojugular reflex

S3 heart sound

Pulmonary congestion, pleural effusion, pulmonary artery pressure changes; blood pressure changes

Change in mental status; restlessness

Specific gravity changes

Decreased Hb/Hct, azotemia, altered electrolytes

Desired Outcomes/Evaluation Criteria—Client Will:

- Stabilize fluid volume as evidenced by balanced I&O, vital signs within client's normal limits, stable weight, and free of signs of edema.

Information that appears in brackets has been added by the authors to clarify and enhance the use of nursing diagnoses.

🌐 Cultural   🔄 Collaborative   🏠 Community/Home Care

- Verbalize understanding of individual dietary and fluid restrictions.
- Demonstrate behaviors to monitor fluid status and reduce recurrence of fluid excess.
- List signs that require further evaluation.

Actions/Interventions

Nursing Priority No. 1.

To assess causative/precipitating factors:

- Note presence of medical conditions or situations that potentiate fluid excess (e.g., cardiac failure, cerebral lesions, renal or adrenal insufficiency, psychogenic polydipsia, acute stress, surgical procedure, anesthesia, excessive or rapid infusion of IV fluids, decrease or loss of serum proteins).
- Note amount and rate of fluid intake from all sources: PO, IV, ventilator humidifier, and so forth.
- Review intake of sodium (dietary, drug, IV) and protein.

Nursing Priority No. 2.

To evaluate degree of excess:

- Compare current weight with admission and/or previously stated weight.
- Measure vital signs and invasive hemodynamic parameters (e.g., CVP, PAP/PCWP), if available.
- Auscultate breath sounds **for presence of crackles, congestion.**
- Record occurrence of dyspnea (exertional, nocturnal, etc.).
- Auscultate heart tones for S_3, **ventricular gallop.**
- Assess for presence of neck vein distention, hepatojugular reflux.
- Note presence of edema (puffy eyelids, dependent swelling of ankles and feet if ambulatory or up in chair; sacrum and posterior thighs when recumbent), anasarca.
- Measure abdominal girth **for changes that may indicate increasing fluid retention/edema.**
- Note patterns and amount of urination (e.g., nocturia, oliguria).
- Evaluate mentation **for confusion, personality changes.**
- Assess neuromuscular reflexes **to evaluate for presence of electrolyte imbalances such as hypernatremia.**
- Assess appetite; note presence of nausea, vomiting.
- Observe skin and mucous membranes **for presence of decubitus or ulceration.**
- Note fever. **Client could be at increased risk of infection.**

Information that appears in brackets has been added by the authors to clarify and enhance the use of nursing diagnoses.

- Review laboratory data (e.g., BUN/Cr, Hb/Hct, serum albumin, proteins, and electrolytes; urine specific gravity and osmolality, sodium excretion) and chest x-ray **to evaluate degree of fluid and electrolyte imbalance and response to therapies.**

Nursing Priority No. 3.
To promote mobilization/elimination of excess fluid:

- Restrict sodium and fluid intake, as indicated.
- Record I&O accurately; calculate 24-hour fluid balance noting plus or minus.
- Set an appropriate rate of fluid intake or infusion throughout 24-hour period **to prevent peaks and valleys in fluid level and thirst.**
- Weigh daily or on a regular schedule, as indicated. **Provides a comparative baseline and evaluates the effectiveness of diuretic therapy when used (i.e., if I & O is 1 liter negative, weight loss of 2.2 pounds should be noted).**
- Administer medications (e.g., diuretics, cardiotonics, steroid replacement, plasma or albumin volume expanders).
- Elevate edematous extremities, change position frequently **to reduce tissue pressure and risk of skin breakdown.**
- Place in semi-Fowler's position, as appropriate, **to facilitate movement of diaphragm, thus improving respiratory effort.**
- Promote early ambulation.
- Provide quiet environment, limiting external stimuli.
- Use safety precautions if confused or debilitated.
- Assist with procedures, as indicated (e.g., dialysis).

Nursing Priority No. 4.
To maintain integrity of skin and oral mucous membranes:

- Refer to NDs impaired/risk for impaired Skin Integrity; impaired Oral Mucous Membrane.

Nursing Priority No. 5.
To promote wellness (Teaching/Discharge Considerations):

- Review dietary restrictions and safe substitutes for salt (e.g., lemon juice or spices such as oregano).
- Discuss importance of fluid restrictions and "hidden sources" of intake (such as foods high in water content).
- Instruct client/family in use of voiding record, I&O.
- Consult dietitian, as needed.
- Suggest interventions, such as frequent oral care, chewing gum/hard candy, use of lip balm, **to reduce discomfort of fluid restrictions.**

Information that appears in brackets has been added by the authors to clarify and enhance the use of nursing diagnoses.

- Review drug regimen (and side effects) used to increase urine output and/or manage hypertension, kidney disease, or heart failure.
- Stress need for mobility and/or frequent position changes **to prevent stasis and reduce risk of tissue injury.**
- Identify "danger" signs requiring notification of healthcare provider **to ensure timely evaluation/intervention.**

Documentation Focus

Assessment/Reassessment
- Assessment findings, noting existing conditions contributing to and degree of fluid retention (vital signs; amount, presence, and location of edema; and weight changes).
- I&O, fluid balance.
- Results of laboratory tests and diagnostic studies.

Planning
- Plan of care and who is involved in the planning.
- Teaching plan.

Implementation/Evaluation
- Response to interventions, teaching, and actions performed.
- Attainment or progress toward desired outcome(s).
- Modifications to plan of care.

Discharge Planning
- Long-range needs, noting who is responsible for actions to be taken.

Sample Nursing Outcomes & Interventions Classifications (NOC/NIC) NIC

NOC—Fluid Balance
NIC—Hypervolemia Management

risk for deficient Fluid Volume

Taxonomy II: Nutrition—Class 5 Hydration (00028)
[Diagnostic Division: Food/Fluid]
Submitted 1978

Definition: At risk for experiencing vascular, cellular, or intracellular dehydration

Information that appears in brackets has been added by the authors to clarify and enhance the use of nursing diagnoses.

Risk Factors

Extremes of age or weight
Loss of fluid through abnormal routes (e.g., indwelling tubes)
Knowledge deficiency
Factors influencing fluid needs (e.g., hypermetabolic state)
Medication (e.g., diuretics)
Excessive losses through normal routes (e.g., diarrhea)
Deviations affecting access, intake, or absorption of fluids

> **NOTE:** A risk diagnosis is not evidenced by signs and symptoms as the problem has not occurred; rather, nursing interventions are directed at prevention.

Desired Outcomes/Evaluation Criteria—Client Will:

• Identify individual risk factors and appropriate interventions.
• Demonstrate behaviors or lifestyle changes to prevent development of fluid volume deficit.

Actions/Interventions

Nursing Priority No. 1.

To assess causative/contributing factors:

• Note possible conditions or processes that may lead to deficits: (1) fluid loss (e.g., fever, diarrhea, vomiting, excessive sweating; heat stroke; diabetic ketoacidosis; burns, other draining wounds; gastrointestinal obstruction; salt-wasting diuretics; rapid breathing, mechanical ventilation; surgical drains); (2) limited intake (e.g., sore throat or mouth; client dependent on others for eating and drinking; NPO status); (3) fluid shifts (e.g., ascites, effusions, burns, sepsis); and (4) environmental factors (e.g., isolation, restraints, malfunctioning air conditioning, exposure to extreme heat).
∞• Determine effects of age. **Very young and extremely elderly individuals are quickly affected by fluid volume deficit, and are least able to express need. For example, elderly people often have a decreased thirst reflex and/or may not be aware of water needs. Infants, young children and other nonverbal persons cannot describe thirst.**
• Note client's level of consciousness and mentation **to evaluate ability to express needs.**
• Evaluate nutritional status, noting current intake, type of diet (e.g., client is NPO or is on a restricted diet). Note problems

---

Information that appears in brackets has been added by the authors to clarify and enhance the use of nursing diagnoses.

⊕ Cultural 🐾 Collaborative 🏠 Community/Home Care

(e.g., impaired mentation, nausea, fever, facial injuries, immobility, insufficient time for intake) **that can negatively affect fluid intake.**

• Review laboratory data (e.g., Hb/Hct, electrolytes, BUN/Cr).

Nursing Priority No. 2.
To prevent occurrence of deficit:

• Monitor I&O balance, being aware of altered intake or output **to ensure accurate picture of fluid status.**
• Weigh client and compare with recent weight history. Perform serial weights **to determine trends.**
• Assess skin turgor and oral mucous membranes.
• Monitor vital signs for changes (e.g., orthostatic hypotension, tachycardia, fever).
• Establish individual fluid needs and replacement schedule. Distribute fluids over 24-hour period.
• Encourage oral intake:

Provide water and other fluid needs to a minimum amount daily (up to 2.5 L/day or amount determined by healthcare provider for client's age, weight, and condition).

Offer fluids between meals and regularly throughout the day.

Provide fluids in manageable cup, bottle, or with drinking straw.

Allow for adequate time for eating and drinking at meals.

Ensure that immobile or restrained client is assisted.

Encourage a variety of fluids in small frequent offerings, attempting to incorporate client's preferred beverages and temperature (e.g., iced or hot).

Limit fluids that tend to exert a diuretic effect (e.g., caffeine, alcohol).

Promote intake of high-water content foods (e.g., popsicles, gelatin, soup, eggnog, watermelon) and/or electrolyte replacement drinks (e.g., Smartwater, Gatorade, Pedialyte), as appropriate.

• Provide supplemental fluids (e.g., enteral, parenteral), as indicated. **Fluids may be given in this manner if client is unable to take oral fluid, is NPO for procedures, or when rapid fluid resuscitation is required.**
• Administer medications as indicated (e.g., anti-emetics, anti-diarrheals, antipyretics).

Nursing Priority No. 3.
To promote wellness (Teaching/Discharge Considerations):

Information that appears in brackets has been added by the authors to clarify and enhance the use of nursing diagnoses.

🏠 • Discuss individual risk factors, potential problems and specific interventions (e.g., proper clothing and bedding for infants and elderly during hot weather, use of room cooler or fan for comfortable ambient environment, fluid replacement options and schedule).

• Encourage client to increase fluid intake when exercising or during hot weather.

💊 • Review appropriate use of medications **that have potential for causing or exacerbating dehydration.**

🏠 • Encourage client to maintain diary of food/fluid intake; number and amount of voidings and stools; and so forth.

• Refer to NDs [deficient Fluid Volume: hyper/hypotonic] or [isotonic].

Documentation Focus

Assessment/Reassessment
• Individual findings, including individual factors influencing fluid needs or requirements.
• Baseline weight, vital signs.
• Results of laboratory tests.
• Specific client preferences for fluids.

Planning
• Plan of care and who is involved in planning.
• Teaching plan.

Implementation/Evaluation
• Responses to interventions, teaching, and actions performed.
• Attainment or progress toward desired outcome(s).
• Modifications to plan of care.

Discharge Planning
• Individual long-term needs, noting who is responsible for actions to be taken.
• Specific referrals made.

Sample Nursing Outcomes & Interventions Classifications (NOC/NIC) NIC

NOC—Fluid Balance
NIC—Fluid Monitoring

Information that appears in brackets has been added by the authors to clarify and enhance the use of nursing diagnoses.

risk for imbalanced Fluid Volume

Taxonomy II: Nutrition—Class 5 Hydration (00025)
[Diagnostic Division: Food/Fluid]
Submitted 1998; revised 2008

Definition: At risk for a decrease, increase, or rapid shift from one to the other of intravascular, interstitial, and/or intracellular fluid. This refers to body fluid loss, gain, or both.

Risk Factors

Abdominal surgery; intestinal obstruction
Pancreatitis; ascites
Burns; sepsis
Traumatic injury (e.g., fractured hip)
Receiving apheresis

NOTE: A risk diagnosis is not evidenced by signs and symptoms, as the problem has not occurred; rather, nursing interventions are directed at prevention.

Desired Outcomes/Evaluation Criteria—Client Will:

• Demonstrate adequate fluid balance as evidenced by stable vital signs, palpable pulses of good quality, normal skin turgor, moist mucous membranes, individual appropriate urinary output, lack of excessive weight fluctuation (loss or gain), and no edema present.

Actions/Interventions

Nursing Priority No. 1.
To determine risk/contributing factors:

• Note potential sources of fluid loss and intake (e.g., presence of conditions, such as diabetes insipidus, hyperosmolar non-ketotic syndrome, bowel obstruction, heart/kidney/liver failure, sepsis), major invasive procedures [e.g., surgery], use of anesthesia, preoperative vomiting and dehydration, draining wounds, use or overuse of certain medications [e.g., diuretics, laxatives, anitcoagulants], use of IV fluids and delivery device, administration of total parenteral nutrition [TPN]).

Information that appears in brackets has been added by the authors to clarify and enhance the use of nursing diagnoses.

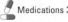

- Note client's age, current level of hydration, and mentation. **Provides information regarding ability to tolerate fluctuations in fluid level and risk for creating or failing to respond to problem (e.g., confused client may have inadequate intake, disconnect tubings, or readjust IV flow rate).**
- Review laboratory data, chest x-ray **to determine changes indicative of electrolyte and/or fluid status.**

Nursing Priority No. 2.

To prevent fluctuations/imbalances in fluid levels:

- Measure and record intake:

   Include all sources (e.g., PO, IV, antibiotic additives, liquids with medications).

- Measure and record output:

   Monitor urine output hourly or as needed. Report urine output less than 30 mL/hr or 0.5 mL/kg/hr **because this may indicate deficient fluid volume or cardiac or kidney failure.**

   Observe color of all excretions **to evaluate for bleeding.**

   Measure or estimate amount of liquid stool; weigh diapers or continence pads, when indicated.

   Measure emesis and output from drainage devices (e.g., gastric, wound, chest).

   Estimate or calculate insensible fluid losses **to include in replacement calculations.**

   Calculate 24-hour fluid balance (intake > output or output > intake).

- Weigh daily, or as indicated, and evaluate changes **as they relate to fluid status.**
- Auscultate blood pressure, calculate pulse pressure. **Pulse pressure widens before systolic blood pressure drops in response to fluid loss.**
- Monitor vital sign responses to activities. **Blood pressure and heart and respiratory rate often increase initially when either fluid deficit or excess is present.**
- Assess for clinical signs of dehydration (e.g., hypotension, dry skin and mucous membranes, delayed capillary refill) or fluid excess (e.g., peripheral/dependent edema, adventitious breath sounds, distended neck veins).
- Note increased lethargy, hypotension, muscle cramping. **Electrolyte imbalances may be present.**
- Establish fluid oral intake, incorporating beverage preferences when possible.
- Maintain fluid and sodium restrictions, when needed.

Information that appears in brackets has been added by the authors to clarify and enhance the use of nursing diagnoses.

Cultural Collaborative Community/Home Care

- Administer IV fluids, as prescribed, using infusion pumps **to deliver fluids accurately and at desired rates to prevent either under- or overinfusion.**
- Tape tubing connections longitudinally **to reduce risk of disconnection and loss of fluids.**
- Administer diuretics, antiemetics, antidiarrheals, as prescribed.
- Assist with rotating tourniquets (if used while awaiting response to pharmacological therapies); dialysis; or ultrafiltration **to correct fluid overload situation.**

Nursing Priority No. 3.

To promote wellness (Teaching/Discharge Considerations):

- Discuss individual risk factors, potential problems, and specific interventions **to prevent or limit occurrence of fluid deficit or excess.**
- Instruct client/SO(s) in how to measure and record I&O, if indicated.
- Review or instruct in medication or nutritional regimen (e.g., enteral/parenteral feedings) **to alert to potential complications and appropriate management.**
- Identify signs and symptoms indicating need for prompt evaluation/follow-up care.
- Refer to NDs [deficient Fluid Volume: hyper/hypotonic] or [isotonic]; excess Fluid Volume; risk for deficient Fluid Volume for additional interventions.

Documentation Focus ————————

Assessment/Reassessment

- Individual findings, including individual factors influencing fluid needs/requirements.
- Baseline weight, vital signs.
- Results of laboratory test and diagnostic studies.
- Specific client preferences for fluids.

Planning

- Plan of care and who is involved in planning.
- Teaching plan.

Implementation/Evaluation

- Responses to interventions, teaching, and actions performed.
- Attainment or progress toward desired outcome(s).
- Modifications to plan of care.

———————

Information that appears in brackets has been added by the authors to clarify and enhance the use of nursing diagnoses.

Discharge Planning

- Individual long-term needs, noting who is responsible for actions to be taken.
- Specific referrals made.

Sample Nursing Outcomes & Interventions Classifications (NOC/NIC) ⟨NIC⟩

NOC—Fluid Balance
NIC—Fluid Monitoring

impaired Gas Exchange

Taxonomy II: Elimination and Exchange—Class 4 Respiratory Function (00030)
[Diagnostic Division: Respiration]
Submitted 1980; Revised 1996, 1998 by Nursing Diagnosis Extension and Classification (NDEC)

Definition: Excess or deficit in oxygenation and/or carbon dioxide elimination at the alveolar-capillary membrane [This may be an entity of its own, but it also may be an end result of other pathology with an interrelatedness between airway clearance and/or breathing pattern problems.]

Related Factors

Ventilation perfusion imbalance [as in altered blood flow (e.g., pulmonary embolus, increased vascular resistance), vasospasm, heart failure, hypovolemic shock]

Alveolar-capillary membrane changes [e.g., acute respiratory distress syndrome; chronic conditions, such as restrictive/obstructive lung disease, pneumoconiosis, asbestosis/silicosis]

Altered oxygen supply (e.g., altitude sickness)

Altered oxygen-carrying capacity of blood (e.g., sickle cell or other anemia, carbon monoxide poisoning)

Defining Characteristics

Subjective
Dyspnea
Visual disturbances
Headache upon awakening
Sense of impending doom

Information that appears in brackets has been added by the authors to clarify and enhance the use of nursing diagnoses.

⊕ Cultural ⊗ Collaborative ⌂ Community/Home Care

Objective

Confusion [decreased mental acuity]

Restlessness; irritability; [agitation]

Somnolence; [lethargy]

Abnormal ABGs/arterial pH; hypoxia/hypoxemia; hypercapnia; hypercarbia; decreased carbon dioxide

Cyanosis (in neonates only); abnormal skin color (e.g., pale, dusky)

Abnormal breathing (e.g., rate, rhythm, depth); nasal flaring

Tachycardia; [development of dysrhythmias]

Diaphoresis

Polycythemia

Desired Outcomes/Evaluation Criteria— Client Will:

• Demonstrate improved ventilation and adequate oxygenation of tissues by ABGs within client's normal limits and absence of symptoms of respiratory distress (as noted in Defining Characteristics).

• Verbalize understanding of causative factors and appropriate interventions.

• Participate in treatment regimen (e.g., breathing exercises, effective coughing, use of oxygen) within level of ability or situation.

Actions/Interventions

Nursing Priority No. 1.

To assess causative/contributing factors:

• Note presence of factors listed in Related Factors. Refer to NDs ineffective Airway Clearance; ineffective Breathing Pattern, as appropriate.

Nursing Priority No. 2.

To evaluate degree of compromise:

• Note respiratory rate, depth, use of accessory muscles, pursed-lip breathing; and areas of pallor/cyanosis: for example, peripheral (nailbeds) versus central (circumoral) or general duskiness.

• Auscultate breath sounds, note areas of decreased/adventitious breath sounds as well as fremitus.

• Note character and effectiveness of cough mechanism (e.g, ability to clear airways of secretions).

Information that appears in brackets has been added by the authors to clarify and enhance the use of nursing diagnoses.

- Assess level of consciousness and mentation changes. Note somnolence, restlessness, reports of headache on arising.
- Monitor vital signs and cardiac rhythm.
- Evaluate pulse oximetry **to determine oxygenation and levels of carbon dioxide retention;** and evaluate lung volumes and forced vital capacity **to assess for respiratory insufficiency.**
- Review other pertinent laboratory data (e.g., ABGs, CBC); chest x-rays.
- Assess energy level and activity tolerance.
- Note effect of illness on self-esteem and body image.

Nursing Priority No. 3.

To correct/improve existing deficiencies:

- Elevate head of bed and position client appropriately, provide airway adjuncts and suction, as indicated, **to maintain airway.**
- Encourage frequent position changes and deep-breathing and coughing exercises. Use incentive spirometer, chest physiotherapy, intermittent positive-pressure breathing (IPPB), and so forth, as indicated. **Promotes optimal chest expansion and drainage of secretions.**
- Provide supplemental oxygen at lowest concentration indicated by laboratory results and client symptoms or situation.
- Monitor for carbon dioxide narcosis (e.g., change in level of consciousness, changes in O_2 and CO_2 blood gas levels, flushing, decreased respiratory rate, headaches), **which may occur in client receiving long-term oxygen therapy.**
- Maintain adequate I&O **for mobilization of secretions,** but avoid fluid overload.
- Use sedation judiciously **to avoid depressant effects on respiratory functioning.**
- Ensure availability of proper emergency equipment, including ET/tracheostomy set and suction catheters appropriate for age and size of infant, child, or adult.
- Avoid use of face mask in elderly emaciated client **as oxygen can leak out around the mask because of poor fit, and mask can increase client's agitation.**
- Encourage adequate rest and limit activities to within client tolerance. Promote calm, restful environment. **Helps limit oxygen needs and consumption.**
- Provide psychological support, active-listen questions/concerns **to reduce anxiety.**

Information that appears in brackets has been added by the authors to clarify and enhance the use of nursing diagnoses.

- Administer medications, as indicated (e.g., inhaled and systemic glucocorticosteroids, antibiotics, bronchodilators, methylxanthines, expectorants), **to treat underlying conditions.**
- Monitor and instruct client in therapeutic and adverse effects as well as interactions of drug therapy.
- Minimize blood loss from procedures (e.g., tests, hemodialysis) **to limit adverse affects of anemia.**
- Assist with procedures as individually indicated (e.g., transfusion, phlebotomy, bronchoscopy) **to improve respiratory function/oxygen-carrying capacity.**
- Monitor and adjust ventilator settings (e.g., fractional concentration of inspired oxygen [FiO_2], tidal volume, inspiratory/expiratory ratio, sigh, positive end-expiratory pressure [PEEP]), as indicated, when mechanical support is being used.
- Keep environment allergen and pollutant free **to reduce irritant effect of dust and chemicals on airways.**

Nursing Priority No. 4.

To promote wellness (Teaching/Discharge Considerations):

- Review risk factors, particularly environmental/employment-related, **to promote prevention or management of risk.**
- Discuss implications of smoking related to the illness/condition.
- Encourage client and SO(s) to stop smoking; recommend smoking cessation programs **to reduce health risks and/or prevent further decline in lung function.**
- Discuss reasons for allergy testing when indicated. Review individual drug regimen and ways of dealing with side effects.
- Instruct in the use of relaxation, stress-reduction techniques, as appropriate.
- Reinforce need for adequate rest, while encouraging activity and exercise (e.g., upper and lower extremity strength and flexibility training, and endurance) **to decrease dyspnea and improve quality of life.**
- Emphasize the importance of nutrition **in improving stamina and reducing the work of breathing.**
- Review oxygen-conserving techniques (e.g., sitting instead of standing to perform tasks; eating small meals; performing slower, purposeful movements).
- Review job description and work activities **to identify need for job modifications or vocational rehabilitation.**
- Discuss home oxygen therapy and safety measures, as indicated, when home oxygen implemented.

Information that appears in brackets has been added by the authors to clarify and enhance the use of nursing diagnoses.

- Identify and refer to specific suppliers for supplemental oxygen/necessary respiratory devices, as well as other individually appropriate resources, such as home care agencies, Meals on Wheels, and so on, **to facilitate independence.**

Documentation Focus

Assessment/Reassessment
- Assessment findings, including respiratory rate, character of breath sounds; frequency, amount, and appearance of secretions; presence of cyanosis; laboratory findings; and mentation level.
- Conditions that may interfere with oxygen supply.

Planning
- Plan of care, specific interventions, and who is involved in the planning.
- Ventilator settings, liters of supplemental oxygen.
- Teaching plan.

Implementation/Evaluation
- Client's responses to treatment, teaching, and actions performed.
- Attainment or progress toward desired outcome(s).
- Modifications to plan of care.

Discharge Planning
- Long-term needs, identifying who is responsible for actions to be taken.
- Community resources for equipment and supplies postdischarge.
- Specific referrals made.

Sample Nursing Outcomes & Interventions Classifications (NOC/NIC) NIC

NOC—Respiratory Status: Gas Exchange
NIC—Respiratory Monitoring

Information that appears in brackets has been added by the authors to clarify and enhance the use of nursing diagnoses.

Cultural   Collaborative   Community/Home Care

risk for unstable blood Glucose Level

Taxonomy II: Nutrition—Class 4 Metabolism (00179)
[Diagnostic Division: Food/Fluid]
Submitted 2006

Definition: Risk for variation of blood glucose/sugar levels from the normal range

Risk Factors

Lack of acceptance of diagnosis; deficient knowledge of diabetes management (e.g., action plan)

Lack of diabetes management or adherence to diabetes management (e.g., action plan); inadequate blood glucose monitoring; medication management

Dietary intake; weight gain or loss; rapid growth periods; pregnancy

Physical health status or activity level

Stress; mental health status

Developmental level

> **NOTE:** A risk diagnosis is not evidenced by signs and symptoms, as the problem has not occurred; rather, nursing interventions are directed at prevention.

Desired Outcomes/Evaluation Criteria— Client/Caregivers Will:

* Acknowledge factors that may lead to unstable glucose.
* Verbalize understanding of body and energy needs.
* Verbalize plan for modifying factors to prevent or minimize shifts in glucose level.
* Maintain glucose in satisfactory range.

Actions/Interventions

Nursing Priority No. 1.

To assess risk/contributing factors:

* Determine individual factors that may contribute to unstable glucose as listed in risk factors. **Client or family history of diabetes; known diabetic with poor glucose control; eating disorders (e.g., morbid obesity); poor exercise habits; failure to recognize changes in glucose needs or control due**

Information that appears in brackets has been added by the authors to clarify and enhance the use of nursing diagnoses.

to adolescent growth spurts or pregnancy can result in problems with glucose stability.

- Ascertain client's/SO's knowledge and understanding of condition and treatment needs.
- Identify individual perceptions and expectations of treatment regimen.
- Note influence of cultural or religious factors impacting dietary practices, taking responsibility for own care, expectations of outcomes.
- Determine client's awareness and ability to be responsible for dealing with situation. Age, maturity, current health status, and developmental stage affect client's ability to provide for own safety.
- Assess family/SO(s) support of client. Client may need assistance with lifestyle changes (e.g., food preparation or consumption, timing of intake and/or exercise, administration of medications).
- Note availability and use of resources.

Nursing Priority No. 2.

To assist client to develop preventive strategies to avoid glucose instability:

- Ascertain whether client/SO(s) are adept at operating client's home glucose monitoring device. **All available machines will provide satisfactory readings if properly used and maintained and routinely calibrated.**
- Provide information on balancing food intake, antidiabetic agents, and energy expenditure.
- Review medical necessity for regularly scheduled lab screening tests for diabetes. **Tests, including fasting and daily glucose and HgbA1c, help identify acute and long-term glucose control.**
- Discuss home glucose monitoring according to individual parameters (e.g., six times a day for normal day and more frequently during times of stress) **to identify and manage glucose variations.**
- Review client's common situations that contribute to glucose instability on daily, occasional, or crisis basis. **Multiple factors can play a role at any time, such as missing meals, adolescent growth spurt, or infection or other illness.**
- Review client's diet, especially carbohydrate intake. **Glucose balance is determined by the amount of carbohydrates consumed, which should be determined in needed grams per day.**

Information that appears in brackets has been added by the authors to clarify and enhance the use of nursing diagnoses.

Cultural   Collaborative   Community/Home Care

- Encourage client to read labels and choose foods described as having a low glycemic index, higher fiber, and low fat content. **These foods produce a slower rise in blood glucose.**
- Discuss how client's antidiabetic medication(s) work. **Drugs and combinations of drugs work in varying ways with different blood glucose control and side effects. Understanding drug actions can help client avoid or reduce risk of potential for hypoglycemic reactions.**

For Client Receiving Insulin

- Emphasize importance of checking expiration dates of medications, inspecting insulin for cloudiness if it is normally clear, and monitoring proper storage and preparation (when mixing required). **Affects insulin absorbability.**
- Review type(s) of insulin used (e.g., rapid, short, intermediate, long-acting, premixed) and delivery method (e.g., subcutaneous, intramuscular injection; inhaled, pump). Note time when short- and long-acting insulins are administered. Remind client that only short-acting insulin is used in pump. **Affects timing of effects and provides clues to potential timing of glucose instability.**
- Check injection sites periodically. **Insulin absorption can vary from day to day in healthy sites and is less absorbable in lipohypertrophic (lumpy) tissues.**
- Ascertain that all injections are being given. **Children, adolescents, and elderly clients may forget injections or be unable to self-inject and may need reminders and supervision.**

Nursing Priority No. 3.

To promote wellness (Teaching/Discharge Considerations):

- Review individual risk factors and provide information to assist client in efforts to avoid complications, such as those caused by chronic hyperglycemia and acute hypoglycemia. **Note: Hyperglycemia is most commonly caused by alterations in nutrition needs, inactivity, and/or inadequate use of antidiabetic medications. Hypoglycemia is the most common complication of antidiabetic therapy, stress, and exercise.**
- Emphasize consequences of actions and choices—both immediate and long-term.
- Engage client/family/caregiver in formulating plan to manage blood glucose level incorporating lifestyle, age and

---

Information that appears in brackets has been added by the authors to clarify and enhance the use of nursing diagnoses.

developmental level, physical and psychological ability to manage condition.

- Consult with dietitian about specific dietary needs based on individual situation (e.g., growth spurt, pregnancy, change in activity level following injury).
- Encourage client to develop a system for self-monitoring to provide a sense of control and enable client to follow own progress and assist with making choices.
- Refer to appropriate community resources, diabetic educator, and/or support groups, as needed, **for lifestyle modification, medical management, referral for insulin pump or glucose monitor, financial assistance for supplies, and so forth.**

Documentation Focus

Assessment/Reassessment

- Findings related to individual situation, risk factors, current caloric intake and dietary pattern; prescription medication use; monitoring of condition.
- Client's/caregiver's understanding of individual risks and potential complications.
- Results of laboratory tests and fingerstick testing.

Planning

- Plan of care and who is involved in planning.
- Teaching plan.

Implementation/Evaluation

- Individual responses to interventions, teaching, and actions performed.
- Specific actions and changes that are made.
- Attainment or progress toward desired outcomes.
- Modifications to plan of care.

Discharge Planning

- Long-term plans for ongoing needs, monitoring and management of condition, and who is responsible for actions to be taken.
- Sources for equipment/supplies.
- Specific referrals made.

Information that appears in brackets has been added by the authors to clarify and enhance the use of nursing diagnoses.

⊕ Cultural   ⊛ Collaborative   🏠 Community/Home Care

Sample Nursing Outcomes & Interventions
Classifications (NOC/NIC) `NIC`

NOC—Blood Glucose Level
NIC—Hyperglycemia Management

Grieving

Taxonomy II: Coping/Stress Tolerance—Class 2 Coping
   Responses (00136)
[Diagnostic Division: Ego Integrity]
Submitted as anticipatory Grieving 1980; Revised 1996,
   2006

Definition: A normal complex process that includes
emotional, physical, spiritual, social, and intellectual
responses and behaviors by which individuals, families,
and communities incorporate an actual, anticipated, or
perceived loss into their daily lives

Related Factors

Anticipatory loss or loss of significant object (e.g., possessions,
   job, status, home, parts and processes of body)
Anticipatory loss or death of a significant other

Defining Characteristics

Subjective

Anger; pain; suffering; despair; blame
Alteration in activity level, sleep or dream patterns
Making meaning of the loss; personal growth
Experiencing relief

Objective

Detachment; disorganization; psychological distress; panic be-
   havior
Maintaining the connection to the deceased
Alterations in immune or neuroendocrine function

Desired Outcomes/Evaluation Criteria—
Client Will:

• Identify and express feelings (e.g., sadness, guilt, fear) freely
   and effectively.

Information that appears in brackets has been added by the authors to clarify
and enhance the use of nursing diagnoses.

 Diagnostic Studies   Pediatric/Geriatric/Lifespan   Medications **395**

- Acknowledge impact or effect of the grieving process (e.g., physical problems of eating, sleeping) and seek appropriate help.
- Look toward and plan for future, one day at a time.

Community Will:

- Recognize needs of citizens, including underserved population.
- Activate or develop plan to address identified needs.

Actions/Interventions

Nursing Priority No. 1.
To identify causative/contributing factors:

- Determine circumstances of current situation (e.g., sudden death, prolonged fatal illness, loved one kept alive by extreme medical interventions). **Grief can be anticipatory (mourning the loss of loved one's former self before actual death), or actual. Both types of grief can provoke a wide range of intense and often conflicting feelings. Grief also follows losses other than death (e.g., traumatic loss of a limb, or loss of home by a tornado, loss of known self due to brain injury).**
- Evaluate client's perception of anticipated or actual loss and meaning to him or her: "What are your concerns?" "What are your fears?" "Your greatest fear?" "How do you see this affecting you or your lifestyle?"
- Identify cultural or religious beliefs that may impact sense of loss.
- Ascertain response of family/SO(s) to client's situation and concerns.
- Determine significance of loss to community (e.g., school bus accident with loss of life, major tornado damage to infrastructure, financial failure of major employer).

Nursing Priority No. 2.
To determine current response:

- Note emotional responses, such as withdrawal, angry behavior, crying.
- Observe client's body language and check out meaning with the client. Note congruency with verbalizations.
- Note cultural and religious expectations that may dictate client's responses **to assess appropriateness of client's reaction to the situation.**

Information that appears in brackets has been added by the authors to clarify and enhance the use of nursing diagnoses.

Cultural Collaborative Community/Home Care

- Identify problems with eating, activity level, sexual desire, role performance (e.g., work, parenting). **Indicators of severity of feelings client is experiencing and need for specific interventions to address these issues.**
- Determine impact on general well-being (e.g., increased frequency of minor illnesses, exacerbation of chronic condition).
- Note family communication and interaction patterns.
- Determine availability and use of community resources and support groups.
- Note community plans in place to deal with major loss (e.g., team of crisis counselors stationed at a school to address the loss of classmates, vocational counselors or retraining programs, outreach of services from neighboring communities).

Nursing Priority No. 3.

To assist client/community to deal with situation:

- Provide open environment and trusting relationship. **Promotes a free discussion of feelings and concerns.**
- Use therapeutic communication skills of active-listening, silence, acknowledgment. Respect client desire/request not to talk.
- Inform children about death or anticipated loss in age-appropriate language. **Providing accurate information about impending loss or change in life situation will help child begin mourning process.**
- Provide puppets or play therapy for toddlers and young children. **May help them more readily express grief and deal with loss.**
- Permit appropriate expressions of anger, fear. Note hostility toward, or feelings of abandonment by, spiritual power. (Refer to appropriate NDs, e.g., Spiritual Distress.)
- Provide information about normalcy of individual grief reaction.
- Be honest when answering questions, providing information. **Enhances sense of trust and nurse-client relationship.**
- Provide assurance to child that cause for situation is not own doing, bearing in mind age and developmental level. **May lessen sense of guilt and affirm there is no need to assign blame to self or any family member.**
- Provide hope within parameters of specific situation. Refrain from giving false reassurance.
- Review past life experiences and previous loss(es), role changes, and coping skills, noting strengths and successes.

Information that appears in brackets has been added by the authors to clarify and enhance the use of nursing diagnoses.

 Diagnostic Studies ∞ Pediatric/Geriatric/Lifespan Medications **397**

May be useful in dealing with current situation and problem solving existing needs.

- Discuss control issues, such as what is in the power of the individual to change and what is beyond control. **Recognition of these factors helps client focus energy for maximal benefit and outcome.**
- Incorporate family/SO(s) in problem solving. **Encourages family to support and assist client to deal with situation while meeting needs of family members.**
- Determine client's status and role in family (e.g., parent, sibling, child) and address loss of family member role.
- Instruct in use of visualization and relaxation techniques.
- Use sedatives or tranquilizers with caution. **May retard passage through the grief process, although short-term use may be beneficial to enhance sleep.**
- Encourage community members or groups to engage in talking about event or loss and verbalizing feelings. Seek out underserved populations to include in process.
- Encourage individuals to participate in activities to deal with loss, rebuild community.

Nursing Priority No. 4.

To promote wellness (Teaching/Discharge Considerations):

- Give information that feelings are okay and are to be expressed appropriately. **Expression of feelings can facilitate the grieving process, but destructive behavior can be damaging.**
- Provide information that on birthdays, major holidays, at times of significant personal events, or anniversary of loss, client may experience (needs to be prepared for) intense grief reactions. **If these reactions start to disrupt day-to-day functioning, client may need to seek help.** (Refer to NDs complicated Grieving; ineffective community Coping, as appropriate.)
- Encourage continuation of usual activities or schedule and involvement in appropriate exercise program.
- Identify and promote family and social support systems.
- Discuss and assist with planning for future or funeral, as appropriate.
- Refer to additional resources, such as pastoral care, counseling, psychotherapy, community or organized support groups (including hospice), as indicated, for both client and family/SO(s), **to meet ongoing needs and facilitate grief work.**

Information that appears in brackets has been added by the authors to clarify and enhance the use of nursing diagnoses.

⊕ Cultural 🐱 Collaborative 🏠 Community/Home Care

• Support community efforts to strengthen support or develop plan to foster recovery and growth.

Documentation Focus

Assessment/Reassessment
- Assessment findings, including client's perception of anticipated loss and signs/symptoms that are being exhibited.
- Responses of family/SO(s) or community members, as indicated.
- Availability and use of resources.

Planning
- Plan of care and who is involved in planning.
- Teaching plan.

Implementation/Evaluation
- Client's response to interventions, teaching, and actions performed.
- Attainment or progress toward desired outcome(s).
- Modifications to plan of care.

Discharge Planning
- Long-term needs and who is responsible for actions to be taken.
- Specific referrals made.

Sample Nursing Outcomes & Interventions Classifications (NOC/NIC) NIC

NOC—Grief Resolution
NIC—Grief Work Facilitation

---

complicated Grieving

Taxonomy II: Coping/Stress Tolerance—Class 2 Coping Responses (00135)
[Diagnostic Division: Ego Integrity]
Submitted as dysfunctional Grieving 1980; Revised 1996, 2004, 2006

Definition: A disorder that occurs after the death of a significant other, in which the experience of distress accompanying bereavement fails to follow normative expectations and manifests in functional impairment

---

Information that appears in brackets has been added by the authors to clarify and enhance the use of nursing diagnoses.

Related Factors

General
Death/sudden death of a significant other
Emotional instability
Lack of social support
Loss of significant object (e.g., possessions, job, status, home, parts and processes of body)

Defining Characteristics

Subjective
Verbalizes anxiety, lack of acceptance of the death, persistent painful memories, distressful feelings about the deceased, self-blame
Verbalizes feelings of anger, disbelief, detachment from others
Verbalizes feeling dazed, empty, stunned, in shock
Decreased sense of well-being, fatigue, low levels of intimacy, depression
Yearning

Objective
Decreased functioning in life roles
Persistent emotional distress; separation or traumatic distress
Preoccupation with thoughts of the deceased, longing for the deceased, searching for the deceased, self-blame
Experiencing somatic symptoms of the deceased
Rumination
Grief avoidance

Desired Outcomes/Evaluation Criteria—Client Will:

- Acknowledge presence and impact of dysfunctional situation.
- Demonstrate progress in dealing with stages of grief at own pace.
- Participate in work and self-care activities of daily living (ADLs) as able.
- Verbalize a sense of progress toward grief resolution, hope for the future.

Information that appears in brackets has been added by the authors to clarify and enhance the use of nursing diagnoses.

  Cultural Collaborative Community/Home Care

Nursing Priority No. 1.

To determine causative/contributing factors:

- Identify loss that is present. Note circumstances of death, such as sudden or traumatic (e.g., fatal accident, suicide, homicide), related to socially sensitive issue (e.g., AIDS, suicide, murder), or associated with unfinished business (e.g., spouse died during time of crisis in marriage; son has not spoken to parent for years). **These situations can sometimes cause individual to become stuck in grief and unable to move forward with life.**
- Determine significance of the loss to client (e.g., presence of chronic condition leading to divorce or disruption of family unit and change in lifestyle, financial security).
- Identify cultural or religious beliefs and expectations that may impact or dictate client's response to loss.
- Ascertain response of family/SO(s) to client's situation (e.g., sympathetic or urging client to "just get over it").

Nursing Priority No. 2.

To determine degree of impairment/dysfunction:

- Observe for cues of sadness (e.g., sighing; faraway look; unkempt appearance; inattention to conversation; somatic complaints, such as exhaustion, headaches).
- Listen to words/communications indicative of renewed or intense grief (e.g., constantly bringing up death or loss even in casual conversation long after event; outbursts of anger at relatively minor events; expressing desire to die), **indicating person is possibly unable to adjust or move on from feelings of severe grief.**
- Identify stage of grief being expressed: denial, isolation, anger, bargaining, depression, acceptance.
- Determine level of functioning, ability to care for self.
- Note availability and use of support systems and community resources.
- Be aware of avoidance behaviors (e.g., anger, withdrawal, long periods of sleeping, or refusing to interact with family; sudden or radical changes in lifestyle; inability to handle everyday responsibilities at home, work, or school; conflict).
- Determine if client is engaging in reckless or self-destructive behaviors (e.g., substance abuse, heavy drinking, promiscuity, aggression) **to identify safety issues.**

Information that appears in brackets has been added by the authors to clarify and enhance the use of nursing diagnoses.

- Identify cultural factors and ways individual has dealt with previous loss(es) **to put current behavior and responses in context.**
- Refer to mental health providers for specific diagnostic studies and intervention in issues associated with debilitating grief.
- Refer to ND Grieving for additional interventions, as appropriate.

Nursing Priority No. 3.

To assist client to deal appropriately with loss:

- Encourage verbalization without confrontation about realities. **Helps to begin resolution and acceptance.**
- Encourage client to talk about what he or she chooses and refrain from forcing the client to "face the facts."
- Active-listen to feelings and be available for support and assistance. Speak in soft, caring tone.
- Encourage expression of anger, fear, and anxiety. Refer to appropriate NDs.
- Permit verbalization of anger with acknowledgment of feelings and setting of limits regarding destructive behavior. **Enhances client safety and promotes resolution of grief process.**
- Acknowledge reality of feelings of guilt or blame, including hostility toward spiritual power. Do not minimize loss, avoid clichés and easy answers. (Refer to ND Spiritual Distress.) Assist client to take steps toward resolution.
- Respect the client's needs and wishes for quiet, privacy, talking, or silence.
- Give "permission" to be at this point when the client is depressed.
- Provide comfort and availability as well as caring for physical needs.
- Reinforce use of previously effective coping skills. Instruct in, or encourage use of, visualization and relaxation techniques.
- Assist SO(s) to cope with client's response and include age-specific interventions. **Family/SO(s) may not understand or be intolerant of client's distress and inadvertently hamper client's progress.**
- Include family/SO(s) in setting realistic goals for meeting needs of family members.
- Use sedatives or tranquilizers with caution **to avoid retarding resolution of grief process.**

Information that appears in brackets has been added by the authors to clarify and enhance the use of nursing diagnoses.

Cultural Collaborative Community/Home Care

Nursing Priority No. 4.

To promote wellness (Teaching/Discharge Considerations):

- Discuss with client/SO(s) healthy ways of dealing with difficult situations.
- Have client identify familial, religious, and cultural factors that have meaning for him or her. **May help bring loss into perspective and promote grief resolution.**
- Encourage involvement in usual activities, exercise, and socialization within limits of physical ability and psychological state.
- Advocate planning for the future, as appropriate, to individual situation (e.g., staying in own home after death of spouse, returning to sporting activities following traumatic amputation, choice to have another child or to adopt, rebuilding home following a disaster).
- Refer to other resources (e.g., pastoral care, family counseling, psychotherapy, organized support groups). **Provides additional help, when needed, to resolve situation/continue grief work.**

Documentation Focus

Assessment/Reassessment
- Assessment findings, including meaning of loss to the client, current stage of the grieving process, and responses of family/SO(s).
- Cultural or religious beliefs and expectations.
- Availability and use of resources.

Planning
- Plan of care and who is involved in the planning.
- Teaching plan.

Implementation/Evaluation
- Client's response to interventions, teaching, and actions performed.
- Attainment or progress toward desired outcome(s).
- Modifications to plan of care.

Discharge Planning
- Long-term needs and who is responsible for actions to be taken.
- Specific referrals made.

Information that appears in brackets has been added by the authors to clarify and enhance the use of nursing diagnoses.

Sample Nursing Outcomes & Interventions Classifications (NOC/NIC) `NIC`

NOC—Grief Resolution
NIC—Grief Work Facilitation

risk for complicated Grieving

Taxonomy II: Coping/Stress Tolerance – Class 2 Coping
   Responses (00172)
[Diagnostic Division: Ego Integrity]
Submitted as risk for dysfunctional Grieving 2004;
   Revised 2006

Definition: At risk for a disorder that occurs after the
death of a significant other, in which the experience of
distress accompanying bereavement fails to follow
normative expectations and manifests in functional
impairment

Risk Factors

Death of a significant other
Emotional instability
Lack of social support
Loss of significant object (e.g., possessions, job, status, home,
   parts and processes of body)

NOTE: A risk diagnosis is not evidenced by signs and
symptoms, as the problem has not occurred; rather
nursing interventions are directed at prevention.

Desired Outcomes/Evaluation Criteria— Client Will:

- Acknowledge awareness of individual factors affecting client
  in this situation. (See Risk Factors.)
- Identify emotional responses and behaviors occurring after
  the death or loss.
- Participate in therapy to learn new ways of dealing with an-
  xiety and feelings of inadequacy.
- Discuss meaning of loss to individual/family.
- Verbalize a sense of beginning to deal with grief process.

Information that appears in brackets has been added by the authors to clarify
and enhance the use of nursing diagnoses.

⊕ Cultural   Ⓐ Collaborative   🏠 Community/Home Care

Actions/Interventions ———————————

risk for complicated GRIEVING

Nursing Priority No. 1.

To identify risk/contributing factors:

- Determine loss that has occurred and meaning to client. Note whether loss was sudden or expected.
- ∞ Ascertain gestational age of fetus at time of loss, or length of life of infant or child. **Death of child may be more difficult for parents/family to deal with based on individual values and sense of life unlived.**
- Note stage of grief client is experiencing. **Stages of grief may progress in a predictable manner or stages may be random or revisited.**
- Assess client's ability to manage activities of daily living and period of time since loss has occurred. **Periods of crying, feelings of overwhelming sadness, and loss of appetite and insomnia can occur with grieving; however, when they persist and interfere with normal activities, client may need additional assistance.**
- Note availability and use of support systems, community resources.
- Identify cultural or religious beliefs and expectations that may impact or dictate client's response to loss.
- Assess status of relationships, marital difficulties, and adjustments to loss.

Nursing Priority No. 2.

To assist client to deal appropriately with loss:

- Discuss meaning of loss to client, Active-listen responses without judgment.
- Encourage expression of feelings, including anger, fear, or anxiety. Let client know that all feelings are okay, while setting limits on destructive behavior.
- Respect client's desire for quiet, privacy, talking, or silence.
- Acknowledge client's sense of relief or guilt at feeling relief when death follows a long and debilitating course. **Sadness and loss are still there, but the death may be a release; or, client may feel guilty about having a sense of relief.**
- ∞ Discuss the circumstances surrounding the death of a fetus or child. Was it sudden or expected? Have other children been lost (multiple miscarriages)? Was a congenital anomaly present? **Repeated losses increase sense of futility and compromise resolution of grieving process.**

Information that appears in brackets has been added by the authors to clarify and enhance the use of nursing diagnoses.

- Meet with both members of the couple **to determine how they are dealing with the loss.**
• Encourage client/SOs to honor cultural practices through funerals, wakes, sitting shiva, and so forth.
- Assist SO(s)/family to understand and be tolerant of client's feelings and behavior.

Nursing Priority No. 3.

To promote wellness (Teaching/Discharge Considerations):

- Encourage client/SO(s) to identify healthy coping skills they have used in the past. **These can be used in current situation to facilitate dealing with grief.**
- Assist in setting goals for meeting needs of client and family members to move beyond the grieving process.
- Suggest resuming involvement in usual activities, exercise, and socialization within physical and psychological abilities.
- Discuss planning for the future, as appropriate to individual situation (e.g., staying in own home after death of spouse, returning to sporting activities following traumatic amputation, choosing to have another child or to adopt, rebuilding home following a disaster).
- Refer to other resources, as needed, such as counseling, psychotherapy, spiritual advisor, grief support group. **Depending upon meaning of the loss, individual may require ongoing support to work through grief.**

Documentation Focus

Assessment/Reassessment
- Assessment findings, including meaning of loss to the client, current stage of the grieving process, psychological status, and responses of family/SO(s).
- Availability and use of resources.

Planning
- Plan of care and who is involved in the planning.
- Teaching plan.

Implementation/Evaluation
- Client's response to interventions, teaching, and actions performed.
- Attainment or progress toward desired outcome(s).
- Modifications to plan of care.

Information that appears in brackets has been added by the authors to clarify and enhance the use of nursing diagnoses.

Cultural   Collaborative   Community/Home Care

Discharge Planning
• Long-term needs and who is responsible for actions to be taken.
• Specific referrals made.

Sample Nursing Outcomes & Interventions Classifications (NOC/NIC) NIC

NOC—Grief Resolution
NIC—Grief Work Facilitation

---

risk for disproportionate Growth

Taxonomy II: Growth/Development—Class 1 Growth (00113)
[Diagnostic Division: Teaching/Learning]
Nursing Diagnosis Extension and Classification (NDEC) Submission 1998

Definition: At risk for growth above the 97th percentile or below the 3rd percentile for age, crossing two percentile channels

---

Risk Factors ————————————————————

Prenatal
Maternal nutrition, infection; multiple gestation
Substance use or abuse; teratogen exposure
Congenital or genetic disorders [e.g., dysfunction of endocrine gland, tumors]

Individual
Prematurity
Malnutrition; caregiver's or individual's maladaptive feeding behaviors; insatiable appetite; anorexia [impaired metabolism, greater than normal energy requirements]
Infection; chronic illness [e.g., chronic inflammatory diseases]
Substance [use or] abuse [including anabolic steroids]

Environmental
Deprivation; poverty
Violence; natural disasters
Teratogen; lead poisoning

Information that appears in brackets has been added by the authors to clarify and enhance the use of nursing diagnoses.

Diagnostic Studies   ∞ Pediatric/Geriatric/Lifespan   Medications **407**

Caregiver

Abuse

Mental illness

Learning difficulties (mental handicap); severe learning disability

> **NOTE:** A risk diagnosis is not evidenced by signs and symptoms, as the problem has not occurred; rather nursing interventions are directed at prevention.

Desired Outcomes/Evaluation Criteria— Client Will:

* Receive appropriate nutrition as indicated by individual needs.
* Demonstrate weight and growth stabilizing or progress toward age-appropriate size.
* Participate in plan of care as appropriate for age and ability.

Caregiver Will:

* Verbalize understanding of potential for growth delay or deviation and plans for prevention.

Actions/Interventions

Nursing Priority No. 1.

To assess causative/contributing factors:

* Determine factors or condition(s) existing that could contribute to growth deviation as listed in Risk Factors, including familial history of pituitary tumors, Marfan's syndrome, genetic anomalies, use of certain drugs or substances during pregnancy, maternal diabetes or other chronic illness, poverty or inability to attend to nutritional issues, eating disorders, and so forth.
* Identify nature and effectiveness of parenting/caregiving activities (e.g., inadequate, inconsistent, unrealistic or insufficient expectations; lack of stimulation, limit setting, responsiveness).
* Note severity and pervasiveness of situation (e.g., individual showing effects of long-term physical or emotional abuse or neglect versus individual experiencing recent-onset situational disruption or inadequate resources during period of crisis or transition).

Information that appears in brackets has been added by the authors to clarify and enhance the use of nursing diagnoses.

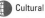 Cultural Collaborative Community/Home Care

- Perform nutritional assessment. **Overfeeding or malnutrition (protein and other basic nutrients) on a constant basis prevents child from reaching healthy growth potential, even if no disorder/disease exists.** (Refer to ND imbalanced Nutrition: [specify].)
- Note results of laboratory tests.
- Determine cultural, familial, and societal issues that may impact situation (e.g., childhood obesity now a risk for American children; parental concern for amount of food intake; expectations for "normal growth").
- Assess significant stressful events, losses, separation, and environmental changes (e.g., abandonment, divorce, death of parent/sibling, aging, move).
- Assess cognition, awareness, orientation, behavior (e.g., withdrawal or aggression), reaction to environment and stimuli.
- Active-listen concerns about body size, ability to perform competitively (e.g., sports, body building) **to ascertain the potential for use of anabolic steroids or other drugs.**

Nursing Priority No. 2.

To prevent/limit deviation from growth norms:

- Determine chronological age, familial factors (body build and stature) **to determine growth expectations.** Note reported losses or alterations in functional level. **Provides comparative baseline.**
- Identify present age and growth stage. Review expectations for current height and weight percentiles and any degree of deviation.
- Investigate deviations from normal (e.g., height and weight, head circumference, hand and feet size, facial features). **Deviations can be multifactorial and require varying interventions (e.g., weight deviation only [increased or decreased] may be remedied by changes in nutrition and exercise; other deviations may require in-depth evaluation and long-term treatment).**
- Determine if child's growth is above 97th percentile (very tall and large) for age. **Suggests need for evaluation for endocrine or other disorders.**
- Determine if child's growth is below 3rd percentile (very short and small) for age. **May require evaluation for failure to thrive.**
- Note reports of changes in facial features, joint pain, lethargy, sexual dysfunction, and/or progressive increase in hat, glove, ring, or shoe size in adults, especially after age 40. **Individual**

Information that appears in brackets has been added by the authors to clarify and enhance the use of nursing diagnoses.

 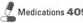

should be referred for further evaluation for **hyperpitui-tarism, growth hormone imbalance, or acromegaly.**

• Review results of x-rays, bone scans, MRIs **to determine bone age; extent of bone and soft-tissue overgrowth; presence of tumors;** note laboratory studies (e.g., growth hormone levels or other endocrine studies) **to identify pathology.**

• Assist with therapy to treat or correct underlying conditions (e.g., Crohn's disease, cardiac problems, renal disease); endocrine problems (e.g., hyperpituitarism, hypothyroidism, type 1 diabetes mellitus, growth hormone abnormalities); genetic or intrauterine growth retardation; infant feeding problems; nutritional deficits.

• Include nutritionist and other specialists (e.g., physical and occupational therapist) in developing plan of care.

• Determine need for medications (e.g., appetite stimulants or antidepressants, growth hormones).

• Monitor growth periodically. **Aids in evaluating effectiveness of interventions and promotes early identification of need for additional actions.**

Nursing Priority No. 3.

To promote wellness (Teaching/Discharge Considerations):

• Provide information regarding normal growth, as appropriate, including pertinent reference materials and credible Web sites.

• Address caregiver issues (e.g., parental abuse, learning deficiencies, environment of poverty) **that could impact client's ability to thrive.**

• Discuss appropriateness of appearance, grooming, touching, language, and other associated developmental issues. (Refer to NDs delayed Growth and Development; Self-Care Deficit [specify].)

• Recommend involvement in regular exercise or sports medicine program **to enhance muscle tone and strength, and appropriate body building.**

• Promote lifestyle that prevents or limits complications (e.g., management of obesity, hypertension, sensory or perceptual impairments); regular medical follow-up; nutritionally balanced meals; socialization for age and development **to maintain functional independence and enhance quality of life.**

• Discuss consequences of substance use or abuse with girls and women of childbearing age, and provide pregnant women with information regarding known teratogenic agents. **Edu-**

Information that appears in brackets has been added by the authors to clarify and enhance the use of nursing diagnoses.

⊕ Cultural ◉ Collaborative 🏠 Community/Home Care

cation can influence mother to abstain from use of drugs or agents that may cause birth defects.

- Refer for genetic screening, as appropriate.
- Identify available community resources, as appropriate (e.g., public health programs, such as WIC; medical equipment supplies; nutritionists; substance-abuse programs; specialists in endocrine problems/genetics).

Documentation Focus

Assessment/Reassessment
- Assessment findings, individual needs, including current growth status, and trends.
- Caregiver's understanding of situation and individual role.

Planning
- Plan of care and who is involved in the planning.
- Teaching plan.

Implementation/Evaluation
- Client's responses to interventions, teaching, and actions performed.
- Caregiver response to teaching.
- Attainment or progress toward desired outcome(s).
- Modifications to plan of care.

Discharge Planning
- Identified long-term needs and who is responsible for actions to be taken.
- Specific referrals made, sources for assistive devices, educational tools.

Sample Nursing Outcomes & Interventions Classifications (NOC/NIC) **NIC**

NOC—Growth
NIC—Nutritional Monitoring

delayed Growth and Development

Taxonomy II: Growth/Development—Class 1 Growth/
   Class 2 Development (00111)
[Diagnostic Division: Teaching/Learning]
Submitted 1986

Definition: Deviations from age-group norms

Information that appears in brackets has been added by the authors to clarify and enhance the use of nursing diagnoses.

Related Factors

Inadequate caretaking; [physical or emotional neglect or abuse]
Indifference; inconsistent responsiveness; multiple caretakers
Separation from SOs
Environmental or stimulation deficiencies
Effects of physical disability [handicapping condition]
Prescribed dependence [insufficient expectations for self-care]
Physical or emotional illness (chronic, traumatic) (e.g., chronic inflammatory disease, pituitary tumors, impaired nutrition or metabolism, greater than normal energy requirements, prolonged or painful treatments, prolonged or repeated hospitalizations)
Sexual abuse
Substance use or abuse

Defining Characteristics

Subjective
Inability to perform self-care or self-control activities appropriate for age

Objective
Delay or difficulty in performing skills typical of age group [loss of previously acquired skills]
Altered physical growth
Flat affect; listlessness; decreased responses
Sleep disturbances; negative mood or response

Desired Outcomes/Evaluation Criteria— Client Will:

- Perform motor, social, and/or expressive skills typical of age group within scope of present capabilities.
- Perform self-care and self-control activities appropriate for age.
- Demonstrate weight and growth stabilization or progress toward age-appropriate size.

Parents/Caregivers Will:

- Verbalize understanding of growth or developmental delay or deviation and plan(s) for intervention.
- (Refer to ND risk for delayed Development for additonal actions or interventions.)

Information that appears in brackets has been added by the authors to clarify and enhance the use of nursing diagnoses.

 Cultural · Collaborative · Community/Home Care

Actions/Interventions

Nursing Priority No. 1.

To assess causative/contributing factors:

- Determine existing condition(s) contributing to growth or developmental deviation, such as limited intellectual capacity, physical disabilities, chronic illness, genetic anomalies, substance use or abuse, multiple birth (e.g., twins), minimal length of time between pregnancies.
- Determine nature of parenting/caretaking activities (e.g., inadequate, inconsistent, unrealistic or insufficient expectations; lack of stimulation, limit setting, responsiveness).
- Note severity and pervasiveness of situation (e.g., long-term physical or emotional abuse versus situational disruption or inadequate assistance during period of crisis or transition).
- Assess occurrence and frequency of significant stressful events, losses, separation, and environmental changes (e.g., abandonment; divorce; death of parent/sibling; aging; unemployment; new job; moves; new baby or sibling; marriage; new stepparent).
- Determine presence of environmental risk factors (e.g., child of parent[s] with active substance abuse issues, or who are abusive, neglectful, or mentally disabled).
- Active-listen to SO's concerns about client's body size, ability to communicate or perform desired/needed activites or participate competitively (e.g., sports, body building).
- Determine use of drugs, **which may affect body growth.**
- Evaluate usual care setting (e.g., home, day care, institutional environment) **to determine adequacy of care provided, including nourishing meals, healthy sleep or rest time, stimulation, diversional or play activities.**

Nursing Priority No. 2.

To determine degree of deviation from norms:

- Record height and weight over time **to determine trends, identify needs, and evaluate effectiveness of therapies.**
- Review expectations for current height and weight percentile. **Compares measurements to "standard" or normal range for children of same age and gender to determine degree of deviation.**
- Note chronological age, familial factors (e.g., including body build and stature), and cultural concerns **to determine individual growth and developmental expectations.**

Information that appears in brackets has been added by the authors to clarify and enhance the use of nursing diagnoses.

- Identify present age and developmental stage. Note reported deficits in functional level or evidence of precocious development. **Provides comparative baseline.**
- Review expected skills/activities, using authoritative text (e.g., Gesell, Mussen-Conger) or assessment tools (e.g., Draw-a-Person, Denver Developmental Screening Test, Bender's Visual Motor Gestalt Test).
- Note degree of individual deviation, multiple skills affected (e.g., speech, motor activity, socialization), versus a single area of difficulty, such as toileting.
- Note whether difficulty is temporary or permanent (e.g., setback or delay versus irreversible condition, such as brain damage, stroke, dementia).
- Investigate sexual acting-out behaviors inappropriate for age. **May indicate sexual abuse.**
- Note findings of psychological evaluation of client and family **to determine factors that may impact development of client or impair psychological health of family.**

Nursing Priority No. 3.

To correct/minimize growth deviations and associated complications:

- Participate in treatment of underlying medical or psychological conditions (e.g., malnourishment, kidney failure, congenital heart disease, cystic fibrosis, inflammatory bowel disease, bone or cartilage conditions, endocrine disorders, adverse effects of medications, mental illness, substance abuse), as appropriate.
- Review medication regimen given to stimulate or suppress growth, as appropriate, or possibly to shrink pituitary tumor when present.
- Emphasize necessity of not stopping medications without approval of healthcare provider.
- Discuss appropriateness and potential complications of bone-lengthening procedures.
- Review consequences of substance use or abuse.
- Include nutritionist and other specialists (e.g., physical or occupational therapists) in developing plan of care. Encourage "early intervention services" for children birth to 3 years of age with developmental delays. **Federally funded entitlement program for qualified child (e.g., Down syndrome or cerebral palsy; prematurity; deprived physical or social environment) aimed at maximizing child's development. Services include nursing, occupational, physical, or speech**

Information that appears in brackets has been added by the authors to clarify and enhance the use of nursing diagnoses.

Cultural   Collaborative   Community/Home Care

therapy, service coordination, social work, and assistive technologies.

- Monitor growth and development factors periodically. **Aids in evaluating effectiveness of interventions over time and promotes early identification of need for additional actions.**

Nursing Priority No. 4.

To assist client (and/or caregivers) to prevent, minimize, or overcome delay or regressed development:

- Provide anticipatory guidance for parents/caregivers regarding expectations for client's development **to clarify misconceptions and assist them in dealing with reality of situation.**
- Consult appropriate professional resources (e.g., occupational, rehabilitation, or speech therapists, special-education teacher, job counselor) **to address specific individual needs.**
- Encourage recognition that certain deviations or behaviors are appropriate for a specific developmental age level (e.g., 14-year-old is functioning at level of 6-year-old is not able to anticipate the consequences of his or her actions). **Promotes acceptance of client, as presented, and helps shape expectations reflecting actual situation.**
- Avoid blame when discussing contributing factors.
- Maintain positive, hopeful attitude. Support self-actualizing nature of the individual and attempts to maintain or return to optimal level of self-control or self-care activities.
- Refer family/client for counseling/psychotherapy **to deal with issues of abuse or neglect.**
- Encourage setting of short-term, realistic goals for achieving developmental potential.
- Involve client in opportunities to practice new behaviors (e.g., role playing, group activities). **Strengthens learning process.**
- Identify equipment needs (e.g., adaptive or growth-stimulating computer programs, communication devices).
- Evaluate progress on continual basis **to increase complexity of tasks and goals, as appropriate.**
- Provide positive feedback for efforts, successes, and adaptation while minimizing failures. **Encourages continuation of efforts, thus improving outcome.**
- Assist client/caregivers to accept and adjust to irreversible developmental deviations (e.g., Down syndrome).
- Provide support for caregiver during transitional crises (e.g., residential schooling, institutionalization).

Information that appears in brackets has been added by the authors to clarify and enhance the use of nursing diagnoses.

Nursing Priority No. 5.

To promote wellness (Teaching/Discharge Considerations):

- Provide information regarding normal growth and development process, as appropriate. Suggest genetic counseling for family/client dependent on causative factors.

- Determine reasonable expectations for individual without restricting potential (i.e., set realistic goals that, if met, can be advanced). **Provides hope for achievement and promotes continued personal growth.**

- Discuss appropriateness of appearance, grooming, touching, language, and other associated developmental issues. (Refer to ND Self-Care Deficit [specify].)

- Recommend involvement in regular exercise or sports medicine program **to enhance muscle tone and strength, and appropriate body building.**

- Discuss actions to take to avoid preventable complications **(e.g., periodic laboratory studies monitoring hormone levels or nutritional status).**

- Recommend that client wears medical alert bracelet when taking replacement growth hormones **to alert care providers in case client is injured or ill.**

- Encourage attendance at appropriate educational programs (e.g., parenting and expectant parent classes; infant stimulation sessions; seminars on life stresses, aging process).

- Provide pertinent reference materials and pamphlets. **Enhances learning at own pace.**

- Discuss community responsibilities (e.g., services required to be provided to school-age child). Include social worker or special-education team in planning process **for meeting educational, physical, psychological, and monitoring needs of child.**

- Identify community resources, as appropriate: public health programs, such as WIC; well-baby care provider; nutritionist; substance abuse programs; early-intervention programs; seniors' activity or support groups; gifted and talented programs; sheltered workshop; disabled children's services; medical equipment supplier. **Provides additional assistance to support family efforts in treatment program.**

- Refer to social services, as indicated, **to determine safety of client and consideration of placement in foster care.**

- Refer to the NDs impaired Parenting; interrupted Family Processes.

Information that appears in brackets has been added by the authors to clarify and enhance the use of nursing diagnoses.

Cultural   Collaborative   Community/Home Care

Documentation Focus

Assessment/Reassessment
- Assessment findings individual needs, current growth status and trends, and developmental level, evidence of regression.
- Caregiver's understanding of situation and individual role.
- Safety of individual, need for placement.

Planning
- Plan of care and who is involved in the planning.
- Teaching plan.

Implementation/Evaluation
- Client's responses to interventions, teaching, and actions performed.
- Caregiver response to teaching.
- Attainment or progress toward desired outcome(s).
- Modifications to plan of care.

Discharge Planning
- Identified long-term needs and who is responsible for actions to be taken.
- Specific referrals made; sources for assistive devices, educational tools.

Sample Nursing Outcomes & Interventions Classifications (NOC/NIC) NIC

NOC—Child Development: [specify age group]
NIC—Developmental Enhancement: Child [or] Adolescent

---

ineffective Health Maintenance

Taxonomy II: Health Promotion—Class 2 Health Management (00099)
[Diagnostic Division: Safety]
Submitted 1982

Definition: Inability to identify, manage, and/or seek out help to maintain health

---

Information that appears in brackets has been added by the authors to clarify and enhance the use of nursing diagnoses.

 Diagnostic Studies Pediatric/Geriatric/Lifespan Medications **417**

This diagnosis contains components of other NDs. We recommend subsuming health maintenance interventions under the "basic" nursing diagnosis when a single causative factor is identified (e.g., deficient Knowledge [specify]; ineffective self Health Management; chronic Confusion; impaired verbal Communication; disturbed Thought Processes; ineffective Coping; compromised family Coping; delayed Growth and Development).

Related Factors

Deficient communication skills [written, verbal, and/or gestural]
Unachieved developmental tasks
Inability to make appropriate judgments
Perceptual or cognitive impairment
Diminished or lack of gross or fine motor skills
Ineffective individual or family coping; complicated grieving; spiritual distress
Insufficient resources (e.g., equipment, finances); [lack of psychosocial supports]

Defining Characteristics

Subjective
Lack of expressed interest in improving health behaviors
Reported compulsive behaviors

Objective
Demonstrated lack of knowledge regarding basic health practices
Inability to take the responsibility for meeting basic health practices; history of lack of health-seeking behavior
Demonstrated lack of adaptive behaviors to environmental changes
Impairment of personal support system
Observed compulsive behaviors

Desired Outcomes/Evaluation Criteria— Client Will:

• Identify necessary health maintenance activities.
• Verbalize understanding of factors contributing to current situation.

Information that appears in brackets has been added by the authors to clarify and enhance the use of nursing diagnoses.

  Cultural Collaborative Community/Home Care

- Assume responsibility for own healthcare needs within level of ability.
- Adopt lifestyle changes supporting individual healthcare goals.

SO/Caregiver Will:

- Verbalize ability to cope adequately with existing situation, provide support/monitoring as indicated.

Actions/Interventions

Nursing Priority No. 1.

To assess causative/contributing factors:

- Identify risk factors in client's personal and family history. Note health values, religious or cultural beliefs and expectations regarding healthcare.
- Assess level of client's cognitive, emotional, physical functioning. Determine presence of developmental disabilities.
- Determine whether impairment is an acute or sudden onset situation, a progressive illness, long-term health problem, or exacerbation or complication of chronic illness. **Requires more intensive or long-lasting support and interventions with progressive or chronic conditions.**
- Note client's age (e.g., very young or elderly) and level of dependence and independence. **May range from complete dependence (dysfunctional) to partial or relative independence requiring support in a single area.**
- Evaluate for substance use or abuse (e.g., alcohol or other drugs). **Affects client's desire and ability to help self.**
- Ascertain recent changes in lifestyle (e.g., widowed man who has no skills for taking care of his own/family's health needs; loss of independence; changing support systems).
- Note setting where client lives (e.g., long-term care facility, homebound, homeless).
- Note desire and level of ability to meet health maintenance needs, as well as self-care ADLs.
- Determine level of adaptive behavior, knowledge, and skills about health maintenance, environment, and safety. **Determines beginning point for planning and interventions to assist client in addressing needs.**
- Assess client's ability and desire to learn. Determine barriers to learning (e.g., can't read, speaks or understands different

Information that appears in brackets has been added by the authors to clarify and enhance the use of nursing diagnoses.

language than is used in the present setting, is overcome with grief or stress, has no interest in subject).
- Assess communication skills and ability, or need for interpreter. Identify support person requesting or willing to accept information.
- Note client's use of professional services and resources (e.g., appropriate or inappropriate/nonexistent).

Nursing Priority No. 2.

To assist client/caregiver(s) to maintain and manage desired health practices:
- Discuss with client/SO(s) beliefs about health and reasons for not following prescribed plan of care. **Determines client's view about current situation and potential for change.**
- Evaluate environment **to note individual adaptation needs.**
- Develop plan with client/SO(s) for self-care. **Allows for incorporating existing disabilities with client's/SO's desires and ability to adapt and organize care activites.**
- Involve comprehensive specialty health teams when indicated (e.g., pulmonary, psychiatric, enterostomal, IV therapy, nutritional support, substance-abuse counselors).
- Provide anticipatory guidance **to maintain and manage effective health practices during periods of wellness and identify ways client can adapt when progressive illness/ long-term health problems occur.**
- Encourage socialization and personal involvement **to enhance support system, provide pleasant stimuli, and prevent permanent regression.**
- Provide for communication and coordination between the healthcare facility team and community healthcare providers **to provide continuation of care.**
- Monitor adherence to prescribed medical regimen **to problem-solve difficulties in adherence and alter the plan of care, as needed.**

Nursing Priority No. 3.

To promote wellness (Teaching/Discharge Considerations):
- Provide information about individual healthcare needs, using client's/SO's preferred learning style (e.g., pictures, words, video, Internet) **to assist client in understanding own situation and enhance interest/involvement in meeting own health needs.**
- Limit amount of information presented at one time, especially when dealing with elderly, or cognitively or developmentally

Information that appears in brackets has been added by the authors to clarify and enhance the use of nursing diagnoses.

impaired client. Present new material through self-paced instruction when possible. **Allows client time to process and store new information.**

 • Help client/SO(s) develop realistic healthcare goals. Provide a written copy to those involved in planning process **for future reference and revision, as appropriate.**

• Assist client/SO(s) to develop stress management skills.

• Identify ways to adapt things in current circumstances **to meet client's changing needs and abilities, and environmental concerns.**

• Identify signs and symptoms requiring further medical screening, evaluation, and follow-up care.

• Make referral, as needed, for community support services (e.g., homemaker/home attendant, Meals on Wheels, skilled nursing care, well-baby clinic, senior citizen healthcare activities).

• Refer to social services, as indicated, **for assistance with financial, housing, or legal concerns (e.g., conservatorship).**

• Refer to support groups, as appropriate (e.g., senior citizens, Salvation Army shelter, homeless clinic, Alcoholics or Narcotics Anonymous).

• Arrange for hospice service for client with terminal illness.

Documentation Focus

Assessment/Reassessment
• Assessment findings, including individual abilities; family involvement; support factors, and availability of resources.
• Cultural or religious beliefs and healthcare values.

Planning
• Plan of care and who is involved in planning.
• Teaching plan.

Implementation/Evaluation
• Responses of client/SO(s) to plan, specific interventions, teaching, and actions performed.
• Attainment or progress toward desired outcome(s).
• Modifications to plan of care.

Discharge Planning
• Long-range needs and who is responsible for actions to be taken.
• Specific referrals made.

Information that appears in brackets has been added by the authors to clarify and enhance the use of nursing diagnoses.

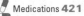

Sample Nursing Outcomes & Interventions Classifications (NOC/NIC) [NIC]

NOC—Health Promoting Behavior
NIC—Health System Guidance

ineffective self Health Management

Taxonomy II: Health Promotion—Class 2 Health Management (00078)
[Diagnostic Division: Teaching/Learning]
Submitted as ineffective Therapeutic Regimen Management 1992; revised 2008

Definition: Pattern of regulating and integrating into daily living a therapeutic regimen for treatment of illness and its sequelae that is unsatisfactory for meeting specific health goals

Related Factors

Complexity of healthcare system or therapeutic regimen
Decisional conflicts
Economic difficulties
Excessive demands made (e.g., individual, family); family conflict
Family patterns of healthcare
Inadequate number of cues to action
Knowledge deficit
Regimen; perceived seriousness, susceptibility, barriers, or benefits
Powerlessness
Social support deficits

Defining Characteristics

Subjective
Verbalizes desire to manage the illness
Verbalizes difficulty with prescribed regimen

Objective
Failure to include treatment regimens in daily living or take action to reduce risk factors
Makes choices in daily living ineffective for meeting the health goals
Unexpected acceleration of illness symptoms

Information that appears in brackets has been added by the authors to clarify and enhance the use of nursing diagnoses.

Desired Outcomes/Evaluation Criteria— Client Will:

- Verbalize acceptance of need and desire to change actions to achieve agreed-on health goals.
- Verbalize understanding of factors or blocks involved in individual situation.
- Participate in problem solving of factors interfering with integration of therapeutic regimen.
- Demonstrate behaviors and changes in lifestyle necessary to maintain therapeutic regimen.
- Identify and use available resources.

Actions/Interventions

Nursing Priority No. 1.
To identify causative/contributing factors:

- Ascertain client's knowledge and understanding of condition and treatment needs **so that he or she can make informed decisions about managing self-care.**
- Determine client's/family's health goals and patterns of healthcare.
- Identify cultural values or religious beliefs affecting client's view of situation and willingness to make necessary changes.
- Identify client locus of control: internal (expressions of responsibility for self and ability to control outcomes: "I didn't quit smoking") or external (expressions of lack of control over self and environment: "Nothing ever works out"; "What bad luck to get lung cancer").
- Identify individual perceptions and expectations of treatment regimen.
- Review complexity of treatment regimen (e.g., number of expected tasks, such as taking medication four times/day or once/day) and evaluate how difficult tasks might be for client (e.g., must stop smoking, must follow strict dialysis diet even when feeling well). **These factors are often involved in lack of participation in treatment plan.**
- Note availability and use of resources for assistance, caregiving and respite care.

Nursing Priority No. 2.
To assist client/SO(s) to develop strategies to improve management of therapeutic regimen:

- Use therapeutic communication skills **to assist client to problem solve solution(s).**

Information that appears in brackets has been added by the authors to clarify and enhance the use of nursing diagnoses.

- Explore client involvement in or lack of mutual goal setting.
- Use client's locus of control to develop individual plan to adapt regimen (e.g., for client with internal control, encourage client to take control of own care and for those with external control, begin with small tasks and add, as tolerated).
- Identify steps necessary to reach desired goal(s).
- Contract with the client for participation in care.
- Accept client's evaluation of own strengths and limitations while working together to improve abilities. State belief in client's ability to cope and/or adapt to situation.
- Provide positive reinforcement for efforts **to encourage continuation of desired behaviors.**
- Provide information and encourage client to seek out resources on own. Reinforce previous instructions and rationale, using a variety of learning modalities, including role playing, demonstration, and written materials.

Nursing Priority No. 3.
To promote wellness (Teaching/Discharge Considerations):

- Emphasize importance of client knowledge and understanding of the need for treatment or medication as well as consequences of actions and choices.
- Promote client/caregiver/SO(s) participation in planning and evaluating process. **Enhances commitment to plan, optimizing outcomes.**
- Assist client to develop strategies for monitoring therapeutic regimen. **Promotes early recognition of changes, allowing proactive response.**
- Mobilize support systems, including family/SO(s), social, and financial.
- Refer to counseling or therapy (group and individual), as indicated.
- Identify home- and community-based nursing services **for assessment, follow-up care, and education in client's home.**

Documentation Focus ———————————————

Assessment/Reassessment
- Findings, including underlying dynamics of individual situation, client's perception of problem or needs, locus of control.
- Cultural values, religious beliefs.
- Family involvement and needs.

Information that appears in brackets has been added by the authors to clarify and enhance the use of nursing diagnoses.

    Cultural   Collaborative   Community/Home Care

- Individual strengths and limitations.
- Availability and use of resources.

Planning
- Plan of care and who is involved in planning.
- Teaching plan.

Implementation/Evaluation
- Response to interventions, teaching, and actions performed.
- Attainment or progress toward desired outcome(s).
- Modifications to plan of care.

Discharge Planning
- Long-term needs and who is responsible for actions to be taken.
- Available resources, specific referrals made.

Sample Nursing Outcomes & Interventions Classifications (NOC/NIC) NIC

NOC—Treatment Behavior: Illness or Injury
NIC—Self-Modification Assistance

---

readiness for enhanced self Health Management

Taxonomy II: Health Promotion—Class 2 Health Management (00162)
[Diagnostic Division: Teaching/Learning]
Submitted as readiness for enhanced Therapeutic Regimen Management 2002; name change 2008

Definition: A pattern of regulating and integrating into daily living a therapeutic regimen for treatment of illness and its sequelae that is sufficient for meeting health-related goals and can be strengthened

---

Related Factors

To be developed

Defining Characteristics

Subjective
Expresses desire to manage the illness (e.g., treatment, prevention of sequelae)

Information that appears in brackets has been added by the authors to clarify and enhance the use of nursing diagnoses.

Expresses little difficulty with prescribed regimens
Describes reduction of risk factors

Objective

Choices of daily living are appropriate for meeting goals (e.g., treatment, prevention)
No unexpected acceleration of illness symptoms

Desired Outcomes/Evaluation Criteria— Client Will:

* Assume responsibility for managing treatment regimen.
* Demonstrate proactive management by anticipating and planning for eventualities of condition or potential complications.
* Identify and use additional resources as appropriate.
* Remain free of preventable complications, progression of illness and sequelae.

Actions/Interventions

Nursing Priority No. 1.

To determine motivation for continued growth:

* Verify client's level of knowledge and understanding of therapeutic regimen. Note specific health goals. **Provides opportunity to ensure accuracy and completeness of knowledge base for future learning.**
* Determine client's current health status and perception of possible threats to health.
* Active-listen concerns to identify underlying issues (e.g., physical or emotional stressors, external factors such as environmental pollutants or other hazards) **that could impact client's ability to control own health.**
* Ascertain client's beliefs about health and his or her ability to maintain health. **Belief in ability to accomplish desired action is predictive of performance.**
* Identify individual's expectations of long-term treatment needs and anticipated changes.
* Determine present resources used by client **to note whether changes can be arranged (e.g., increased hours of home care assistance; access to case manager to support complex or long-term program).**

Nursing Priority No. 2.

To assist client/SO(s) to develop plan to meet individual needs:

Information that appears in brackets has been added by the authors to clarify and enhance the use of nursing diagnoses.

🌐 Cultural 🔬 Collaborative 🏠 Community/Home Care

- Acknowledge client's strengths in present health management and build on in planning for future.
- Identify steps necessary to reach desired health goal(s). **Understanding the process enhances commitment and the likelihood of achieving the goals.**
- Explore with client/SO(s) areas of health over which each individual has control and discuss barriers to healthy practices (e.g., chooses fast food instead of cooking for one; lack of time or access to convenient facility or safe environment in which to exercise). **Identifies actions individual can take to plan for improving health practices.**
- Accept client's evaluation of own strengths and limitations while working together to improve abilities. **Promotes sense of self-esteem and confidence to continue efforts.**
- Incorporate client's cultural values or religious beliefs that support attainment of health goals.
- Provide information and bibliotherapy. Help client/SO(s) identify and evaluate resources they can access on their own. **When referencing the Internet or nontraditional, unproven resources, the individual must exercise some restraint and determine the reliability of the source and information provided before acting on it.**
- Acknowledge individual efforts and capabilities to reinforce movement toward attainment of desired outcomes. **Provides positive reinforcement encouraging continued progress toward desired goals.**

Nursing Priority No. 3.
To promote optimum wellness:

- Promote client/caregiver choices and involvement in planning for and implementing added tasks and responsibilities.
- Encourage use of exercise, relaxation skills, yoga, meditation, visualization, and guided imagery **to assist in management of stress and promote general health and well-being.**
- Assist in implementing strategies for monitoring progress and responses to therapeutic regimen. **Promotes proactive problem solving.**
- Identify additional community resources/support groups (e.g., nutritionist/weight control program, smoking cessation program). **Provides further opportunities for role modeling, skill training, anticipatory problem solving, and so forth.**
- Instruct in individually appropriate wellness behaviors such as breast self-examination and mammogram, testicular

Information that appears in brackets has been added by the authors to clarify and enhance the use of nursing diagnoses.

self-examination and prostate examination, immunizations and flu shots, regular medical and dental examinations.

Documentation Focus

Assessment/Reassessment
- Findings, including dynamics of individual situation.
- Individual strengths, additional needs.
- Cultural values, religious beliefs.

Planning
- Plan of care and who is involved in planning.
- Teaching plan.

Implementation/Evaluation
- Response to interventions, teaching, and actions performed.
- Attainment or progress toward desired outcome(s).
- Modifications to plan of care.

Discharge Planning
- Short- and long-term needs and who is responsible for actions.
- Available resources, specific referrals made.

Sample Nursing Outcomes & Interventions Classifications (NOC/NIC) NIC

NOC—Health Seeking Behavior
NIC—Self-Modification Assistance

impaired Home Maintenance

Taxonomy II: Health Promotion—Class 2 Health Management (00098)
[Diagnostic Division: Safety]
Submitted 1980

Definition: Inability to independently maintain a safe growth-promoting immediate environment

Related Factors

Disease; injury
Insufficient family organization or planning
Insufficient finances

Information that appears in brackets has been added by the authors to clarify and enhance the use of nursing diagnoses.

Cultural Collaborative Community/Home Care

Impaired functioning
Lack of role modeling
Unfamiliarity with neighborhood resources
Deficient knowledge
Inadequate support systems

Defining Characteristics

Subjective
Household members express difficulty in maintaining their home in a comfortable [safe] fashion
Household members request assistance with home maintenance
Household members describe outstanding debts, financial crises

Objective
Disorderly or unclean surroundings; offensive odors
Inappropriate household temperature
Presence of vermin
Repeated unhygienic disorders or infections
Lack of necessary equipment; unavailable cooking equipment
Insufficient or lack of clothes or linen
Overtaxed family members

Desired Outcomes/Evaluation Criteria—Client/Caregiver Will:

- Identify individual factors related to difficulty in maintaining a safe environment.
- Verbalize plan to eliminate health and safety hazards.
- Adopt behaviors reflecting lifestyle changes to create and sustain a healthy, growth-promoting environment.
- Demonstrate appropriate, effective use of resources.

Actions/Interventions

Nursing Priority No. 1.
To assess causative/contributing factors:

- Identify presence of, or potential for, physical or mental conditions (e.g., advanced age, chronic illnesses, brain/other traumatic injuries; severe depression or other mental illness; multiple persons in one home incapable of handling home tasks) **that compromise client's/SO's functional abilities in taking care of home.**

Information that appears in brackets has been added by the authors to clarify and enhance the use of nursing diagnoses.

- Note presence of personal and/or environmental factors (e.g., family member with multiple care tasks; substance abuse; absence of family/support systems; lifestyle of self-neglect; client comfortable with home environment, has no desire for change).
- Determine problem in household and degree of discomfort and unsafe conditons noted by client/SO(s). **Safety problems may be obvious (e.g., lack of heat or water; unsanitary rooms), while other problems may be more subtle and difficult to manage (e.g., lack of finances for home repair, or lack of knowledge about food storage, rodent control).**
- Assess client/SO's level of cognitive, emotional, or physical functioning **to ascertain needs and capabilities in handling tasks of home management.**
- Identify lack of knowledge, misinformation.
- Discuss home environment or perform home visit, as appropriate, **to determine ability to care for self and to identify potential health and safety hazards.**
- Identify support systems available to client/SO(s) **to determine needs and initiate referrals (e.g., companionship, daily care, household cleaning or homemaking, running errands).**
- Determine financial resources to meet needs of individual situation.

Nursing Priority No. 2.
To help client/SO(s) create/maintain a safe, growth-promoting environment:

- Coordinate planning with multidisciplinary team, as appropriate.
- Assist client/SO(s) to develop plan for maintaining a clean, healthful environment (e.g., sharing of household tasks and repairs between family members, contract services, exterminators, trash removal).
- Assist client/SO(s) to identify and acquire necessary equipment (e.g., lifts, commode chair, safety grab bars, cleaning supplies, structural adaptations) **to meet individual needs.**
- Identify resources available for appropriate assistance (e.g., visiting nurse, budget counseling, homemaker, Meals on Wheels, physical or occupational therapy, social services).

Nursing Priority No. 3.
To promote wellness (Teaching/Discharge Considerations):

Information that appears in brackets has been added by the authors to clarify and enhance the use of nursing diagnoses.

  Cultural Collaborative Community/Home Care

• Discuss environmental hazards **that may negatively affect health or ability to perform desired activities.**
• Develop long-term plan for taking care of environmental needs (e.g., assistive personnel to clean house, do laundry; trash removal; and pest control services).
• Identify ways to access and use community resources and support systems (e.g., extended family, neighbors).
• Refer to NDs deficient Knowledge (specify); Self-Care Deficit [specify]; ineffective Coping; compromised family Coping; Caregiver Role Strain; risk for Injury.

Documentation Focus

Assessment/Reassessment
• Assessment findings include individual and environmental factors.
• Availability and use of support systems.

Planning
• Plan of care and who is involved in planning; support systems and community resources identified.
• Teaching plan.

Implementation/Evaluation
• Client's/SO's responses to interventions, teaching, and actions performed.
• Attainment or progress toward desired outcome(s).
• Modifications to plan of care.

Discharge Planning
• Long-term needs and who is responsible for actions to be taken.
• Specific referrals made, equipment needs/resources.

Sample Nursing Outcomes & Interventions Classifications (NOC/NIC) NIC

NOC—Self-Care: Instrumental Activities of Daily Living (IADL)
NIC—Home Maintenance Assistance

Information that appears in brackets has been added by the authors to clarify and enhance the use of nursing diagnoses.

Taxonomy II: Life Principles—Class 1 Values Class 2
   Beliefs/Self-Perception—Class 1 Self-Concept (00185)
[Diagnostic Division: Ego Integrity]
Submitted 2006

Definition: A pattern of expectations and desires that is
sufficient for mobilizing energy on one's own behalf and
can be strengthened

Related Factors

To be developed

Defining Characteristics

Subjective
Expresses desire to enhance hope; belief in possibilities; congruency of expectations with desires; ability to set achievable
   goals; problem solving to meet goals
Expresses desire to enhance sense of meaning to life; interconnectedness with others; spirituality

Desired Outcomes/Evaluation Criteria—
Client Will:

* Identify and verbalize feelings related to expectations and de-
   sires.
* Verbalize belief in possibilities for the future.
* Discuss current situation and desire to enhance hope.
* Set short-term goals that will lead to behavioral changes to
   meet desire for enhanced hope.

Actions/Interventions

Nursing Priority No. 1.
To determine needs and desire for improvement:
* Review familial and social history to identify past situations
   (e.g., illness, emotional conflicts, alcoholism) that have led to
   decision to improve life.
* Determine current physical condition of client/SO(s). **Treatment regimen can influence ability to promote positive
   feelings of hope.**

Information that appears in brackets has been added by the authors to clarify
and enhance the use of nursing diagnoses.

  Cultural Collaborative Community/Home Care

- Ascertain client's perception of current state and expectations/goals for the future (e.g., general well-being, prosperity, independence).
- Identify spiritual beliefs and cultural values that influence sense of hope and connectedness and give meaning to life.
- Note degree of involvement in activities and relationships with others. **Superficial interactions with others can limit sense of connectedness and reduce enjoyment of relationships.**
- Determine level of commitment and expectations for change and congruency of expectations with desires.

Nursing Priority No. 2.

To assist client to achieve goals and strengthen sense of hope:

- Establish a therapeutic relationship, showing positive regard and sense of hope for the client. **Enhances feelings of worth and comfort, inspiring client to continue pursuit of goals.**
- Help client recognize areas that are in his or her control versus those that are not. **To be most effective, client needs to expend energy in those areas where he or she has control/can make changes and let the others go.**
- Assist client to develop manageable short-term goals.
- Identify activities to achieve goals and facilitate contingency planning. **Helps client deal with situation in manageable steps, enhancing chances for success and sense of control.**
- Explore interrelatedness of unresolved emotions, anxieties, fears, and guilt. **Provides opportunity to address issues that may be limiting individual's ability to improve life situation.**
- Assist client to acknowledge current coping behaviors and defense mechanisms that are not helping client move toward goals. **Allows client to focus on coping mechanisms that are more successful in problem solving.**
- Encourage client to concentrate on progress not perfection. **If client can accept that perfection is difficult and generally not the focus—rather achieving the desired goal is—then he or she may be able to view own accomplishments with pride.**
- Involve client in care and explain all procedures thoroughly, answering questions truthfully. **Enhances trust and relationship, promoting hope for a positive outcome.**
- Express hope to client and encourage SO(s) and other heath team members to do so. **Enhances client's sense of hope and belief in possibility of a positive outcome.**

Information that appears in brackets has been added by the authors to clarify and enhance the use of nursing diagnoses.

🏠 • Identify ways to strengthen sense of interconnectedness or harmony with others **to support sense of belonging and connection that promotes feelings of wholeness and hopefulness.**

Nursing Priority No. 3.

To promote optimum wellness:

🏠 • Demonstrate and encourage use of relaxation techniques, guided imagery, and meditation activities.

🏠 • Provide positive feedback for actions taken to improve problem-solving skills and for setting achievable goals. **Acknowledges client's efforts and reinforces gains.**

🏠 • Explore how beliefs give meaning and value to daily living. **As client's understanding of these issues improves, hope for the future is strengthened.**

🏠 • Encourage life-review by client **to acknowledge own successes, identify opportunity for change, and clarify meaning in life.**

🏠 • Identify ways for client to express and strengthen spirituality. **There are many options for enhancing spirituality through connectedness with self/others (e.g., volunteering, mentoring, involvement in religious activities).** (Refer to ND readiness for enhanced Spiritual Well-Being.)

🏠 • Encourage client to join groups with similar or new interests. **Expanding knowledge and making friendships with new people will broaden horizons for the individual.**

🅐 • Refer to community resources and support groups, spiritual advisor, as indicated.

Documentation Focus ─────────────────

Assessment/Reassessment
• Assessment findings, including client's perceptions of current situation, relationships, sense of desire for enhancing life.
• Motivation and expectations for improvement.

Planning
• Plan of care and who is involved in planning.
• Teaching plan.

Implementation/Evaluation
• Responses to interventions, teaching, and actions performed.
• Attainment or progress toward desired outcome(s).
• Modifications to plan of care.

───────────────

Information that appears in brackets has been added by the authors to clarify and enhance the use of nursing diagnoses.

Discharge Planning

- Long-term needs and goals for change, and who is responsible for actions to be taken.
- Specific referrals made.

Sample Nursing Outcomes & Interventions Classifications (NOC/NIC) NIC

NOC—Hope
NIC—Spiritual Growth Facilitation

Hopelessness

Taxonomy II: Self-Perception—Class 1 Self-Concept (00124)
[Diagnostic Division: Ego Integrity]
Submitted 1986

Definition: Subjective state in which an individual sees limited or no alternatives or personal choices available and is unable to mobilize energy on own behalf

Related Factors

Prolonged activity restriction creating isolation
Deteriorating physiological condition
Long-term stress; abandonment
Lost belief in spiritual power or transcendent values

Defining Characteristics

Subjective
Verbal cues (despondent content, "I can't," sighing) [believes things will not change, problems will always be there]

Objective
Passivity; decreased verbalization
Decreased affect, appetite, or response to stimuli
Depressed cognitive functions; problems with decisions, thought processes; regression
Lack of initiative or involvement in care
Sleep pattern disturbance [increased or decreased sleep]
Turning away from speaker; shrugging in response to speaker; [withdrawal from environs; closing eyes]

Information that appears in brackets has been added by the authors to clarify and enhance the use of nursing diagnoses.

HOPELESSNESS

Lack of involvement or interest in SO(s) (children, spouse)
Angry outbursts
Substance abuse

Desired Outcomes/Evaluation Criteria— Client Will:

- Recognize and verbalize feelings.
- Identify and use coping mechanisms to counteract feelings of hopelessness.
- Involve self in and control (within limits of the individual situation) own self-care and ADLs.
- Set progressive short-term goals that develop and sustain behavioral changes, and foster positive outlook.
- Participate in diversional activities of own choice.

Actions/Interventions

Nursing Priority No. 1.
To identify causative/contributing factors:

- Review familial and social history and physiological history for problems, such as history of poor coping abilities, disorder of familial relating patterns, emotional problems, recent or long-term illness of client or family member, multiple social and/or physiological traumas to individual or family members.
- Note current familial, social, or physical situation of client (e.g., newly diagnosed with chronic or terminal disease, lack of support system, recent job loss, loss of spiritual or religious faith, recent multiple traumas, alcoholism or other substance abuse).
- Identify cultural or spiritual values and language barriers **that can impact beliefs in own ability to change situation.**
- Determine coping behaviors and defense mechanisms displayed.
- Discuss problem of alcohol or drug abuse. **Client may feel hopeless, believing behavior is impossible to stop.**
- Determine suicidal thoughts and if the client has a plan. **Hopelessness is a symptom of suicidal ideation.**

Nursing Priority No. 2.
To assess level of hopelessness:

- Note behaviors indicative of hopelessness. (Refer to Defining Characteristics.)

Information that appears in brackets has been added by the authors to clarify and enhance the use of nursing diagnoses.

Cultural Collaborative Community/Home Care

- Determine coping behaviors previously used and client's perception of effectiveness then and now.
- Evaluate and discuss use of defense mechanisms (useful or not), such as increased sleeping, use of drugs (including alcohol), illness behaviors, eating disorders, denial, forgetfulness, daydreaming, ineffectual organizational efforts, exploiting own goal setting, regression.

Nursing Priority No. 3.

To assist client to identify feelings and to begin to cope with problems as perceived by the client:

- Establish a therapeutic and facilitative relationship showing positive regard for the client. **Client may then feel safe to disclose feelings and feel understood and listened to.**
- Complete Beck's Depression Scale. Explain all tests and procedures. Involve client in planning schedule for care. Answer questions truthfully. **Enhances trust and therapeutic relationship, enabling client to talk freely about concerns.**
- Discuss initial signs of hopelessness (e.g., procrastination, increasing need for sleep, decreased physical activity, and withdrawal from social or familial activities).
- Encourage client to verbalize and explore feelings and perceptions (e.g., anger, helplessness, powerlessness, confusion, despondency, isolation, grief).
- Provide opportunity for children to "play out" feelings (e.g., puppets or art for preschooler, peer discussions for adolescents). **Provides insight into perceptions and may give direction for coping strategies.**
- Engage teens in discussions and arrange to do activities with them. **Parents can make a difference in their children's lives by being with them, discussing sensitive topics, and going different places with them.**
- Express hope to client and encourage SO(s) and other health-team members to do so. **Client may not identify positives in own situation.**
- Assist client to identify short-term goals. Encourage activities to achieve goals; facilitate contingency planning. **Promotes dealing with situation in manageable steps, enhancing chances for success and sense of control.**
- Discuss current options and list actions that may be taken to gain some control of situation. Correct misconceptions expressed by the client.
- Endeavor to prevent situations that might lead to feelings of isolation or lack of control in client's perception.

Information that appears in brackets has been added by the authors to clarify and enhance the use of nursing diagnoses.

- Promote client control in establishing time, place, and frequency of therapy sessions. Involve family members in the therapy situation, as appropriate.
- Help client recognize areas in which he or she has control versus those that are not within his or her control.
- Encourage risk taking in situations in which the client can succeed.
- Help client begin to develop coping mechanisms that can be learned and used effectively **to counteract hopelessness.**
- Encourage structured and controlled increase in physical activity. **Enhances sense of well-being.**
- Demonstrate and encourage use of relaxation exercises, guided imagery.
- Discuss safe use of prescribed antidepressants, including expected effects, adverse side effects, and interactions with other drugs.

Nursing Priority No. 4.

To promote wellness (Teaching/Discharge Considerations):

- Provide positive feedback for actions taken to deal with and overcome feelings of hopelessness. **Encourages continuation of desired behaviors.**
- Assist client/family to become aware of factors/situations leading to feelings of hopelessness. **Provides opportunity to avoid/modify situation.**
- Facilitate client's incorporation of personal loss. **Enhances grief work and promotes resolution of feelings.**
- Encourage client/family to develop support systems in the immediate community.
- Help client to become aware of, nurture, and expand spiritual self. (Refer to ND Spiritual Distress.)
- Introduce the client into a support group before the individual therapy is terminated **for continuation of therapeutic process.**
- Stress need for continued monitoring of medication regimen by healthcare provider.
- Refer to other resources for assistance, as indicated (e.g., clinical nurse specialist, psychiatrist, social services, spiritual advisor, Alcoholics or Narcotics Anonymous, Al-Anon or Alateen).

Documentation Focus

Assessment/Reassessment

- Assessment findings, including degree of impairment, use of coping skills, and support systems.

Information that appears in brackets has been added by the authors to clarify and enhance the use of nursing diagnoses.

⊕ Cultural   Ⓐ Collaborative   🏠 Community/Home Care

Planning
- Plan of care and who is involved in planning.
- Teaching plan.

Implementation/Evaluation
- Responses to interventions, teaching, and actions performed.
- Attainment or progress toward desired outcome(s).
- Modifications to plan of care.

Discharge Planning
- Identified long-term needs, client's goals for change and who is responsible for actions to be taken.
- Specific referrals made.

Sample Nursing Outcomes & Interventions Classifications (NOC/NIC) `NIC`

NOC—Depression Self-Control
NIC—Hope Inspiration

Hyperthermia

Taxonomy II: Safety/Protection—Class 6 Thermoregulation (00007)
[Diagnostic Division: Safety]
Submitted 1986

Definition: Body temperature elevated above normal range

Related Factors

Exposure to hot environment; inappropriate clothing
Vigorous activity; dehydration
Decreased perspiration
Medications; anesthesia
Increased metabolic rate; illness; trauma

Defining Characteristics

Subjective
Headache

Information that appears in brackets has been added by the authors to clarify and enhance the use of nursing diagnoses.

Objective

Increase in body temperature above normal range

Flushed skin; warm to touch

Tachypnea; tachycardia; [unstable blood pressure]

Seizures; convulsions; [muscle rigidity, fasciculations]

Confusion

Desired Outcomes/Evaluation Criteria— Client Will:

- Maintain core temperature within normal range.
- Be free of complications such as irreversible brain or neurological damage, acute renal failure.
- Identify underlying cause or contributing factors and importance of treatment, as well as signs/symptoms requiring further evaluation or intervention.
- Demonstrate behaviors to monitor and promote normothermia.
- Be free of seizure activity.

Actions/Interventions

Nursing Priority No. 1.

To assess causative/contributing factors:

- Identify underlying cause (e.g., excessive heat production, such as hyperthyroid state; malignant hyperpyrexia; impaired heat dissipation, such as heatstroke; dehydration; autonomic dysfunction as occurs with spinal cord transection; hypothalamic dysfunction, such as CNS infection; brain lesions; drug overdose; infection).
- ∞ Note chronological and developmental age of client. **Children are more susceptible to heatstroke; elderly or impaired individuals may not be able to recognize and/or act on symptoms of hyperthermia.**

Nursing Priority No. 2.

To evaluate effects/degree of hyperthermia:

- Monitor core temperature. Note: Rectal and tympanic temperatures most closely approximate core temperature; however, abdominal temperature monitoring may be done in the premature neonate.
- Assess neurological response, noting level of consciousness and orientation, reaction to stimuli, reaction of pupils, presence of posturing or seizures.

Information that appears in brackets has been added by the authors to clarify and enhance the use of nursing diagnoses.

Cultural   Collaborative   Community/Home Care

- Monitor BP and invasive hemodynamic parameters if available (e.g., MAP, CVP, PAP, PCWP). **Central hypertension or postural hypotension can occur.**
- Monitor heart rate and rhythm. **Dysrhythmias and ECG changes are common due to electrolyte imbalance, dehydration, specific action of catecholamines, and direct effects of hyperthermia on blood and cardiac tissue.**
- Monitor respirations. **Hyperventilation may initially be present, but ventilatory effort may eventually be impaired by seizures, hypermetabolic state (shock and acidosis).**
- Auscultate breath sounds, noting adventitious sounds such as crackles (rales).
- Monitor and record all sources of fluid loss such as urine **(oliguria and/or renal failure may occur due to hypotension, dehydration, shock, and tissue necrosis);** vomiting and diarrhea; wounds, fistulas; and insensible losses, **which can potentiate fluid and electrolyte losses.**
- Note presence or absence of sweating as body attempts to increase heat loss by evaporation, conduction, and diffusion. **Evaporation is decreased by environmental factors of high humidity and high ambient temperature, as well as body factors producing loss of ability to sweat or sweat gland dysfunction (e.g., spinal cord transection, cystic fibrosis, dehydration, vasoconstriction).**
- Monitor laboratory studies, such as ABGs, electrolytes, cardiac and liver enzymes **(may reveal tissue degeneration);** glucose; urinalysis **(myoglobinuria, proteinuria, and hemoglobinuria can occur as products of tissue necrosis);** and coagulation profile **(for presence of disseminated intravascular coagulation [DIC]).**

Nursing Priority No. 3.

To assist with measures to reduce body temperature/restore normal body/organ function:

- Administer antipyretics, orally or rectally (e.g., aspirin, acetaminophen), as ordered. Refrain from use of aspirin products in children **(may cause Reye's syndrome)** or individuals with a clotting disorder or receiving anticoagulant therapy.
- Promote surface cooling by means of undressing **(heat loss by radiation and conduction);** cool environment and/or fans **(heat loss by convection);** cool, tepid sponge baths or immersion **(heat loss by evaporation and conduction);** local ice packs, especially in groin and axillae **(areas of high blood flow).** *Note:* In pediatric clients, tepid water is preferred.

Information that appears in brackets has been added by the authors to clarify and enhance the use of nursing diagnoses.

Alcohol sponge baths are contraindicated because they increase peripheral vascular constriction and CNS depression; cold-water sponges or immersion can increase shivering, producing heat.

- Monitor use of hypothermia blanket and wrap extremities with bath towels **to minimize shivering.** Turn off hypothermia blanket when core temperature is within 1 to 3 degrees of desired temperature **to allow for downward drift.**
- Administer medications (e.g., chlorpromazine or diazepam), as ordered, **to control shivering and seizures.**
- Assist with internal cooling methods to treat malignant hyperthermia **to promote rapid core cooling.**
- Promote client safety (e.g., maintain patent airway; padded side rails; skin protection from cold, such as when hypothermia blanket is used; observation of equipment safety measures).
- Provide supplemental oxygen **to offset increased oxygen demands and consumption.**
- Administer medications, as indicated, **to treat underlying cause,** such as antibiotics **(for infection),** dantrolene **(for malignant hyperthermia),** beta-adrenergic blockers **(for thyroid storm).**
- Administer replacement fluids and electrolytes **to support circulating volume and tissue perfusion.**
- Maintain bedrest **to reduce metabolic demands and oxygen consumption.**
- Provide high-calorie diet, enteral or parenteral nutrition **to meet increased metabolic demands.**

Nursing Priority No. 4.

To promote wellness (Teaching/Discharge Considerations):

- Review specific risk factor or cause, such as underlying conditions (hyperthyroidism, dehydration, neurological diseases, nausea, vomiting, sepsis); use of certain medications (diuretics, blood pressure medications, alcohol or other drugs [cocaine, amphetamines]); environmental factors (exercise or labor in hot environment, lack of air conditioning, lack of acclimatization); reaction to anesthesia (malignant hyperthermia); other risk factors (salt or water depletion, elderly living alone).
- Identify those factors that client can control (if any), such as treating underlying disease process (e.g., thyroid control medication), protecting oneself from excessive exposure to

Information that appears in brackets has been added by the authors to clarify and enhance the use of nursing diagnoses.

Cultural Collaborative Community/Home Care

environmental heat (e.g., proper clothing, restriction of activity, scheduling outings during cooler part of day, use of fans/air-conditioning where possible), and understanding of family traits (e.g., malignant hyperthermia reaction to anesthesia is often familial).

- Instruct parents to avoid leaving young children in unattended car **to prevent heat injury and death.**
- Discuss importance of adequate fluid intake **to prevent dehydration.**
- Review signs/symptoms of hyperthermia (e.g., flushed skin, increased body temperature, increased respiratory and heart rate, fainting, loss of consciousness, seizures). **Indicates need for prompt intervention.**
- Recommend avoidance of hot tubs and saunas, as appropriate **(e.g., clients with MS, cardiac conditions, pregnancy that may affect fetal development or increase cardiac workload).**
- Identify community resources, especially for elderly clients, to address specific needs **(e.g., provision of fans for individual use, location of cooling rooms—usually in a community center—during heat waves, daily telephone contact to assess wellness).**

Documentation Focus

Assessment/Reassessment
- Temperature and other assessment findings, including vital signs and state of mentation.

Planning
- Plan of care, specific interventions, and who is involved in the planning.
- Teaching plan.

Implementation/Evaluation
- Responses to interventions, teaching, and actions performed.
- Attainment or progress toward desired outcome(s).
- Modifications to plan of care.

Discharge Planning
- Referrals that are made, those responsible for actions to be taken.

Information that appears in brackets has been added by the authors to clarify and enhance the use of nursing diagnoses.

Sample Nursing Outcomes & Interventions Classifications (NOC/NIC) <u>NIC</u>

NOC—Thermoregulation
NIC—Temperature Regulation

Hypothermia

Taxonomy II: Safety/Protection—Class 6 Thermoregulation (00006)
[Diagnostic Division: Safety]
Submitted 1986; Revised 1988

Definition: Body temperature below normal range

Related Factors

Exposure to cool environment [prolonged exposure, e.g., homeless, immersion in cold water, near-drowning, induced hypothermia, cardiopulmonary bypass]
Inadequate clothing
Evaporation from skin in cool environment
Decreased ability to shiver
Aging [or very young]
Debilitating illness; trauma; damage to hypothalamus
Malnutrition; decreased metabolic rate, inactivity
Consumption of alcohol; medications; [drug overdose]

Defining Characteristics

Objective
Body temperature below normal range
Shivering; piloerection
Cool skin
Pallor; slow capillary refill; cyanotic nailbeds
Hypertension; tachycardia
Core temperature 95°F (35°C): increased respirations, poor judgment, shivering
Core temperature 95°F to 93.2°F (35°C–34°C): bradycardia or tachycardia, myocardial irritability and dysrhythmias, muscle rigidity, shivering, lethargy, confusion, decreased coordination
Core temperature 93.2°F to 86°F (34°C–30°C): hypoventilation, bradycardia, generalized rigidity, metabolic acidosis, coma

---

Information that appears in brackets has been added by the authors to clarify and enhance the use of nursing diagnoses.

🌐 Cultural   Ⓐ Collaborative   🏠 Community/Home Care

[Core temperature below 86°F (30°C): no apparent vital signs, heart rate unresponsive to drug therapy, coma, cyanosis, dilated pupils, apnea, areflexia, no shivering (appears dead)]

Desired Outcomes/Evaluation Criteria—Client Will:

- Display core temperature within normal range.
- Be free of complications, such as cardiac failure, respiratory infection or failure, thromboembolic phenomena.
- Identify underlying cause or contributing factors that are within client control.
- Verbalize understanding of specific interventions to prevent hypothermia.
- Demonstrate behaviors to monitor and promote normothermia.

Actions/Interventions

Nursing Priority No. 1.
To assess causative/contributing factors:

- Note underlying cause (e.g., exposure to cold weather, winter outdoor activities; cold-water immersion; surgery; open wounds, exposed viscera; large burns; multiple rapid transfusions of banked blood; cooling therapy for hyperthermia).
- Note contributing factors: age of client (e.g., premature neonate, child, elderly person); concurrent or coexisting medical problems (e.g., brainstem injury, CNS trauma, near-drowning, sepsis, hypothyroidism); other factors (e.g., alcohol or other drug use or abuse; homelessness); living condition; relationship status (e.g., mentally impaired client alone).

Nursing Priority No. 2.
To prevent further decrease in body temperature:

- Remove wet clothing. Wrap in warm blankets, extra clothing, as appropriate.
- Place knit cap on infant's head.
- Prevent pooling of antiseptic and irrigating solutions under client in operating room. Cover skin areas outside of operative field.
- Prevent drafts in room; raise ambient temperature.
- Place infant under radiant warmer or in isolet and monitor temperature closely.

Information that appears in brackets has been added by the authors to clarify and enhance the use of nursing diagnoses.

- Avoid use of heat lamps or hot water bottles. **Surface rewarming can result in rewarming shock due to surface vasodilation.**
- Provide warm liquids if client can swallow.
- Warm IV solutions, as appropriate.

Nursing Priority No. 3.

To evaluate effects of hypothermia:

- Measure core temperature with low-register thermometer (measuring below 94°F [34°C]).
- Assess respiratory effort (**rate and tidal volume are reduced when metabolic rate decreases and respiratory acidosis occurs**).
- Auscultate lungs, noting adventitious sounds—**pulmonary edema, respiratory infection, and pulmonary embolus are possible complications of hypothermia.**
- Monitor heart rate and rhythm. **Cold stress reduces pacemaker function, and causes bradycardiaunresponsive to atropine, atrial fibrillation, atrioventricular blocks, and ventricular tachycardia can occur. Ventricular fibrillation occurs most frequently when core temperature is 82°F (28°C) or below.**
- Monitor BP, noting hypotension. **Can occur due to vasoconstriction and shunting of fluids as a result of cold injury effect on capillary permeability.**
- Measure urine output. **Oliguria and renal failure can occur due to low flow state and/or following hypothermic osmotic diuresis.**
- Note CNS effects (e.g., mood changes, sluggish thinking, amnesia, complete obtundation) and peripheral CNS effects (e.g., paralysis—87.7°F [31°C], dilated pupils—below 86°F [30°C], flat EEG—68°F [20°C]).
- Monitor laboratory studies, such as ABGs (**respiratory and metabolic acidosis**); electrolytes; CBC (**increased hematocrit, decreased white blood cell count**); cardiac enzymes (**myocardial infarct may occur owing to electrolyte imbalance, cold-stress catecholamine release, hypoxia, or acidosis**); coagulation profile; glucose; pharmacological profile (**for possible cumulative drug effects**).

Nursing Priority No. 4.

To restore normal body temperature/organ function:

- Assist with measures to normalize core temperature, such as warmed IV solutions and warm solution lavage of body

Information that appears in brackets has been added by the authors to clarify and enhance the use of nursing diagnoses.

cavities (gastric, peritoneal, bladder) or cardiopulmonary bypass, if indicated.

- Rewarm no faster than 1 to 2 degrees per hour **to avoid sudden vasodilation, increased metabolic demands on heart, and hypotension (rewarming shock).**

- Assist with surface warming by means of warmed blankets, warm environment or radiant heater, electronic warming devices. Cover head, neck and thorax, leaving extremities uncovered, as appropriate, **to maintain peripheral vasoconstriction.** Refrain from instituting surface rewarming prior to core rewarming in severe hypothermia **as it may cause after drop of temperature by shunting cold blood back to heart in addition to rewarming shock as a result of surface vasodilation).**

- Protect skin and tissues by repositioning, applying lotion or lubricants, and avoiding direct contact with heating appliance or blanket. **Impaired circulation can result in severe tissue damage.**

- Keep client quiet; handle gently **to reduce potential for fibrillation in cold heart.**

- Provide CPR, as necessary, with compressions initially at one-half normal heart rate **(severe hypothermia causes slowed conduction, and cold heart may be unresponsive to medications, pacing, and defibrillation).**

- Maintain patent airway. Assist with intubation, if indicated.

- Provide heated, humidified oxygen when used.

- Turn off warming blanket when temperature is within 1 to 3 degrees of desired temperature **to avoid hyperthermia situation.**

- Administer IV fluids with caution **to prevent overload as the vascular bed expands (cold heart is slow to compensate for increased volume).**

- Avoid vigorous drug therapy. **As rewarming occurs, organ function returns, correcting endocrine abnormalities, and tissues become more receptive to the effects of drugs previously administered.**

- Immerse hands and feet in warm water, or apply warm packs once body temperature is stabilized. Place sterile cotton between digits and wrap hands and feet with a bulky gauze wrap.

- Perform range-of-motion exercises, provide support hose, reposition, encourage coughing and deep-breathing exercises, avoid restrictive clothing or restraints **to reduce circulatory stasis.**

- Provide well-balanced, high-calorie diet or feedings **to replenish glycogen stores and nutritional balance.**

Information that appears in brackets has been added by the authors to clarify and enhance the use of nursing diagnoses.

 Diagnostic Studies ∞ Pediatric/Geriatric/Lifespan Medications **447**

Nursing Priority No. 5.

To promote wellness (Teaching/Discharge Considerations):

• Review specific risk factors or causes of hypothermia. Note that hypothermia can be *accidental* (see Related Factors) or *intentional* (such as occurs when induced-hypothermia therapy is used after cardiac arrest or brain injury), requiring interventions to protect client from adverse effects.

• Discuss signs/symptoms of early hypothermia (e.g., changes in mentation, poor judgment, somnolence, impaired coordination, slurred speech) **to facilitate recognition of problem and timely intervention.**

• Identify factors that client can control (if any), such as protection from environment/adequate heat in home; layering clothing and blankets; minimizing heat loss from head with hat/scarf; appropriate cold-weather clothing; avoidance of alcohol/other drugs if anticipating exposure to cold; potential risk for future hypersensitivity to cold, and so forth.

Documentation Focus

Assessment/Reassessment
• Findings, noting degree of system involvement, respiratory rate, ECG pattern, capillary refill, and level of mentation.
• Graph temperature.

Planning
• Plan of care and who is involved in planning.
• Teaching plan.

Implementation/Evaluation
• Responses to interventions, teaching, and actions performed.
• Attainment or progress toward desired outcome(s).
• Modifications to plan of care.

Discharge Planning
• Long-term needs, identifying who is responsible for each action.

Sample Nursing Outcomes & Interventions Classifications (NOC/NIC) NIC

NOC—Thermoregulation
NIC—Hypothermia Treatment

Information that appears in brackets has been added by the authors to clarify and enhance the use of nursing diagnoses.

disturbed personal Identity

Taxonomy II: Self-Perception—Class 1 Self-Concept
(00121)
[Diagnostic Division: Ego Integrity]
Submitted 1978; revised 2008

Definition: Inability to maintain an integrated and
complete perception of self

Related Factors

Low self-esteem; dysfunctional family processes
Situational crises; stages of growth or development; social role
change
Ingestion or inhalation of toxic chemicals; use of psychoactive
drugs
Cultural discontinuity; discrimination or prejudice
Manic states; multiple personality disorder; psychiatric disorders (e.g., psychoses, depression, dissociative disorder); organic brain syndromes
Cult indoctrination

Defining Characteristics

Subjective

Disturbed body image; delusional description of self
Fluctuating feelings about self; feelings of strangeness, emptiness
Uncertainty about goals, cultural or ideological values (e.g., beliefs, religious and moral questions)
Gender confusion
Unable to distinguish between inner and outer stimuli

Objective

Contradictory personal traits
Disturbed relationships
Ineffective coping or role performance

Desired Outcomes/Evaluation Criteria— Client Will:

- Acknowledge threat to personal identity.
- Integrate threat in a healthy, positive manner (e.g., states anxiety is reduced, makes plans for the future).

Information that appears in brackets has been added by the authors to clarify
and enhance the use of nursing diagnoses.

- Verbalize acceptance of changes that have occurred.
- State ability to identify and accept self (long-term outcome).

Actions/Interventions

Nursing Priority No. 1.

To assess causative/contributing factors:

- Ascertain client's perception of the extent of the threat to self and how client is handling the situation.
- Determine speed of occurrence of threat. **An event that has happened quickly may be more threatening (e.g., a traumatic event resulting in change in body image).**
- Have client define own body image. **Body image is the basis of personal identity and client's perception will affect how changes are viewed, may prevent achievement of ideals and expectations, and have a negative effect.**
- Identify physical signs of panic state such as palpitations, diaphoresis, trembling, chest or abdominal pain, nausea. (Refer to ND Anxiety.)
- ∞ Note age of client. **An adolescent may struggle with the developmental task of personal or sexual identity, whereas an older person may have more difficulty accepting or dealing with a threat to identity, such as progressive loss of memory.**
- Assess availability and use of support systems. Note response of family/SO(s).
- ∞ Note withdrawn or automatic behavior, regression to earlier developmental stage, general behavioral disorganization, or display of self-mutilation behaviors in adolescent or adult; delayed development, preference for solitary play, unusual display of self-stimulation in child.
- Determine presence of hallucinations, delusions, distortions of reality.

Nursing Priority No. 2.

To assist client to manage/deal with threat:

- Make time to listen to client, encouraging appropriate expression of feelings, including anger and hostility.
- Provide calm environment. **Helps client to remain calm and able to discuss important issues related to the identity crisis.**
- Use crisis-intervention principles **to restore equilibrium when possible.**

Information that appears in brackets has been added by the authors to clarify and enhance the use of nursing diagnoses.

⊕ Cultural   Ⓒ Collaborative   🏠 Community/Home Care

- Discuss client's commitment to an identity. **Those who have made a strong commitment to an identity tend to be more comfortable with self and happier than those who have not.**
- Assist client to develop strategies to cope with threat to identity. **Helps reduce anxiety and promotes self-awareness and self-esteem.**
- Engage client in activities to help in identifying self as an individual (e.g., use of mirror for visual feedback, tactile stimulation).
- Provide for simple decisions, concrete tasks, calming activities.
- Allow client to deal with situation in small steps. **May be unable to cope with larger picture when in stress overload.**
- Encourage client to develop and participate in an individualized exercise program (walking is an excellent beginning).
- Provide concrete assistance, as needed (e.g., help with ADLs, preparing food).
- Take advantage of opportunities to promote growth. Realize that client will have difficulty learning while in a dissociative state.
- Maintain reality orientation without confronting client's irrational beliefs. **Client may become defensive, blocking opportunity to look at other possibilities.**
- Use humor judiciously, when appropriate.
- Discuss options for dealing with issues of sexual gender (e.g., therapy, gender-change surgery when client is a transsexual).
- Refer to NDs disturbed Body Image; Self-Esteem [specify]; Spiritual Distress.

Nursing Priority No. 3.
To promote wellness (Teaching/Discharge Considerations):

- Provide accurate information about threat to and potential consequences for individual. **Helps client to make positive decisions for future.**
- Assist client and SO(s) to acknowledge and integrate threat into future planning (e.g., wearing ID bracelet when prone to mental confusion; change of lifestyle to accommodate change of gender for transsexual client).
- Refer to appropriate support groups (e.g., day-care program, counseling/psychotherapy, gender identity).

Information that appears in brackets has been added by the authors to clarify and enhance the use of nursing diagnoses.

 Diagnostic Studies ∞ Pediatric/Geriatric/Lifespan   Medications **451**

Documentation Focus

Assessment/Reassessment
- Findings, noting degree of impairment.
- Nature of and client's perception of the threat.
- Degree of commitment to own identity.

Planning
- Plan of care and who is involved in the planning.
- Teaching plan.

Implementation/Evaluation
- Client's response to interventions/teaching and actions performed.
- Attainment or progress toward desired outcome(s).
- Modifications to plan of care.

Discharge Planning
- Long-term needs and who is responsible for actions to be taken.
- Specific referrals made.

Sample Nursing Outcomes & Interventions Classifications (NOC/NIC) NIC

NOC—Identity
NIC—Self-Esteem Enhancement

---

readiness for enhanced **Immunization Status**

Taxonomy II: Health Promotion—Class 2 Health Management (00186)
Safety/Protection—Class 1 Infection/Class 5 Defensive Protection
[Diagnostic Division: Safety]
Submitted 2006

Definition: A pattern of conforming to local, national, and/or international standards of immunization to prevent infectious disease(s) that is sufficient to protect a person, family, or community and can be strengthened

---

Related Factors

To be developed

Information that appears in brackets has been added by the authors to clarify and enhance the use of nursing diagnoses.

Defining Characteristics

Subjective

Expresses desire to enhance:
Knowledge of immunization standards
Immunization status
Identification of providers of immunizations
Record-keeping of immunizations
Identification of possible problems associated with immunizations
Behavior to prevent infectious diseases

Desired Outcomes/Evaluation Criteria— Client Will:

- Express understanding of immunization recommendations.
- Develop plan to obtain appropriate immunizations.
- Identify and adopt behaviors to reduce risk of infectious disease.
- Maintain and update immunization records.

Community Will:

- Provide information to community regarding immunization requirements or recommendations.
- Identify underserved populations requiring immunization support and ways to meet their needs.
- Develop plan to provide mass immunizations in time of major threat or disease outbreak.

Actions/Interventions

Nursing Priority No. 1.

To determine current immunization status:

- Assess client's history of immunizations. **Response may vary widely depending on client's age (infant to adult), cultural influences, travel history, family beliefs about immunization, and medical conditions (e.g., some vaccines should not be given to children with certain cancers, persons taking immunosuppressant drugs, or those with serious allergies to eggs).**
- Ascertain motivation and expectations for change.
- Determine if adult client works in or frequents high-risk areas (e.g., doctor's office, home care, homeless or immigrant shelters or clinics, correctional facility) **to review potential**

Information that appears in brackets has been added by the authors to clarify and enhance the use of nursing diagnoses.

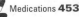

exposures and determine new vaccines or boosters client may need.

- Address client's/SO's concerns (e.g., client may wonder if annual flu shots are truly beneficial, or whether adult boosters may be needed for particular immunizations received in childhood; parent may be concerned about safety of vaccine supply). **Helps to clarify plans and deal with misconceptions or myths.**
- Identify conditions that may preclude client receiving specific immunizations **such as history of prior adverse reaction, currrent fever illness, pregnancy, and current cancer or other immunosuppressant treatments.**
- Review community plan for dealing with immunizations and disease outbreak. **Identifies community strengths and limitations.**

Nursing Priority No. 2.

To assist client/SO/community to develop/strengthen plan to meet identified needs:

- Review parents' knowledge regarding immunizations recommended or required to enter school (e.g., hepatitis B, rotavirus, *Haemophilus influenzae,* mumps/measles/rubella (MMR), varicella, and hepatitis A prior to kindergarten; tetanus/diphtheria/pertussis (TDP), human papillomavirus by middle-school age; meningitis for college freshmen planning to live in dorm) **to document status, plan for boosters, and/or discuss appropriate intervals for follow-up.**
- Review protective benefit of each vaccine, route of administration, expected side effects, and potential adverse reactions **so that client/SO(s) can make informed decisions**.
- Discuss appropriate time intervals for all recommended immunizations, as well as catch-up and booster options for children birth to 18 years.
- Identify requirements for client preparing for international travel **to ascertain potential for contracting vaccine-preventable disease in geographical area of client's travel, so that vaccines can be provided, if needed.**
- Inform of exemptions when client/SO desires. **Some states permit medical, religious, personal, and philosophical exemptions when parent does not want child to participate in immunization programs.** Refer to appropriate care providers for further discussion or intervention.
- Define and discuss current needs and anticipated or projected concerns of community health promotion programs. **Agreement**

Information that appears in brackets has been added by the authors to clarify and enhance the use of nursing diagnoses.

　⊕ Cultural　⊛ Collaborative　🏠 Community/Home Care

on scope and parameters of needs is essential for effective planning.
- Prioritize goals **to facilitate accomplishment.**
- Identify available community resources (**e.g., persons, groups, financial, governmental, as well as other communities**).
- Seek out and involve underserved and at-risk groups within the community. **Supports communication and commitment of community as a whole.**

Nursing Priority No. 3.
To promote optimum wellness:

- Review reasons to continue immunization programs. **Viruses and bacteria that cause vaccine-preventable disease and death still exist and can be passed on to people who are not protected, thus increasing medical, social, and economic costs.**
- Provide reliable vaccine information in written form or Internet Web sites (**e.g., brochures or fact sheets from the CDC, American Academy of Pediatrics, National Network for Immunization Information**).
- Identify community resources for obtaining immunizations, such as Public Health Department, family physician.
- Discuss management of common side effects (e.g., muscle pain, rash, fever, site swelling).
- Support development of community plans for maintaining and enhancing efforts **to increase immunization level of population.**
- Establish mechanism for self-monitoring of community needs and evaluation of efforts.
- Use multiple formats: for example, TV, radio, print media, billboards and computer bulletin boards, speakers' bureau, reports to community leaders and groups on file and accessible to the public, **to keep community informed regarding immunization needs, disease prevention.**

Documentation Focus

Assessment/Reassessment
- Assessment findings of immunization status, potential risks or disease exposure.
- Identified areas of concern, strengths and limitations.
- Understanding of immunization needs, safety concerns, and disease prevention.
- Motivation and expectations for change.

Information that appears in brackets has been added by the authors to clarify and enhance the use of nursing diagnoses.

Diagnostic Studies   Pediatric/Geriatric/Lifespan   Medications **455**

Planning
- Action plan and who is involved in planning.
- Teaching plan.

Implementation/Evaluation
- Individual/family responses to interventions, teaching, and actions performed.
- Response of community entities to the actions performed.
- Attainment or progress toward desired outcome(s).
- Modifications to plan.

Discharge Planning
- Identified needs, referrals for follow-up care, support systems.
- Short- and long-term plans to deal with current, anticipated, and potential community needs and who is responsible for follow-through.
- Specific referrals made, coalitions formed.

Sample Nursing Outcomes & Interventions Classifications (NOC/NIC) NIC

NOC—Immunization Behavior
NIC—Immunization/Vaccination Management

---

disorganized Infant Behavior

Taxonomy II: Coping/Stress Tolerance—Class 3 Neurobehavioral Stress (00116)
[Diagnostic Division: Neurosensory]
Submitted 1994; Nursing Diagnosis Extension and Classification (NDEC) Revision 1998

Definition: Disintegrated physiological and neurobehavioral responses of infant to the environment

---

Related Factors

Prenatal
Congenital or genetic disorders; teratogenic exposure; [exposure to drugs]

Postnatal
Prematurity; oral or motor problems; feeding intolerance; malnutrition
Invasive procedures; pain

Information that appears in brackets has been added by the authors to clarify and enhance the use of nursing diagnoses.

Individual

Gestational or postconceptual age; immature neurological system

Illness; [infection]; [hypoxia, birth asphyxia]

Environmental

Physical environment inappropriateness

Sensory inappropriateness, overstimulation, deprivation

Lack of containment or boundaries

Caregiver

Cue misreading; cue knowledge deficit

Environmental stimulation contribution

Defining Characteristics

Objective

Regulatory Problems

Inability to inhibit startle; irritability

State-Organization System

Active-awake (fussy, worried gaze); quiet-awake (staring, gaze aversion)

Diffuse sleep, state-oscillation

Irritable crying

Attention-Interaction System

Abnormal response to sensory stimuli (e.g., difficult to soothe, inability to sustain alert status)

Motor System

Finger splaying, fisting; hands to face; hyperextension of extremities

Tremors, startles, twitches; jittery; uncoordinated movement

Changes to motor tone; altered primitive reflexes

Physiological

Bradycardia, tachycardia, arrhythmias

Skin color changes; desaturation

"Time-out signals" (e.g., gaze, grasp, hiccough, cough, sneeze, sigh, slack jaw, open mouth, tongue thrust)

Feeding intolerances

Information that appears in brackets has been added by the authors to clarify and enhance the use of nursing diagnoses.

Desired Outcomes/Evaluation Criteria— Infant Will:

- Exhibit organized behaviors that allow the achievement of optimal potential for growth and development as evidenced by modulation of physiological, motor, state, and attentional-interactive functioning.

Parent/Caregiver Will:

- Recognize individual infant cues.
- Identify appropriate responses (including environmental modifications) to infant's cues.
- Verbalize readiness to assume caregiving independently.

Actions/Interventions

Nursing Priority No. 1.
To assess causative/contributing factors:

- Determine infant's chronological and developmental age; note length of gestation.
- Observe for cues suggesting presence of situations that may result in pain/discomfort.
- Determine adequacy of physiological support.
- Evaluate level and appropriateness of environmental stimuli.
- Ascertain parents' understanding of infant's needs and abilities.
- Listen to parents' concerns about their capabilities to meet infant's needs.

Nursing Priority No. 2.
To assist parents in providing co-regulation to the infant:

- Provide a calm, nurturant physical and emotional environment.
- Encourage parents to hold infant, including skin-to-skin contact (kangaroo care [KC]), as appropriate. **Research suggests KC may have a positive effect on infant development by enhancing neurophysiological organization as well as an indirect effect by improving parental mood, perceptions, and interactive behavior.**
- Model gentle handling of baby and appropriate responses to infant behavior. **Provides cues to parent.**
- Support and encourage parents to be with infant and participate actively in all aspects of care. **Situation may be**

Information that appears in brackets has been added by the authors to clarify and enhance the use of nursing diagnoses.

Cultural Collaborative Community/Home Care

overwhelming, and support may enhance coping and strengthen attachment.

* Provide positive feedback for progressive parental involvement in caregiving process. **Transfer of care from staff to parents progresses along a continuum as parents' confidence level increases and they are able to take on more complex care activities.**

* Discuss infant growth and development, pointing out current status and progressive expectations, as appropriate. **Augments parents' knowledge of co-regulation.**

* Incorporate the parents' observations and suggestions into plan of care. **Demonstrates valuing of parents' input and encourages continued involvement.**

Nursing Priority No. 3.

To deliver care within the infant's stress threshold:

* Provide a consistent caregiver. **Facilitates recognition of infant cues or changes in behavior.**

* Identify infant's individual self-regulatory behaviors (e.g., sucking, mouthing, grasp, hand-to-mouth, face behaviors, foot clasp, brace, limb flexion, trunk tuck, boundary seeking).

* Support hands to mouth and face; offer pacifier or non-nutritive sucking at the breast with gavage feedings. **Provides opportunities for infant to suck.**

* Avoid aversive oral stimulation, such as routine oral suctioning; suction ET tube only when clinically indicated.

* Use Oxyhood large enough to cover the infant's chest so arms will be inside the hood. **Allows for hand-to-mouth activities during this therapy.**

* Provide opportunities for infant to grasp.

* Provide boundaries and/or containment during all activities. Use swaddling, nesting, bunting, caregiver's hands as indicated.

* Allow adequate time and opportunities to hold infant. Handle infant very gently, move infant smoothly, slowly, and contained, avoiding sudden or abrupt movements.

* Maintain normal alignment, position infant with limbs softly flexed, shoulders and hips adducted slightly. Use appropriate-sized diapers.

* Evaluate chest for adequate expansion, placing rolls under trunk if prone position indicated.

* Avoid restraints, including at IV sites. If IV board is necessary, secure to limb positioned in normal alignment.

Information that appears in brackets has been added by the authors to clarify and enhance the use of nursing diagnoses.

- Provide a sheepskin, egg-crate mattress, water bed, and/or gel pillow or mattress for infant who does not tolerate frequent position changes. **Minimizes tissue pressure, lessens risk of tissue injury.**
- Visually assess color, respirations, activity, invasive lines without disturbing infant. Assess with "hands on" every 4 hours as indicated and prn. **Allows for undisturbed rest and quiet periods.**
- Schedule daily activities, time for rest, and organization of sleep and wake states to maximize tolerance of infant. Defer routine care when infant in quiet sleep.
- Provide care with baby in side-lying position. Begin by talking softly to the baby, then placing hands in containing hold on baby, **allows baby to prepare.** Proceed with least-invasive manipulations first.
- Respond promptly to infant's agitation or restlessness. Provide "time out" when infant shows early cues of overstimulation. Comfort and support the infant after stressful interventions.
- Remain at infant's bedside for several minutes after procedures and caregiving **to monitor infant's response and provide necessary support.**
- Administer analgesics as individually appropriate.

Nursing Priority No. 4.

To modify the environment to provide appropriate stimulation:

- Introduce stimulation as a single mode and assess individual tolerance.

Light/Vision

- Reduce lighting perceived by infant; introduce diurnal lighting (and activity) when infant achieves physiological stability. (Daylight levels of 20–30 candles and night light levels of less than 10 candles are suggested.) Change light levels gradually **to allow infant time to adjust.**
- Protect the infant's eyes from bright illumination during examinations and procedures, as well as from indirect sources, such as neighboring phototherapy treatments, **to prevent retinal damage.**
- Deliver phototherapy (when required) with biliblanket devices if available **(alleviates need for eye patches).**
- Provide caregiver face (preferably parent's) as visual stimulus when infant shows readiness (awake, attentive).

Information that appears in brackets has been added by the authors to clarify and enhance the use of nursing diagnoses.

⊕ Cultural   🐾 Collaborative   🏠 Community/Home Care

Sound

- Identify sources of noise in environment and eliminate or re-duce (e.g., speak in a low voice; reduce volume on alarms and telephones to safe but not excessive volume; pad metal trash can lids; open paper packages (such as IV tubing and suction catheters), slowly and at a distance from bedside; con-duct rounds or report away from bedside; place soft, thick fabric, such as blanket rolls and toys, near infant's head to absorb sound).
- Keep all incubator portholes closed, closing with two hands **to avoid loud snap with closure and associated startle re-sponse.**
- Refrain from playing musical toys or tape players inside in-cubator.
- Avoid placing items on top of incubator; if necessary to do so, pad surface well.
- Conduct regular decibel (dB) checks of interior noise level in incubator (recommended not to exceed 60 dB).
- Provide auditory stimulation **to console, support infant be-fore and through handling or to reinforce restfulness.**

Olfactory

- Be cautious in exposing infant to strong odors (e.g., alcohol, Betadine, perfumes), **as olfactory capability of the infant is very sensitive.**
- Place a cloth or gauze pad scented with milk near the infant's face during gavage feeding. **Enhances association of milk with act of feeding and gastric fullness.**
- Invite parents to leave a handkerchief that they have scented by wearing close to their body near infant. **Strengthens infant recognition of parents.**

Vestibular

- Move and handle the infant slowly and gently. Do not restrict spontaneous movement.
- Provide vestibular stimulation **to console, stabilize breathing and heart rate, or enhance growth.** Use a water bed (with or without oscillation), a motorized or moving bed or cradle, or rocking in the arms of a caregiver.

Gustatory

- Dip pacifier in milk and offer to infant during gavage feeding **for sucking and to stimulate tasting.**

Information that appears in brackets has been added by the authors to clarify and enhance the use of nursing diagnoses.

Tactile
- Maintain skin integrity and monitor closely. Limit frequency of invasive procedures.
- Minimize use of chemicals on skin (e.g., alcohol, Betadine, solvents) and remove afterward with warm water **because skin is very sensitive/fragile.**
- Limit use of tape and adhesives directly on skin. Use DuoDerm under tape **to prevent dermal injury.**
- Touch infant with a firm containing touch, avoid light stroking. Provide a sheepskin pad, soft linen. *Note:* **Tactile experience is the primary sensory mode of the infant.**
- Encourage frequent parental holding of infant (including skin-to-skin). Supplement activity with extended family, staff, volunteers.

Nursing Priority No. 5.
To promote wellness (Teaching/Discharge Considerations):

🏠• Evaluate home environment **to identify appropriate modifications.**

🔬• Identify community resources (e.g., early stimulation program, qualified childcare facilities, respite care, visiting nurse, home-care support, specialty organizations).

🏠• Determine sources for equipment and therapy needs.

🔬• Refer to support or therapy groups, as indicated, **to provide role models, facilitate adjustment to new roles/ responsibilities, and enhance coping.**

🏠• Provide contact number, as appropriate (e.g., primary nurse), **to support adjustment to home setting.**

- Refer to additional NDs, such as risk for impaired Attachment; compromised/disabled or readiness for enhanced family Coping; delayed Growth and Development; risk for Caregiver Role Strain.

Documentation Focus ─────────────

Assessment/Reassessment
- Findings, including infant's cues of stress, self-regulation, and readiness for stimulation; chronological and developmental age.
- Parents' concerns, level of knowledge.

Planning
- Plan of care and who is involved in the planning.
- Teaching plan.

─────────────────

Information that appears in brackets has been added by the authors to clarify and enhance the use of nursing diagnoses.

🌐 Cultural   🔬 Collaborative   🏠 Community/Home Care

Implementation/Evaluation
* Infant's responses to interventions and actions performed.
* Parents' participation and response to interactions and teaching.
* Attainment or progress toward desired outcome(s).
* Modifications of plan of care.

Discharge Planning
* Long-term needs and who is responsible for actions to be taken.
* Specific referrals made.

Sample Nursing Outcomes & Interventions Classifications (NOC/NIC) NIC

NOC—Preterm Infant Organization
NIC—Environmental Management

readiness for enhanced organized Infant Behavior

Taxonomy II: Coping/Stress Tolerance—Class 3 Neurobehavioral (00117)
[Diagnostic Division: Neurosensory]
Submitted 1994

Definition: A pattern of modulation of the physiological and behavioral systems of functioning (i.e., autonomic, motor, state-organizational, self-regulators, and attentional-interactional systems) in an infant that is satisfactory but that can be improved

Related Factors

Prematurity
Pain

Defining Characteristics

Objective
Stable physiological measures
Definite sleep-wake states
Use of some self-regulatory behaviors
Response to stimuli (e.g., visual, auditory)

Information that appears in brackets has been added by the authors to clarify and enhance the use of nursing diagnoses.

Desired Outcomes/Evaluation Criteria— Infant Will:

- Continue to modulate physiological and behavioral systems of functioning.
- Achieve higher levels of integration in response to environmental stimuli.

Parent/Caregiver Will:

- Identify cues reflecting infant's stress threshold and current status.
- Develop or modify responses (including environment) to promote infant adaptation and development.

Actions/Interventions

Nursing Priority No. 1.
To assess infant status and parental skill level:

- Determine infant's chronological and developmental age; note length of gestation.
- Identify infant's individual self-regulatory behaviors: suck, mouth, grasp, hand-to-mouth, face behaviors, foot clasp, brace, limb flexion, trunk tuck, boundary seeking.
- Observe for cues suggesting presence of situations that may result in pain/discomfort.
- Evaluate level and appropriateness of environmental stimuli.
- Ascertain parents' understanding of infant's needs and abilities.
- Listen to parents' perceptions of their capabilities to promote infant's development.

Nursing Priority No. 2.
To assist parents to enhance infant's integration:

- Review infant growth and development, pointing out current status and progressive expectations. Identify cues reflecting infant stress.
- Discuss possible modifications of environmental stimuli, activity schedule, sleep, and pain control needs.
- Provide positive feedback for parental involvement in caregiving process. **Transfer of care from staff to parents progresses along a continuum as parents' confidence level increases and they are able to take on more responsibility.**
- Discuss use of skin-to-skin contact (kangaroo care [KC]), as appropriate. **Research suggests KC may have a positive**

Information that appears in brackets has been added by the authors to clarify and enhance the use of nursing diagnoses.

🌐 Cultural 🔬 Collaborative 🏠 Community/Home Care

effect on infant development by enhancing neurophysiological organization as well as an indirect effect by improving parental mood, perceptions, and interactive behavior.

- Incorporate parents' observations and suggestions into plan of care. **Demonstrates value of and regard for parents' input and enhances sense of ability to deal with situation.**

Nursing Priority No. 3.
To promote wellness (Teaching/Learning Considerations):

- Identify community resources (e.g., visiting nurse, home-care support, child care).
- Refer to support group or individual role model **to facilitate adjustment to new roles/responsibilities.**
- Refer to additional NDs; for example, readiness for enhanced family Coping.

Documentation Focus

Assessment/Reassessment
- Findings, including infant's self-regulation and readiness for stimulation; chronological and developmental age.
- Parents' concerns, level of knowledge.

Planning
- Plan of care and who is involved in the planning.
- Teaching plan.

Implementation/Evaluation
- Infant's responses to interventions and actions performed.
- Parents' participation and response to interactions and teaching.
- Attainment or progress toward desired outcome(s).
- Modifications of plan of care.

Discharge Planning
- Long-term needs and who is responsible for actions to be taken.
- Specific referrals made.

Sample Nursing Outcomes & Interventions Classifications (NOC/NIC) NIC

NOC—Neurological Status
NIC—Developmental Care

Information that appears in brackets has been added by the authors to clarify and enhance the use of nursing diagnoses.

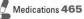

risk for disorganized **Infant Behavior**

Taxonomy II: Coping/Stress Tolerance—Class 3
  Neurobehavioral Stress (00115)
[Diagnostic Division: Neurosensory]
Submitted 1994

Definition: Risk for alteration in integration and modulation of the physiological and behavioral systems of functioning (i.e., autonomic, motor, state, organizational, self-regulatory, and attentional-interactional systems)

Risk Factors

Pain; invasive or painful procedures
Oral or motor problems
Environmental overstimulation
Lack of containment within environment
Prematurity; [immaturity of the CNS; genetic problems that alter neurological and/or physiological functioning; conditions resulting in hypoxia or birth asphyxia]
Malnutrition; infection; drug addiction
Environmental events or conditions, such as separation from parents, exposure to loud noise, excessive handling, bright lights

NOTE: A risk diagnosis is not evidenced by signs and symptoms, as the problem has not occurred; rather nursing interventions are directed at prevention.

Desired Outcomes/Evaluation Criteria— Infant Will:

- Exhibit organized behaviors that allow the achievement of optimal potential for growth and development as evidenced by modulation of physiological, motor, state, and attentional-interactive functioning.

Parent/Caregiver Will:

- Identify cues reflecting infant's stress threshold and current status.
- Develop or modify responses (including environment) to promote infant adaptation and development.
- Verbalize readiness to assume caregiving independently.

Information that appears in brackets has been added by the authors to clarify and enhance the use of nursing diagnoses.

🌐 Cultural   🐾 Collaborative   🏠 Community/Home Care

Refer to ND disorganized Infant Behavior for Actions/ Interventions and Documentation Focus.

Sample Nursing Outcomes & Interventions Classifications (NOC/NIC) NIC

NOC—Neurological Status
NIC—Environmental Management

> ### risk for Infection
>
> Taxonomy II: Safety/Protection—Class 1 Infection (00004)
> [Diagnostic Division: Safety]
> Submitted 1986
>
> **Definition:** At increased risk for being invaded by pathogenic organisms

Risk Factors

Inadequate primary defenses (broken skin, traumatized tissue, decrease in ciliary action, stasis of body fluids, change in pH secretions, altered peristalsis)

Inadequate secondary defenses (e.g., decreased hemoglobin, leukopenia, suppressed inflammatory response)

Inadequate acquired immunity; immunosuppression

Tissue destruction; increased environmental exposure to pathogens; invasive procedures

Chronic disease; malnutrition; trauma

Pharmaceutical agents (e.g., immunosuppressants, [antibiotic therapy])

Rupture of amniotic membranes

Insufficient knowledge to avoid exposure to pathogens

> **NOTE:** A risk diagnosis is not evidenced by signs and symptoms, as the problem has not occurred; rather, nursing interventions are directed at prevention.

Desired Outcomes/Evaluation Criteria— Client Will:

• Verbalize understanding of individual causative or risk factor(s).

Information that appears in brackets has been added by the authors to clarify and enhance the use of nursing diagnoses.

- Identify interventions to prevent or reduce risk of infection.
- Demonstrate techniques, lifestyle changes to promote safe environment.
- Achieve timely wound healing; be free of purulent drainage or erythema; be afebrile.

Actions/Interventions

Nursing Priority No. 1.
To assess causative/contributing factors:

- Note risk factors for occurrence of infection (e.g., extremes of age; immunocompromised host; skin/tissue wounds; communities or persons sharing close quarters and/or equipment [e.g., college dorm, group home, long-term-care facility, day care, correctional facility]; prolonged illness or hospitalization; multiple surgeries or invasive procedures; indwelling catheters; IV drug use; accidental or intentional environmental exposure [e.g., act of bioterrorism]).
- Observe for localized signs of infection at insertion sites of invasive lines, sutures, surgical incisions, wounds.
- Assess and document skin conditions around insertions of pins, wires, and tongs, noting inflammation and drainage.
- Note signs and symptoms of sepsis (systemic infection): fever, chills, diaphoresis, altered level of consciousness, positive blood cultures.
- Obtain appropriate tissue or fluid specimens for observation and culture and sensitivities testing.

Nursing Priority No. 2.
To reduce/correct existing risk factors:

- Stress proper hand hygiene by all caregivers between therapies and clients. **A first-line defense against healthcare-associated infections (HAIs).**
- Monitor client's visitors and caregivers for respiratory illnesses. Offer masks and tissues to client or visitors who are coughing or sneezing **to limit exposures, thus reducing cross-contamination.**
- Post visual alerts in healthcare settings instructing clients/SO(s) to inform healthcare providers if they have symptoms of respiratory infections or influenza-like symptoms.
- Encourage parents of sick children to keep them away from childcare settings and school until afebrile for 24 hours.

Information that appears in brackets has been added by the authors to clarify and enhance the use of nursing diagnoses.

Cultural Collaborative Community/Home Care

- Provide for isolation, as indicated (e.g., wound and skin, respiratory, or reverse). Educate staff in infection control procedures. **Reduces risk of cross-contamination.**
- Emphasize proper use of personal protective equipment (PPE) by staff and visitors, as dictated by agency policy.
- Perform or instruct in daily mouth care. Include use of antiseptic mouthwash for individuals in acute or long-term-care settings **at high-risk for nosocomial or HAIs.**
- Recommend routine or preoperative body shower or scrubs, when indicated (e.g., orthopedic, plastic surgery) **to reduce bacterial colonization.**
- Maintain sterile technique for all invasive procedures (e.g., IV, urinary catheter, pulmonary suctioning).
- Fill bubbling humidifiers and nebulizers with *sterile* water, not distilled or tap water. Avoid use of room-air humidifiers unless unit is sterilized daily and filled with sterile water.
- Use heat and moisture exchangers (HME) instead of heated humidifier with mechanical ventilator.
- Assist with weaning from mechanical ventilator as soon as possible **to reduce risk of ventilator-associated pneumonia (VAP).**
- Choose proper vascular access device based on anticipated treatment duration and solution/medication to be infused and best available aseptic insertion techniques; cleanse incisions and insertion sites per facility protocol with appropriate solution **to reduce potential for catheter-related bloodstream infections.**
- Change surgical or other wound dressings, as indicated, using proper technique for changing/disposing of contaminated materials.
- Separate touching surfaces when skin is excoriated, such as in herpes zoster. Use gloves when caring for open lesions **to minimize autoinoculation or transmission of viral diseases (e.g., herpes simplex virus, hepatitis, AIDS).**
- Cover perineal and pelvic region dressings or casts with plastic when using bedpan **to prevent contamination.**
- Encourage early ambulation, deep breathing, coughing, position changes, and early removal of ET tube or nasal or oral feeding tubes **for mobilization of respiratory secretions and prevention of aspiration/respiratory infections.**
- Encourage or assist with use of adjuncts (e.g., respiratory aids, such as incentive spirometry) **to prevent pneumonia.**
- Maintain adequate hydration, stand or sit to void, and catheterize, if necessary, **to avoid bladder distention and urinary stasis.**

Information that appears in brackets has been added by the authors to clarify and enhance the use of nursing diagnoses.

• Provide regular urinary catheter and perineal care. **Reduces risk of ascending urinary tract infection.**

• Assist with medical procedures (e.g., wound or joint aspiration, incision and drainage of abscess, bronchoscopy), as indicated.

• Administer/monitor medication regimen (e.g., antimicrobials, drip infusion into osteomyelitis, subeschar clysis, topical antibiotics) and note client's response **to determine effectiveness of therapy or presence of side effects.**

• Administer prophylactic antibiotics and immunizations, as indicated.

Nursing Priority No. 3.

To promote wellness (Teaching/Discharge Considerations):

• Review individual nutritional needs, appropriate exercise program, and need for rest.

• Instruct client/SO(s) in techniques to protect the integrity of skin, care for lesions, and prevention of spread of infection.

• Emphasize necessity of taking antivirals or antibiotics, as directed (e.g., dosage and length of therapy). **Premature discontinuation of treatment when client begins to feel well may result in return of infection and potentiation of drug-resistant strains.**

• Discuss importance of not taking antibiotics or using "leftover" drugs unless specifically instructed by healthcare provider. **Inappropriate use can lead to development of drug-resistant strains or secondary infections.**

• Discuss the role of smoking in respiratory infections.

• Promote safer-sex practices and report sexual contacts of infected individuals **to prevent the spread of HIV and other sexually transmitted diseases.**

• Provide information and involve in appropriate community and national education programs **to increase awareness of and prevention of communicable diseases.**

• Discuss precautions with client engaged in international travel, and refer for immunizations **to reduce incidence and transmission of global infections.**

• Promote childhood immunization program. Encourage adults to obtain/update immunizations as appropriate.

• Include information in preoperative teaching about ways to reduce potential for postoperative infection (e.g., respiratory measures to prevent pneumonia, wound and dressing care, avoidance of others with infection).

Information that appears in brackets has been added by the authors to clarify and enhance the use of nursing diagnoses.

Cultural   Collaborative   Community/Home Care

- Review use of prophylactic antibiotics if appropriate (e.g., prior to dental work for clients with history of rheumatic fever or valvular heart disease).
- Encourage contacting healthcare provider for prophylactic therapy, as indicated, following exposure to individuals with infectious disease (e.g., tuberculosis, hepatitis, influenza).
- Identify resources available to the individual (e.g., substance abuse rehabilitation or needle exchange program, as appropriate; free condoms).
- Refer to NDs readiness for enhanced Immunization Status; risk for Disuse Syndrome; impaired Home Maintenance; ineffective Health Maintenance.

Documentation Focus

Assessment/Reassessment
- Individual risk factors including recent or current antibiotic therapy.
- Wound and/or insertion sites, character of drainage or body secretions.
- Signs and symptoms of infectious process.

Planning
- Plan of care, specific interventions, and who is involved in planning.
- Teaching plan.

Implementation/Evaluation
- Responses to interventions, teaching, and actions performed.
- Attainment or progress toward desired outcome(s).
- Modifications to plan of care.

Discharge Planning
- Discharge needs, referrals made, and who is responsible for actions to be taken.
- Specific referrals made.

Sample Nursing Outcomes & Interventions Classifications (NOC/NIC) NIC

NOC—Immune Status
NIC—Infection Protection

Information that appears in brackets has been added by the authors to clarify and enhance the use of nursing diagnoses.

 Diagnostic Studies ∞ Pediatric/Geriatric/Lifespan 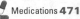 Medications **471**

risk for Injury

Taxonomy II: Safety/Protection—Class 2 Physical Injury
(00035)
[Diagnostic Division: Safety]
Submitted 1978

Definition: At risk of injury as a result of environmental
conditions interacting with the individual's adaptive and
defensive resources

Risk Factors

Internal

Physical (e.g., broken skin, altered mobility); tissue hypoxia;
malnutrition

Abnormal blood profile (e.g., leukocytosis, leukopenia, altered
clotting factors, thrombocytopenia, sickle cell, thalassemia,
decreased hemoglobin)

Biochemical dysfunction; sensory dysfunction

Integrative or effector dysfunction; immune-autoimmune dysfunction

Psychological (affective, orientation); developmental age
(physiological, psychosocial)

External

Biological (e.g., immunization level of community, microor-
ganism)

Chemical (e.g., pollutants, poisons, drugs, pharmaceutical
agents, alcohol, nicotine, preservatives, cosmetics, dyes); nutritional (e.g., vitamins, food types)

Physical (e.g., design, structure, and arrangement of community, building, and/or equipment), mode of transport

Human (e.g., nosocomial agents, staffing patterns; cognitive,
affective, psychomotor factors)

> **NOTE:** A risk diagnosis is not evidenced by signs
> and symptoms, as the problem has not occurred;
> rather, nursing interventions are directed at pre-
> vention.

Information that appears in brackets has been added by the authors to clarify
and enhance the use of nursing diagnoses.

Cultural Collaborative Community/Home Care

Desired Outcomes/Evaluation Criteria— Client/Caregivers Will:

- Verbalize understanding of individual factors that contribute to possibility of injury.
- Demonstrate behaviors, lifestyle changes to reduce risk factors and protect self from injury.
- Modify environment as indicated to enhance safety.
- Be free of injury.

Actions/Interventions

In reviewing this ND, it is apparent there is much overlap with other diagnoses. We have chosen to present generalized interventions. Although there are commonalities to injury situations, we suggest that the reader refer to other primary diagnoses as indicated, such as Activity Intolerance; risk for Aspiration; risk for imbalanced Body Temperature; decreased Cardiac Output; acute or chronic Confusion; risk for Contamination; risk for Falls; impaired Environmental Interpretation; impaired Gas Exchange; impaired Home Maintenance; impaired Mobility [specify]; impaired/risk for impaired Parenting; imbalanced Nutrition [specify]; risk for Poisoning; disturbed Sensory Perception; impaired/risk for impaired Skin Integrity; Sleep Deprivation; risk for Suffocation; disturbed Thought Processes; ineffective tissue Perfusion [specify]; risk for Infection; risk for Trauma; risk for other-directed/self-directed Violence; Wandering.

Nursing Priority No. 1.

To evaluate degree/source of risk inherent in the individual situation:

- Perform thorough assessments regarding safety issues when planning for client care and/or preparing for discharge from care. **Failure to accurately assess and intervene or refer these issues can place the client at needless risk and creates negligence issues for the healthcare practitioner.**
- Ascertain knowledge of safety needs, injury prevention, and motivation to prevent injury at home, in community, and work setting.
- ∞ Note client's age, gender, developmental stage, decision-making ability, level of cognition/competence. **Affects client's ability to protect self and/or others, and influences choice of interventions and teaching.**

Information that appears in brackets has been added by the authors to clarify and enhance the use of nursing diagnoses.

Diagnostic Studies ∞ Pediatric/Geriatric/Lifespan Medications **473**

- Assess mood, coping abilities, personality styles (e.g., temperament, aggression, impulsive behavior, level of self-esteem) **that may result in carelessness or increased risk-taking without consideration of consequences.**
- Assess client's muscle strength, gross and fine motor coordination **to identify risk for falls.**
- Note socioeconomic status and availability and use of resources.
- Evaluate individual's emotional and behavioral response to violence in environmental surroundings (e.g., home, neighborhood, peer group, media). **May affect client's view of and regard for own/others' safety.**
- Determine potential for abusive behavior by family members/SO(s)/peers.
- Observe for signs of injury and age (current, recent, and past such as old or new bruises, history of fractures, frequent absences from school or work **to determine need for evaluation of intentional injury or abuse in client relationship or living environment.**

Nursing Priority No. 2.

To assist client/caregiver to reduce or correct individual risk factors:

- Provide healthcare within a culture of safety (e.g., adherence to nursing standards of care and facility safe-care policies) **to prevent errors resulting in client injury, promote client safety, and model safety behaviors for client/SO(s):**

  Maintain bed or chair in lowest position with wheels locked.

  Ensure that pathway to bathroom is unobstructed and properly lighted.

  Place assistive devices (e.g., walker, cane, glasses, hearing aid) within reach.

  Instruct client/SO(s) to request assistance as needed; make sure call light is within reach and client knows how to operate.

  Monitor environment for potentially unsafe conditions and modify as needed.

   Administer medications and infusions using "6 rights" system (right patient, right medication, right route, right dose, right time, right reason).

- Inform and educate client/SO(s) regarding all treatments and medications and so forth.
- Refer to NDs previously listed for additional interventions.
- Develop plan of care with family to meet client's and SO's individual needs.

Information that appears in brackets has been added by the authors to clarify and enhance the use of nursing diagnoses.

- Provide information regarding disease or condition(s) that may result in increased risk of injury (e.g., weakness, dementia, head injury, immunosuppression, use of multiple medications, use of alcohol or other drugs, exposure to environmental chemicals or other hazards).
- Identify interventions and safety devices **to promote safe physical environment and individual safety.** Refer to physical or occupational therapist, as appropriate.
- Demonstrate and encourage use of techniques to reduce or manage stress and vent emotions, such as anger, hostility.
- Review consequences of previously determined risk factors that client is reluctant to modify (e.g., oral cancer in teenager using smokeless tobacco, occurrence of spontaneous abortion, fetal alcohol syndrome or neonatal addiction in prenatal woman using drugs, fall related to failure to use assistive equipment, toddler getting into medicine cabinet, binge drinking while skiing, health and legal implications of illicit drug use, working too many hours for safe operation of machinery or vehicles).
- Discuss importance of self-monitoring of condition or emotions **that can contribute to occurrence of injury (e.g., fatigue, anger, irritability).**
- Encourage participation in self-help programs, such as assertiveness training, positive self-image, to enhance self-esteem and sense of self-worth.
- Perform home assessment and identify safety issues, such as locking up medications and poisonous substances, locking exterior doors **to prevent client from wandering off while SO is engaged in other household activities,** or removing matches and smoking material and knobs from the stove **so confused client does not start a fire or turn on burner and leave it unattended.**
- ∞ Review expectations caregivers have of children, cognitively impaired, and/or elderly family members.
- ∞ Discuss need for and sources of supervision (e.g., before- and after-school programs, elderly day care).
- ∞ Discuss concerns about childcare, discipline practices.

Nursing Priority No. 3.
To promote wellness (Teaching/Discharge Considerations):

- Identify individual needs and resources for safety education such as first-aid/CPR classes, babysitter class, water or gun safety, smoking cessation, substance-abuse program, weight and exercise management, industry and community safety courses.

Information that appears in brackets has been added by the authors to clarify and enhance the use of nursing diagnoses.

- Provide telephone numbers and other contact numbers, as individually indicated (e.g., doctor, 911, poison control, police, lifeline, hazardous materials handler).
- Refer to other resources, as indicated (e.g., counseling, psychotherapy, budget counseling, parenting classes).
- Provide bibliotherapy or written resources **for later review and self-paced learning.**
- Promote community education programs geared to increasing awareness of safety measures and resources available to the individual (e.g., correct use of child safety seats, bicycle helmets, home hazard information, firearm safety, fall prevention, CPR and first aid).
- Promote community awareness about the problems of design of buildings, equipment, transportation, and workplace practices that contribute to accidents.
- Identify community resources/neighbors/friends to assist elderly/handicapped individuals in providing such things as structural maintenance and removal of snow and ice from walks and steps.

Documentation Focus

Assessment/Reassessment
- Individual risk factors, noting current physical findings (e.g., bruises, cuts).
- Client's/caregiver's understanding of individual risks and safety concerns.
- Availability and use of resources.

Planning
- Plan of care and who is involved in planning.
- Teaching plan.

Implementation/Evaluation
- Individual responses to interventions, teaching, and actions performed.
- Specific actions and changes that are made.
- Attainment or progress toward desired outcome(s).
- Modifications to plan of care.

Discharge Planning
- Long-range plans for discharge needs, lifestyle and community changes, and who is responsible for actions to be taken.
- Specific referrals made.

Information that appears in brackets has been added by the authors to clarify and enhance the use of nursing diagnoses.

Cultural   Collaborative   Community/Home Care

Sample Nursing Outcomes & Interventions Classifications (NOC/NIC) `NIC`

NOC—Safety Behavior: Personal
NIC—Surveillance: Safety

> ### risk for perioperative positioning Injury
>
> Taxonomy II: Safety/Protection—Class 2 Physical Injury (00087)
> [Diagnostic Division: Safety]
> Submitted 1994; Revised 2006
>
> **Definition:** At risk for injury as a result of the environmental conditions found in the perioperative setting

Risk Factors

Disorientation; sensory or perceptual disturbances due to anesthesia
Immobilization, muscle weakness; [preexisting musculoskeletal conditions]
Obesity; emaciation; edema
Elderly

> **NOTE:** A risk diagnosis is not evidenced by signs and symptoms, as the problem has not occurred; rather, nursing interventions are directed at prevention.

Desired Outcomes/Evaluation Criteria— Client Will:

- Be free of injury related to perioperative disorientation.
- Be free of untoward skin and tissue injury or changes lasting beyond 24 to 48 hours postprocedure.
- Report resolution of localized numbness, tingling, or changes in sensation related to positioning within 24 to 48 hours, as appropriate.

Actions/Interventions

Nursing Priority No. 1.

To identify individual risk factors/needs:

- Review client's history, noting age, weight and height, nutritional status, physical limitations or preexisting conditions

---

Information that appears in brackets has been added by the authors to clarify and enhance the use of nursing diagnoses.

(e.g., elderly person with arthritis; extremes of weight; diabetes or other conditions affecting peripheral vascular health; nutrition and hydration impairments). **Affects choice of perioperative positioning and affects skin and tissue integrity during surgery.**

- Evaluate and document client's preoperative reports of neurological, sensory, or motor deficits **for comparative baseline of perioperative and postoperative sensations.**

- Note anticipated length of procedure and customary position **to increase awareness of potential postoperative complications (e.g., supine position may cause low back pain and skin pressure at heels, elbows, and sacrum; lateral chest position can cause shoulder and neck pain, or eye and ear injury on the client's downside).**

- Assess the individual's responses to preoperative sedation/medication, noting level of sedation and/or adverse effects (e.g., drop in blood pressure) and report to surgeon, as indicated.

- Evaluate environmental conditions and safety issues surrounding the sedated client (e.g., client holding area, side rails up on bed or cart, someone staying with or close observation of client).

Nursing Priority No. 2.

To position client to provide protection for anatomical structures and to prevent client injury:

- Lock cart or bed in place; support client's body and limbs; use adequate number of personnel during transfer **to prevent shear and friction injuries.**

- Place safety strap strategically to secure client for specific procedure **to prevent unintended movement.**

- Maintain body alignment as much as possible using pillows, padding, and safety straps **to reduce potential for neurovascular complications associated with compression, overstretching, or ischemia of nerve(s).**

- Apply and reposition padding of pressure points and bony prominences (e.g., arms, elbows, sacrum, ankles, heels) and neurovascular pressure points (e.g., breasts, knees) **to maintain position of safety, especially when repositioning client and/or table attachments.**

- Check peripheral pulses and skin color and temperature periodically **to monitor circulation.**

- Protect body from contact with metal parts of the operating table, **which could produce burns or electric shock injury.**

Information that appears in brackets has been added by the authors to clarify and enhance the use of nursing diagnoses.

Cultural   Collaborative   Community/Home Care

- Reposition slowly at transfer and in bed (especially halothane-anesthetized client) **to prevent severe drop in blood pressure, dizziness, or unsafe transfer.**
- Protect airway and facilitate respiratory effort following extubation.
- Determine specific position reflecting procedure guidelines (e.g., head of bed elevated following spinal anesthesia, turn to unoperated side following pneumonectomy).
- Identify potential hazards in the surgical suite and implement corrections, as appropriate.

Nursing Priority No. 3.

To promote wellness (Teaching/Discharge Considerations):

- Provide perioperative teaching relative to client safety issues, including not crossing legs during procedures performed under local or light anesthesia, postoperative needs and limitations, and signs/symptoms requiring medical evaluation.
- Inform client and postoperative caregivers of expected/transient reactions (such as low backache, localized numbness, and reddening or skin indentations, all of which should disappear in 24 hours).
- Assist with therapies and routine nursing actions, including skin care measures, application of elastic stockings, early mobilization **to promote skin and tissue integrity.**
- Encourage and assist with frequent range-of-motion exercises, especially when joint stiffness occurs.
- Refer to appropriate resources, as needed.

Documentation Focus

Assessment/Reassessment
- Findings, including individual risk factors for problems in the perioperative setting, or need to modify routine activities or positions.
- Periodic evaluation of monitoring activities.

Planning
- Plan of care and who is involved in planning.
- Teaching plan.

Implementation/Evaluation
- Response to interventions and actions performed.
- Attainment or progress toward desired outcome(s).
- Modifications to plan of care.

Information that appears in brackets has been added by the authors to clarify and enhance the use of nursing diagnoses.

Discharge Planning

- Long-term needs and who is responsible for actions to be taken.

Sample Nursing Outcomes & Interventions Classifications (NOC/NIC) NIC

NOC—Risk Control
NIC—Positioning: Intraoperative

Insomnia

Taxonomy II: Activity/Rest—Class 1 Sleep/Rest (00095)
[Diagnostic Division: Activity/Rest]
Submitted 2006

Definition: A sustained disruption in amount and quality of sleep that impairs functioning

Related Factors

Intake of stimulants or alcohol; medications; gender-related hormonal shifts

Stress (e.g., ruminative presleep pattern); depression, fear, anxiety, grief

Impairment of normal sleep pattern (e.g., travel, shift work, parental responsibilities, interruptions for interventions); inadequate sleep hygiene (current)

Activity pattern (e.g., timing, amount)

Physical discomfort (e.g., body temperature, pain, shortness of breath, cough, gastroesophageal reflux, nausea, incontinence/urgency)

Environmental factors (e.g., ambient noise, daylight/darkness exposure, ambient temperature/humidity, unfamiliar setting)

Defining Characteristics

Subjective

Difficulty falling or staying asleep

Waking up too early

Dissatisfaction with sleep (current); nonrestorative sleep

Sleep disturbances that produce next-day consequences; lack of energy; difficulty concentrating; changes in mood

---

Information that appears in brackets has been added by the authors to clarify and enhance the use of nursing diagnoses.

Cultural Collaborative Community/Home Care

Decreased health status or quality of life
Increased accidents

Objective
Observed lack of energy
Observed changes in affect
Increased work or school absenteeism

Desired Outcomes/Evaluation Criteria—Client Will:

- Verbalize understanding of sleep impairment.
- Identify individually appropriate interventions to promote sleep.
- Adjust lifestyle to accommodate chronobiological rhythms.
- Report improvement in sleep-rest pattern.
- Report increased sense of well-being and feeling rested.

Actions/Interventions

Nursing Priority No. 1.
To identify causative/contributing factors:

- Identify presence of Related Factors such as chronic pain, arthritis, dyspnea, movement disorders, dementia, obesity, pregnancy, menopause, psychiatric disorders; metabolic diseases (e.g., hyperthyroidism, diabetes); prescribed and OTC drugs; alcohol, stimulant or other recreational drug use; circadian rhythm disorders (e.g., shift work, jet lag); environmental factors (e.g., noise, no control over thermostat, uncomfortable bed); major life stressors (e.g., grief, loss, finances) **that can contribute to insomnia.**
- Note age **(high percentage of elderly individuals are affected by sleep problems).**
- Observe parent-infant interaction and /provision of emotional support. Note mother's sleep-wake pattern. **Lack of knowledge of infant cues or problem relationships may create tension interfering with sleep. Structured sleep routines based on adult schedules may not meet child's needs.**
- Ascertain presence and frequency of enuresis, incontinence, or need for frequent nighttime voidings, **interrupting sleep.**
- Review psychological assessment, noting individual and personality characteristics **if anxiety disorders or depression could be affecting sleep.**
- Determine recent traumatic events in client's life (e.g., death in family, loss of job).

Information that appears in brackets has been added by the authors to clarify and enhance the use of nursing diagnoses.

- Review client's medications, including prescription (e.g., beta-adrenergic blockers, bronchodilators, weight-loss drugs, thyroid preparations); OTC products; herbals; **to determine if adjustments may be needed (such as change in dose or time medication is taken).**
- Evaluate use of caffeine and alcoholic beverages **(overindulgence interferes with rapid eye movement [REM] sleep).**
- Assist with diagnostic testing (e.g., EEG, full-night sleep studies) **to determine cause and type of sleep disturbance.**

Nursing Priority No. 2.
To evaluate sleep pattern and dysfunction(s):

- Observe and/or obtain feedback from client/SO(s) regarding client's sleep problems, usual bedtime, rituals and routines, number of hours of sleep, time of arising, and environmental needs **to determine usual sleep pattern and provide comparative baseline.**
- Listen to subjective reports of sleep quality (e.g., client never feels rested, or feels sleepy during day).
- Identify circumstances that interrupt sleep and the frequency at which they occur.
- Determine client's/SO's expectations of adequate sleep. **Provides opportunity to address misconceptions or unrealistic expectations.**
- Investigate whether client snores and in what position(s) this occurs **to determine if further evaluation is needed to rule out obstructive sleep disorder.**
- Note alteration of habitual sleep time, such as change of work pattern, rotating shifts, change in normal bedtime (hospitalization).
- Observe physical signs of fatigue (e.g., restlessness, hand tremors, thick speech).
- Develop a chronological chart **to determine peak performance rhythm.**
- Graph "circadian" rhythms of individual's biological internal chemistry per protocol, as indicated. *Note:* **Studies have shown sleep cycles are affected by body temperature at onset of sleep.**

Nursing Priority No. 3.
To assist client to establish optimal sleep/rest patterns:

- Arrange care to provide for uninterrupted periods for rest, especially allowing for longer periods of sleep at night when possible. Do as much care as possible without waking client.

Information that appears in brackets has been added by the authors to clarify and enhance the use of nursing diagnoses.

Cultural Collaborative Community/Home Care

- Explain necessity of disturbances for monitoring vital signs and/or other care when client is hospitalized.
- Provide quiet environment and comfort measures (e.g., back rub, washing hands/face, cleaning and straightening sheets) in preparation for sleep.
∞ • Discuss and implement effective age-appropriate bedtime rituals (e.g., going to bed at same time each night, drinking warm milk, rocking, story reading, cuddling, favorite blanket or toy) **to enhance client's ability to fall asleep, reinforce that bed is a place to sleep, and promote sense of security for child.**
- Recommend limiting intake of chocolate and caffeinated or alcoholic beverages, especially prior to bedtime.
- Limit fluid intake in evening if nocturia is a problem **to reduce need for nighttime elimination.**
- Explore other sleep aids (e.g., warm bath, protein intake before bedtime).
💊 • Administer pain medications (if required) 1 hour before sleep **to relieve discomfort and take maximum advantage of sedative effect.**
💊 • Monitor effects of drug regimen—amphetamines or stimulants (e.g., methylphenidate—Ritalin used in narcolepsy).
💊 • Use barbiturates and/or other sleeping medications sparingly. **Research indicates long-term use of these medications can actually induce sleep disturbances.**
🅰 • Encourage routine use of continuous positive airway pressure (CPAP) therapy, when indicated, **to obtain optimal benefit of treatment for sleep apnea.**
🏠 • Develop behavioral program for insomnia, such as:
  Establishing routine bedtime and arising
  Thinking relaxing thoughts when in bed
  Not napping in the daytime
  Not reading or watching TV in bed
  Getting out of bed if not asleep in 15 minutes
  Limiting sleep to 7 hours a night
  Getting up the same time each day—even on weekends and days off
  Getting adequate exposure to bright light during day
  Individually tailoring stress reduction program, music therapy, relaxation routine
🅰 • Collaborate in treatment of underlying medical problem (e.g., obstructive sleep apnea, pain, gastroesophageal reflux disease [GERD], lower urinary tract infection [UTI], prostatic hypertrophy, depression, complicated grief).

Information that appears in brackets has been added by the authors to clarify and enhance the use of nursing diagnoses.

⚕️ • Refer to sleep specialist, as indicated or desired. **Follow-up evaluation or intervention may be needed when insomnia is seriously impacting client's quality of life, productivity, and safety (e.g., on the job, at home, on the road).**

Nursing Priority No. 4.
To promote wellness (Teaching/Discharge Considerations):

🏠 • Assure client that occasional sleeplessness should not threaten health. **Worrying about not sleeping can perpetuate or exacerbate the problem.**

🏠 • Assist client to develop individual program of relaxation. Demonstrate techniques (e.g., biofeedback, self-hypnosis, visualization, progressive muscle relaxation).

🏠 • Encourage participation in regular exercise program during day **to aid in stress control and release of energy. Exercise at bedtime may stimulate rather than relax client and actually interfere with sleep.**

🏠 • Recommend inclusion of bedtime snack (e.g., milk or mild juice, crackers, protein source such as cheese/peanut butter) in dietary program **to reduce sleep interference from hunger or hypoglycemia.**

🏠 • Suggest that bed and bedroom be used only for sleep, not for working, watching TV.

∞ • Provide for child's (or impaired individual's) sleep time safety (e.g., infant placed on back, bedrails or bed in low position, nonplastic sheets).

🏠 • Investigate use of aids to block out light and noise, such as sleep mask, darkening shades or curtains, earplugs, monotonous sounds such as low-level background noise (white noise).

🏠 • Participate in program to "reset" the body's sleep clock (chronotherapy) **when client has delayed-sleep-onset insomnia.**

🏠 • Assist individual to develop schedules that take advantage of peak performance times as identified in chronobiological chart.

🏠 • Recommend midmorning nap if one is required. **Napping, especially in the afternoon, can disrupt normal sleep patterns.**

🏠 • Assist client to deal with grieving process when loss has occurred. (Refer to ND Grieving.)

Information that appears in brackets has been added by the authors to clarify and enhance the use of nursing diagnoses.

Documentation Focus

Assessment/Reassessment
- Assessment findings, including specifics of sleep pattern (current and past) and effects on lifestyle and level of functioning.
- Medications or interventions used, previous therapies tried.

Planning
- Plan of care and who is involved in planning.
- Teaching plan.

Implementation/Evaluation
- Client's response to interventions, teaching, and actions performed.
- Attainment or progress toward desired outcome(s).
- Modifications to plan of care.

Discharge Planning
- Long-term needs and who is responsible for actions to be taken.
- Specific referrals made.

Sample Nursing Outcomes & Interventions Classifications (NOC/NIC) NIC

NOC—Sleep
NIC—Sleep Enhancement

---

decreased Intracranial Adaptive Capacity

Taxonomy II: Coping/Stress Tolerance—Class 3
  Neurobehavioral Stress (00049)
[Diagnostic Division: Circulation]
Submitted 1994

Definition: Intracranial fluid dynamic mechanisms that normally compensate for increases in intracranial volume are compromised, resulting in repeated disproportionate increases in intracranial pressure (ICP) in response to a variety of noxious and non-noxious stimuli

---

Information that appears in brackets has been added by the authors to clarify and enhance the use of nursing diagnoses.

 Diagnostic Studies   ∞ Pediatric/Geriatric/Lifespan   Medications **485**

Related Factors

Brain injuries
Sustained increase in ICP of 10 to 15 mm Hg
Decreased cerebral perfusion pressure (≤50–60 mm Hg)
Systemic hypotension with intracranial hypertension

Defining Characteristics

Objective

Repeated increases of ICP >10 mm Hg for more than 5 minutes
   following a variety of external stimuli
Disproportionate increase in ICP following stimulus
Elevated P_2 ICP waveform
Volume pressure response test variation (volume-pressure ratio
   2, pressure-volume index <10)
Baseline ICP ≤10 mm Hg
Wide amplitude ICP waveform
[Altered level of consciousness—coma]
[Changes in vital signs, cardiac rhythm]

Desired Outcomes/Evaluation Criteria— Client Will:

- Demonstrate stable ICP as evidenced by normalization of
  pressure waveforms and appropriate response to stimuli.
- Display improved neurological signs.

Actions/Interventions

Nursing Priority No. 1.

To assess causative/contributing factors:

- Determine factors related to individual situation (e.g., cause
  of loss of consciousness or coma; accompanying symptoms;
  early Glasgow Coma Scale).
- Monitor and document changes in ICP; monitor waveform
  and corresponding event (e.g., suctioning, position change,
  monitor alarms, family visit) **to alter care appropriately.**

Nursing Priority No. 2.

To note degree of impairment:

- Assess and document client's eye opening, position, and
  movement; size, shape, equality, light reactivity of pupils; and

---

Information that appears in brackets has been added by the authors to clarify
and enhance the use of nursing diagnoses.

🌐 Cultural 🔬 Collaborative 🏠 Community/Home Care

consciousness and mental status (Glasgow Coma Scale) **to determine client's baseline neurological status and monitor changes over time.**

- Note purposeful and nonpurposeful motor response (posturing, etc.), comparing right and left sides.
- Test for presence of reflexes (e.g., blink, cough, gag, Babinski's reflex), nuchal rigidity.
- Monitor vital signs and cardiac rhythm before, during, after activity.
- Review results of diagnostic imaging (e.g., CT scans) **to note location, type, and severity of tissue injury.**

Nursing Priority No. 3.
To minimize/correct causative factors/maximize perfusion:

- Elevate head of bed, as individually appropriate. **Although some researchers recommend head elevation up to 45 degrees, recent studies suggest a 30-degree head elevation for maximum benefit.**
- Maintain head and neck in neutral position, support with small towel rolls or pillows **to maximize venous return.** Avoid placing head on large pillow or causing hip flexion of 90 degrees or more.
- Decrease extraneous stimuli and provide comfort measures (e.g., quiet environment, soft voice, tapes of familiar voices played through earphones, back massage, gentle touch as tolerated) **to reduce CNS stimulation and promote relaxation.**
- Limit painful procedures (e.g., venipunctures, redundant neurological evaluations) to those that are absolutely necessary.
- Provide rest periods between care activities and limit duration of procedures. Lower lighting and noise level, schedule and limit activities **to provide restful environment and promote regular sleep patterns (i.e., day or night pattern).**
- Limit or prevent activities that increase intrathoracic or abdominal pressures (e.g., coughing, vomiting, straining at stool). Avoid or limit use of restraints. **These factors markedly increase ICP.**
- Suction with caution—only when needed—to just beyond end of endotracheal tube without touching tracheal wall or carina. Administer lidocaine intratracheally per protocol **to reduce cough reflex,** and hyperoxygenate before suctioning as appropriate **to minimize hypoxia.**
- Maintain patency of urinary drainage system **to reduce risk of hypertension, increased ICP, and associated dysreflexia**

decreased INTRACRANIAL ADAPTIVE CAPACITY

Information that appears in brackets has been added by the authors to clarify and enhance the use of nursing diagnoses.

 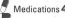

when spinal cord injury is also present and spinal cord shock is past. (Refer to ND Autonomic Dysreflexia.)

- Weigh, as indicated. Calculate fluid balance every shift or daily **to determine fluid needs, maintain hydration, and prevent fluid overload.**
- Restrict fluid intake, as necessary, administer IV fluids via pump or control device **to prevent inadvertent fluid bolus or vascular overload.**
- Regulate environmental temperature; use cooling blanket as indicated **to decrease metabolic and O_2 needs when fever present or therapeutic hypothermia therapy is used.**
- Investigate increased restlessness **to determine causative factors and initiate corrective measures as early as possible.**
- Provide appropriate safety measures and initiate treatment for seizures **to prevent injury and increased ICP or hypoxia.**
- Administer supplemental oxygen, as indicated, **to prevent cerebral ischemia;** hyperventilate (as indicated per protocol) when on mechanical ventilation. **Therapeutic hyperventilation may be used ($PaCO_2$ of 30–35 mm) to reduce intracranial hypertension for a short period of time, while other methods of ICP control are initiated.**
- Administer medications (e.g., antihypertensives, diuretics, analgesics, sedatives, antipyretics, vasopressors, antiseizure drugs, neuromuscular blocking agents, and corticosteroids), as appropriate, **to maintain cerebral homeostasis and manage symptoms associated with neurological injury.**
- Prepare client for surgery, as indicated (e.g., evacuation of hematoma or space-occupying lesion), **to reduce ICP and enhance circulation.**

Nursing Priority No. 4.

To promote wellness (Teaching/Discharge Considerations):

- Discuss with caregivers specific situations (e.g., if client choking or experiencing pain, needing to be repositioned, constipated, blocked urinary flow) and review appropriate interventions **to prevent or limit episodic increases in ICP.**
- Identify signs/symptoms suggesting increased ICP (in client at risk without an ICP monitor); for example, restlessness, deterioration in neurological responses. Review appropriate interventions.

Information that appears in brackets has been added by the authors to clarify and enhance the use of nursing diagnoses.

Cultural Collaborative Community/Home Care

Assessment/Reassessment
- Neurological findings noting right and left sides separately (such as pupils, motor response, reflexes, restlessness, nuchal rigidity); Glasgow Coma Scale.
- Response to activities and events (e.g., changes in pressure waveforms or vital signs).
- Presence and characteristics of seizure activity.

Planning
- Plan of care and who is involved in planning.
- Teaching plan.

Implementation/Evaluation
- Response to interventions and actions performed.
- Attainment or progress toward desired outcome(s).
- Modifications to plan of care.

Discharge Planning
- Future needs, plan for meeting them, and determining who is responsible for actions.
- Referrals as identified.

Sample Nursing Outcomes & Interventions Classifications (NOC/NIC) NIC

NOC—Neurological Status
NIC—Cerebral Edema Management

---

neonatal Jaundice

Taxonomy II: Nutrition Class 4 Metabolism (00194)
[Diagnostic Division: Safety]
Submitted 2008

Definition: The yellow orange tint of the neonate's skin and mucous membranes that occurs after 24 hours of life as a result of unconjugated bilirubin in the circulation

Related Factors

Neonate age 1 to 7 days
Feeding pattern not well established

Information that appears in brackets has been added by the authors to clarify and enhance the use of nursing diagnoses.

Abnormal weight loss (>7%–8% in breastfeeding newborn; 15% in term infant)

Stool (meconium) passage delayed

Infant experiences difficulty making transition to extrauterine life

Defining Characteristics

Objective

Yellow-orange skin; yellow sclera

Abnormal skin bruising

Abnormal blood profile (hemolysis; total serum bilirubin >2 mg/dL; inherited disorder; total serum bilirubin in high risk range [for] age in hour-specific nomogram)

Sample Clinical Applications:

Newborn, premature infant

Desired Outcomes/Evaluation Criteria

Infant Will: (Include Specific Time Frame)

• Display decreasing bilirubin levels with resolution of jaundice.

• Be free of central nervous system (CNS) involvement, or complications associated with therapeutic regimen.

Parent/Caregiver Will: (Include Specific Time Frame)

• Verbalize understanding of cause, treatment, and possible outcomes of hyperbilirubinemia.

• Demonstrate appropriate care of infant.

Actions/Interventions

Nursing Priority No. 1.

To assess causative/contributing factors:

• Determine infant and maternal blood groups and blood types. **ABO incompatibilities affect 20% of all pregnancies.**

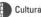 • Note gender, race, and place of birth. **Risk of developing jaundice is higher in males, infants of East Asian or American Indian descent, and those living at high altitudes.**

Information that appears in brackets has been added by the authors to clarify and enhance the use of nursing diagnoses.

- Review intrapartal record for specific risk factors, such as low birth weight (LBW) or intrauterine growth retardation (IUGR), prematurity, abnormal metabolic processes, vascular injuries, abnormal circulation, sepsis, or polycythemia.
- Note use of instruments or vacuum extractor for delivery. Assess infant for presence of birth trauma, cephalohematoma, and excessive ecchymosis or petechiae. **Resorption of blood trapped in fetal scalp tissue and excessive hemolysis may increase the amount of bilirubin being released.**
- Review infant's condition at birth, noting need for resuscitation or evidence of excessive ecchymosis or petechiae, cold stress, asphyxia, or acidosis. **Asphyxia and acidosis reduce affinity of bilirubin to albumin increasing the amount of unbound circulating (indirect) bilirubin, which may cross the blood-brain barrier, causing CNS toxicity.**
- Evaluate maternal and prenatal nutritional levels; note possible neonatal hypoproteinemia, especially in preterm infant. **One gram of albumin carries 16 mg of unconjugated bilirubin; therefore, lack of sufficient albumin (hypoproteinemia) in the newborn increases risk of jaundice.**
- Assess infant for signs of hypoglycemia such as jitteriness, irritability, and lethargy. Obtain healstick glucose levels as indicated. **Hypoglycemia necessitates use of fat stores for energy-releasing fatty acids, which compete with bilirubin for binding sites on albumin.**
- Determine successful initiation and adequacy of breastfeeding. **Poor caloric intake and dehydration associated with ineffective breastfeeding increases risk of developing hyperbilirubinemia.**
- Evaluate infant for pallor, edema, or hepatosplenomegaly. **These signs may be associated with hydrops fetalis, Rh incompatibility, and in utero hemolysis of fetal RBCs.**
- Evaluate for jaundice in natural light, noting sclera and oral mucosa, yellowing of skin immediately after blanching, and specific body parts involved. Assess oral mucosa, posterior portion of hard palate, and conjunctival sacs in dark-skinned newborns.
- Note infant's age at onset of jaundice. Aids in differentiating type of jaundice (i.e., physiological, breast milk-induced, or pathological). **Physiological jaundice usually appears between the second and third day of life, breast milk jaundice between the fourth and the seventh day of life, and pathological jaundice occurs within the first 24 hours of**

Information that appears in brackets has been added by the authors to clarify and enhance the use of nursing diagnoses.

life, or when the total serum bilirubin level rises by more than 5 mg/dL per day.

Nursing Priority No. 2.

To evaluate degree of compromise:

- Review laboratory studies including total serum bilirubin and albumin levels, hemoglobin and hematocrit, reticulocyte count.
- Calculate plasma bilirubin-albumin binding capacity. **Aids in determining risk of kernicterus and treatment needs.**
- Assess infant for progression of signs and behavioral changes associated with bilirubin toxicity. **Early-stage toxicity involves neuro-depression-lethargy, poor feeding, high-pitched cry, diminished or absent reflexes; late-stage hypotonia, neuro-hyperreflexia-twitching, convulsions, opisthotonos, fever.**
- Evaluate appearance of skin and urine, noting brownish-black color. **An uncommon side effect of phototherapy involves exaggerated pigment changes (bronze baby syndrome) that may last for 2 to 4 months but is not associated with harmful sequelae.**

Nursing Priority No. 3.

To correct hyperbilirubinemia and prevent associated complications:

- Keep infant warm and dry; monitor skin and core temperature frequently. **Prevents cold stress and the release of fatty acids that compete for binding sites on albumin, thus increasing the level of freely circulating bilirubin.**
- Initiate early oral feedings within 4 to 6 hours following birth, especially if infant is to be breastfed. **Establishes proper intestinal flora necessary for reduction of bilirubin to urobilinogen and decreases reabsorption of bilirubin from bowel.**
- Encourage frequent breastfeeding—8 to 12 times per day. Assist mother with pumping of breasts as needed **to maintain milk production.**
- Administer small amounts of breast milk substitute (L-aspartic acid or enzymatically hydrolyzed casein [EHC]) for 24 to 48 hours if indicated. **Use of feeding additives is under investigation for inhibition of beta-glucuronidase leading to increased fecal excretion of bilirubin; results have been mixed.**

Information that appears in brackets has been added by the authors to clarify and enhance the use of nursing diagnoses.

⊕ Cultural ⊛ Collaborative 🏠 Community/Home Care

- Apply transcutaneous jaundice meter. **Provides noninvasive screening of jaundice.**
- Initiate phototherapy per protocol, using fluorescent bulbs placed above the infant, or fiberoptic pad or blanket (except for newborns with Rh disease). **Primary therapy for neonates with unconjugated hyperbilirubinemia.**
- Apply eye patches, ensuring correct fit during periods of phototherapy, to prevent retinal injury. Remove eye covering during feedings or other care activities as appropriate **to provide visual stimulation and interaction with caregivers/parents.**
- Avoid application of lotion or oils to skin of infant receiving phototherapy **to prevent dermal irritation or injury.**
- Reposition infant every 2 hours **to ensure that all areas of skin are exposed to bili light when fiberoptic pad or blanket is not used.**
- Cover male groin with small pad **to protect from heat-related injury to testes.**
- Monitor infant's weight loss, urine output and specific gravity, and fecal water loss from loose stools associated with phototherapy **to determine adequacy of fluid intake.** *Note: Infant may sleep for longer periods in conjunction with phototherapy, increasing risk of dehydration.*
- Administer intravenous immunoglobulin (IVIG) to neonates with Rh or ABO isoimmunization. **Rate of hemolysis in Rh disease or other cases of immune hemolytic jaundice usually exceeds the rate of bilirubin reduction related to phototherapy. IVIG inhibits antibodies that cause red cell destruction, helping to limit the rise in bilirubin levels.**
- Administer enzyme induction agent (phenobarbital) as appropriate. **May be used on occasion to stimulate hepatic enzymes to enhance clearance of bilirubin.**
- Assist with preparation and administration of exchange transfusion. **Exchange transfusions are occasionally required in cases of severe hemolytic anemia unresponsive to other treatment options, or in presence of acute bilirubin encephalopathy as evidenced by hypertonia, arching, retrocollis, opisthotonos, fever, high-pitched cry.**
- Document events during transfusion, carefully recording amount of blood withdrawn and injected (usually 7–20 mL at a time).

Nursing Priority No. 4.
To promote wellness (Teaching/Discharge Considerations):

Information that appears in brackets has been added by the authors to clarify and enhance the use of nursing diagnoses.

🏠 • Provide information about types of jaundice and pathophys-iological factors and future implications of hyperbilirubine-mia. **Promotes understanding, corrects misconceptions, and can reduce fear and feelings of guilt.**

🏠 • Review means of assessing infant status (feedings, intake and ouptut [I&O], stools, temperature, and serial weights if scale available) and for monitoring increasing bilirubin levels (e.g., observing blanching of skin over bony prominence or behav-ior changes), especially if infant is to be discharged early. *Note:* **Persistence of jaundice in formula-fed infant beyond 2 weeks, or 3 weeks in breast-fed infant, requires further evaluation.**

🔵 • Provide parents with 24-hour emergency telephone number and name of contact person, stressing importance of reporting increased jaundice or changes in behavior.

🔵 • Refer to lactation specialist **to enhance or reestablish breast-feeding process.**

🔵 • Arrange appropriate referral for home phototherapy program if necessary.

🏠 • Provide written explanation of home phototherapy, safety pre-cautions, and potential problems. **Home phototherapy is rec-ommended only for full-term infants after the first 48 hours of life, if serum bilirubin levels are between 14 and 18 mg/dL, with no increase in direct reacting bilirubin concentration.**

🧪 • Make appropriate arrangements for follow-up testing of serum bilirubin at same laboratory facility. **Treatment is discontin-ued once serum bilirubin concentrations fall below 14 mg/dL. Untreated or chronic hyperbilirubinemia can lead to permanent damage such as high-pitch hearing loss, cere-bral palsy, or mental retardation.**

🏠 • Discuss possible long-term effects of hyperbilirubinemia and the need for continued assessment and early intervention. **Neurolog-ical damage associated with kernicterus includes cerebral palsy, mental retardation, sensory difficulties, delayed speech, poor muscle coordination, learning difficulties, death.**

Documentation Focus

Assessment/Reassessment

• Assessment findings, risk or related factors.
• Adequacy of intake—hydration level, character and number of stools.
• Laboratory results and bilirubin trends.

Information that appears in brackets has been added by the authors to clarify and enhance the use of nursing diagnoses.

⊕ Cultural   🔵 Collaborative   🏠 Community/Home Care

Planning

- Plan of care, specific interventions, and who is involved in the planning.
- Teaching plan and resources provided.

Implementation/Evaluation

- Client's responses to treatment and actions performed.
- Parents' understanding of teaching.
- Attainment or progress toward desired outcome(s).
- Modifications to plan of care.

Discharge Planning

- Long-range needs, identifying who is responsible for actions to be taken.
- Community resources for equipment and supplies postdischarge.
- Specific referrals made.

Sample Nursing Outcomes & Interventions Classifications (NOC/NIC) NIC

NOC—Newborn Adaptation
NIC—Phototherapy: Neonate

---

deficient Knowledge [Learning Need] (specify)

Taxonomy II: Perception/Cognition—Class 4 Cognition (00126)
[Diagnostic Division: Teaching/Learning]
Submitted 1980

Definition: Absence or deficiency of cognitive information related to specific topic [Lack of specific information necessary for clients/SO(s) to make informed choices regarding condition, treatment, and/or lifestyle changes]

Related Factors

Lack of exposure or recall
Information misinterpretation [inaccurate or incomplete information presented]
Unfamiliarity with information resources
Cognitive limitation
Lack of interest in learning [client's request for no information]

Information that appears in brackets has been added by the authors to clarify and enhance the use of nursing diagnoses.

Defining Characteristics

Subjective
Verbalization of the problem
Request for information
Statements reflecting misconceptions

Objective
Inaccurate follow-through of instruction or performance of test
Inappropriate or exaggerated behaviors (e.g., hysterical, hostile, agitated, apathetic)
Development of preventable complication

Desired Outcomes/Evaluation Criteria—Client Will:

- Participate in learning process.
- Identify interferences to learning and specific action(s) to deal with them.
- Exhibit increased interest and assume responsibility for own learning by beginning to look for information and ask questions.
- Verbalize understanding of condition, disease process, and treatment.
- Identify relationship of signs/symptoms to the disease process and correlate symptoms with causative factors.
- Perform necessary procedures correctly and explain reasons for the actions.
- Initiate necessary lifestyle changes and participate in treatment regimen.

Actions/Interventions

Nursing Priority No. 1.
To assess readiness to learn and individual learning needs:

- Ascertain level of knowledge, including anticipatory needs.
- Determine client's ability, readiness, and barriers to learning. **Individual may not be physically, emotionally, or mentally capable at this time.**
- Be alert to signs of avoidance. **Client may need to suffer consequences of lack of knowledge before he or she is ready to accept information.**
- Identify support persons/SO(s) requiring information (e.g., parent, caregiver, spouse).

Information that appears in brackets has been added by the authors to clarify and enhance the use of nursing diagnoses.

Cultural   Collaborative   Community/Home Care

Nursing Priority No. 2.

To determine other factors pertinent to the learning process:

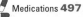 • Note personal factors (e.g., age and developmental level, gender, social and cultural influences, religion, life experiences, level of education, emotional stability).
* Determine blocks to learning: language barriers (e.g., client can't read; speaks or understands a different language than healthcare provider); physical factors (e.g., cognitive impairment, aphasia, dyslexia); physical stability (e.g., acute illness, activity intolerance); difficulty of material to be learned.
* Assess the level of the client's capabilities and the possibilities of the situation. **May need to help SO(s) and/or caregivers to learn.**

Nursing Priority No. 3.

To assess the client's/SO's motivation:

* Identify motivating factors for the individual (e.g., client needs to stop smoking because of advanced lung cancer, or client wants to lose weight because family member died of complications of obesity). **Motivation may be a negative stimulus (e.g., smoking caused lung cancer); or positive (e.g., client wants to promote health and prevent disease).**
* Provide information relevant only to the situation **to prevent overload.**
* Provide positive reinforcement. **Can encourage continuation of efforts.** Avoid use of negative reinforcers (e.g., criticism, threats).

Nursing Priority No. 4.

To establish priorities in conjunction with client:

* Determine client's most urgent need from both client's and nurse's viewpoint **(which may differ and require adjustments in teaching plan).**
* Discuss client's perception of need. Relate information to client's personal desires, needs, values, and beliefs **so that client feels competent and respected.**
* Differentiate "critical" content from "desirable" content. **Identifies information that can be addressed at a later time.**

Nursing Priority No. 5.

To establish the content to be included:

* Identify information that needs to be remembered (cognitive).

Information that appears in brackets has been added by the authors to clarify and enhance the use of nursing diagnoses.

- Identify information having to do with emotions, attitudes, and values (affective).
- Identify psychomotor skills that are necessary for learning.

Nursing Priority No. 6.
To develop learner's objectives:
- State objectives clearly in learner's terms **to meet learner's (not instructor's) needs.**
- Identify outcomes (results) to be achieved.
- Recognize level of achievement, time factors, and short- and long-term goals.
- Include the affective goals (e.g., reduction of stress).

Nursing Priority No. 7.
To identify teaching methods to be used:
- Determine client's method of accessing information (visual, auditory, kinesthetic, gustatory/olfactory) and include in teaching plan **to facilitate learning or recall.**
- Involve the client/SO(s) by using age-appropriate materials tailored to client's literacy skills, questions, and dialogue.
- Involve with others who have same problems, needs, or concerns (e.g., group presentations, support groups). **Provides role model and sharing of information.**
- Provide mutual goal setting and learning contracts. **Clarifies expectations of teacher and learner.**
- Use team and group teaching as appropriate.

Nursing Priority No. 8.
To facilitate learning:
- Use short, simple sentences and concepts. Repeat and summarize as needed.
- Use gestures and facial expressions that help convey meaning of information.
- Discuss one topic at a time; avoid giving too much information in one session.
- Provide written information or guidelines and self-learning modules for client to refer to as necessary. **Reinforces learning process; allows client to proceed at own pace.**
- Pace and time learning sessions and learning activities to individual's needs. Evaluate effectiveness of learning activities with client.
- Provide an environment that is conducive to learning.

Information that appears in brackets has been added by the authors to clarify and enhance the use of nursing diagnoses.

Cultural   Collaborative   Community/Home Care

- Be aware of factors related to teacher in the situation (e.g., vocabulary, dress, style, knowledge of the subject, and ability to impart information effectively).
- Begin with information the client already knows and move to what the client does not know, progressing from simple to complex. **Can arouse interest/limit sense of being over-whelmed.**
- Deal with the client's anxiety or other strong emotions. Present information out of sequence, if necessary, dealing first with material that is most anxiety producing **when the anxiety is interfering with the client's ability to learn.**
- Provide active role for client in learning process. **Promotes sense of control over situation and is means for determining that client is assimilating and using new information.**
- Provide for feedback (positive reinforcement) and evaluation of learning and acquisition of skills.
- Be aware of informal teaching and role modeling that takes place on an ongoing basis (e.g., answering specific questions and reinforcing previous teaching during routine care).
- Assist client to use information in all applicable areas (e.g., situational, environmental, personal).

Nursing Priority No. 9.
To promote wellness (Teaching/Discharge Considerations):

- Provide access information for contact person **to answer questions and validate information postdischarge.**
- Identify available community resources and support groups.
- Provide information about additional learning resources (e.g., bibliography, Web sites, tapes). **May assist with further learning and promote learning at own pace.**

Documentation Focus ——————————————

Assessment/Reassessment
- Individual findings including learning style, identified needs, presence of learning blocks (e.g., hostility, inappropriate behavior).

Planning
- Plan for learning, methods to be used, and who is involved in the planning.
- Teaching plan.

Information that appears in brackets has been added by the authors to clarify and enhance the use of nursing diagnoses.

Implementation/Evaluation

* Responses of the client/SO(s) to the learning plan and actions performed. How the learning is demonstrated.
* Attainment or progress toward desired outcome(s).
* Modifications to plan of care.

Discharge Planning

* Additional learning and referral needs.

Sample Nursing Outcomes & Interventions Classifications (NOC/NIC) NIC

NOC—Knowledge: [specify—42 choices]
NIC—Teaching: [specify—30 choices]

---

readiness for enhanced **Knowledge** (specify)

Taxonomy II: Perception/Cognition—Class 4 Cognition (00161)
[Diagnostic Division: Teaching/Learning]
Submitted 2002

Definition: The presence or acquisition of cognitive information related to a specific topic is sufficient for meeting health-related goals and can be strengthened

---

Related Factors

To be developed

Defining Characteristics

Subjective

Expresses an interest in learning
Explains knowledge of the topic; describes previous experiences pertaining to the topic

Objective

Behaviors congruent with expressed knowledge

Desired Outcomes/Evaluation Criteria— Client Will:

* Exhibit responsibility for own learning by seeking answers to questions.

Information that appears in brackets has been added by the authors to clarify and enhance the use of nursing diagnoses.

- Verify accuracy of informational resources.
- Verbalize understanding of information gained.
- Use information to develop individual plan to meet healthcare needs and goals.

Actions/Interventions

Nursing Priority No. 1.
To develop plan for learning:

- Verify client's level of knowledge about specific topic. **Provides opportunity to ensure accuracy and completeness of knowledge base for future learning.**
- Determine motivation and expectations for learning. **Provides insight useful in developing goals and identifying information needs.**
- Assist client to identify learning goals. **Helps to frame or focus content to be learned and provides measure to evaluate learning process.**
- Ascertain preferred methods of learning (e.g., auditory, visual, interactive, or "hands-on"). **Identifies best approaches to facilitate learning process.**
- Note personal factors (e.g., age/developmental level, gender, social/cultural influences, religion, life experiences, level of education) **that may impact learning style, choice of informational resources.**
- Determine any challenges to learning: language barriers (e.g., client can't read, speaks or understands language other than that of care provider, dyslexia); physical factors (e.g., sensory deficits, such as vision or hearing deficits, aphasia); physical stability (e.g., acute illness, activity intolerance); difficulty of material to be learned. **Identifies special needs to be addressed if learning is to be successful.**

Nursing Priority No. 2.
To facilitate learning:

- Identify and provide information in varied formats appropriate to client's learning style (e.g., audiotapes, print materials, videos, classes or seminars, Internet). **Use of multiple formats increases learning and retention of material.**
- Provide information about additional or outside learning resources (e.g., bibliography, pertinent Web sites). **Promotes ongoing learning at own pace.**
- Discuss ways to verify accuracy of informational resources. **Encourages independent search for learning opportunities**

Information that appears in brackets has been added by the authors to clarify and enhance the use of nursing diagnoses.

while reducing likelihood of acting on erroneous or unproven data that could be detrimental to client's wellbeing.

- Identify available community resources/support groups. **Provides additional opportunities for role modeling, skill training, anticipatory problem solving, and so forth.**
- Be aware of informal teaching and role modeling that takes place on an ongoing basis (e.g., community and peer role models, support group feedback, print advertisements, popular music or videos). **Incongruencies may exist, creating questions and potentially undermining learning process.**

Nursing Priority No. 3.

To enhance optimum wellness:

- Assist client to identify ways to integrate and use information in all applicable areas (e.g., situational, environmental, personal). **Ability to apply or use information increases desire to learn and retain information.**
- Encourage client to journal, keep a log, or graph as appropriate. **Provides opportunity for self-evaluation of effects of learning, such as better management of chronic condition, reduction of risk factors, acquisition of new skills.**

Documentation Focus ——————————

Assessment/Reassessment
- Individual findings including learning style and identified needs, presence of challenges to learning.
- Motivation and expectations for learning.

Planning
- Plan for learning, methods to be used, and who is involved in the planning.
- Educational plan.

Implementation/Evaluation
- Responses of the client/SO(s) to the learning plan and actions performed.
- How the learning is demonstrated.
- Attainment or progress toward desired outcome(s).
- Modifications to lifestyle and treatment plan.

Discharge Planning
- Additional learning/referral needs.

———————————

Information that appears in brackets has been added by the authors to clarify and enhance the use of nursing diagnoses.

Sample Nursing Outcomes & Interventions Classifications (NOC/NIC) (NIC)

NOC—Knowledge: [specify—42 choices]
NIC—Teaching: Individual

sedentary **Lifestyle**

Taxonomy II: Activity/Rest—Class 2 Activity/Exercise (00168)
[Diagnostic Division: Activity/Rest]
Submitted 2004

Definition: Reports a habit of life that is characterized by a low physical activity level

Related Factors

Lack of interest, motivation, or resources (time, money, companionship, facilities)
Lack of training for accomplishment of physical exercise
Deficient knowledge of health benefits of physical exercise

Defining Characteristics

Subjective
Verbalizes preference for activities low in physical activity

Objective
Chooses a daily routine lacking physical exercise
Demonstrates physical deconditioning

Desired Outcomes/Evaluation Criteria— Client Will:

- Verbalize understanding of importance of regular exercise to general well-being.
- Identify necessary precautions or safety concerns and self-monitoring techniques.
- Formulate realistic exercise program with gradual increase in activity.

Nursing Priority No. 1.
To assess precipitating/etiological factors:
- Identify conditions that may contribute to immobility or the onset and continuation of inactivity or sedentary lifestyle

---

Information that appears in brackets has been added by the authors to clarify and enhance the use of nursing diagnoses.

 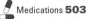

(e.g., obesity, depression, MS, arthritis, Parkinson's disease, surgery, hemiplegia or paraplegia, chronic pain, brain injury).

- Assess client's developmental level, motor skills, ease and capability of movement, posture, and gait.
- Note emotional and behavioral responses to problems associated with self- or condition-imposed sedentary lifestyle. **Feelings of frustration and powerlessness may impede attainment of goals.**
- Determine usual exercise and dietary habits, physical limitations, work environment, family dynamics, available resources.

Nursing Priority No. 2.
To motivate and stimulate client involvement:

- Establish therapeutic relationship acknowledging reality of situation and client's feelings. **Changing a lifelong habit can be difficult, and client may be feeling discouragement with body and hopelessness (i.e., unable to turn situation around into a positive experience).**
- Ascertain client's perception of current activity/exercise patterns, impact on life, and cultural expectations of client/others.
- Determine client's actual ability to participate in exercise or activities, noting attention span, physical limitations and tolerance, level of interest or desire, and safety needs. **Identifies barriers that need to be addressed.**
- Discuss motivation for change. **Concerns of SO(s) regarding threats to personal health and longevity, or acceptance by teen peers may be sufficient to cause client to initiate change; to sustain change, however, client must want to change for himself or herself.**
- Review necessity for, and benefits of, regular exercise. **Research confirms that exercise has benefits for the whole body (e.g., can boost energy, enhance coordination, reduce muscle deterioration, improve circulation, lower blood pressure, produce healthier skin and a toned body, prolong youthful appearance). Exercise has also been found to boost cardiac fitness in both conditioned and out-of-shape individuals.**
- Involve client, SO, parent, or caregiver in developing exercise plan and goals to meet individual needs, desires, and available resources.
- Introduce activities at client's current level of functioning, progressing to more complex activities, as tolerated.
- Recommend mix of age and gender appropriate activities or stimuli (e.g., movement classes, walking, hiking, jazzercise

Information that appears in brackets has been added by the authors to clarify and enhance the use of nursing diagnoses.

or other dance, swimming, biking, skating, bowling, golf, weight training). **Activities need to be personally meaningful for client to derive the most enjoyment and to sustain motivation to continue with program.**

 • Encourage change of scenery (indoors and out, where possible), and periodic changes in the personal environment when client is confined inside.

Nursing Priority No. 3.

To promote optimal level of function and prevent exercise failure:

• Assist with treatment of underlying condition impacting participation in activities **to maximize function within limitations of situation.**

• Collaborate with physical medicine specialist or occupational/physical therapist in providing active or passive range-of-motion exercises, isotonic muscle contractions. **Techniques such as gait training, strength training, and exercise to improve balance and coordination can be helpful in rehabilitating client.**

 • Schedule ample time to perform exercise activities balanced with adequate rest periods.

 • Provide for safety measures as indicated by individual situation, including environmental management/fall prevention. (Refer to ND risk for Falls.)

 • Reevaluate ability/commitment periodically. **Changes in strength/endurance signal readiness for progression of activities or possibly to decrease exercise if overly fatigued. Wavering commitment may require change in types of activities, addition of a workout buddy to reenergize involvement.**

 • Discuss discrepancies in planned and performed activities with client aware and unaware of observation. Suggest methods for dealing with identified problems. **May be necessary when client is using avoidance or controlling behavior, or is not aware of own abilities due to anxiety/fear.**

 • Review importance of adequate intake of fluids, especially during hot weather/strenuous activity.

Nursing Priority No. 4.

To promote wellness (Teaching/Discharge Considerations):

 • Review components of physical fitness: (1) muscle strength and endurance, (2) flexibility, (3) body composition (muscle mass, percentage of body fat), and (4) cardiovascular health.

Information that appears in brackets has been added by the authors to clarify and enhance the use of nursing diagnoses.

Fitness routines need to include all elements to attain maximum benefits and prevent deconditioning.

🏠 • Instruct in safety measures as individually indicated (e.g., warm-up and cool-down activities; taking pulse before, during, and after activity; wearing reflective clothing when jogging, reflectors on bicycle; locking wheelchair before transfers; judicious use of medications; supervision as indicated).

🏠 • Recommend keeping an activity or exercise log, including physical and psychological responses, changes in weight, endurance, body mass. **Provides visual evidence of progress or goal attainment and encouragement to continue with program.**

🏠 • Encourage client to involve self in exercise as part of wellness management for the whole person; encourage parents to set a positive example for children by participating in exercise and an active lifestyle.

🏠 • Identify community resources, charity activities, support groups. **Community walking or hiking trails, sports leagues, and so on, provide free or low-cost options. Activities such as 5K walks for charity, participation in Special Olympics, or age-related competitive games provide goals to work toward.** *Note:* **Some individuals may prefer solitary activities; however, most individuals enjoy supportive companionship when exercising.**

🏠 • Discuss alternatives for exercise program in changing circumstances (e.g., walking the mall during inclement weather, using exercise facilities at hotel when traveling, water aerobics at local swimming pool, joining a gym).

🏠 • Promote individual participation in community awareness of problem and discussion of solutions. **Physical inactivity (and associated diseases) is a major public health problem that affects huge numbers of people in all regions of the world. Recognizing the problem and future consequences may empower the global community to develop effective measures to promote physical activity and improve public health.**

🏠 • Introduce and promote established goals for increasing physical activity, such as Sports, Play, and Active Recreation for Kids (SPARK) and Physician-Based Assessment and Counseling for Exercise (PACE) **to address national concerns about obesity and major barriers to physical activity, such as time constraints, lack of training in physical activity or behavioral change methods, and lack of standard protocols.**

Information that appears in brackets has been added by the authors to clarify and enhance the use of nursing diagnoses.

Documentation Focus

Assessment/Reassessment
- Individual findings, including level of function and ability to participate in specific or desired activities.
- Motivation for change.

Planning
- Plan of care and who is involved in the planning.
- Teaching plan.

Implementation/Evaluation
- Responses to interventions, teaching, and actions performed.
- Attainment or progress toward desired outcome(s).
- Modifications to plan of care.

Discharge Planning
- Discharge and long-range needs, noting who is responsible for each action to be taken.
- Specific referrals made.
- Sources of, and maintenance for, assistive devices.

Sample Nursing Outcomes & Interventions Classifications (NOC/NIC) NIC

NOC—Knowledge: Prescribed Activity
NIC—Exercise Promotion

risk for impaired Liver Function

Taxonomy II: Nutrition—Class 4 Metabolism (0000178)
[Diagnostic Division: Food/Fluid]
Submitted 2006

Definition: At risk for a decrease in liver function that may compromise health

Risk Factors

Viral infection (e.g., hepatitis A, hepatitis B, hepatitis C, Epstein-Barr); HIV co-infection
Hepatotoxic medications (e.g., acetaminophen, statins)
Substance abuse (e.g., alcohol, cocaine)

Information that appears in brackets has been added by the authors to clarify and enhance the use of nursing diagnoses.

> **NOTE:** A risk diagnosis is not evidenced by signs and symptoms, as the problem has not occurred; rather, nursing interventions are directed at prevention.

Desired Outcomes/Evaluation Criteria—Client Will:

- Verbalize understanding of individual risk factors that contribute to possibility of liver damage/failure.
- Demonstrate behaviors, lifestyle changes to reduce risk factors and protect self from injury.
- Be free of signs of liver failure as evidenced by liver function studies within normal levels, and absence of jaundice, hepatic enlargement, or altered mental status.

Actions/Interventions

Nursing Priority No. 1.
To identify individual risk factors/needs:

- Determine presence of condition(s) as listed in Risk Factors, noting whether problem is acute (e.g., viral hepatitis, acetaminophen overdose) or chronic (e.g., alcoholic cirrhosis). **Influences choice of interventions.**
- Note if client works in high-risk occupation (e.g., performs tasks that involve contact with blood, blood-contaminated body fluids, other body fluids, or sharps/needles). **Carries high risk for exposure to hepatitis B and C.**
- Assess for exposure to contaminated food or poor sanitation practices by food service workers. **Poses risk for exposure to enteric viruses (hepatitis A and E).**

Nursing Priority No. 2.
To assist client to reduce or correct individual risk factors:

- Educate client on way(s) to prevent exposure **to reduce incidence of hepatitis B and C (HBV and HCV) infections/limit damage to liver.**
- Review results of laboratory tests (e.g., abnormal liver function studies, drug toxicity, HVB positive) and diagnostic studies **that indicate presence of hepatotoxic condition and need for medical treatment.**
- Assist with medical treatment of underlying condition **to support organ function and minimize liver damage.**

Information that appears in brackets has been added by the authors to clarify and enhance the use of nursing diagnoses.

Cultural Collaborative Community/Home Care

- Emphasize importance of responsible drinking or avoiding alcohol, when indicated, **to reduce incidence of cirrhosis or severity of liver damage/failure**.
- Encourage client with liver dysfunction to avoid fatty foods. Fat interferes with normal function of liver cells and can cause additional damage and permanent scarring to liver cells when they can no longer regenerate.
- Refer to nutritionist, as indicated, for dietary needs, including intake of proteins, vitamins, etc., to promote healing.
- Discuss safe use and concerns about client's medication regimen (e.g., acetaminophen; NSAIDs; herbal or vitamin supplements; phenobarbitol; cholesterol-lowering drugs, such as "statins"; some antibiotics [e.g., sulfonamides, INH]; certain cardiovascular drugs [e.g., amiodarone, hydralazine]; antidepressants [e.g., tricyclics]) **known to cause hepatotoxicity, either alone or in combination, or in overdose situation.**
- Identify signs/symptoms that warrant prompt notification of healthcare provider (e.g., increased abdominal girth; rapid weight loss or gain; increased peripheral edema; dyspnea, fever; blood in stool or urine; excess bleeding of any kind; jaundice). **Indicators of severe liver dysfunction, possible organ failure.**
- Refer to specialist or liver treatment center, as indicated. **May be beneficial for person with chronic liver disease when decompensating, or client with hepatitis and other coexisting disease condition (e.g., HIV), or intolerance to treatment due to side effects.**

Nursing Priority No. 3.
To promote wellness (Teaching/Discharge Considerations):

- Encourage client routinely taking acetaminophen for pain management to read labels, determine strength of medication, note safe number of doses over 24 hours, become familiar with "hidden" sources of acetaminophen (e.g., Nyquil, Vicodin), limit alcohol intake **to avoid/limit risk of liver damage.**
- Emphasize importance of hand hygiene and avoidance of fresh produce, use of bottled water and avoidance of raw meat and seafood (**if client is traveling to area where hepatitis A is endemic or food or waterborne illness is a risk**).
- Instruct in measures including protection from blood and other body fluids, sharps safety, safer sex practices, avoiding needle sharing, avoiding body tattoos or piercings **to prevent occupational and nonoccupational exposures to hepatitis.**

Information that appears in brackets has been added by the authors to clarify and enhance the use of nursing diagnoses.

- Discuss need and refer for vaccination, as indicated (e.g., healthcare and public safety worker, children under 18, international traveler, recreational drug user, men who have sexual relationships with other men, client with clotting disorders or liver disease, anyone sharing household with an infected person), **to prevent exposure and transmission of blood or body fluid hepatitis and limit risk of liver injury.**
- Discuss appropriateness of prophylactic immunizations. **Although the best way to protect against hepatitis B and C infections is to prevent exposure to viruses, postexposure prophylaxis (PEP) should be initiated promptly to prevent or limit severity of infection.**
- Provide information regarding availability of gamma globulin, immune serum globulin (ISG), HepB immunoglobulin (H-BIG), HepB vaccine (Recombivax HB, Engerix-B) through health department or family physician.
- Stress necessity of follow-up care (in client with chronic liver disease) and adherence to therapeutic regimen.
- Refer to community resources, drug and alcohol treatment program, as indicated.

Documentation Focus

Assessment/Reassessment
- Assessment findings, including individual risk factors.
- Results of laboratory tests and diagnostic studies.

Planning
- Plan of care and who is involved in planning.
- Teaching plan.

Implementation/Evaluation
- Response to interventions, teaching, and actions performed.
- Attainment or progress toward desired outcome(s).
- Modifications to plan of care.

Discharge Planning
- Long-term needs, plan for follow-up, and who is responsible for actions to be taken.
- Specific referrals made.

Information that appears in brackets has been added by the authors to clarify and enhance the use of nursing diagnoses.

Sample Nursing Outcomes & Interventions Classifications (NOC/NIC) NIC

NOC—Treatment Behavior: Illness or Injury
NIC—Substance Use Treatment

---

risk for Loneliness

Taxonomy II: Self-Perception—Class 1 Self-Concept (00054)
[Diagnostic Division: Social Interaction]
Submitted 1994

Definition: At risk for experiencing discomfort associated with a desire or need for more contact with others

---

Risk Factors

Affectional deprivation
Physical or social isolation
Cathectic deprivation
Problems of attachment for infants or adolescents
Chaotic family relationships

NOTE: A risk diagnosis is not evidenced by signs and symptoms, as the problem has not occurred; rather, nursing interventions are directed at prevention.

Desired Outcomes/Evaluation Criteria— Client Will:

• Identify individual difficulties and ways to address them.
• Engage in social activities.
• Report involvement in interactions and relationship client views as meaningful.

Parent/Caregiver Will:

• Provide infant with consistent and loving caregiving.
• Participate in programs for adolescents and families.

Information that appears in brackets has been added by the authors to clarify and enhance the use of nursing diagnoses.

 Diagnostic Studies   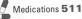 Pediatric/Geriatric/Lifespan   Medications **511**

Actions/Interventions

Nursing Priority No. 1.

To identify causative/precipitating factors:

- Differentiate between ordinary loneliness and a state or constant sense of dysphoria. **Influences type of and intensity of interventions.**
- Note client's age and duration of problem; that is, situational (such as leaving home for college) or chronic. **Adolescents may experience lonely feelings related to the changes that are happening as they become adults. Elderly individuals incur multiple losses associated with aging, loss of spouse, decline in physical health, and changes in roles that intensify feelings of loneliness.**
- Determine degree of distress, tension, anxiety, restlessness present. Note history of frequent illnesses, accidents, crises. **Most people feel lonely at some time in their lives related to situational occurrences that engender these feelings, which are normal in the circumstances.**
- Note presence and proximity of family, SO(s), and whether they are helpful or not.
- Discuss with client whether there is a person or persons in his or her life who can be trustworthy and who will listen with empathy to the feelings that are expressed.
- Determine how individual perceives and deals with solitude. **A person may feel alone in a crowd or may choose to be alone and enjoy the quiet.**
- Review issues of separation from parents as a child, loss of SO(s)/spouse.
- Assess sleep and appetite disturbances, ability to concentrate. **Indicators of distress related to feelings of loneliness and low self-esteem.**
- Note expressions of "yearning" for an emotional partnership.

Nursing Priority No. 2.

To assist client to identify feelings and situations in which he or she experiences loneliness:

- Establish nurse-client relationship. **Client may feel free to talk about feelings in context of an empathetic relationship.**
- Discuss individual concerns about feelings of loneliness and relationship between loneliness and lack of SO(s). Note desire and willingness to change situation. **Motivation can impede—or facilitate—achieving desired outcomes.**

Information that appears in brackets has been added by the authors to clarify and enhance the use of nursing diagnoses.

 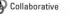 🌐 Cultural 🐾 Collaborative 🏠 Community/Home Care

- Support expression of negative perceptions of others and note whether client agrees. **Provides opportunity for client to clarify reality of situation, recognize own denial.**
- Accept client's expressions of loneliness as a primary condition and not necessarily as a symptom of some underlying condition.

Nursing Priority No. 3.

To assist client to become involved:

- Discuss reality versus perceptions of situation.
- Discuss importance of emotional bonding (attachment) between infants or young children and parents/caregivers when appropriate.
- Involve in classes, such as assertiveness, language and communication, social skills, **to address individual needs and potential for enhanced socialization.**
- Role-play situations **to develop interpersonal skills.**
- Discuss positive health habits, including personal hygiene, exercise activity of client's choosing.
- Identify individual strengths, areas of interest **that provide opportunities for involvement with others.**
- Encourage attendance at support group activities to meet individual needs (e.g., therapy, separation/grief, religious).
- Help client establish plan for progressive involvement, beginning with a simple activity (e.g., call an old friend, speak to a neighbor) and leading to more complicated interactions and activities.
- Provide opportunities for interactions in a supportive environment (e.g., have client accompanied, as in a "buddy system") during initial attempts to socialize. **Helps reduce stress, provides positive reinforcement, and facilitates successful outcome.**

Nursing Priority No. 4.

To promote wellness (Teaching/Discharge Considerations):

- Let client know that loneliness can be overcome. **It is up to the individual to build self-esteem and learn to feel good about self.**
- Encourage involvement in special-interest groups (e.g., computers, gardening club, reading circles, bird-watchers); charitable services (e.g., serving in a soup kitchen, youth groups, animal shelter).
- Suggest volunteering for church committee or choir; attending community events with friends and family; becoming

---

Information that appears in brackets has been added by the authors to clarify and enhance the use of nursing diagnoses.

 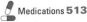

involved in political issues or campaigns; enrolling in classes at local college or continuing education programs.

• Refer to appropriate counselors for help with relationships and so on.
• Refer to NDs Hopelessness; Anxiety; Social Isolation.

Documentation Focus

Assessment/Reassessment
• Assessment findings, including client's perception of problem, availability of resources and support systems.
• Client's desire and commitment to change.

Planning
• Plan of care and who is involved in planning.
• Teaching plan.

Implementation/Evaluation
• Response to interventions, teaching, and actions performed.
• Attainment or progress toward desired outcome(s).
• Modifications to plan of care.

Discharge Planning
• Long-term needs, plan for follow-up, and who is responsible for actions to be taken.
• Specific referrals made.

Sample Nursing Outcomes & Interventions Classifications (NOC/NIC) **NIC**

NOC—Loneliness
NIC—Socialization Enhancement

---

risk for disturbed **Maternal/Fetal Dyad**

Taxonomy II: Sexuality—Class 3 Reproduction (00209)
[Diagnostic Division: Safety]
Submitted 2008

Definition: At risk for disruption of the symbiotic maternal/fetal dyad as a result of comorbid or pregnancy-related complications

---

Information that appears in brackets has been added by the authors to clarify and enhance the use of nursing diagnoses.

🌐 Cultural 🅐 Collaborative 🏠 Community/Home Care

Related Factors

Complications of pregnancy (e.g., premature rupture of membranes, placenta previa or abruption, late prenatal care, multiple gestation)

Compromised O_2 transport (e.g., anemia, asthma, hypertension, seizures, premature labor, hemorrhage; [sickle cell anemia])

Impaired glucose metabolism (e.g., diabetes, steroid use)

Physical abuse

Substance abuse (e.g., tobacco, alcohol, drugs)

Treatment-related side effects (e.g., medications, surgery, chemotherapy)

> **NOTE:** A risk diagnosis is not evidenced by signs and symptoms, as the problem has not occurred; rather, nursing interventions are directed at prevention.

Desired Outcomes/Evaluation Criteria—Client Will: (Include Specific Time Frame)

- Verbalize understanding of individual risk factors or condition(s) that may impact pregnancy.
- Engage in necessary alterations in lifestyle and daily activities to manage risks.
- Participate in screening procedures as indicated.
- Identify signs/symptoms requiring medical evaluation or intervention.
- Display fetal growth within normal limits (WNL) and carry pregnancy to term.

Actions/Interventions

Nursing Priority No. 1.

To identify individual risk/contributing factors:

- Review history of previous pregnancies for presence of complications, such as premature rupture of membranes (PROM), placenta previa, miscarriage or pregnancy losses due to premature dilation of the cervix, preterm labor or deliveries, previous birth defects, hyperemesis gravidarum, or repeated urinary tract or vaginal infections.
- Obtain history about prenatal screening and amount and timing of care. **Lack of prenatal care can place both mother and fetus at risk.**

Information that appears in brackets has been added by the authors to clarify and enhance the use of nursing diagnoses.

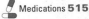

- Note conditions potentiating vascular changes/reduced placental circulation (e.g., diabetes, pregnancy-induced hypertension [PIH], cardiac problems, smoking) or those that alter oxygen-carrying capacity (e.g., asthma, anemia, Rh incompatibility, hemorrhage). **Extent of maternal vascular involvement and reduction of oxygen-carrying capacity have a direct influence on uteroplacental circulation and gas exchange.**
- Note maternal age. **Maternal age above 35 years is associated with increased risk of spontaneous abortions, preterm delivery or stillbirths, fetal chromosomal abnormalities and malformations, and IUGR. In pregnant adolescents (younger than 15), the most common high-risk conditions include PIH, anemia, labor dysfunction, cephalopelvic disproportion and low birth weight, and preterm delivery.**
- Ascertain current/past dietary patterns and practices. **Client may be malnourished, obese, or underweight (weight <100 lb or >200 lb).**
- Assess for severe, unremitting nausea and vomiting, especially when it persists after the first trimester (hyperemesis gravidarum).
- Note history of exposure to teratogenic agents, infectious diseases (e.g., tuberculosis, influenza, measles); high-risk occupations; exposure to toxic substances such as lead, organic solvents, carbon monoxide; use of certain OTC or prescription medications; substance use or abuse (including illicit drugs and alcohol).
- Identify family or cultural influences in pregnancy. **Family history may include multiple births or congenital diseases, or generational abuse or lack of support or finances. Cultural background may identify health risks associated with nationality (e.g., sickle cell in people of African descent or Tay-Sachs disease in people of eastern European Jewish ancestry); or religious practices (e.g., exclusion of dairy products, or no maternal immunizations for rubella) which can impact health of mother or fetal development.**
- Review laboratory studies. **Low hemoglobin suggests anemia, which is associated with hypoxia. Blood type and Rh group may reveal incompatibility risks; elevated serum glucose may be seen in gestational diabetes mellitus (GDM); elevated liver function studies suggest hypertensive liver involvement; drop in platelet count may be associated with PIH and HELLP (hemolysis, elevated liver enzymes, and low platelet) syndrome. Nutritional studies**

Information that appears in brackets has been added by the authors to clarify and enhance the use of nursing diagnoses.

Cultural   Collaborative   Community/Home Care

may reveal decreased levels of serum proteins, electrolytes, minerals, or vitamins essential to maternal health and fetal development.

• Review vaginal, cervical, or rectal cultures and serology results. **May reveal presence of sexually transmitted diseases (STDs), or identify active or carrier state of hepatitis, HIV, AIDS.**

• Assist in screening for and identifying genetic or chromosomal disorders. **Disorders such as phenylketonuria (PKU) or sickle cell disease necessitate special treatment to prevent negative effects on fetal growth.**

• Investigate current home situation. **May have history of unstable relationship, or inadequate/lack of housing that affects safety as well as general well-being.**

Nursing Priority No. 2.
To monitor maternal/fetal status:

• Weigh client and compare current weight with pregravid weight. Have client record weight between visits. **Underweight clients are at risk for anemia, inadequate protein and calorie intake, vitamin or mineral deficiencies, and PIH. Overweight women are at increased risk for development of PIH, GDM, and hyperinsulinemia of the fetus.**

• Assess fetal heart rate (FHR), noting rate and regularity. Have client monitor fetal movement daily as indicated. Tachycardia in a term infant may indicate a compensatory mechanism to reduced oxygen levels and/or presence of sepsis. A reduction in fetal activity occurs before bradycardia.

• Test urine for presence of ketones. **Indicates inadequate glucose utilization and breakdown of fats for metabolic processes.**

• Provide information and assist with procedures as indicated, for example:

Amniocentesis: **May be performed for genetic purposes or to assess fetal lung maturity. Spectrophotometric analysis of the fluid may be done to detect bilirubin after 26 weeks gestation.**

Ultrasonography: **Assesses gestational age of fetus, detects presence of multiples, or fetal abnormalities. Locates placenta (and amniotic fluid pockets before amniocentesis, if performed), monitors clients at risk for reduced or inadequate placental perfusion (such as adolescents, clients older than 35 years, and clients with diabetes, PIH, cardiac or kidney disease, anemia, or respiratory disorders).**

Information that appears in brackets has been added by the authors to clarify and enhance the use of nursing diagnoses.

Biophysical profile (BPP): **Assesses fetal well-being through ultrasound evaluation to measure amniotic fluid index (AFI), FHR, nonstress test (NST) reactivity, fetal breathing movement, body movement (large limbs), and muscle tone (flexion and extension).**

Contraction stress test (CST): **A positive CST with late decelerations indicates a high-risk client and fetus with possible reduced uteroplacental reserves.**

- Screen for abuse during pregnancy. **Prenatal abuse is correlated with a low maternal weight gain, infections, anemia, delay in seeking prenatal care until the third trimester, and preterm delivery.**
- Screen for preterm uterine contractions, which may or may not be accompanied by cervical dilatation.

Nursing Priority No. 3.

To correct/improve maternal/fetal well-being:

- Instruct client in reportable symptoms, and monitor for unusual symptoms at each prenatal visit (e.g., vaginal bleeding, headache along with blurred vision and ankle swelling, faintness, persistent vomiting). **Provides opportunity for early intervention in event of developing complications.**
- Assist in treatment of underlying medical condition(s) that have potential for causing maternal or fetal harm.
- Assess perceived impact of complication on client and family members. Encourage verbalization of concerns. **Family stress is amplified in a high-risk pregnancy, where concerns focus on the health of both the client and the fetus.**
- Facilitate positive adaptation to situation, through active-listening, acceptance, and problem solving. **Helps in successful accomplishment of the psychological tasks of pregnancy.**
- Develop dietary plan with client that provides necessary nutrients (calories, protein, vitamins and minerals).
- Promote fluid intake of at least 2 quarts of noncaffeinated fluid per day **to prevent dehydration which may compromise optimal uterine and placental functioning and increase uterine irritability.**
- Encourage client to participate in individually appropriate adaptations and self-care techniques, such as scheduling rest periods two to three times a day, avoiding overexertion or heavy lifting, or maintaining contact with family and daily life if bedrest is required.
- Review medication regimen. **Prepregnancy treatment for chronic conditions may require alteration for maternal and fetal safety.**

Information that appears in brackets has been added by the authors to clarify and enhance the use of nursing diagnoses.

 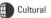 Cultural Collaborative Community/Home Care

- Review availability and use of resources.
- Administer Rh immunoglobulin (RhIgG) to client at 28 weeks gestation in Rh-negative clients with Rh-positive partners, or following amniocentesis, if indicated.
- Encourage modified or complete bedrest as indicated. **Activity level may need modification, depending on symptoms of uterine activity, cervical changes, or bleeding. Side-lying position increases renal and placental perfusion, which is effective in preventing supine hypotensive syndrome.**
- Provide supplemental oxygen as appropriate. **Increases the oxygen available for fetal uptake, especially in presence of severe anemia or sickle cell crisis.**
- Prepare for and assist with intrauterine fetal exchange transfusion as indicated by titers (Kleihauer-Betke test).

Nursing Priority No. 4.
To promote wellness (Teaching/Discharge Considerations):

- Emphasize the normalcy of pregnancy, focus on pregnancy milestones, "countdown to birth." **Avoids or limits perception of "sick role"; promotes sense of hope that modifications or restrictions serve a worthwhile purpose.**
- Discuss implications of preexisting condition and possible impact on pregnancy. **Pregnancy may have no effect, or may reduce or exacerbate severity of symptoms of chronic conditions.**
- Provide information about risks of weight reduction during pregnancy and about nourishment needs of client and fetus. **Prenatal calorie restriction and resultant weight loss may result in nutrient deficiency or ketonemia, with negative effects on fetal CNS and possible IUGR.**
- Encourage smoking cessation, refer to community program or support group as indicated. **Severe adverse effects of smoking on the fetus may be reduced if mother quits smoking early in pregnancy, and pregnancy outcomes can still be improved if mother stops smoking as late as 32 weeks gestation.**
- Help client/couple plan restructuring of roles and activities necessitated by complication of pregnancy.
- Have client demonstrate new behaviors and therapeutic techniques. **During pregnancy, control of condition may require specific modified or new behaviors.**
- Recommend client assess uterine tone and contractions for 1 hour, once or twice a day as indicated **to monitor uterine irritability or early indication of premature labor.**

Information that appears in brackets has been added by the authors to clarify and enhance the use of nursing diagnoses.

- Encourage close monitoring of blood glucose levels, as appropriate. **Type I or insulin-dependent diabetes mellitus (IDDM) clients generally need to check blood glucose levels 4 to 12 times/day because insulin needs may increase two to three times above pregravid baseline.**
- Demonstrate technique and specific equipment used when FHR monitoring is done in the home setting.
- Identify danger signals requiring immediate notification of healthcare provider (e.g., PROM, preterm labor, vaginal drainage or bleeding).
- Review availability and use of resources. **Presence or absence of supportive resources can make the difference for the client and family in being able to manage the situation.**
- Refer to community service agencies (e.g., visiting nurse, social service) or resources, such as Sidelines. **Community supports may be needed for ongoing assessment of medical problem, family status, coping behaviors, and financial stressors.** *Note:* **Sidelines is a national telephone support group for pregnant women on bedrest.**
- Refer for counseling if family does not sustain positive coping and growth. **May be necessary to promote growth and to prevent family disintegration.**

Documentation Focus

Assessment/Reassessment
- Assessment findings including weight, signs of pregnancy, safety concerns.
- Specific risk factors, comorbidities and treatment regimen.
- Results of screening laboratory tests and diagnostic studies.
- Participation in prenatal care.
- Cultural beliefs and practices.

Planning
- Plan of care, specific interventions, and who is involved in the planning.
- Community resources for equipment and supplies.
- Specific referrals made.
- Teaching plan.

Implementation/Evaluation
- Client/fetal response to treatment and actions performed.
- Client's response to teaching provided.

Information that appears in brackets has been added by the authors to clarify and enhance the use of nursing diagnoses.

⊕ Cultural   Ⓐ Collaborative   🏠 Community/Home Care

- Attainment or progress toward desired outcome(s).
- Modifications to plan of care.

Sample Nursing Outcomes & Interventions Classifications (NOC/NIC) NIC

NOC—Prenatal Health Behavior
NIC—High-Risk Pregnancy Care

---

impaired Memory

Taxonomy II: Perception/Cognition—Class 4 Cognition (00131)
[Diagnostic Division: Neurosensory]
Submitted 1994

Definition: Inability to remember or recall bits of information or behavioral skills [Impaired memory may be attributed to physiopathological or situational causes that are either temporary or permanent.]

Related Factors

Hypoxia; anemia
Fluid and electrolyte imbalance; decreased cardiac output
Neurological disturbances [e.g., brain injury, concussion]
Excessive environmental disturbances; [manic state, fugue, traumatic event]
Substance use or abuse; effects of medications
Age

Defining Characteristics

Subjective
Reported experience of forgetting
Inability to recall events or factual information [or familiar persons, places, items]

Objective
Observed experience of forgetting
Inability to determine if a behavior was performed
Inability to learn or retain new skills and information
Inability to perform a previously learned skill
Forgets to perform a behavior at a scheduled time

Information that appears in brackets has been added by the authors to clarify and enhance the use of nursing diagnoses.

Desired Outcomes/Evaluation Criteria—Client Will:

- Verbalize awareness of memory problems.
- Establish methods to help in remembering essential things when possible.
- Accept limitations of condition and use resources effectively.

Actions/Interventions

Nursing Priority No. 1.

To assess causative factor(s)/degree of impairment:

- Determine physical, biochemical, and environmental factors (e.g, systemic infections; brain injury; pulmonary disease with hypoxia; use of multiple medications; exposure to toxic substances; use or abuse of alcohol or other drugs; traumatic event; removal from known environment) that may be associated with confusion and loss of memory.
- Note client's age and potential for depression. **Depressive disorders affecting memory and concentration are particularly prevalent in older adults; however, impairments can occur in depressed persons of any age.**
- Collaborate with medical and psychiatric providers in evaluating orientation, attention span, ability to follow directions, send/receive communication, appropriateness of response **to determine presence and/or severity of impairment.**
- Perform or review results of cognitive testing (e.g., Blessed Information-Memory-Concentration [BIMC] test, Mini-Mental Status Examination [MMSE]), **to complete picture of client's overall condition and prognosis.**
- Evaluate skill proficiency levels, including self-care activities and driving ability.
- Ascertain how client/family view the problem (e.g., practical problems of forgetting and/or role and responsibility impairments related to loss of memory and concentration) **to determine significance and impact of problem.**

Nursing Priority No. 2.

To maximize level of function:

- Assist with treatment of underlying conditions (e.g., electrolyte imbalances, reaction to medications, drug intoxication) **where treatment can improve memory processes.**

Information that appears in brackets has been added by the authors to clarify and enhance the use of nursing diagnoses.

🌐 Cultural Collaborative 🏠 Community/Home Care

- Orient/reorient client as needed. Introduce self with each client contact **to meet client's safety and comfort needs.** (Refer to NDs acute/chronic Confusion, for additional interventions.)
- Implement appropriate memory-retraining techniques (e.g., keeping calendars, writing lists, memory cue games, mnemonic devices, using computers).
- Assist with and instruct client and family in associate-learning tasks, such as practice sessions recalling personal information, reminiscing, locating a geographic location (Stimulation Therapy).
- Encourage ventilation of feelings of frustration, helplessness, and so on. Refocus attention to areas of control and progress **to diminish feelings of powerlessness/hopelessness.**
- Provide for and emphasize importance of pacing learning activities and getting sufficient rest **to avoid fatigue that may further impair cognitive abilities.**
- Monitor client's behavior and assist in use of stress-management techniques (e.g., music therapy, reading, television, games, socialization) **to reduce frustration and enhance enjoyment of life.**
- Structure teaching methods and interventions to client's level of functioning and/or potential for improvement.
- Determine client's response to and effects of medications prescribed to improve attention, concentration, memory processes and to lift spirits or modify emotional responses. **Medication for cognitive enhancement can be effective, but benefits need to be weighed against whether quality of life is improved after side effects and cost of drugs are considered.**

Nursing Priority No. 3.
To promote wellness (Teaching/Discharge Considerations):

- Assist client/SO(s) to establish compensation strategies (e.g., menu planning with a shopping list, timely completion of tasks on a daily planner, checklists at the front door to ascertain that lights and stove are off before leaving) **to improve functional lifestyle and safety.** (Refer to NDs acute/chronic Confusion for additional interventions.)
- Refer for follow-up with counselors, rehabilitation programs, job coaches, social or financial support systems **to help deal with persistent or difficult problems.**

Information that appears in brackets has been added by the authors to clarify and enhance the use of nursing diagnoses.

🏠 • Assist client to deal with functional limitations (such as loss of driving privileges) and identify resources **to meet individual needs, maximizing independence.**

Documentation Focus

Assessment/Reassessment
- Individual findings, testing results, and perceptions of significance of problem.
- Actual impact on lifestyle and independence.

Planning
- Plan of care and who is involved in planning process.
- Teaching plan.

Implementation/Evaluation
- Responses to interventions, teaching, and actions performed.
- Attainment or progress toward desired outcome(s).
- Modifications to plan of care.

Discharge Planning
- Long-term needs and who is responsible for actions to be taken.
- Specific referrals made.

Sample Nursing Outcomes & Interventions Classifications (NOC/NIC) [NIC]

NOC—Memory
NIC—Memory Training

---

impaired bed **Mobility**

Taxonomy II: Activity/Rest—Class 2 Activity/Exercise (00091)
[Diagnostic Division: Safety]
Submitted 1998; Revised 2006

Definition: Limitation of independent movement from one bed position to another

---

Related Factors

Neuromuscular or musculoskeletal impairment
Insufficient muscle strength; deconditioning; obesity

Information that appears in brackets has been added by the authors to clarify and enhance the use of nursing diagnoses.

Environmental constraints (i.e., bed size and type, treatment equipment, restraints)

Pain; sedating medications

Deficient knowledge

Cognitive impairment

Defining Characteristics

Subjective
[Reported difficulty performing activities]

Objective
Impaired ability to: turn side to side; move from supine to sitting, sitting to supine; "scoot" or reposition self in bed; move from supine to prone, prone to supine; move from supine to long-sitting, long-sitting to supine

Desired Outcomes/Evaluation Criteria— Client/Caregiver Will:

- Verbalize willingness to participate in repositioning program.
- Verbalize understanding of situation and risk factors, individual therapeutic regimen, and safety measures.
- Demonstrate techniques and behaviors that enable safe repositioning.
- Maintain position of function and skin integrity as evidenced by absence of contractures, footdrop, decubitus, and so forth.
- Maintain or increase strength and function of affected and/or compensatory body part.

Actions/Interventions

Nursing Priority No. 1.
To identify causative/contributing factors:

- Determine diagnoses that contribute to immobility (e.g., MS, arthritis, Parkinson's disease, hemi-/para-/tetraplegia, fractures, multiple trauma, burns, head injury, depression, dementia).
- Note individual risk factors and current situation, such as surgery, casts, amputation, traction, pain, age, general weakness or debilitation.
- Determine degree of perceptual or cognitive impairment and/or ability to follow directions.

Information that appears in brackets has been added by the authors to clarify and enhance the use of nursing diagnoses.

 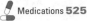

Nursing Priority No. 2.

To assess functional ability:

- Determine functional level classification 1 to 4 (1 = requires use of equipment or device, 2 = requires help from another person for assistance, 3 = requires help from another person and equipment device, 4 = dependent, does not participate in activity).
- Note cognitive, emotional, or behavioral conditions or concerns impacting mobility.
- Note presence of complications related to immobility. (Refer to ND Disuse Syndrome.)

Nursing Priority No. 3.

To promote optimal level of function and prevent complications:

- Ascertain that dependent client is placed in best bed for situation (e.g., correct size, support surface, and mobility functions) **to promote mobility and enhance environmental safety.**
- Turn dependent client frequently, utilizing bed and mattress positioning settings to assist movements; reposition in good body alignment, using appropriate supports.
- Instruct client and caregivers in methods of moving client relative to specific situations and mobility needs.
- Observe skin for reddened areas or shearing injury. Provide appropriate pressure relief and surface support mattress **to reduce friction, maintain safe skin and tissue pressures, and wick away moisture**. Provide regular skin care, as appropriate.
- Assist on and off bedpan and into sitting position (or use cardioposition bed or foot-egress bed) **to facilitate elimination.**
- Administer medication prior to activity as needed for pain relief **to permit maximal effort and involvement in activity.**
- Observe for change in strength to do more or less self-care **to adjust care as indicated.**
- Assist with activities of hygiene, toileting, feeding, as indicated.
- Provide diversional activities, as appropriate.
- Ensure telephone and call bell is within reach **to promote safety and timely response**.
- Provide individually appropriate methods to communicate adequately with client.

Information that appears in brackets has been added by the authors to clarify and enhance the use of nursing diagnoses.

- Provide extremity protection (padding, exercises, etc.). (Refer to NDs impaired Skin Integrity; risk for Peripheral Neurovascular Dysfunction, for additional interventions.)
- Include physical and occupational therapists and rehabilitation providers in creating movement program and identifying assistive devices.

Nursing Priority No. 4.
To promote wellness (Teaching/Discharge Considerations):
- Involve client/SO(s) in determining activity schedule. **Promotes commitment to plan, maximizing outcomes.**
- Encourage continuation of exercises **to maintain and enhance gains in strength and muscle control.**
- Obtain, or identify sources for, assistive devices. Demonstrate safe use and proper maintenance.

Documentation Focus

Assessment/Reassessment
- Individual findings, including level of function, ability to participate in specific or desired activities.

Planning
- Plan of care and who is involved in the planning.

Implementation/Evaluation
- Responses to interventions, teaching, and actions performed.
- Attainment or progress toward desired outcome(s).
- Modification to plan of care.

Discharge Planning
- Discharge and long-term needs, noting who is responsible for each action to be taken.
- Specific referrals made.
- Sources for, and maintenance of, assistive devices.

Sample Nursing Outcomes & Interventions Classifications (NOC/NIC) [NIC]

NOC—Body Position: Self-Initiated
NIC—Bed Rest Care

Information that appears in brackets has been added by the authors to clarify and enhance the use of nursing diagnoses.

impaired physical **Mobility**

Taxonomy II: Activity/Rest—Class 2 Activity/Exercise
  (00085)
[Diagnostic Division: Safety]
Submitted 1973; Nursing Diagnosis Extension and
  Classification (NDEC) Revision 1998

Definition: Limitation in independent, purposeful physical movement of the body or of one or more extremities

Related Factors

Sedentary lifestyle; activity intolerance; disuse; deconditioning; decreased endurance; limited cardiovascular endurance

Decreased muscle strength, control, or mass; joint stiffness; contractures; loss of integrity of bone structures

Pain; discomfort

Neuromuscular or musculoskeletal impairment

Sensoriperceptual or cognitive impairment; developmental delay

Depressive mood state; anxiety

Malnutrition; altered cellular metabolism; body mass index above 75th age-appropriate percentile

Deficient knowledge regarding value of physical activity; cultural beliefs regarding age-appropriate activity; lack of environmental supports (e.g., physical or social)

Prescribed movement restrictions; medications

Reluctance to initiate movement

Defining Characteristics

Subjective

Report of pain or discomfort on movement; unwillingness to move

Objective

Limited range of motion; limited ability to perform gross or fine motor skills; difficulty turning

Slowed movement; uncoordinated or jerky movements; movement-induced tremor; decreased [slower] reaction time

Postural instability; gait changes

Engages in substitutions for movement (e.g., increased attention to other's activity, controlling behavior, focus on pre-illness disability/activity)

Information that appears in brackets has been added by the authors to clarify and enhance the use of nursing diagnoses.

Cultural Collaborative Community/Home Care

Suggested Functional Level Classification:

0—Completely independent
1—Requires use of equipment or device
2—Requires help from another person for assistance, supervision, or teaching
3—Requires help from another person and equipment device
4—Dependent, does not participate in activity

Desired Outcomes/Evaluation Criteria— Client Will:

- Verbalize understanding of situation and individual treatment regimen and safety measures.
- Demonstrate techniques or behaviors that enable resumption of activities.
- Participate in ADLs and desired activities.
- Maintain position of function and skin integrity as evidenced by absence of contractures, footdrop, decubitus, and so forth.
- Maintain or increase strength and function of affected and/or compensatory body part.

Actions/Interventions

Nursing Priority No. 1.

To identify causative/contributing factors:

- Determine diagnosis that contributes to immobility (e.g., MS, arthritis, Parkinson's disease, hemi- or paraplegia, depression).
- Note situations such as surgery, fractures, amputation, tubings (chest, catheter, etc.) **that may restrict movement.**
- Assess degree of pain, listening to client's description.
- Ascertain client's perception of activity and exercise needs.
- Note decreased motor agility or essential tremor related to age.
- Determine degree of perceptual or cognitive impairment and ability to follow directions.
- Assess nutritional status and client's report of energy level.

Nursing Priority No. 2.

To assess functional ability:

- Determine degree of immobility in relation to previously suggested scale.
- Observe movement when client is unaware of observation **to note any incongruencies with reports of abilities.**

Information that appears in brackets has been added by the authors to clarify and enhance the use of nursing diagnoses.

- Note emotional/behavioral responses to problems of immobility. **Feelings of frustration or powerlessness may impede attainment of goals.**
- Determine presence of complications related to immobility (e.g., pneumonia, elimination problems, contractures, decubitus, anxiety). (Refer to ND risk for Disuse Syndrome.)

Nursing Priority No. 3.

To promote optimal level of function and prevent complications:

- Assist or have client reposition self on a regular schedule as dictated by individual situation (including frequent shifting of weight when client is wheelchair bound).
- Instruct in use of siderails, overhead trapeze, roller pads **for position changes and transfers.**
- Support affected body parts or joints using pillows, rolls, foot supports or shoes, air mattress, water bed, and so forth **to maintain position of function and reduce risk of pressure ulcers.**
- Assist with treatment of underlying condition causing pain and/or dysfunction.
- Administer medications prior to activity as needed for pain relief **to permit maximal effort and involvement in activity.**
- Provide regular skin care to include pressure area management.
- Schedule activities with adequate rest periods during the day **to reduce fatigue.**
- Encourage participation in self-care; occupational, diversional, or recreational activities. **Enhances self-concept and sense of independence.**
- Provide client with ample time to perform mobility-related tasks.
- Identify energy-conserving techniques for ADLs. **Limits fatigue, maximizing participation.**
- Discuss discrepancies in movement when client aware and unaware of observation, and methods for dealing with identified problems.
- Provide for safety measures as indicated by individual situation, including environmental management and fall prevention.
- Consult with physical or occupational therapist, as indicated, **to develop individual exercise and mobility program, and identify appropriate mobility devices.**

Information that appears in brackets has been added by the authors to clarify and enhance the use of nursing diagnoses.

 Cultural 🐾 Collaborative 🏠 Community/Home Care

- Encourage adequate intake of fluids and nutritious foods. **Promotes well-being and maximizes energy production.**

Nursing Priority No. 4.
To promote wellness (Teaching/Discharge Considerations):

- Encourage client's/SO's involvement in decision making as much as possible. **Enhances commitment to plan, optimizing outcomes.**
- Review safety measures as individually indicated (e.g., use of heating pads, locking wheelchair before transfers, removal or securing of scatter/area rugs).
- Involve client and SO(s) in care, assisting them to learn ways of managing problems of immobility.
- Demonstrate use of standing aids and mobility devices (e.g., walkers, strollers, scooters, braces, prosthetics), and have client/care provider demonstrate knowledge about, and safe use of device. Identify appropriate resources for obtaining and maintaining appliances and equipment. **Promotes independence and enhances safety.**
- Review individual dietary needs. Identify appropriate vitamin or herbal supplements.

Documentation Focus

Assessment/Reassessment
- Individual findings, including level of function, ability to participate in specific or desired activities.

Planning
- Plan of care and who is involved in the planning.
- Teaching plan.

Implementation/Evaluation
- Responses to interventions, teaching, and actions performed.
- Attainment or progress toward desired outcome(s).
- Modifications to plan of care.

Discharge Planning
- Discharge and long-term needs, noting who is responsible for each action to be taken.
- Specific referrals made.
- Sources for, and maintenance of, assistive devices.

Information that appears in brackets has been added by the authors to clarify and enhance the use of nursing diagnoses.

Sample Nursing Outcomes & Interventions Classifications (NOC/NIC) NIC

NOC—Mobility Level
NIC—Exercise Therapy: [specify]

impaired wheelchair Mobility

Taxonomy II: Activity/Rest—Class 2 Activity/Exercise (00089)
[Diagnostic Division: Safety]
Submitted 1998; Revised 2006

Definition: Limitation of independent operation of wheelchair within environment

Related Factors

Neuromuscular or musculoskeletal impairments (e.g., contractures)
Insufficient muscle strength; limited endurance; deconditioning; obesity
Impaired vision
Pain
Depressed mood; cognitive impairment
Deficient knowledge
Environmental constraints (e.g., stairs, inclines, uneven surfaces, unsafe obstacles, distances, lack of assistive devices or persons, wheelchair type)

Defining Characteristics

Impaired ability to operate manual or power wheelchair on even or uneven surface, an incline or decline, or curbs

NOTE: Specify level of independence using a standardized functional scale. [Refer to ND impaired physical Mobility.]

Desired Outcomes/Evaluation Criteria—Client Will:

• Move safely within environment, maximizing independence.
• Identify and use resources appropriately.

Information that appears in brackets has been added by the authors to clarify and enhance the use of nursing diagnoses.

Cultural   Collaborative   Community/Home Care

Caregiver Will:

• Provide safe mobility within environment and community.

Actions/Interventions

Nursing Priority No. 1.

To identify causative/contributing factors:

• Determine diagnosis that contributes to immobility (e.g., ALS, SCI, spastic cerebral palsy, brain injury) and client's functional level and individual abilities.
• Identify factors in environments frequented by the client that contribute to inaccessibility (e.g., uneven floors or surfaces, lack of ramps, steep incline or decline, narrow doorways or spaces).
• Ascertain access to and appropriateness of public and/or private transportation.

Nursing Priority No. 2.

To promote optimal level of function and prevent complications:

• Determine that client's underlying cognitive, emotional, and physical impairment(s) (e.g., brain injury, pain, depression, vision deficits) are treated or being managed **to maximize desire and motivation to participate in wheelchair activities.**
• Ascertain that wheelchair provides the base mobility to maximize function.
• Provide for, and instruct client in, safety while in a wheelchair (e.g., adaptive cushions, supports for all body parts, repositioning and transfer assistive devices, and height adjustment).
• Note evenness of surfaces client would need to negotiate and refer to appropriate sources for modifications. Clear pathways of obstructions.
• Recommend or refer for modifications to home, work or school, and recreational settings frequented by client **to provide safe and suitable environment.**
• Determine need for and capabilities of assistive persons. Provide training and support as indicated.
• Monitor client's use of joystick, sip and puff, sensitive mechanical switches, and so forth, **to provide necessary equipment if condition or capabilities change.**
• Monitor client for adverse effects of immobility (e.g., contractures, muscle atrophy, DVT, pressure ulcers). (Refer to

NDs Disuse Syndrome; risk for Peripheral Vascular Dysfunction, for additional interventions.)

Nursing Priority No. 3.

To promote wellness (Teaching/Discharge Considerations):

- Identify or refer to medical equipment suppliers **to customize client's wheelchair for size, proper seating angle, positioning aids, incline and decline stability, accessories (e.g., side guards, head rests, heel loops, brake extensions, tool packs) and electronics suited to client's ability (e.g., sip and puff, head movement, sensitive switches).**
- Encourage client's/SO's involvement in decision making as much as possible. **Enhances commitment to plan, optimizing outcomes.**
- Involve client/SO(s) in care, assisting them in managing immobility problems. **Promotes independence.**
- Demonstrate or provide information regarding individually appropriate safety measures.
- Refer to support groups relative to specific medical condition or disability; independence or political action groups. **Provides role modeling, assistance with problem solving and social change.**
- Identify community resources **to provide ongoing support.**

Documentation Focus

Assessment/Reassessment
- Individual findings, including level of function, ability to participate in specific or desired activities.
- Type of wheelchair and equipment needs.

Planning
- Plan of care and who is involved in the planning.
- Teaching plan.

Implementation/Evaluation
- Responses to interventions, teaching, and actions performed.
- Attainment or progress toward desired outcome(s).
- Modifications to plan of care.

Discharge Planning
- Discharge and long-term needs, noting who is responsible for each action to be taken.

Information that appears in brackets has been added by the authors to clarify and enhance the use of nursing diagnoses.

- Specific referrals made.
- Sources for, and maintenance of, assistive devices.

Sample Nursing Outcomes & Interventions Classifications (NOC/NIC) ⬛NIC

NOC—Ambulation: Wheelchair
NIC—Positioning: Wheelchair

dysfunctional gastrointestinal Motility

Taxonomy II: Elimination and Exchange—Class 2 Gastrointestinal Function (00196)
[Diagnostic Division: Elimination]
Submitted 2008

Definition: Increased, decreased, ineffective, or lack of peristaltic activity within the gastrointestinal system

Related Factors

Aging; prematurity
Surgery
Malnutrition; enteral feedings
Pharmaceutical agents (e.g., narcotics/opiates, laxatives, antibiotics, anesthesia)
Food intolerance (e.g., gluten, lactose); ingestion of contaminants (e.g., food, water)
Sedentary lifestyle; immobility
Anxiety

Defining Characteristics

Subjective
Absence of flatus
Abdominal cramping, pain
Diarrhea
Difficulty passing stool
Nausea; regurgitation

Objective
Change in bowel sounds (e.g., absent, hypoactive, hyperactive)
Abdominal distortion
Accelerated gastric emptying; diarrhea
Increased gastric residual; bile-colored gastric residual

Information that appears in brackets has been added by the authors to clarify and enhance the use of nursing diagnoses.

Dry stool
Vomiting

Desired Outcomes/Evaluation Criteria— Client Will:

- Reestablish and maintain normal pattern of bowel functioning.
- Verbalize understanding of causative factors and rationale for treatment regimen.
- Demonstrate appropriate behaviors to assist with resolution of causative factors.

Actions/Interventions:

Nursing Priority No. 1.

To assess causative/contributing factors:

- Note presence of conditions (e.g., congestive heart failure, major trauma, chronic conditions, sepsis) affecting systemic circulation/perfusion **that can result in GI hypoperfusion, and short- and/or long-term GI dysfunction.**
- Determine presence of disorders causing localized or diffuse reduction in GI blood flow, such as esophageal varices, GI hemorrhage, pancreatitis, intraperitoneal hemorrhage, **to identify client at higher risk for ineffective tissue perfusion.**
- Note presence of chronic/long-term disorders, such as gastrointestinal reflux disease (GERD), hiatal hernia, inflammatory bowel (e.g., ulcerative colitis, Crohn's disease), malabsorption (e.g., dumping syndrome, celiac disease), short-bowel syndrome, as may occur after surgical removal of portions of the small intestine. **These conditions are associated with increased, decreased, or ineffective peristaltic activity.**
- Note client's age and developmental concerns. **Children are prone to infections causing gastroenteritis manifested by vomiting and diarrhea. The elderly have problems associated with decreased motility, such as constipation. Premature or low-birth-weight neonates are at risk for developing necrotizing enterocolitis (NEC).**
- Review client's medication regimen. **Medications (e.g., laxatives, antibiotics, opiates, sedatives, iron preparations) may cause or exacerbate intestinal issues. In addition, likelihood of bleeding increases from use of medications such as NSAIDs, Coumadin, Plavix.**

Information that appears in brackets has been added by the authors to clarify and enhance the use of nursing diagnoses.

⊕ Cultural   🔬 Collaborative   🏠 Community/Home Care

- Note lifestyle issues that can affect GI function: for example, people who regularly engage in competitive sports such as long-distance running, cycling; persons with poor sanitary living conditions; people who travel to areas with contaminated food or water.
- Ascertain whether client is experiencing anxiety, stress or other psychogenic factors (e.g., anorexia or bulimia) **that can affect GI function.**
- Review laboratory and other diagnostic studies **to evaluate for GI problems, such as bleeding, inflammation, toxicity, and infection; or to help identify masses, dilation/obstruction, abnormal stool and gas patterns, and so forth.**

Nursing Priority No. 2.
To note degree of dysfunction/organ involvement:

- Assess vital signs, noting presence of low blood pressure, elevated heart rate, fever. **May suggest hypoperfusion or developing sepsis. Fever in presence of bright red blood in stool may indicate ischemic colitis.**
- Ascertain presence and characteristics of abdominal pain. **Pain is a common symptom of GI disorders and can vary in location, duration, and intensity.**
- Investigate reports of pain out of proportion to degree of traumatic injury. **May reflect developing abdominal compartment syndrome.**
- Inspect abdomen, noting contour. **Distention of bowel results in accumulation of fluids (salivary, gastric, pancreatic, biliary, and intestinal) and gases formed from bacteria, swallowed air, or any food or fluid the client has consumed.**
- Auscultate abdomen. **Hypoactive bowel sounds may indicate ileus. Hyperactive bowels sounds may indicate early intestinal obstruction or irritable bowel, or GI bleeding.**
- Palpate abdomen **to note masses, enlarged organs (e.g., spleen, liver, or portions of colon); elicitation of pain with touch; pulsation of aorta.**
- Measure abdominal girth and compare with clients customary waist size or belt length **to monitor development or progression of distention.**
- Note frequency and characteristics of bowel movements. **Bowel movements need to be considered in total assessment as they may reveal underlying problem or effect of pathology.**
- Note presence of nausea, with or without vomiting, and relationship to food intake or other events, if indicated. **History**

Information that appears in brackets has been added by the authors to clarify and enhance the use of nursing diagnoses.

can provide important information about cause (e.g., pregnancy, gastroenteritis, cancers, myocardial infarction, hepatitis, systemic infections, contaminated food, drug toxicity).

- Evaluate clients current nutritional status, noting ability to ingest and digest food. **Health depends on the intake, digestion and absorption of nutrients, which both affect and are affected by GI function.**

- Measure intra-abdominal pressure as indicated. **Tissue edema or free fluid collecting in the abdominal cavity leads to intra-abdominal hypertension which if untreated can cause abdominal compartment syndrome with end-stage organ failure.**

Nursing Priority No. 3.

To correct/improve existing dysfunction:

- Collaborate in treatment of underlying conditions **to correct or treat disorders associated with clients current GI dysfunction.**

- Maintain GI rest when indicated—NPO, fluids only, gastric or intestinal decompression **to reduce intestinal bloating and risk of vomiting.**

- Measure GI output periodically, and note characteristics of drainage **to manage fluid losses and replacement needs.**

- Administer fluids and electrolytes as indicated **to replace losses and to improve GI circulation and function.**

- Encourage ambulation if able. **Promotes general circulation, stimulates peristalsis and intestinal function.**

- Collaborate with dietician or nutritionist **to provide diet sufficient in nutrients by best possible route—oral, enteral, parenteral.**

- Provide small servings of easily digested food and fluids when oral intake tolerated.

- Encourage rest after meals **to maximize blood flow to digestive system.**

- Manage pain with medications as ordered, and nonpharmacological interventions such as positioning, back rub, heating pad (unless contraindicated) **to enhance muscle relaxation and reduce discomfort.**

- Report changes in nature or intensity of pain to physician, **as this may indicate worsening of condition, requiring interventions that are more intensive.**

- Collaborate with physician for medication management. **Dose modification, discontinuation of certain drugs, or**

Information that appears in brackets has been added by the authors to clarify and enhance the use of nursing diagnoses.

🌐 Cultural 🅐 Collaborative 🏠 Community/Home Care

alternative route of administration may be required to improve client's GI tolerance and/or function.

 Prepare client for procedures and surgery, as indicated. **May require a variety of interventions to treat problem causing or contributing to severe GI dysfunction.**

Nursing Priority No. 4.

To promote wellness (Teaching/Discharge Considerations):

• Provide information regarding cause of GI dysfunction and treatment plans, utilizing best learning methods for client, and including written information, bibliography, and other resources for postdischarge learning.

• Discuss normal variations in bowel patterns **to help alleviate unnecessary concern, initiate planned interventions, or seek timely medical care—may prevent overuse of laxatives, or help client understand when food, fluid, or drug modifications are needed to prevent constipation.**

• Encourage discussion of feelings regarding prognosis and long-term effects of condition. **Stress, anxiety, depression can affect food and fluid intake, exercise, and GI function.**

• Discuss value of relaxation and distraction techniques **if anxiety is suspected to play a role in GI dysfunction.**

• Identify necessary changes in lifestyle and assist client to incorporate disease management into ADLs. **Promotes independence and ability to manage own needs.**

• Review specific dietary changes and restrictions with client.

• Suggest healthier variations in preparation of foods, as indicated—broiled instead of fried, spices added to foods instead of salt, addition of higher fiber foods, use of lactose-free dairy products—**when these factors are affecting GI health.**

• Discuss fluid intake appropriate to individual situation. **Water is necessary to general health and GI function; client may need encouragement to increase intake or to make appropriate fluid choices if intake restricted for certain medical conditions.**

• Recommend maintenance of normal weight, or weight loss if client obese, **to decrease risk associated with GI disorders such as GERD or gallbladder disease.**

• Emphasize benefits of regular exercise in promoting normal GI function.

• Recommend smoking cessation. **Risk for acquiring or exacerbating certain GI disorders (e.g., Crohn's disease) may be increased with smoking.**

Information that appears in brackets has been added by the authors to clarify and enhance the use of nursing diagnoses.

- Discuss medication regimen, including reasons for and consequences of failure to take prescribed long-term maintenance. **Nonadherance can negatively affect treatment efficacy and client's quality of life.**
- Emphasize importance of avoiding use of NSAIDs, including aspirin; corticosteroids; some OTC drugs; vitamins containing potassium; mineral oil; or alcohol when taking anticoagulants. **These medications can be harmful to GI mucosa and increase risk of bleeding.**
- Refer to NDs, Constipation, Diarrhea, Bowel Incontinence for additional interventions.

Documentation Focus

Assessment/Reassessment
- Individual findings, noting nature, extent, and duration of problem, effect on independence and lifestyle.
- Dietary pattern, recent intake, food intolerances.
- Frequency and characteristics of stools.
- Characteristics of abdominal tenderness or pain, precipitators, and what relieves pain.

Planning
- Plan of care and who is involved in planning.
- Teaching plan.

Implementation/Evaluation
- Response to interventions, teaching, and actions performed.
- Attainment or progress toward desired outcome(s).
- Modifications to plan of care.

Discharge Planning
- Long-term needs and who is responsible for actions to be taken.
- Available resources, specific referrals made.

Sample Nursing Outcomes & Interventions Classifications (NOC/NIC) NIC

NOC—Gastrointestinal Function
NIC—Bowel Management

Information that appears in brackets has been added by the authors to clarify and enhance the use of nursing diagnoses.

risk for dysfunctional gastrointestinal Motility

Taxonomy II: Elimination and Exchange—Class 2
 Gastrointestinal Function (00197)
[Diagnostic Division: Elimination]
Submitted 2008

Definition: Risk for increased, decreased, ineffective, or lack of peristaltic activity within the gastrointestinal system

Risk Factors

Aging

Abdominal surgery; decreased gastrointestinal circulation

Food intolerance (e.g., gluten, lactose); change in food or water; unsanitary food preparation

Pharmaceutical agents (e.g., antibiotics, laxatives, narcotics/opiates, proton pump inhibitors)

Gastrointestinal reflux disease

Diabetes mellitus

Infection (e.g., bacterial, parasitic, viral)

Sedentary lifestyle; immobility

Stress; anxiety

> **NOTE:** A risk diagnosis is not evidenced by signs and symptoms, as the problem has not occurred; rather, nursing interventions are directed at prevention.

Desired Outcomes/Evaluation Criteria—Client Will (Include Specific Time Frame)

- Maintain normal pattern of bowel functioning.
- Verbalize understanding of individual risk factors and benefits of managing condition.
- Identify preventive interventions to reduce risk and promote normal bowel pattern.

Actions/Interventions

- Note presence of conditions affecting systemic circulation or perfusion such as congestive heart failure, major trauma with

---

Information that appears in brackets has been added by the authors to clarify and enhance the use of nursing diagnoses.

 Diagnostic Studies ∞ Pediatric/Geriatric/Lifespan 🔴 Medications **541**

blood loss, sepsis, shock, **which can result in GI hypoperfusion dysfunction.**

- Determine presence of disorders (e.g., esophageal varices, pancreatitis), foreign body ingestion, or prior abdominal surgery with adhesions, **which can impact peristaltic activity.**
- Assess client's current situation in conjunction with prior GI history. **Client may have an isolated incident putting him or her at risk (e.g., blunt force trauma to abdomen, prior history of strangulated hernia).**
- Auscultate abdomen **to evaluate peristaltic activity and note developing bowel disorders.**
- Palpate abdomen for masses, enlarged organs (e.g., spleen, liver, or portions of colon), elicitation of pain with touch, or pulsation of aorta, **which could identify problem in GI system.**
- Note frequency and characteristics of bowel movements. **Bowel movements by themselves are not necessarily diagnostic, but they can help make a differential diagnosis.**
- Ascertain presence and characteristics of abdominal pain. **Pain is a common symptom of GI disorders, with location and type aiding in identifying underlying problems.**
- Assess vital signs, noting presence of low blood pressure, elevated heart rate, fever. **May suggest hypoperfusion or other developing problems.**
- Evaluate client's current nutritional status, noting ability to ingest and digest food.
- ∞ Note client's age and developmental concerns. **Children are prone to infections causing gastroenteritis manifested by vomiting and diarrhea. The elderly have problems associated with decreased motility (e.g., constipation related to slower peristalsis, lack of sufficient fiber and fluid intake, or chronic use of laxatives). Premature/low-birth-weight neonates are at risk for developing NEC.**
- Note lifestyle issues **that can affect GI function (e.g., people who regularly engage in competitive sports such as long-distance running, cycling; or anorexia and bulimia).**
- Ascertain whether client is experiencing anxiety, stress, or other psychogenic factors.
- Review client's drug regimen. **Medications such as laxatives, antibiotics, anticholesterol agents, opiates, sedatives, iron preparations, and NSAIDs may cause or exacerbate intestinal issues.**
- Review laboratory and other diagnostic studies **to identify factors that may affect GI function.**

Information that appears in brackets has been added by the authors to clarify and enhance the use of nursing diagnoses.

Cultural   Collaborative   Community/Home Care

Nursing Priority No. 2.

To reduce or correct individual risk factors:

- Discuss normal variations in bowel patterns **so client can initiate planned interventions, or seek timely medical care.**
- Collaborate in treatment of underlying conditions.
- Practice and promote hand hygiene and other infection precautions **to prevent transmission of infections that may cause or spread gastrointestinal illnesses.**
- Maintain GI rest when indicated (e.g., NPO, fluids only, gastric or intestinal decompression after abdominal surgery) **to reduce intestinal bloating and reduce risk of vomiting.**
- Administer fluids and electrolytes as indicated.
- Administer prescribed prophylactic medications **to reduce potential for GI complications such as bleeding, ulceration of stomach mucosa, viral diarrheas.**
- Collaborate with dietician or nutritionist **to provide diet sufficient in nutrients and provided by best possible route (e.g., oral, enteral, parenteral).**
- Emphasize importance and assist with early ambulation, especially following surgery, **to stimulate peristalsis and help reduce GI complications associated with immobility.**
- Encourage relaxation and distraction techniques if anxiety is suspected to play a role in GI dysfunction.

Nursing Priority No. 3.

To promote wellness (Teaching/Discharge Considerations):

- Review measures to maintain bowel health:

  Use of dietary fiber and/or stool softeners.

  Fluid intake appropriate to individual.

  Establish or maintain regular bowel evacuation habits, incorporating privacy needs, assistance to bathroom on regular schedule, and so forth as indicated

  Emphasize benefits of regular exercise in promoting normal GI function.

- Discuss dietary recommendations with client/SO. **The client may elect to make adaptations in food choices and eating habits to avoid GI complications.**
- Instruct in healthier variations in preparation of foods, as indicated **when these factors may affect GI health.**
- Recommend maintenance of normal weight, or weight loss if client obese, **to decrease risk associated with GI disorders such as GERD or gallbladder disease.**

Information that appears in brackets has been added by the authors to clarify and enhance the use of nursing diagnoses.

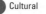

- Collaborate with physician in medication management. **Dose modification, discontinuation of certain drugs (e.g., laxatives, opioids, antidepressants, iron supplements), or alternative route of administration may be required to improve client's GI function.**
- Emphasize importance of discussing with physician current and new prescribed medications, and/or planned use of certain medications (e.g., NSAIDs, including aspirin; corticosteroids, some OTC drugs, herbals supplements) **that can be harmful to GI mucosa.**
- Recommend smoking cessation. **Smoking is a risk factor for acquiring or exacerbating certain GI disorders such as Crohn's disease.**
- Review food- and waterborne illnesses, contamination and hygiene issues, as indicated, and make needed follow-up referrals.
- Refer to appropriate resources (e.g., Social Services, Public Health Services) **for follow-up if client at risk for ingestion of contaminated water or food sources, or would benefit from teaching concerning food preparation and storage.**
- Recommend and/or refer to physician for vaccines as indicated. **The CDC makes recommendations for travelers and/or persons in high-risk areas or situations in which person might be exposed to contaminated food or water.**

Documentation Focus

Assessment/Reassessment
Individual findings, noting specific risk factors.
Dietary pattern, recent intake, food intolerances.
Frequency and characteristics of stools.

Planning
Plan of care and who is involved in planning.
Teaching plan.

Implementation/Evaluation
Response to interventions, teaching, and actions performed.
Attainment or progress toward desired outcome(s).
Modifications to plan of care.

Discharge Planning
Long-term needs and who is responsible for actions to be taken.
Available resources, specific referrals made.

Information that appears in brackets has been added by the authors to clarify and enhance the use of nursing diagnoses.

⊕ Cultural 🔅 Collaborative 🏠 Community/Home Care

Sample Nursing Outcomes & Interventions Classifications (NOC/NIC) NIC

NOC—Gastrointestinal Function
NIC—Bowel Management

Nausea

Taxonomy II: Comfort—Class 1 Physical Comfort (00134)
[Diagnostic Division: Food/Fluid]
Submitted 1998; Revised 2002

Definition: A subjective unpleasant, wavelike sensation in the back of the throat, epigastrium, or abdomen that may lead to the urge or need to vomit

Related Factors

Treatment
Gastric irritation [e.g., alcohol, blood]
Gastric distention
Pharmaceuticals [e.g., analgesics—aspirin, , NSAIDs, opioids; anesthesia, antiviral for HIV, steroids, antibiotics, chemotherapeutic agents]
Radiation therapy or exposure

Biophysical
Biochemical disorders (e.g., uremia, diabetic ketoacidosis, pregnancy)
Localized tumors (e.g., acoustic neuroma, primary or secondary brain tumors, bone metastases at base of the skull); intra-abdominal tumors
Toxins (e.g., tumor-produced peptides, abdominal metabolites due to cancer)
Esophageal or pancreatic disease; liver or splenetic capsule stretch
Gastric distention [e.g., delayed gastric emptying, pyloric intestinal obstruction, external compression of the stomach, other organ enlargement that slows stomach functioning (squashed stomach syndrome)]
Gastric irritation [e.g., pharyngeal and/or peritoneal inflammation]
Motion sickness; Ménière's disease; labyrinthitis
Increased intracranial pressure; meningitis

Information that appears in brackets has been added by the authors to clarify and enhance the use of nursing diagnoses.

Situational
Noxious odors or taste; unpleasant visual stimulation
Pain
Psychological factors; anxiety; fear

Defining Characteristics

Subjective
Report of nausea ["sick to my stomach"]

Objective
Aversion toward food
Increased salivation; sour taste in mouth
Increased swallowing; gagging sensation

Desired Outcomes/Evaluation Criteria— Client Will:

* Be free of nausea.
* Manage chronic nausea, as evidenced by acceptable level of dietary intake.
* Maintain or regain weight as appropriate.

Actions/Interventions

Nursing Priority No. 1.
To determine causative/contributing factors:

* Assess for presence of conditions of the GI tract (e.g., peptic ulcer disease, cholecystitis, gastritis, ingestion of "problem" foods). **Dietary changes may be sufficient to decrease frequency of nausea.**
* Note systemic conditions that may result in nausea (e.g., pregnancy, cancer treatment, myocardial infarction [MI], hepatitis, systemic infections, drug toxicity, presence of neurogenic causes [stimulation of the vestibular system], CNS trauma/tumor). **Helps in determining appropriate interventions or need for treatment of underlying condition.**
* Identify situations that client perceives as anxiety-inducing, threatening, or distasteful (e.g., "This is nauseating"). **May be able to limit or control exposure to situations or take medication prophylactically.**
* Note psychological factors, including those that are culturally determined (e.g., eating certain foods considered repulsive in one's own culture).

Information that appears in brackets has been added by the authors to clarify and enhance the use of nursing diagnoses.

- Determine if nausea is potentially self-limiting and/or mild (e.g., first trimester of pregnancy, 24-hour GI viral infection) or is severe and prolonged (e.g., cancer treatment, hyperemesis gravidarum). **Suggests severity of effect on fluid and electrolyte balance and nutritional status.**
- Check vital signs, especially for children and older clients, and note signs of dehydration. **Nausea may occur in the presence of postural hypotension and fluid volume deficit.**

Nursing Priority No. 2.

To promote comfort and enhance intake:

- Administer and monitor response to medications used to treat underlying cause of nausea (e.g., vestibular, bowel obstruction, dysmotility of upper gut, infection, inflammation, toxins). *Note:* **Older individuals are more prone to side effects of antiemetic and anti-anxiety or antipsychotic medications (e.g., excessive sedation, extrapyramidal movements), and there is increased risk of aspiration in the sedated client.**
- Select route of medication administration best suited to client's needs (i.e., oral, sublingual, injectable, rectal, transdermal).
- Review pain control regimen. **Converting to long-acting opioids or combination drugs may decrease stimulation of the chemotactic trigger zone (CTZ), reducing the occurrence of narcotic-related nausea.**
- Have client try dry foods such as toast, crackers, dry cereal before arising when nausea occurs in the morning, or throughout the day, as appropriate.
- Encourage client to begin with ice chips or sips/small amounts of fluids—4 to 8 ounces for adult; 1 ounce or less for child.
- Advise client to drink liquids 30 minutes before or after meals, instead of with meals.
- Provide diet and snacks of preferred or bland foods when available (including bland, caffeine-free nondiet carbonated beverages, clear soup broth, nonacidic fruit juice, gelatin, sherbet or ices, skinless cooked chicken) **to reduce gastric acidity and improve nutrient intake.**
- Avoid milk/dairy products, overly sweet or fried and fatty foods, gas-forming vegetables (e.g., broccoli, cauliflower, cucumbers) **that may increase nausea or be more difficult to digest.**
- Encourage client to eat small meals spaced throughout the day instead of large meals **so stomach does not feel excessively full.**

Information that appears in brackets has been added by the authors to clarify and enhance the use of nursing diagnoses.

- Instruct client to eat slowly, chewing food well **to enhance digestion.**
- Recommend client remain seated after meal, or with head well elevated above feet if in bed.
- Provide clean, peaceful environment and fresh air with fan or open window. Avoid offending odors, such as cooking smells, smoke, perfumes, mechanical emissions when possible, **as they may stimulate or worsen nausea.**
- Provide frequent oral care (especially after vomiting) **to cleanse mouth and minimize "bad tastes."**
- Encourage deep, slow breathing **to promote relaxation and refocus attention away from nausea.**
- Use distraction with music, chatting with family/friends, watching TV **to limit dwelling on unpleasant sensation.**
- Administer antiemetic on regular schedule before, during and after administration of antineoplastic agents **to prevent or control side effects of medication.**
- Time chemotherapy doses **for least interference with food intake.**
- Investigate use of accupressure point therapy (e.g., elastic band worn around wrist with small, hard bump that presses against accupressure point). **Some individuals with chronic nausea or history of motion sickness report this to be helpful; without sedative effect of medication.**

Nursing Priority No. 3.
To promote wellness (Teaching/Discharge Considerations):

- Review individual factors or triggers causing nausea and ways to avoid problem. **Provides necessary information for client to manage own care. Some individuals develop anticipatory nausea (a conditioned reflex) that recurs each time he or she encounters the situation that triggers the reflex.**
- Instruct in proper use, side effects, and adverse reactions of antiemetic medications. **Enhances client safety and effective management of condition.**
- Discuss appropriate use of OTC medications and herbal products (e.g., Dramamine, antacids, antiflatulents, ginger), or the use of THC (Marinol).
- Encourage use of nonpharmacological interventions. **Activities such as self-hypnosis, progressive muscle relaxation, biofeedback, guided imagery, and systemic desensitization promote relaxation, refocus client's attention, increase sense of control, and decrease feelings of helplessness.**

Information that appears in brackets has been added by the authors to clarify and enhance the use of nursing diagnoses.

• Advise client to prepare and freeze meals in advance, have someone else cook, or use microwave or oven instead of stove-top cooking **for days when nausea is severe or cooking is impossible.**

 • Suggest wearing loose-fitting clothing **to reduce external pressure on abdomen.**

• Recommend recording weight weekly, if appropriate, **to help monitor fluid and nutritional status.**

• Discuss potential complications and possible need for medical follow-up or alternative therapies. **Timely recognition and intervention may limit severity of complications (e.g., dehydration).**

• Review signs of dehydration and stress importance of replacing fluids and/or electrolytes (with products such as Gatorade or other electrolyte drinks for adults, or Pedialyte for children). **Increases likelihood of preventing potentially serious electrolyte depletion.**

• Identify signs (e.g., emesis appears bloody, black, or like coffee grounds; feeling faint) requiring immediate notification of healthcare provider.

Documentation Focus

Assessment/Reassessment
• Individual findings, including individual factors causing nausea.
• Baseline and periodic weight, vital signs.
• Specific client preferences for nutritional intake.
• Response to medication.

Planning
• Plan of care and who is involved in planning.
• Teaching plan.

Implementation/Evaluation
• Response to interventions, teaching, and actions performed.
• Attainment or progress toward desired outcome(s).
• Modifications to plan of care.

Discharge Planning
• Individual long-term needs, noting who is responsible for actions to be taken.
• Specific referrals made.

Information that appears in brackets has been added by the authors to clarify and enhance the use of nursing diagnoses.

Sample Nursing Outcomes & Interventions Classifications (NOC/NIC) NIC

NOC—Nausea and Vomiting Control
NIC—Nausea Management

self Neglect

Taxonomy II: Health Promotion—Class 2 Health Management (00193)
[Diagnostic Division: Hygiene]
Submitted 2008

Definition: A constellation of culturally framed behaviors involving one or more self-care activities in which there is a failure to maintain a socially accepted standard of health and well-being

Related Factors

Major life stressor; depression
Obsessive-compulsive disorder; schizotypal or paranoid personality disorders
Frontal lobe dysfunction and executive processing ability; cognitive impairment (e.g. dementia); Capgras syndrome
Functional impairment; learning disability
Lifestyle/choice; substance abuse; malingering
Maintaining control; fear of institutionalization

Defining Characteristics

Objective
Inadequate personal or environmental hygiene
Nonadherence to health activities

Desired Outcomes/Evaluation Criteria: Client Will (Include Specific Time Frame)

- Acknowledge difficulty maintaining hygiene practices.
- Demonstrate ability to manage lifestyle changes and medication regimen.
- Perform activities of daily living within level of own ability.

Information that appears in brackets has been added by the authors to clarify and enhance the use of nursing diagnoses.

Caregiver Will:

- Assist individual with personal and environmental hygiene as needed.
- Identify and assist client with medical, dental, and other healthcare appointments as indicated.

Actions/Interventions

Nursing Priority No. 1.

To identify causative or precipitating factors:

- Determine existing health problems, age, developmental level, and cognitive psychological factors including presence of delusions affecting ability to care for own needs. **A wide variety of impairments can cause a person to neglect hygiene needs, particularly aging, homelessness, and dementia.**
- Use an appropriate screening instrument, such as the Elder Assessment Instrument (EAI). **Neglect and elder abuse is underreported, and the use of a good tool can help identify presence.**
- Identify other problems that may interfere with ability to care for self such as visual or hearing impairment, language barrier, emotional instability or lability.
- Note recent life events or changes in circumstances. **Losses such as of a loved one, financial security, or physical independence can trigger or exacerbate self-neglect behaviors.**
- Review circumstances of client illness, possible monetary rewards, sympathy or attention from family. **On occasion self-neglect may be malingering as an attempt to gain something from others or relinquish unwanted responsibilities.**
- Perform mental status examination. **Mental illness (e.g., psychosis, depression, dementia) can affect individual's ability or desire to maintain self-care activities or care for home surroundings.**
- Evaluate for frontal lobe dysfunction, possibility of Diogenes syndrome.
- Assess economic factors and living arrangements. **May live alone or with family members who are not helpful, or may be homeless; may have little or no financial resources, resulting in inability to achieve or lack of concern about personal well-being.**
- Determine availability and use of resources.
- Interview SO/family members to determine level of involvement and support. **Client may be exhibiting acting-out/ paranoid behaviors, stressing caregivers, who may not**

Information that appears in brackets has been added by the authors to clarify and enhance the use of nursing diagnoses.

realize that cognitive impairment prevents individual from exercising self-control.

Nursing Priority No. 2.

To determine degree of impairment:

- Perform head-to-toe assessment inspecting scalp and skin noting personal hygiene, body odor, rashes, bruising, skin tears, lesions, burns, presence of vermin; inspecting oral cavity for gum disease, inflammation, lesions, loose or broken teeth, fit of dentures. **Identifies specific needs and may reveal signs of trauma or abuse.**
- Perform nutritional assessment as indicated. **Neglecting oneself often includes not eating meals regularly or not eating nutritionally balanced foods, especially when alcoholism or drug abuse is present.**
- Review medication regimen. **In addition to neglecting self-care activities, client will likely not pay attention to taking prescriptions as ordered, resulting in exacerbation of medical problem. Some psychotropic medications may cause individual to "feel different" or not in control of self, resulting in reluctance to take drug.**
- Determine client's willingness to change situation.

Nursing Priority No. 3.

To assist in correcting/dealing with situation:

- Develop multidisciplinary team specific to individual needs, such as case manager, physician, dietitian, physical or occupational therapist, rehabilitation specialist. **To develop a plan appropriate to the individual situation, making use of client's capabilities and maximizing potential.**
- Establish therapeutic relationship with client and with family, if available and willing to be involved.
- Identify specific priorities and goals of client/SOs. **Helps client to look at possibilities for dealing with difficult situation of no longer being able to maintain lifestyle and moving on to a new way of managing.**
- Promote client/SO's participation in problem identification and decision making.
- Evaluate need for safety balancing client's need for autonomy. **The ethical challenge of providing individual safety within the current laws for client's right to refuse care in face of self-neglect and self-destructive behaviors, which can impact others as well as the client, is difficult to manage.**

Information that appears in brackets has been added by the authors to clarify and enhance the use of nursing diagnoses.

🌐 Cultural   🅐 Collaborative   🏠 Community/Home Care

- Perform home assessment **to determine safety issues, cleanliness, compulsive hoarding, neglected property concerns.**
- Demonstrate or review skills necessary for caring for self, using terms appropriate to client's level of understanding.
- Plan time for listening to client's/SO's concerns. **Provides opportunity to determine whether plan is being followed and identify the barriers to participation.**
- Refer to NDs Self-Care Deficit, ineffective Health Maintenance, impaired Home Maintenance, and disturbed Sensory Perception for additional interventions as appropriate.

Nursing Priority No. 4.
To promote wellness (Discharge/Evaluation Criteria):

- Establish remotivation or resocialization program when indicated. **Depending on where the client is residing, isolation may become a problem as individual withdraws from contact with others.**
- Assist with setting up medication regimen as indicated.
- Discuss dietary needs and client's ability to provide nutritious meals. **May require support such as food stamps, community pantry, elder meal program, Meals on Wheels.**
- Provide for ongoing evaluation of self-care program. **Helps to identify whether client is managing effectively or whether cognitive functioning is deteriorating and a new plan needs to be developed.**
- Evaluate for appropriateness of providing a companion animal. **Taking responsibility for another life and sharing unconditional love can provide purpose and motivation for client to take more interest in own situation.**
- Refer to support services such as home care, day care program, social services, food stamps, community clinic, physical/occupational therapy, senior services as indicated.
- Investigate alternative placements as indicated.
- Discuss need for respite for family members. **Care of cognitively impaired member can be wearing, and time away allows for renewing oneself and enhancing ability to cope with continued care responsibilities.**
- Refer for counseling as indicated.

Documentation Focus

Assessment/Reassessment
- Individual findings, functional level and limitations, mental status.

Information that appears in brackets has been added by the authors to clarify and enhance the use of nursing diagnoses.

- Personal safety issues.
- Needed resources, possible need for placement.

Planning
- Plan of care and who is involved in planning.
- Teaching plan.

Implementation/Evaluation
- Response to interventions, teaching, and actions performed.
- Attainment or progress toward desired outcomes.
- Modifications of plan of care.

Discharge Planning
- Long-term needs and who is responsible for actions to be taken.
- Type of assistance and resources needed.
- Specific referrals made.

Sample Nursing Outcomes & Interventions Classifications (NOC/NIC) NIC

NOC—Self-Care Status
NIC—Self-Responsibility Facilitation

unilateral Neglect

Taxonomy II: Perception/Cognition—Class 1 Attention (00123)
[Diagnostic Division: Neurosensory]
Submitted 1986; Revised 2006

Definition: Impairment in sensory and motor response, mental representation, and spatial attention to body and the corresponding environment characterized by inattention to one side and overattention to the opposite side. Left-side neglect is more severe and persistent than right-side neglect.

Related Factors

Brain injury from: cerebrovascular problems; neurological illness; trauma; tumor
Left hemiplegia from CVA of the right hemisphere
Hemianopsia

Information that appears in brackets has been added by the authors to clarify and enhance the use of nursing diagnoses.

🌐 Cultural   🅐 Collaborative   🏠 Community/Home Care

Defining Characteristics

Subjective
Reports feeling that part does not belong to own self

Objective
Marked deviation of the eyes, head, or trunk (as if drawn magnetically) to the non-neglected side to stimuli and activities on that side

Failure to move eyes, head, limbs, or trunk in the neglected hemisphere despite being aware of a stimulus in that space; failure to notice people approaching from the neglected side

Displacement of sounds to the non-neglected side

Appears unaware of positioning of neglected limb

Lack of safety precautions with regard to the neglected side

Failure to: eat food from portion of the plate on the neglected side; dress or groom neglected side

Difficulty remembering details of internally represented familiar scenes that are on the neglected side

Use of only vertical half of page when writing; failure to cancel lines on the half of the page on the neglected side; substitution of letters to form alternative words that are similar to the original in length when reading

Distortion or omission of drawing on the half of the page on the neglected side

Perseveration of visual motor tasks on non-neglected side

Transfer of pain sensation to the non-neglected side

Desired Outcomes/Evaluation Criteria— Client/Caregiver Will:

- Acknowledge presence of sensory-perceptual impairment.
- Identify adaptive and protective measures for individual situation.
- Demonstrate behaviors, lifestyle changes necessary to promote physical safety.

Client Will:

- Verbalize positive realistic perception of self incorporating the current dysfunction.
- Perform self-care within level of ability.

Information that appears in brackets has been added by the authors to clarify and enhance the use of nursing diagnoses.

Nursing Priority No. 1.

To assess the extent of altered perception and the related degree of disability:

- Identify underlying reason for alterations in sensory, motor, or behavioral perceptions as noted in Related Factors.
- Ascertain client's/SO's perception of problem/changes, noting differences in perceptions.
- Measure visual acuity and field of vision.
- Assess sensory awareness (e.g., response to stimulus of hot and cold, dull and sharp); note problems with awareness of motion and proprioception.
- Observe client's behavior (as noted in Defining Characteristics) **to determine the extent of impairment.**
- Assess ability to distinguish between right and left.
- Note physical signs of neglect (e.g., disregard for position of affected limb(s), skin irritation/injury).
- Explore and encourage verbalization of feelings **to identify meaning of loss and dysfunction to the client and impact it may have on assuming ADLs.**
- Review results of testing performed to determine cause and/or type of neglect syndrome (e.g., sensory, motor, representational, personal, spatial, behavioral inattention). **Aids in distinguishing neglect from visual field cuts, impaired attention, and planning or visuospatial abilities.**

Nursing Priority No. 2.

To promote optimal comfort and safety for the client in the environment:

- Focus treatment strategies on training of attention to the neglected hemispace:

  Approach client from the unaffected side during acute phase. Explain to client that one side is being neglected; repeat as needed.

  Remove excess stimuli from the environment when working with the client **to reduce distractions.**

  Encourage client to turn head and eyes in full rotation and "scan" the environment **to compensate for visual field loss.**

  Position bedside table and objects (e.g., call bell/telephone, tissues) within functional field of vision.

  Position furniture and equipment so travel path is not obstructed. Keep doors wide open or completely closed.

Information that appears in brackets has been added by the authors to clarify and enhance the use of nursing diagnoses.

 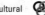 Cultural ⓒⓐ Collaborative 🏠 Community/Home Care

Remove articles in the environment that may create a safety hazard (e.g., footstool, throw rug).

Orient to environment as often as needed and ensure adequate lighting in the environment **to improve client's interpretation of environmental stimuli.**

Monitor affected body part(s) for positioning and anatomical alignment, pressure points, skin irritation or injury, and dependent edema. **Increased risk of injury and ulcer formation necessitates close observation and timely intervention.**

When moving client, describe location of affected areas of body.

Protect affected body part(s) from pressure, injury, and burns, and help client learn to assume this responsibility.

Assist with ADLs, maximizing self-care potential. Help client to bathe, apply lotion, and so forth to affected side.

Refer to ND disturbed Sensory Perception for additional interventions, as needed.

- Collaborate with physical and occupational therapists in promoting task-specific activities (e.g., visual scanning, environmental adaptation, environmental cues, client/family education). **Focuses on functional adaptation.**

Nursing Priority No. 3.

To promote wellness (Teaching/Discharge Considerations):

- Encourage client to look at and handle affected side **to stimulate awareness.**
- Bring the affected limb across the midline **for client to visualize during care.**
- Provide tactile stimuli to the affected side by touching/manipulating, stroking, and communicating about the affected side by itself rather than stimulating both sides simultaneously.
- Provide objects of various weight, texture, and size for client to handle **to provide tactile stimulation.**
- Assist client to position the affected extremity carefully and teach to routinely visualize placement of the extremity. Remind with visual cues. If client completely ignores one side of the body, use positioning **to improve perception (e.g., position client facing/looking at the affected side).**
- Encourage client to accept affected limb or side as part of self even when it no longer feels like it belongs.
- Use a mirror to help client adjust position **by visualizing both sides of the body.**

Information that appears in brackets has been added by the authors to clarify and enhance the use of nursing diagnoses.

- Use descriptive terms to identify body parts rather than "left" and "right"; for example, "Lift this leg" (point to leg) or "Lift your affected leg."
- Encourage client/SO/family members to discuss situation and impact on life/future. **May help verbalize the reality of changes and provides opportunity to explore solutions to problems and special needs.**
- Acknowledge and accept feelings of despondency, grief, and anger. **When feelings are openly expressed, client can deal with them and move forward.** (Refer to ND Grieving, as appropriate.)
- Reinforce to client the reality of the dysfunction and need to compensate.
- Avoid participating in the client's use of denial.
- Encourage family members and SO(s) to treat client normally and not as an invalid, including client in family activities.
- Place nonessential items (e.g., TV, pictures, hairbrush) on affected side during postacute phase once client begins to cross midline **to encourage continuation of behavior.**
- Refer to and encourage client to use rehabilitative services **to enhance independence in functioning.**
- Identify additional community resources to meet individual needs (e.g., Meals on Wheels, home-care services) **to maximize independence, allow client to return to community setting.**
- Provide informational material and Web sites **to reinforce teaching and promote self-paced learning.**

Documentation Focus

Assessment/Reassessment
- Individual findings, including extent of altered perception, degree of disability, effect on independence and participation in ADLs.
- Results of testing.

Planning
- Plan of care and who is involved in the planning.
- Teaching plan.

Implementation/Evaluation
- Responses to intervention, teaching, and actions performed.
- Attainment or progress toward desired outcome(s).
- Modifications to plan of care.

Information that appears in brackets has been added by the authors to clarify and enhance the use of nursing diagnoses.

Cultural   Collaborative   Community/Home Care

Discharge Planning

- Long-term needs and who is responsible for actions to be taken.
- Available resources, specific referrals made.

Sample Nursing Outcomes & Interventions Classifications (NOC/NIC) NIC

NOC—Heedfulness of Affected Side
NIC—Unilateral Neglect Management

Noncompliance [ineffective Adherence] [specify]

Taxonomy II: Life Principles—Class 3 Value/Belief/Action Congruence (00079)
[Diagnostic Division: Teaching/Learning]
Submitted 1973; Revised 1996, 1998

Definition: Behavior of person and/or caregiver that fails to coincide with a health-promoting or therapeutic plan agreed on by the person (and/or family and/or community) and healthcare professional. In the presence of an agreed-on health-promoting or therapeutic plan, person's or caregiver's behavior is fully or partially nonadherent and may lead to clinically ineffective or partially ineffective outcomes.

NOTE: When the plan of care is reviewed with client/SO, use of the term *noncompliance* may create a negative response and sense of conflict between healthcare providers and client. Labeling the client noncompliant may also lead to problems with third-party reimbursement. Where possible, use of the ND ineffective Therapeutic Regimen Management is recommended.

Related Factors

Healthcare Plan
Duration
Cost; financial flexibility of plan; intensity; complexity

Information that appears in brackets has been added by the authors to clarify and enhance the use of nursing diagnoses.

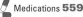

Diagnostic Studies   Pediatric/Geriatric/Lifespan   Medications **559**

Individual
Personal or developmental abilities; knowledge and skill relevant to the regimen behavior; motivational forces

Individual's value system; health beliefs; cultural influences; spiritual values

Altered thought processes, such as depression, paranoia

Difficulty changing behavior, as in addictions

Denial; issues of secondary gain

Health System
Individual health coverage

Credibility of provider; client-provider relationships; provider continuity and regular follow-up; provider reimbursement; communication/teaching skills of the provider

Access or convenience of care; satisfaction with care

Network
Involvement of members in health plan; social value regarding plan

Perceived beliefs of significant others

Defining Characteristics

Objective
Behavior indicative of failure to adhere

Objective tests (e.g., physiological measures, detection of physiological markers)

Failure to progress

Evidence of development of complications or exacerbation of symptoms

Failure to keep appointments

Desired Outcomes/Evaluation Criteria— Client Will:

- Verbalize accurate knowledge of condition and understanding of treatment regimen.
- Make choices at level of readiness based on accurate information.
- Verbalize commitment to mutually agreed upon goals and treatment plan.
- Access resources appropriately.
- Demonstrate progress toward health goals.

Information that appears in brackets has been added by the authors to clarify and enhance the use of nursing diagnoses.

Cultural Collaborative Community/Home Care

Actions/Interventions

Nursing Priority No. 1.

To determine reason for alteration/disregard of therapeutic regimen/instructions:

- Determine client's/SO's perception and understanding of the situation (illness, treatment).
- Listen to/Active-listen client's complaints, comments. **Helps to identify client's thinking about the treatment regimen (e.g., may be concerned about side effects of medications or success of procedures/transplantation).**
- Note language spoken, read, and understood.
- Be aware of developmental level as well as chronological age of client.
- Assess level of anxiety, locus of control, sense of powerlessness, and so forth.
- Determine who (e.g., client, SO, other) manages the medication regimen and whether individual knows what the medications are and why they are prescribed.
- Ascertain how client remembers to take medications and how many doses have been missed in the last 72 hours, last week, last 2 weeks, and last month.
- Identify factors that interfere with taking medications or lead to lack of adherence (e.g., depression, active alcohol or other drug use, low literacy, lack of support, lack of belief in treatment efficacy). **Forgetfulness is the most common reason given for not complying with the treatment plan.**
- Note length of illness. **Individuals tend to become passive and dependent in long-term, debilitating illnesses.**
- Clarify value system: cultural and religious values, health and illness beliefs of the client/SO(s).
- Determine social characteristics, demographic and educational factors, as well as personality of the client.
- Verify psychological meaning of the behavior (e.g., may be denial). Note issues of secondary gain—**family dynamics, school or workplace issues, involvement in legal system may unconsciously affect client's decision making.**
- Assess availability and use of support systems and resources.
- Be aware of nurses'/healthcare providers' attitudes and behaviors toward the client. (Do they have an investment in the client's compliance or recovery? What is the behavior of the client and nurse when client is labeled "noncompliant"?) **Some care providers may be enabling client, whereas others' judgmental attitudes may impede treatment progress.**

Information that appears in brackets has been added by the authors to clarify and enhance the use of nursing diagnoses.

Diagnostic Studies ∞ Pediatric/Geriatric/Lifespan Medications **561**

Nursing Priority No. 2.

To assist client/SO(s) to develop strategies for dealing effectively with the situation:

- Develop therapeutic nurse-client relationship. **Promotes trust, provides atmosphere in which client/SO(s) can freely express views and concerns. Adherence assessment is most successful when conducted in a positive, nonjudgmental atmosphere.**
- Explore client involvement in or lack of mutual goal setting. **Client will be more likely to follow-through on goals he or she participated in developing.**
- Review treatment strategies. Identify which interventions in the plan of care are most important in meeting therapeutic goals and which are least amenable to compliance. **Sets priorities and encourages problem solving areas of conflict.**
- Contract with the client for participation in care. **Enhances commitment to follow through.**
- Encourage client to maintain self-care, providing for assistance when necessary. Accept client's evaluation of own strengths and limitations while working with client to improve abilities.
- Provide for continuity of care in and out of the hospital or care setting, including long-range plans. **Supports trust, facilitates progress toward goals.**
- Provide information and help client to know where and how to find it on own. **Promotes independence and encourages informed decision making.**
- Give information in manageable amounts, using verbal, written, and audiovisual modes at level of client's ability. **Using client's style of learning facilitates learning, enabling client to understand diagnosis and treatment regimen.**
- Have client paraphrase instructions and information heard. **Helps validate client's understanding and reveals misconceptions.**
- Accept the client's choice or point of view, even if it appears to be self-destructive. Avoid confrontation regarding beliefs **to maintain open communication.**
- Establish graduated goals or modified regimen, as necessary (e.g., client with COPD who smokes a pack of cigarettes a day may be willing to reduce that amount). **May improve quality of life, encouraging progression to more advanced goals.**

Information that appears in brackets has been added by the authors to clarify and enhance the use of nursing diagnoses.

🌐 Cultural 🔵 Collaborative 🏠 Community/Home Care

Nursing Priority No. 3.

To promote wellness (Teaching/Discharge Considerations):

• Stress importance of the client's knowledge and understanding of the need for treatment or medication, as well as consequences of actions and choices.

• Develop a system for self-monitoring **to provide a sense of control and enable client to follow own progress and assist with making choices.**

• Suggest using a medication reminder system. **These have been shown to improve client adherence by a significant percentage.**

• Provide support systems **to reinforce negotiated behaviors.** Encourage client to continue positive behaviors, especially if client is beginning to see benefit.

• Refer to counseling, therapy and/or other appropriate resources.

• Refer to NDs ineffective Coping; compromised family Coping; deficient Knowledge, (specify); Anxiety; ineffective self Health Management.

Documentation Focus

Assessment/Reassessment

• Individual findings including deviation from prescribed treatment plan and client's reasons in own words.
• Consequences of actions to date.

Planning

• Plan of care and who is involved in planning.
• Teaching plan.

Implementation/Evaluation

• Response to interventions, teaching, and actions performed.
• Attainment or progress toward desired outcome(s).
• Modifications to plan of care.

Discharge Planning

• Long-term needs and who is responsible for actions to be taken.
• Specific referrals made.

Information that appears in brackets has been added by the authors to clarify and enhance the use of nursing diagnoses.

Sample Nursing Outcomes & Interventions Classifications (NOC/NIC) NIC

NOC—Compliance Behavior
NIC—Mutual Goal Setting

imbalanced Nutrition: less than body requirements

Taxonomy II: Nutrition—Class 1 Ingestion (00002)
[Diagnostic Division: Food/Fluid]
Submitted 1975; Revised 2000

Definition: Intake of nutrients insufficient to meet metabolic needs

Related Factors

Inability to ingest or digest food; inability to absorb nutrients
Biological, psychological, or economic factors
Increased metabolic demands (e.g., burns)
Lack of information, misinformation, misconceptions

Defining Characteristics

Subjective
Reported food intake less than RDA (recommended daily allowances); lack of food
Lack of interest in food; aversion to eating; reported altered taste sensation; perceived inability to digest food
Satiety immediately after ingesting food
Abdominal pain or cramping
Lack of information, misinformation, misconceptions [*Note:* The authors view these as related factors rather than defining characteristics.]

Objective
Body weight 20% or more under ideal [for height and frame]; [decreased subcutaneous fat or muscle mass]
Loss of weight with adequate food intake
Hyperactive bowel sounds; diarrhea; steatorrhea
Weakness of muscles required for swallowing or mastication; poor muscle tone
Sore buccal cavity; pale mucous membranes; capillary fragility

---

Information that appears in brackets has been added by the authors to clarify and enhance the use of nursing diagnoses.

Excessive loss of hair [or increased growth of hair on body (lanugo)]; [cessation of menses]

Abnormal laboratory studies (e.g., decreased albumin, total proteins; iron deficiency; electrolyte imbalances)

Desired Outcomes/Evaluation Criteria— Client Will:

* Demonstrate progressive weight gain toward goal.
* Display normalization of laboratory values and be free of signs of malnutrition as reflected in Defining Characteristics.
* Verbalize understanding of causative factors when known and necessary interventions.
* Demonstrate behaviors, lifestyle changes to regain and/or maintain appropriate weight.

Actions/Interventions

Nursing Priority No. 1.
To assess causative/contributing factors:

* Identify client at risk for malnutrition (e.g., institutionalized elderly; client with chronic illness; child or adult living in poverty/low-income area; client with jaw or facial injuries; intestinal surgery, postmalabsorptive or restrictive surgical interventions for weight loss; hypermetabolic states [e.g., burns, hyperthroidism]; malabsorption syndromes, lactose intolerance; cystic fibrosis; pancreatic disease; prolonged time of restricted intake; prior nutritional deficiencies).
* Determine client's ability to chew, swallow, and taste food. Evaluate teeth and gums for poor oral health, and note denture fit, as indicated. **All factors that can affect ingestion and/or digestion of nutrients.**
* Ascertain understanding of individual nutritional needs **to determine informational needs of client/SO.**
* Note availability and use of financial resources and support systems. Determine ability to acquire and store various types of food.
* Discuss eating habits, including food preferences, intolerances, or aversions **to appeal to client's tastes.**
* Assess drug interactions, disease effects, allergies, use of laxatives, diuretics **that may be affecting appetite, food intake, or absorption.**
* Evaluate impact of cultural, ethnic, or religious desires and influences **that may affect food choices.**

Information that appears in brackets has been added by the authors to clarify and enhance the use of nursing diagnoses.

Diagnostic Studies   ∞ Pediatric/Geriatric/Lifespan   Medications **565**

- Determine psychological factors, perform psychological assessment, as indicated, **to assess body image and congruency with reality.**
- Note occurrence of amenorrhea, tooth decay, swollen salivary glands, and report of constant sore throat, **suggesting bulimia and affecting ability to eat.**
- Review usual activities and exercise program noting repetitive activities (e.g., constant pacing) or inappropriate exercise (e.g., prolonged jogging). **May reveal obsessive nature of weight-control measures.**

Nursing Priority No. 2.
To evaluate degree of deficit:

- Assess weight; measure or calculate body fat and muscle mass via triceps skinfold and midarm muscle circumference or other anthropometric measurements **to establish baseline parameters.**
- Observe for absence of subcutaneous fat and muscle wasting, loss of hair, fissuring of nails, delayed healing, gum bleeding, swollen abdomen, and so on, **which indicate protein-energy malnutrition.**
- Auscultate bowel sounds. Note characteristics of stool (color, amount, frequency, etc.).
- Assist in nutritional assessment, using screening tools (e.g., Mini Nutritional Assessment [MNA]/similar tool).
- Review indicated laboratory data (e.g., serum albumin/prealbumin, transferrin, amino acid profile, iron, BUN, nitrogen balance studies, glucose, liver function, electrolytes, total lymphocyte count, indirect calorimetry).
- Assist with diagnostic procedures (e.g., Schilling's test, D-xylose test, 72-hour stool fat, GI series).

Nursing Priority No. 3.
To establish a nutritional plan that meets individual needs:

- Note age, body build, strength, activity and rest level, and so forth. **Helps determine nutritional needs.**
- Evaluate total daily food intake. Obtain diary of calorie intake, patterns and times of eating, **to reveal possible cause of malnutrition and changes that could be made in client's intake.**
- Calculate basal energy expenditure (BEE) using Harris-Benedict (or similar) formula and estimate energy and protein requirements.

Information that appears in brackets has been added by the authors to clarify and enhance the use of nursing diagnoses.

🌐 Cultural Ⓐ Collaborative 🏠 Community/Home Care

- Assist in treating or managing underlying causative factors (e.g., cancer, malabsorption syndrome, impaired cognition, depression, medications that decrease appetite, fad diets, anorexia).
- Consult dietitian or nutritional team, as indicated, **to implement interdisciplinary team management.**
- Provide diet modifications, as indicated. For example:

  Refer to nutritional resources to determine suitable ways to optimize client's intake of protein, carbohydrates, fats, calories within eating style and needs

  Several small meals and snacks daily

  Mechanical soft or blenderized tube feedings

  Appetite stimulants (e.g., wine), if indicated

  High-calorie, nutrient-rich dietary supplements, such as meal-replacement shake

  Formula tube feedings; parenteral nutrition infusion
- Administer pharmaceutical agents, as indicated:

  Digestive drugs or enzymes

  Vitamin and mineral (iron) supplements, including chewable multivitamin

  Medications (e.g., antacids, anticholinergics, antiemetics, antidiarrheals)
- Determine whether client prefers or tolerates more calories in a particular meal.
- Use flavoring agents (e.g., lemon and herbs) if salt is restricted **to enhance food satisfaction and stimulate appetite.**
- Encourage use of sugar or honey in beverages if carbohydrates are tolerated well.
- Encourage client to choose foods or have family member bring foods that seem appealing **to stimulate appetite.**
- Avoid foods that cause intolerances or increase gastric motility (e.g., foods that are gas-forming, hot/cold, or spicy; caffeinated beverages; milk products), according to individual needs.
- Limit fiber or bulk, if indicated, **because it may lead to early satiety.**
- Promote pleasant, relaxing environment, including socialization when possible **to enhance intake.**
- Prevent or minimize unpleasant odors or sights. **May have a negative effect on appetite and eating.**
- Assist with or provide oral care before and after meals and at bedtime.
- Encourage use of lozenges and so forth **to stimulate salivation when dryness is a factor.**

Information that appears in brackets has been added by the authors to clarify and enhance the use of nursing diagnoses.

 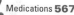

- Promote adequate and timely fluid intake. Limit fluids 1 hour prior to meal **to reduce possibility of early satiety.**
- Weigh regularly and graph results **to monitor effectiveness of efforts.**
- Develop individual strategies when problem is mechanical (e.g., wired jaws or paralysis following stroke). Consult occupational therapist **to identify appropriate assistive devices,** or speech therapist **to enhance swallowing ability.** (Refer to ND impaired Swallowing.)
- Refer to structured (behavioral) program of nutrition therapy (e.g., documented time and length of eating period, blenderized food or tube feeding, administered parenteral nutritional therapy) per protocol, **particularly when problem is anorexia nervosa or bulimia.**
- Recommend and support hospitalization **for controlled environment in severe malnutrition or life-threatening situations.**
- Refer to social services or other community resources **for possible assistance with client's limitations in buying and preparing foods.**

Nursing Priority No. 4.

To promote wellness (Teaching/Discharge Considerations):

- Emphasize importance of well-balanced, nutritious intake. Provide information regarding individual nutritional needs and ways to meet these needs within financial constraints.
- Develop behavior modification program with client involvement appropriate to specific needs.
- Provide positive regard, love, and acknowledgment of "voice within" guiding client with eating disorder.
- Develop consistent, realistic weight goal with client.
- Weigh at regular intervals and document results **to monitor effectiveness of dietary plan.**
- Consult with dietitian or nutritional support team, as necessary, **for long-term needs.**
- Develop regular exercise and stress reduction program.
- Review drug regimen, side effects, and potential interactions with other medications and OTC drugs.
- Review medical regimen and provide information and assistance, as necessary.
- Assist client to identify and access resources, such as way to obtain nutrient-dense, low-budget foods, food stamps, Meals on Wheels, community food banks, and/or other appropriate assistance programs.

Information that appears in brackets has been added by the authors to clarify and enhance the use of nursing diagnoses.

⊕ Cultural Collaborative Community/Home Care

· Refer for dental hygiene or other professional care, including counseling or psychiatric care, family therapy, as indicated.
· Provide and reinforce client teaching regarding preoperative and postoperative dietary needs when surgery is planned.
· Assist client/SO(s) to learn how to blenderize food and/or perform tube feeding.
· Refer to home health resources **for initiation and supervision of home nutrition therapy when used.**

Documentation Focus

Assessment/Reassessment
· Baseline and subsequent assessment findings to include signs/symptoms as noted in Defining Characteristics and laboratory diagnostic findings.
· Caloric intake.
· Individual cultural or religious restrictions, personal preferences.
· Availability and use of resources.
· Personal understanding or perception of problem.

Planning
· Plan of care and who is involved in planning.
· Teaching plan.

Implementation/Evaluation
· Client's responses to interventions, teaching, and actions performed.
· Results of periodic weigh-in.
· Attainment or progress toward desired outcome(s).
· Modifications to plan of care.

Discharge Planning
· Long-term needs, and who is responsible for actions to be taken.
· Specific referrals made.

Sample Nursing Outcomes & Interventions Classifications (NOC/NIC) NIC

NOC—Nutritional Status
NIC—Nutrition Management

Information that appears in brackets has been added by the authors to clarify and enhance the use of nursing diagnoses.

imbalanced Nutrition: more than body requirements

Taxonomy II: Nutrition—Class 1 Ingestion (00001)
[Diagnostic Division: Food/Fluid]
Submitted 1975; Revised 2000

Definition: Intake of nutrients that exceeds metabolic needs

Related Factors

Excessive intake in relationship to metabolic need

Defining Characteristics

Subjective

Dysfunctional eating patterns (e.g., pairing food with other activities)
Eating in response to external cues (e.g., time of day, social situation)
Concentrating food intake at end of day
Eating in response to internal cues other than hunger (e.g., anxiety)
Sedentary activity level

Objective

Weight 20% over ideal for height and frame [obese]
Triceps skin fold >25 mm in women, >15 mm in men
Percentage of body fat greater than 22% for trim women and 15% for trim men

Desired Outcomes/Evaluation Criteria—Client Will:

- Verbalize a realistic self-concept and body image (congruent mental and physical picture of self).
- Demonstrate acceptance of self as is rather than an idealized image.
- Demonstrate appropriate changes in lifestyle and behaviors, including eating patterns, food quantity/quality, and exercise program.
- Attain desirable body weight with optimal maintenance of health.

Information that appears in brackets has been added by the authors to clarify and enhance the use of nursing diagnoses.

🌐 Cultural   ♻ Collaborative   🏠 Community/Home Care

Actions/Interventions

Nursing Priority No. 1.

To identify causative/contributing factors:

- Assess risk or presence of conditions associated with obesity (e.g., familial pattern of obesity; slow metabolism; hypothyroidism; type 2 diabetes; high blood pressure; high cholesterol; or history of stroke, heart attack, gallstones, gout, arthritis, sleep apnea) **to ascertain treatments or interventions that may be needed in addition to weight management.**
- Review daily activity and exercise program. **Sedentary lifestyle is frequently associated with obesity and is a primary focus for modification.**
- Ascertain how client perceives food and the act of eating.
- Review diary of foods and fluids ingested; times and patterns of eating; activities, place; whether alone or with other(s); and feelings before, during, and after eating.
- Calculate total calorie intake.
- Ascertain previous dieting history.
- Discuss client's view of self, including what being heavy does for the client. **Familial traits, cultural beliefs, or life goals may place high importance on food and intake as well as large body size (e.g., Samoan, wrestler/football lineman).**
- Note negative and positive monologues (self-talk) of the individual.
- Obtain comparative body drawing by having client draw self on wall with chalk, then standing against it and having actual body outline drawn. **Determines whether client's view of self-body image is congruent with reality.**
- Ascertain occurrence of negative feedback from SO(s). **May reveal control issues, impact motivation for change.**
- Review results of body fat measurement (e.g., skin calipers, bioelectric impedance analysis [BIA], dual-energy x-ray absorptiometry [DEXA] scanning, hydrostatic weighing) **to determine presence and severity of obesity.**

Nursing Priority No. 2.

To establish weight reduction program:

- Discuss client's motivation for weight loss (e.g., for own satisfaction or self-esteem, or to gain approval from another person). **Helps client determine realistic motivating factors for individual situation (e.g., acceptance of self "as is," improvement of health status).**
- Obtain commitment or contract for weight loss.

Information that appears in brackets has been added by the authors to clarify and enhance the use of nursing diagnoses.

- Record height, weight, body build, gender, and age. **Provides comparative baseline and helps determine nutritional needs.**
- Calculate calorie requirements based on physical factors and activity level.
- Provide information regarding specific nutritional needs. **Obese individual may be deficient in needed nutrients.**
- Set realistic goals for weekly weight loss.
- Discuss eating behaviors (e.g., eating over sink, "nibbling," kinds of activities associated with eating) and identify necessary modifications.
- Encourage client to start with small changes (e.g., adding one more vegetable/day, introducing healthier versions of favorite foods, learning to read/understand nutrition labels) **to slowly change eating habits.**
- Develop carbohydrate and fat portion control and appetite-reduction plan **to support continuation of behavioral changes.**
- Emphasize need for adequate fluid intake and taking fluids between meals rather than with meals **to meet fluid requirements and reduce possibility of early satiety, followed quickly by recurrent hunger.**
- Discuss smart snacks (e.g., low-fat yogurt with fruit, nuts, apple slices with peanut butter, low-fat string cheese) **to assist client in finding healthy options.**
- Collaborate with physician and dietitian or nutrition team **in creating and evaluating effective nutritional program.**
- Encourage involvement in planned exercise program of client's choice and within physical abilities.
- Monitor individual drug regimen (e.g., appetite suppressants, hormone therapy, vitamin and mineral supplements).
- Provide positive reinforcement and encouragement for efforts as well as actual weight loss. **Enhances commitment to program.**
- Refer to bariatric specialist for additional interventions (e.g., extremely low-calorie diet, surgical weight loss procedures).

Nursing Priority No. 3.

To promote wellness (Teaching/Discharge Considerations):

- Discuss reality of obesity and health consequences as well as myths client/SO(s) may believe about weight and weight loss.
- Assist client to choose nutritious foods that reflect personal likes, meet individual needs, and are within financial budget.

Information that appears in brackets has been added by the authors to clarify and enhance the use of nursing diagnoses.

• Encourage parent to model good nutritional choices (e.g., offer vegetables, fruits, and low-fat foods at daily meals and snacks) **to assist child in adopting healthy eating habits.**

• Identify ways to manage stress or tension during meals. **Promotes relaxation to permit focus on act of eating and awareness of satiety.**

• Review and discuss strategies to deal appropriately with stressful events/feelings **instead of overeating.**

• Encourage variety and moderation in dietary plan **to decrease boredom.**

• Advise client to plan for special occasions (birthday/holidays) by reducing intake before event and/or eating "smart" **to redistribute or reduce calories and allow for participation in food events.**

• Discuss importance of an occasional treat by planning for inclusion in diet **to avoid feelings of deprivation arising from self-denial.**

• Recommend client weigh only once per week, same time and clothes, and graph on chart. Measure body fat when possible **(more accurate measure).**

• Discuss normalcy of ups and downs of weight loss: plateauing, set point (at which weight is not being lost), hormonal influences, and so forth. **Prevents discouragement when progress stalls.**

• Encourage buying personal items/clothing as a reward for weight loss or other accomplishments. Suggest disposing of "fat clothes" **to encourage positive attitude of permanent change and remove "safety valve" of having wardrobe available "just in case" weight is regained.**

• Involve SO(s) in treatment plan as much as possible **to provide ongoing support and increase likelihood of success.**

• Refer to community support groups, psychotherapy, as indicated.

• Provide contact number for dietitian, bibliography and Web sites for resources **to address ongoing nutrition concerns/dietary needs.**

• Refer to NDs disturbed Body Image; ineffective Coping.

Documentation Focus

Assessment/Reassessment

• Individual findings, including current weight, dietary pattern; perceptions of self, food, and eating; motivation for loss, support and feedback from SO(s).

Information that appears in brackets has been added by the authors to clarify and enhance the use of nursing diagnoses.

- Results of laboratory and diagnostic testing.
- Results of weekly weigh-in.

Planning

- Plan of care, specific interventions, and who is involved in planning.
- Teaching plan.

Implementation/Evaluation

- Responses to interventions, weekly weight, and actions performed.
- Attainment or progress toward desired outcome(s).
- Modifications to plan of care.

Discharge Planning

- Long-term needs and who is responsible for actions to be taken.
- Specific referrals made.

Sample Nursing Outcomes & Interventions Classifications (NOC/NIC) NIC

NOC—Weight Loss Behavior
NIC—Weight Reduction Assistance

risk for imbalanced Nutrition: more than body requirements

Taxonomy II: Nutrition—Class 1 Ingestion (00003)
[Diagnostic Division: Food/Fluid]
Submitted 1980; Revised 2000

Definition: At risk for an intake of nutrients that exceeds metabolic needs

Risk Factors

Dysfunctional eating patterns; pairing food with other activities; eating in response to external cues (e.g., time of day, social situation) or internal cues other than hunger (e.g., anxiety); concentrating food intake at end of day

Parental obesity

Rapid transition across growth percentiles in children; reported use of solid food as major food source before 5 months of age

---

Information that appears in brackets has been added by the authors to clarify and enhance the use of nursing diagnoses.

🌐 Cultural 🅐 Collaborative 🏠 Community/Home Care

Higher baseline weight at beginning of each pregnancy

Observed use of food as reward or comfort measure

Frequent, repeated dieting

Alteration in usual activity patterns; sedentary lifestyle

Alteration in usual coping patterns; socially or culturally isolated; lacking other outlets

Majority of foods consumed are concentrated, high-calorie or fat sources

Significant or sudden decline in financial resources, lower socioeconomic status

> **NOTE:** A risk diagnosis is not evidenced by signs and symptoms, as the problem has not occurred; rather, nursing interventions are directed at prevention.

Desired Outcomes/Evaluation Criteria— Client Will:

- Verbalize understanding of body and energy needs.
- Identify lifestyle and cultural factors that predispose to obesity.
- Demonstrate behaviors, lifestyle changes to reduce risk factors.
- Acknowledge responsibility for own actions and need to "act, not react" to stressful situations.
- Maintain weight at a satisfactory level for height, body build, age, and gender.

Actions/Interventions

Nursing Priority No. 1.

To assess potential factors for undesired weight gain:

- Note presence of factors as listed in Risk Factors. **A high correlation exists between obesity in parents and their children. When one parent is obese, 40% of the children may be overweight; when both are obese, the proportion may be as high as 80%.**
- Determine age, activity level, and exercise patterns.
- Calculate growth percentiles in infants/children **for comparative baseline and future monitoring.**
- Review laboratory data **for indicators of endocrine or metabolic disorders.**
- Identify cultural factors or lifestyle that may predispose to weight gain. **Socioeconomic group, familial eating**

Information that appears in brackets has been added by the authors to clarify and enhance the use of nursing diagnoses.

patterns, amount of money available for purchasing food, proximity of grocery store, and available storage space for food are all factors that may impact food choices and intake.

- Assess eating patterns in relation to risk factors. Note patterns of hunger and satiety. **Patterns differ in those who are predisposed to weight gain (e.g., client is skipping meals to reduce total calories, but is unaware that this practice decreases the metabolic rate).**
- Determine weight change patterns, history of dieting and kinds of diets used. Determine whether yo-yo dieting or bulimia is a factor.
- Identify personality characteristics that may indicate potential for obesity (e.g., rigid thinking patterns, external locus of control, negative body image or self-concept, negative monologues [self-talk], dissatisfaction with life).
- Determine psychological significance of food to the client.
- Listen to concerns and assess motivation to prevent weight gain.

Nursing Priority No. 2.

To assist client to develop preventive program to avoid weight gain:

- Provide information on balancing calorie intake and energy expenditure.
- Help client develop new eating patterns and habits (e.g., eating slowly, eating only when hungry, controlling portion size, stopping when full, not skipping meals).
- Discuss importance and help client develop a program of exercise and relaxation techniques. **Encourages client to incorporate plan into lifestyle.**
- Assist client to develop strategies for reducing stressful thinking or actions. **Promotes relaxation, reduces likelihood of stress and comfort eating.**

Nursing Priority No. 3.

To promote wellness (Teaching/Discharge Considerations):

- Review individual risk factors and provide information **to assist the client with motivation and decision making.**
- Consult with dietitian or nutritionist about specific nutrition and dietary issues.
- Provide information to new mothers about nutrition for developing babies.

Information that appears in brackets has been added by the authors to clarify and enhance the use of nursing diagnoses.

 Cultural · Collaborative · Community/Home Care

• Encourage client to make a decision to lead an active life and control food habits.

 • Assist client in learning to be in touch with own body and to identify feelings that may provoke "comfort eating," such as anger, anxiety, boredom, sadness.

 • Develop a system for self-monitoring **to provide a sense of control and enable the client to follow own progress and assist with making choices.**

• Refer to support groups and appropriate community resources for education/behavior modification, as indicated.

Documentation Focus

Assessment/Reassessment
• Findings related to individual situation, risk factors, current caloric intake and dietary pattern, activity level.
• Baseline height and weight, growth percentile.
• Results of laboratory tests.
• Motivation to reduce risks and prevent weight problems.

Planning
• Plan of care and who is involved in the planning.
• Teaching plan.

Implementation/Evaluation
• Response to interventions, teaching, and actions performed.
• Attainment or progress toward desired outcome(s).
• Modifications to plan of care.

Discharge Planning
• Long-term needs, noting who is responsible for actions to be taken.
• Specific referrals made.

Sample Nursing Outcomes & Interventions Classifications (NOC/NIC) NIC

NOC—Weight Control
NIC—Weight Management

Information that appears in brackets has been added by the authors to clarify and enhance the use of nursing diagnoses.

readiness for enhanced **Nutrition**

Taxonomy II: Health Promotion—Class 2 Health
Management (00163)
[Diagnostic Division: Food/Fluid]
Submitted 2002

Definition: A pattern of nutrient intake that is sufficient
for meeting metabolic needs and can be strengthened

Related Factors

To be developed

Defining Characteristics

Subjective
Expresses knowledge of healthy food and fluid choices or willingness to enhance nutrition

Eats regularly

Attitude toward eating or drinking is congruent with health
goals

Objective
Consumes adequate food and fluid

Follows an appropriate standard for intake (e.g., the food pyr-
amid or American Diabetic Association Guidelines)

Safe preparation or storage for food and fluids

Desired Outcomes/Evaluation Criteria—
Client Will:

- Demonstrate behaviors to attain or maintain appropriate
weight.
- Be free of signs of malnutrition.
- Be able to safely prepare and store foods.

Actions/Interventions

Nursing Priority No. 1.
To determine current nutritional status and eating patterns:

- Review client's knowledge of current nutritional needs and
ways client is meeting these needs. **Provides baseline for
further teaching and interventions.**

Information that appears in brackets has been added by the authors to clarify
and enhance the use of nursing diagnoses.

Cultural   Collaborative   Community/Home Care

- Assess eating patterns and food and fluid choices in relation to any health risk factors and health goals. **Helps to identify specific strengths and weaknesses that can be addressed.**
- Verify that age-related and developmental needs are met. **These factors are constantly presented throughout the lifespan, although differing for each age group. For example, older adults need same nutrients as younger adults, but in smaller amounts, and with attention to certain components, such as calcium, fiber, vitamins, protein, and water. Infants/children require small meals and constant attention to needed nutrients for proper growth and development while dealing with child's food preferences and eating habits.**
- Evaluate influence of cultural or religious factors **to determine what client considers to be normal dietary practices, as well as to identify food preferences and restrictions, and eating patterns that can be strengthened and/or altered, if indicated.**
- Assess how client perceives food, food preparation, and the act of eating **to determine client's feeling and emotions regarding food and self-image.**
- Ascertain occurrence of, or potential for, negative feedback from SO(s). **May reveal control issues that could impact client's commitment to change.**
- Determine patterns of hunger and satiety. **Helps identify strengths and weaknesses in eating patterns and potential for change (e.g., person predisposed to weight gain may need a different time for a big meal than evening, or need to learn what foods reinforce feelings of satisfaction).**
- Assess client's ability to safely store and prepare foods **to determine if health information or resources might be needed.**

Nursing Priority No. 2.
To assist client/SO(s) to develop plan to meet individual needs:

- Determine motivation and expectation for change.
- Assist in obtaining and review results of individual testing (e.g., weight/height, body fat percent, lipids, glucose, complete blood count, total protein) **to determine that client is healthy and/or identify dietary changes that may be helpful in attaining health goals.**
- Encourage client's beneficial eating patterns/habits (e.g., controlling portion size, eating regular meals, reducing high-fat

---

Information that appears in brackets has been added by the authors to clarify and enhance the use of nursing diagnoses.

 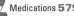

or fast-food intake, following specific dietary program, drinking water and healthy beverages). **Positive feedback promotes continuation of healthy lifestyle habits and new behaviors.**

- Discuss use of nonfood rewards.
- Provide instruction and reinforce information regarding special needs. **Enhances decision-making process and promotes responsibility for meeting own needs.**
- Encourage reading of food labels and instruct in meaning of labeling, as indicated, **to assist client/SO(s) in making healthful choices.**
- Review safe preparation and storage of food **to avoid foodborne illnesses.**
- Consult with, or refer to, dietitian, or physician, as indicated. **Client/SO(s) may benefit from advice regarding specific nutrition and dietary issues or may require regular follow-up to determine that needs are being met when a medically prescribed program is to be followed.**
- Develop a system for self-monitoring **to provide a sense of control and enable the client to follow own progress, and assist in making choices.**

Nursing Priority No. 3.
To promote optimum wellness:

- Review individual risk factors and provide additional information and response to concerns. **Assists the client with motivation and decision making.**
- Provide bibliotherapy and help client/SO(s) identify and evaluate resources they can access on their own. **When referencing the Internet or nontraditional, unproven resources, the individual must exercise some restraint and determine the reliability of the source/information before acting on it.**
- Encourage variety and moderation in dietary plan **to decrease boredom and encourage client in efforts to make healthy choices about eating and food.**
- Discuss use of nutritional supplements, OTC and herbal products. **Confusion may exist regarding the need for and use of these products in a balanced dietary regimen.**
- Assist client to identify and access community resources when indicated. **May benefit from assistance such as food stamps, WIC, budget counseling, Meals on Wheels, community food banks, and/or other assistance programs.**

Information that appears in brackets has been added by the authors to clarify and enhance the use of nursing diagnoses.

Cultural   Collaborative   Community/Home Care

Documentation Focus

Assessment/Reassessment
- Assessment findings, including client perception of needs and desire/expectations for improvement.
- Individual cultural or religious restrictions, personal preferences.
- Availability and use of resources.

Planning
- Individual goals for enhancement.
- Plan for growth and who is involved in planning.

Implementation/Evaluation
- Response to activities and learning, and actions performed.
- Attainment or progress toward desired outcome(s).
- Modifications to plan.

Discharge Planning
- Long-term needs, expectations, and plan of action.
- Available resources and specific referrals made.

Sample Nursing Outcomes & Interventions Classifications (NOC/NIC) NIC

NOC—Weight Maintenance Behavior
NIC—Nutritional Counseling

---

impaired Oral Mucous Membrane

Taxonomy II: Safety/Protection—Class 2 Physical Injury (00045)
[Diagnostic Division: Food/Fluid]
Submitted 1982; Nursing Diagnosis Extension and Classification (NDEC) Revision 1998

Definition: Disruption of the lips and/or soft tissue of the oral cavity

---

Related Factors

Dehydration; NPO for more than 24 hours; malnutrition
Decreased salivation; medication side effects; diminished hormone levels (women); mouth breathing

---

Information that appears in brackets has been added by the authors to clarify and enhance the use of nursing diagnoses.

Deficient knowledge of appropriate oral hygiene

Ineffective oral hygiene; barriers to oral self-care or professional care

Mechanical factors (e.g., ill-fitting dentures, braces, tubes [endotracheal/nasogastric], surgery in oral cavity); loss of supportive structures; trauma; cleft lip or palate

Chemical irritants (e.g., alcohol, tobacco, acidic foods, regular use of inhalers or other noxious agents)

Chemotherapy; immunosuppression; immunocompromised; decreased platelets; infection; radiation therapy

Stress; depression

Defining Characteristics

Subjective

Xerostomia [dry mouth]

Oral pain, discomfort

Reports bad taste in mouth; diminished taste; difficulty eating or swallowing

Objective

Coated tongue; smooth atrophic tongue; geographic tongue

Gingival or mucosal pallor

Stomatitis; hyperemia; gingival hyperplasia; macroplasia; vesicles; nodules; papules

White patches or plaques; spongy patches; white curdlike exudate

Oral lesions or ulcers; fissures; bleeding; cheilitis; desquamation; mucosal denudation

Purulent drainage or exudates; presence of pathogens; enlarged tonsils

Edema

Halitosis; [carious teeth]

Gingival recession, pocketing deeper than 4 mm

Red or bluish masses (e.g., hemangiomas)

Difficult speech

Desired Outcomes/Evaluation Criteria— Client Will:

- Verbalize understanding of causative factors.
- Identify specific interventions to promote healthy oral mucosa.
- Demonstrate techniques to restore/maintain integrity of oral mucosa.

Information that appears in brackets has been added by the authors to clarify and enhance the use of nursing diagnoses.

 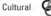

- Report or demonstrate a decrease in symptoms as noted in Defining Characteristics.

Actions/Interventions

Nursing Priority No. 1.
To identify causative/contributing factors affecting oral health:

- Note presence of illness, disease, or trauma (e.g., gingivitis, periodontal disease; presence of oral ulcerations; bacterial, viral, fungal, ororal infections; facial fractures; cancer or cancer therapies; generalized debilitating conditions) **that affect health of oral tissues.**
- Determine nutrition and fluid intake and reported changes (e.g., avoiding eating, change in taste, chews painstakingly, swallows numerous times for even small bites, unexplained weight loss) **that can indicate problems with oral mucosa.**
- Note use of tobacco (including smokeless) and alcohol, **which may predispose mucosa to infection, cell damage, and cancer.**
- Assess for dry mouth, thick or absent saliva, and abnormal tongue surfaces.
- Observe for chipped or sharp-edged teeth. Note fit of dentures or other prosthetic devices when used.
- Assess medication use and possibility of side effects **affecting health or integrity of oral mucous membranes.**
- Determine allergies to food, drugs, other substances.
- Evaluate client's ability to provide self-care and availability of necessary equipment or assistance. **Client's age, as well as current health status, affects ability to provide self-care.**
- Review oral hygiene practices: frequency and type (e.g., brushing, flossing, Water Pik); professional dental care.

Nursing Priority No. 2.
To correct identified/developing problems:

- Routinely inspect oral cavity and throat for inflammation, sores, lesions, and/or bleeding. Determine if client is experiencing pain or painful swallowing.
- Encourage adequate fluids **to prevent dry mouth and dehydration.**
- Encourage use of tart, sour, and citrus foods and drinks; chewing gum; or hard candy **to stimulate saliva.**
- Lubricate lips and provide commercially prepared oral lubricant solution.

Information that appears in brackets has been added by the authors to clarify and enhance the use of nursing diagnoses.

Diagnostic Studies   ∞ Pediatric/Geriatric/Lifespan   Medications **583**

- Provide for increased humidity, if indicated, by vaporizer or room humidifier if client is mouth-breather.
- Provide dietary modifications (e.g., food of comfortable texture, temperature, density) **to reduce discomfort and improve intake,** and adequate nutrients and vitamins **to promote healing.**
- Avoid irritating foods and fluids, temperature extremes. Provide soft or pureed diet as required.
- Use lemon/glycerin swabs with caution; **may be irritating if mucosa is injured.**
- Assist with oral care, as indicated:

   Offer tap water or saline rinses, diluted alcohol-free mouthwashes.

   Provide gentle gum massage and tongue brushing with soft toothbrush or sponge/cotton-tip applicators **(limits mucosal and gum irritation).**

   Assist with or encourage brushing and flossing **when client is unable to do self-care.**

   Review safe use of electric or battery-powered mouth care devices (e.g., toothbrush, plaque remover), as indicated.

   Assist with or provide denture care when indicated (e.g., remove and clean after meals and at bedtime).

- Provide anesthetic lozenges or analgesics such as Stanford solution, viscous lidocaine (Xylocaine), sucralfate slurry, as indicated, **to provide protection or reduce oral discomfort and pain.**
- Administer antibiotics, as ordered, **when infection is present.**
- Reposition ET tubes and airway adjuncts routinely, carefully padding teeth or prosthetics **to minimize pressure on tissues.**
- Emphasize avoiding alcohol, smoking or chewing tobacco especially if periodontal disease present, or if client has xerostomia or other oral discomforts, **which may further irritate and damage mucosa.**
- Refer for evaluation of dentures or other prosthetics, structural defects **when impairments are affecting oral health.**

Nursing Priority No. 3.

To promote wellness (Teaching/Discharge Considerations):

- Review current oral hygiene patterns and provide information about oral health as required or desired **to correct deficiencies and encourage proper care.**
- Instruct parents in oral hygiene techniques and proper dental care for infants/children (e.g., safe use of pacifier, brushing of

---

Information that appears in brackets has been added by the authors to clarify and enhance the use of nursing diagnoses.

teeth and gums, avoidance of sweet drinks and candy, recognition and treatment of thrush). **Encourages early initiation of good oral health practices and timely intervention for treatable problems.**

- Discuss special mouth care required during and after illness or trauma, or following surgical repair (e.g., cleft lip or palate) **to facilitate healing.**
- Identify need for, and demonstrate use of special "appliances" **to perform own oral care.**
- Listen to concerns about appearance and provide accurate information about possible treatments and outcomes. Discuss effect of condition on self-esteem and body image, noting withdrawal from usual social activities or relationships, and/or expressions of powerlessness.
- Review information regarding drug regimen, use of local anesthetics.
- Promote good general health and mental health habits including stress management. (**Altered immune response can affect the oral mucosa.**)
- Provide nutritional information **to correct deficiencies, reduce gum irritation or disease, prevent dental caries.**
- Emphasize importance of limiting nighttime regimen of bottle of milk for infant in bed. Suggest pacifier or use of water during night **to prevent bottle syndrome with decaying of teeth.**
- Recommend regular dental checkups and professional care.
- Identify community resources (e.g., low-cost dental clinics, smoking cessation resources, cancer information services and support group, Meals on Wheels, food stamps, home care aide).

Documentation Focus

Assessment/Reassessment
- Condition of oral mucous membranes, routine oral care habits and interferences.
- Availability of oral care equipment and products.
- Knowledge of proper oral hygiene and care.
- Availability and use of resources.

Planning
- Plan of care and who is involved in planning.
- Teaching plan.

Information that appears in brackets has been added by the authors to clarify and enhance the use of nursing diagnoses.

Implementation/Evaluation
- Responses to interventions, teaching, and actions performed.
- Attainment or progress toward desired outcome(s).
- Modifications to plan of care.

Discharge Planning
- Long-term needs and who is responsible for actions to be taken.
- Specific referrals made, resources for special appliances.

Sample Nursing Outcomes & Interventions Classifications (NOC/NIC) NIC

NOC—Oral Hygiene
NIC—Oral Health Restoration

acute Pain

Taxonomy II: Comfort—Class 1 Physical Comfort (00132)
[Diagnostic Division: Pain/Comfort]
Submitted 1996

Definition: Unpleasant sensory and emotional experience arising from actual or potential tissue damage or described in terms of such damage (International Association for the Study of Pain); sudden or slow onset of any intensity from mild to severe with an anticipated or predictable end and a duration of less than 6 months

Related Factors

Injuring agents (biological, chemical, physical, psychological)

Defining Characteristics

Subjective
Verbal report of pain; coded report [may be less from clients younger than age 40, men, and some cultural groups]
Changes in appetite

Objective
Observed evidence of pain
Guarding behavior; protective gestures; positioning to avoid pain

---

Information that appears in brackets has been added by the authors to clarify and enhance the use of nursing diagnoses.

  Cultural   Collaborative   Community/Home Care

Facial mask; sleep disturbance (eyes lack luster, beaten look, fixed or scattered movement, grimace)

Expressive behavior (e.g., restlessness, moaning, crying, vigilance, irritability, sighing)

Distraction behavior (e.g., pacing, seeking out other people and/or activities, repetitive activities)

Change in muscle tone (may span from listless [flaccid] to rigid)

Diaphoresis; change in blood pressure, heart rate, respiratory rate; pupillary dilation

Self-focusing; narrowed focus (altered time perception, impaired thought process, reduced interaction with people and environment)

Desired Outcomes/Evaluation Criteria— Client Will:

- Report pain is relieved or controlled.
- Follow prescribed pharmacological regimen.
- Verbalize nonpharmacological methods that provide relief.
- Demonstrate use of relaxation skills and diversional activities, as indicated, for individual situation.

Actions/Interventions

Nursing Priority No. 1.

To assess etiology/precipitating contributory factors:

- Note client's age and developmental level and current condition (e.g., infant/child, critically ill, ventilated, sedated, or cognitively impaired client) affecting ability to report pain parameters.
- Determine and document presence of possible pathophysiological and psychological causes of pain (e.g., inflammation; tissue trauma, fractures; surgery; infections; heart attack or angina; abdominal conditions [e.g., appendicitis, cholecystitis]; burns; grief; fear, anxiety; depression; and personality disorders).
- Note location of surgical procedures, **as this can influence the amount of postoperative pain experienced; for example, vertical or diagonal incisions are more painful than transverse or S-shaped. Presence of known or unknown complication(s) may make the pain more severe than anticipated.**
- Assess for referred pain, as appropriate, **to help determine possibility of underlying condition or organ dysfunction requiring treatment.**

Information that appears in brackets has been added by the authors to clarify and enhance the use of nursing diagnoses.

 Diagnostic Studies ∞ Pediatric/Geriatric/Lifespan Medications 587

- Note client's attitude toward pain and use of pain medications, including any history of substance abuse.
- Note client's locus of control (internal or external). **Individuals with external locus of control may take little or no responsibility for pain management.**
- Assist in thorough evaluation, including neurological and psychological factors (pain inventory, psychological interview), as appropriate, when pain persists.

Nursing Priority No. 2.

To evaluate client's response to pain:

- Obtain client's assessment of pain to include location, characteristics, onset and duration, frequency, quality, intensity, and precipitating or aggravating factors. Reassess each time pain occurs/is reported. Note and investigate changes from previous reports **to rule out worsening of underlying condition or development of complications.**
- Use pain rating scale appropriate for age and cognition (e.g., 0–10 scale; facial expression scale [pediatric, nonverbal]; pain assessment scale for dementing elderly [PADE]; behavioral pain scale [BPS]).
- Accept client's description of pain. Acknowledge the pain experience and convey acceptance of client's response to pain. **Pain is a subjective experience and cannot be felt by others.**
- Observe nonverbal cues and pain behaviors (e.g., how client walks, holds body, sits; facial expression; cool fingertips/toes, which can mean constricted blood vessels) and other objective Defining Characteristics, as noted, especially in persons who cannot communicate verbally. **Observations may not be congruent with verbal reports or may be only indicator present when client is unable to verbalize.**
- Ask others who know client well (e.g., spouse, parent) to identify behaviors that may indicate pain **when client is unable to verbalize.**
- Note cultural and developmental influences affecting pain response. **Verbal and/or behavioral cues may have no direct relationship to the degree of pain perceived (e.g., client may deny pain even when feeling uncomfortable, or reactions can be stoic or exaggerated, reflecting cultural or familial norms).**
- Monitor skin color and temperature and vital signs (e.g., heart rate, blood pressure, respirations), **which are usually altered in acute pain.**

Information that appears in brackets has been added by the authors to clarify and enhance the use of nursing diagnoses.

- Ascertain client's knowledge of and expectations about pain management.
- Review client's previous experiences with pain and methods found either helpful or unhelpful for pain control in the past.

Nursing Priority No. 3.

To assist client to explore methods for alleviation/control of pain:

- Determine client's acceptable level of pain and pain control goals. **Varies with individual and situation.**
- **Determine factors in client's lifestyle (e.g., alcohol or other drug use or abuse)** that can affect responses to analgesics and/or choice of interventions for pain management.
- Note when pain occurs (e.g., only with ambulation, every evening) **to medicate prophylactically, as appropriate.**
- Collaborate in treatment of underlying condition or disease processes causing pain and proactive management of pain (e.g., epidural analgesia, nerve blockade for postoperative pain).
- Provide comfort measures (e.g., touch, repositioning, use of heat or cold packs, nurse's presence), quiet environment, and calm activities **to promote nonpharmacological pain management.**
- Instruct in and encourage use of relaxation techniques, such as focused breathing, imaging, CDs/tapes (e.g., "white" noise, music, instructional) **to distract attention and reduce tension.**
- Encourage diversional activities (e.g., TV/radio, socialization with others).
- Review procedures and expectations including when treatment may cause pain **to reduce concern of the unknown and associated muscle tension.**
- Encourage verbalization of feelings about the pain.
- Use puppets to demonstrate procedure for child **to enhance understanding and reduce level of anxiety and fear.**
- Suggest parent be present during procedures **to comfort child.**
- Identify ways of avoiding or minimizing pain (e.g., splinting incision during cough; using firm mattress and proper supporting shoes for low back pain; good body mechanics).
- Work with client to prevent pain. Use flow sheet to document pain, therapeutic interventions, response, and length of time before pain recurs. Instruct client to report pain as soon as it

Information that appears in brackets has been added by the authors to clarify and enhance the use of nursing diagnoses.

begins **as timely intervention is more likely to be successful in alleviating pain.**

🔴 Administer analgesics, as indicated, to maximum dosage, as needed, **to maintain "acceptable" level of pain. Notify physician if regimen is inadequate to meet pain control goal.**

🔴 Demonstrate and monitor use of self-administration/patient-controlled analgesia (PCA) for management of severe, persistent pain.

🔴 Evaluate and document client's response to analgesia, and assist in transitioning or altering drug regimen, based on individual needs and protocols. **Increasing or decreasing dosage, stepped program (switching from injection to oral route, increased time span as pain lessens) helps in self-management of pain.**

🔵 Instruct client in use of transcutaneous electrical stimulation (TENS) unit, when ordered.

Nursing Priority No. 4.
To promote wellness (Teaching/Discharge Considerations):

🏠 Encourage adequate rest periods **to prevent fatigue.**

🏠 Review ways to lessen pain, including techniques such as Therapeutic Touch (TT), biofeedback, self-hypnosis, and relaxation skills.

🏠 Discuss impact of pain on lifestyle/independence and ways to maximize level of functioning.

🔵 Provide for individualized physical therapy or exercise program that can be continued by the client after discharge. **Promotes active, rather than passive, role and enhances sense of control.**

🏠 Discuss with SO(s) ways in which they can assist client and reduce precipitating factors that may cause or increase pain (e.g., participating in household tasks following abdominal surgery).

🔵 Identify specific signs/symptoms and changes in pain characteristics requiring medical follow-up.

Documentation Focus

Assessment/Reassessment
- Individual assessment findings, including client's description of response to pain, specifics of pain inventory, expectations of pain management, and acceptable level of pain.
- Prior medication use; substance abuse.

Information that appears in brackets has been added by the authors to clarify and enhance the use of nursing diagnoses.

🌐 Cultural 🔵 Collaborative 🏠 Community/Home Care

Planning
- Plan of care and who is involved in planning.
- Teaching plan.

Implementation/Evaluation
- Response to interventions, teaching, and actions performed.
- Attainment or progress toward desired outcome(s).
- Modifications to plan of care.

Discharge Planning
- Long-term needs, noting who is responsible for actions to be taken.
- Specific referrals made.

Sample Nursing Outcomes & Interventions Classifications (NOC/NIC) ⬛NIC⬛

NOC—Pain Level
NIC—Pain Management

---

chronic **Pain**

Taxonomy II: Comfort—Class 1 Physical Comfort (00133)
[Diagnostic Division: Pain/Discomfort]
Submitted 1986; Revised 1996

Definition: Unpleasant sensory and emotional experience arising from actual or potential tissue damage or described in terms of such damage (International Association for the Study of Pain); sudden or slow onset of any intensity from mild to severe, constant or recurring without an anticipated or predictable end and a duration of greater than 6 months

---

NOTE: Pain is a signal that something is wrong. Chronic pain can be recurrent and periodically disabling (e.g., migraine headaches) or may be unremitting. While chronic pain syndrome includes various learned behaviors, psychological factors become the primary contribution to impairment. It is a complex entity, combining **elements from other NDs,** such as Powerlessness; deficient Diversional Activity; interrupted Family Processes; Self-Care Deficit; and risk for Disuse Syndrome.

Information that appears in brackets has been added by the authors to clarify and enhance the use of nursing diagnoses.

Related Factors

Chronic physical or psychosocial disability

Defining Characteristics

Subjective
Verbal report of pain; coded report
Fear of reinjury
Altered ability to continue previous activities
Changes in sleep patterns; fatigue; anorexia
Preoccupation with pain
Desperately seeks alternative solutions or therapies for relief or control of pain

Objective
Observed protective or guarding behavior; irritability; restlessness
Facial mask; self-focusing
Reduced interaction with people; depression
Atrophy of involved muscle group
Sympathetic mediated responses (e.g., temperature, cold, changes of body position, hypersensitivity)

Desired Outcomes/Evaluation Criteria— Client Will:

- Verbalize and demonstrate (nonverbal cues) relief and/or control of pain or discomfort.
- Verbalize recognition of interpersonal and family dynamics and reactions that affect the pain situation.
- Demonstrate and initiate behavioral modifications of lifestyle and appropriate use of therapeutic interventions.

Family/SO(s) Will:

- Cooperate in pain management program. (Refer to ND readiness for enhanced family Coping.)

Actions/Interventions

Nursing Priority No. 1.
To assess etiology/precipitating factors:

- Assess for conditions associated with long-term pain (e.g., low back pain, arthritis, fibromyalgia, neuropathies, multiple or slow-healing, traumatic musculoskeletal injuries, amputation

Information that appears in brackets has been added by the authors to clarify and enhance the use of nursing diagnoses.

 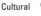 Cultural   Collaborative   Community/Home Care

[phantom limb pain]) **to identify client with potential for pain lasting beyond normal healing period.**

- Assist in thorough diagnosis, including physical, neurological and psychological evaluation (Minnesota Multiphasic Personality Inventory [MMPI], pain inventory, psychological interview), as indicated.
- Evaluate emotionalcomponents of individual situation. Note codependent/enabling behaviors of caregivers and family members **that support continuation of the status quo.**
- Determine cultural factors for the individual situation (e.g., how expression of pain is accepted—moaning aloud or enduring in stoic silence; magnification of symptoms to convince others of reality of pain).
- Note gender and age of client. **Current literature suggests women and men may differ in how they perceive and/or respond to pain. Sensitivity to pain is likely to decline as one gets older.**
- Discuss use of nicotine, sugar, caffeine, white flour, as appropriate **(some holistic practitioners believe these items need to be eliminated from the client's diet to reduce pain).**
- Evaluate current and past analgesic, opioid, other drug use (including alcohol).
- Determine issues of secondary gain for the client/SO(s) (e.g., financial, marital, family concerns, work issues). **May interfere with progress in pain management and resolution of situation.**
- Make home visit when possible, observing such factors as safety equipment, adequate room, colors, plants, family interactions. Note impact of home environment on the client.

Nursing Priority No. 2.

To determine client response to chronic pain situation:

- Acknowledge and assess pain matter-of-factly, avoiding undue expressions of concern while conveying compassionate regard for client's feelings and situation of living with pain and coping with an often ill-defined disability.
- Evaluate pain behaviors. **May be exaggerated because client's perception of pain is not believed or because client believes caregivers are discounting reports of pain.**
- Determine individual client threshold for pain (physical examination, pain profile, etc.).
- Ascertain duration of pain problem, who has been consulted, and what drugs and therapies (including alternative and complementary) have been used **to determine that additional**

Information that appears in brackets has been added by the authors to clarify and enhance the use of nursing diagnoses.

interventions might be beneficial, or that current interventions should be discontinued (either not effective or no longer needed).

- Note lifestyle effects of pain (e.g., decreased activity or deconditioning, severe fatigue, weight loss or gain, sleep difficulties, depression).
- Assess degree of personal maladjustment of the client, such as isolationism, anger, irritability, loss of work time or employment.
- Note availability and use of personal and community resources.

Nursing Priority No. 3.

To assist client to deal with pain:

- Review client pain management goals and expectations versus reality. **Pain may not be completely resolved, but may be significantly lessened to "acceptable level" or managed to the degree that client can participate in desired or needed life activities.**
- Apply pain management interventions, as appropriate (e.g., extended-relief oral pain medications and patches, nerve-blocking injection, implanted pump, electrical stimulation or transcutaneous electrical nerve stimulation [TENS] unit) **to medically intervene, as indicated, in all aspects of long-term pain.**
- Encourage use of nonpharmacological methods of pain control (e.g., heat or cold applications, splinting or exercises, hydrotherapy, deep breathing, meditation, visualization, guided imagery, Therapeutic Touch [TT], posture correction and muscle-strengthening exercises, progressive muscle relaxation, biofeedback, massage).
- Assist client to learn breathing techniques (e.g., diaphragmatic breathing) **to assist in muscle and generalized relaxation.**
- Discuss the physiological dynamics of tension and anxiety and how these affect pain.
- Include client and SO(s) in establishing pattern of discussing pain for specified length of time **to limit focusing on pain.**
- Encourage client to use positive affirmations: "I am healing." "I am relaxed." "I love this life." Have client be aware of internal-external dialogue. Say "cancel" when negative thoughts develop.
- Use tranquilizers, opioids, and analgesics sparingly. **These drugs are physically and psychologically addicting and promote sleep disturbances—especially interfering with**

Information that appears in brackets has been added by the authors to clarify and enhance the use of nursing diagnoses.

⊕ Cultural Ⓐ Collaborative 🏠 Community/Home Care

deep REM (rapid eye movement) sleep. Client may need to be detoxified if many medications are currently used. Note: Antidepressants have an added benefit with analgesic effects because perception of pain decreases as depression is lessened.

* Encourage right-brain stimulation with activities such as love, laughter, and music **to release endorphins, enhancing sense of well-being.**
* Suggest use of subliminal tapes **to bypass logical part of the brain by saying: "I am becoming a more relaxed person." "It is all right for me to relax."**
* Assist family in developing a program of coping strategies (e.g., staying active even when modified activities are required, living a healthy lifestyle, implementing positive reinforcement for all persons, encouraging client to use own control, and diminishing attention given to pain behavior).
* Be alert to changes in pain. **May indicate a new physical problem.**

Nursing Priority No. 4.

To promote wellness (Teaching/Discharge Considerations):

* Provide anticipatory guidance to client with condition in which pain is common and educate about when, where, and how to seek intervention or treatments.
* Assist client and SO(s) to learn how to heal by developing sense of internal control, by being responsible for own treatment, and by obtaining the information and tools to accomplish this.
* Discuss potential for developmental delays in child with chronic pain. Identify current level of function and review appropriate expectations for individual child.
* Review safe use of medications, management of minor side effects, and adverse effects requiring medical intervention.
* Assist client to learn to change pain behavior to wellness behavior: "Act as if you are well."
* Encourage and assist family member/SO(s) to learn massage techniques.
* Recommend that client and SO(s) take time for themselves. **Provides opportunity to reenergize and refocus on tasks at hand.**
* Identify and discuss potential hazards of unproved and/or nonmedical therapies and remedies.
* Identify community support groups and other resources to meet individual needs (e.g., Back Pain Support Group, www .chronicpain.org; yard care, home maintenance, alternative

---

Information that appears in brackets has been added by the authors to clarify and enhance the use of nursing diagnoses.

transportation). **Proper use of resources may reduce negative pattern of "overdoing" heavy activities, then spending several days in bed recuperating.**

- Refer for individual or other therapies (e.g., family counseling, marital therapy, parent effectiveness classes), as needed. **Presence of chronic pain affects all relationships and family dynamics.**
- Refer to NDs ineffective Coping; compromised family Coping.

Documentation Focus

Assessment/Reassessment
- Individual findings, including duration of problem, specific contributing factors, previously and currently used interventions.
- Perception of pain, effects on lifestyle, and expectations of therapeutic regimen.
- Family's/SO's response to client, and support for change.

Planning
- Plan of care and who is involved in planning.
- Teaching plan.

Implementation/Evaluation
- Responses to interventions, teaching, and actions performed.
- Attainment or progress toward desired outcome(s).
- Modifications to plan of care.

Discharge Planning
- Long-term needs and who is responsible for actions to be taken.
- Specific referrals made.

Sample Nursing Outcomes & Interventions Classifications (NOC/NIC) NIC

NOC—Pain Control
NIC—Pain Management

Information that appears in brackets has been added by the authors to clarify and enhance the use of nursing diagnoses.

 Cultural   Collaborative   Community/Home Care

impaired Parenting

Taxonomy II: Role Relationships—Class 1 Caregiving
   Roles (00056)
[Diagnostic Division: Social Interaction]
Submitted 1998; Nursing Diagnosis Extension and
   Classification (NDEC) Revision 1998

Definition: Inability of the primary caretaker to create,
maintain, or regain an environment that promotes the
optimum growth and development of the child

[NOTE: It is important to reaffirm that adjustment to
parenting in general is a normal maturational process
that elicits nursing behaviors to prevent potential
problems and to promote a healthy relationship.]

Related Factors

Infant or Child
Premature birth; multiple births; not desired gender
Illness; separation from parent
Difficult temperament; temperamental conflicts with parental
   expectations
Handicapping condition; developmental delay; altered percep-
   tual abilities; attention-deficit hyperactivity disorder

Knowledge
Deficient knowledge about child development or health main-
   tenance, or parenting skills; inability to respond to infant cues
Unrealistic expectations [for self, infant, partner]
Lack of education; limited cognitive functioning; lack of cog-
   nitive readiness for parenthood
Poor communication skills
Preference for physical punishment

Physiological
Physical illness

Psychological
Young parental age
Lack of prenatal care; difficult birthing process; high number
   of/closely spaced pregnancies

Information that appears in brackets has been added by the authors to clarify
and enhance the use of nursing diagnoses.

Sleep disruption or deprivation; depression
History of mental illness or substance abuse
Disability

Social

Presence of stress (e.g., financial, legal, recent crisis, cultural move [from another country/cultural group within same country]); job problems; unemployment; financial difficulties; relocations; poor home environment

Situational or chronic low self-esteem

Lack of family cohesiveness; marital conflict; change in family unit; inadequate childcare arrangements

Role strain; single parent; father or mother of child not involved

Lack of or poor parental role model; lack of valuing of parenthood; inability to put child's needs before own

Unplanned or unwanted pregnancy

Low socioeconomic class; poverty; lack of resources; lack of transportation

Poor problem-solving skills; maladaptive coping strategies

Lack of social support networks; social isolation

History of being abusive or being abused; legal difficulties

Defining Characteristics

Subjective

Parental

Statements of inability to meet child's needs; verbalization of inability to control child

Negative statements about child

Verbalization of frustration or role inadequacy

Objective

Infant or Child

Frequent accidents or illness; failure to thrive

Poor academic performance or cognitive development

Poor social competence; behavioral disorders

Incidence of trauma (e.g., physical and psychological)/abuse

Lack of attachment or separation anxiety; runaway

Parental

Maternal-child interaction deficit; poor parent-child interaction; little cuddling; inadequate attachment

---

Information that appears in brackets has been added by the authors to clarify and enhance the use of nursing diagnoses.

Cultural Collaborative Community/Home Care

Inadequate child health maintenance; unsafe home environment; inappropriate childcare arrangements; inappropriate stimulation (e.g., visual, tactile, auditory)

Inappropriate caretaking skills; inconsistent care/behavior management

Inflexibility in meeting needs of child

Frequently punitive; rejection of or hostility to child; child abuse or neglect; abandonment

Desired Outcomes/Evaluation Criteria—Parents Will:

- Verbalize realistic information and expectations of parenting role.
- Verbalize acceptance of the individual situation.
- Participate in appropriate classes (e.g., parenting class).
- Identify own strengths, individual needs, and methods and resources to meet them.
- Demonstrate appropriate attachment and parenting behaviors.

Actions/Interventions

Nursing Priority No. 1.

To assess causative/contributing factors:

- Note family constellation; for example, two-parent, single, extended family, or child living with other relative, such as grandparent.
- Determine developmental stage of the family (e.g., new baby, adolescent, child leaving or returning home).
- Assess family relationships between individual members and with others.
- Assess parenting skill level, taking into account the individual's intellectual, emotional, and physical strengths and weaknesses. **Parents with significant impairments may need more education and support.**
- Observe attachment behaviors between parental figure and child. Determine cultural significance of behaviors. (Refer to ND risk for impaired Attachment.)
- Note presence of factors in the child (e.g., birth defects, hyperactivity) **that may affect attachment and caretaking needs.**
- Identify physical challenges or limitations of the parents (e.g., visual or hearing impairment, quadriplegia, severe depression). **May affect ability to care for child and suggest individual needs for assistance and support.**

Information that appears in brackets has been added by the authors to clarify and enhance the use of nursing diagnoses.

 Diagnostic Studies   ∞ Pediatric/Geriatric/Lifespan   Medications **599**

- Determine presence and effectiveness of support systems, role models, extended family, and community resources available to the parent(s).
- Note absence from home setting or lack of child supervision by parent (e.g., working long hours or out of town; multiple responsibilities, such as working and attending educational classes).

Nursing Priority No. 2.
To foster development of parenting skills:

- Create an environment in which relationships can be developed and needs of each individual met. **Learning is more effective when individuals feel safe.**
- Make time for listening to concerns of the parent(s).
- Emphasize positive aspects of the situation, maintaining a hopeful attitude toward the parent's capabilities and potential for improving the situation.
- Note staff attitudes toward parent/child and specific problem or disability; for example, needs of disabled parent(s) to be seen as an individual and to be evaluated apart from a stereotype. **Negative attitudes are detrimental to promoting positive outcomes.**
- Encourage expression of feelings, such as helplessness, anger, frustration. Set limits on unacceptable behaviors. **Individuals who lose control develop feelings of low self-esteem.**
- Acknowledge difficulty of situation and normalcy of feelings. **Enhances feelings of acceptance.**
- Recognize stages of grieving process when the child is disabled or other than anticipated (e.g., girl instead of boy, misshapen head, prominent birthmark). Allow time for parents to express feelings and deal with the "loss."
- Encourage attendance at skill classes (e.g., parent effectiveness). **Assists in improving parenting skills by developing communication and problem-solving techniques.**
- Emphasize parenting functions rather than mothering/fathering skills. **By virtue of gender, each person brings something to the parenting role; however, nurturing tasks can be done by both parents.**

Nursing Priority No. 3.
To promote wellness (Teaching/Discharge Considerations):

- Involve all available members of the family in learning.
- Provide information appropriate to the situation, including time management, limit setting, and stress-reduction techniques.

Information that appears in brackets has been added by the authors to clarify and enhance the use of nursing diagnoses.

🌐 Cultural   🐱 Collaborative   🏠 Community/Home Care

Facilitates satisfactory implementation of plan and new behaviors.

• Discuss parental beliefs about childrearing, punishment and rewards, teaching. **Identifying these beliefs allows opportunity to provide new information regarding not using spanking and/or yelling and what actions can be substituted for more effective parenting.**

• Develop support systems appropriate to the situation (e.g., extended family, friends, social worker, home-care services).

• Assist parent to plan time and conserve energy in positive ways. **Enables individual to cope more effectively with difficulties as they arise.**

• Encourage parents to identify positive outlets for meeting their own needs (e.g., going out for dinner, making time for their own interests and each other, dating). **Promotes general well-being, helps parents to be more effective and reduces burnout.**

• Refer to appropriate support or therapy groups, as indicated.

• Identify community resources (e.g., childcare services, respite house) **to assist with individual needs, provide respite and support.**

• Report and take necessary actions, as legally and professionally indicated, if child's safety is a concern. **Parents/caregivers who engage in corporal punishment as a technique to ensure desired behavior of child are at increased risk for abusive behavior and possibility of childhood depression.**

• Refer to NDs ineffective Coping; compromised family Coping; risk for Violence [specify]; Self-Esteem [specify]; and interrupted Family Processes.

Documentation Focus

Assessment/Reassessment
• Individual findings, including parenting skill level, deviations from normal parenting expectations, family makeup, and developmental stages.
• Availability and use of support systems and community resources.

Planning
• Plan of care and who is involved in planning.
• Teaching plan.

Information that appears in brackets has been added by the authors to clarify and enhance the use of nursing diagnoses.

Diagnostic Studies   ∞ Pediatric/Geriatric/Lifespan   Medications **601**

Implementation/Evaluation

- Responses by parent(s)/child to interventions, teaching, and actions performed.
- Attainment or progress toward desired outcome(s).
- Modification to plan of care.

Discharge Planning

- Long-term needs and who is responsible for actions to be taken.
- Specific referrals made.

Sample Nursing Outcomes & Interventions Classifications (NOC/NIC) NIC

NOC—Parenting Performance
NIC—Parenting Promotion

---

readiness for enhanced Parenting

Taxonomy II: Role Relationships—Class 1 Caregiving
  Roles (00164)
[Diagnostic Division: social interaction]
Submitted 2002

Definition: A pattern of providing an environment for children or other dependent person(s) that is sufficient to nurture growth and development and can be strengthened

---

Related Factors

To be developed

Defining Characteristics

Subjective
Expresses willingness to enhance parenting
Children or other dependent person(s) express(es) satisfaction with home environment

Objective
Emotional support of children[/dependent person(s)]; evidence of attachment
Needs of children[/dependent person(s)] are met (e.g., physical and emotional)

Information that appears in brackets has been added by the authors to clarify and enhance the use of nursing diagnoses.

　🌐 Cultural　🤝 Collaborative　🏠 Community/Home Care

Exhibits realistic expectations of children[/dependent person(s)]

Desired Outcomes/Evaluation Criteria— Parents Will:

- Verbalize realistic information and expectations of parenting role.
- Identify own strengths, individual needs, and methods and resources to meet them.
- Participate in activities to enhance parenting skills.
- Demonstrate improved parenting behaviors.

Actions/Interventions

Nursing Priority No. 1.
To determine need/motivation for improvement:

- Ascertain motivation and expectation for change.
- Note family constellation: two-parent; single parent; extended family; child living with other relative, such as grandparent; or relationship of dependent person. **Understanding makeup of the family provides information about needs to assist individuals in improving their family connections.**
- Determine developmental stage of the family (e.g., new child, adolescent, child leaving/returning home, retirement). **These maturational crises bring changes in the family, which can provide opportunity for enhancing parenting skills and improving family interactions.**
- Assess family relationships and identify needs of individual members, noting any special concerns that exist, such as birth defects, illness, hyperactivity. **The family is a system, and when members make decisions to improve parenting skills, the changes affect all parts of the system. Identifying needs, special situations, and relationships can help in the development of a plan to bring about effective change.**
- Assess parenting skill level, taking into account the individual's intellectual, emotional, and physical strengths and weaknesses. **Identifies areas of need for education, skill training, and information on which to base plan for enhancing parenting skills.**
- Observe attachment behaviors between parent(s) and child(ren), recognizing cultural background that may influence expected behaviors. **Behaviors such as eye-to-eye contact, use of en face position, talking to infant in high-pitched**

Information that appears in brackets has been added by the authors to clarify and enhance the use of nursing diagnoses.

voice, are indicative of attachment behaviors in American culture, but may not be appropriate in another culture. Failure to bond is thought to affect subsequent parent-child interactions.

- Determine presence and effectiveness of support systems, role models, extended family, and community resources available to the parent(s). **Parents desiring to enhance abilities and improve family life can benefit by role models that help them develop their own style of parenting.**
- Note cultural or religious influences on parenting, expectations of self and child, sense of success or failure. **Expectations may vary with different cultures (e.g., Arab-Americans hold children to be sacred, but childrearing is based on negative rather than positive reinforcements, and parents are more strict with girls than with boys). These beliefs may interfere with desire to improve parenting skills when there is conflict between the two.**

Nursing Priority No. 2.

To foster improvement of parenting skills:

- Create an environment in which relationships can be strengthened. **A safe environment in which individuals can freely express their thoughts and feelings optimizes learning and positive interactions among family members, thus enhancing relationships.**
- Make time for listening to concerns of the parent(s). **Promotes sense of importance and of being heard and identifies accurate information regarding needs of the family for enhancing relationships.**
- Encourage expression of feelings, such as frustration or anger, while setting limits on unacceptable behaviors. **Identification of feelings promotes understanding of self and enhances connections with others in the family. Unacceptable behaviors result in diminished self-esteem and can lead to problems in the family relationships.**
- Emphasize parenting functions rather than mothering/fathering skills. **By virtue of gender, each person brings something to the parenting role; however, nurturing tasks can be done by both parents, enhancing family relationships.**
- Encourage attendance at skill classes, such as Parent or Family Effectiveness Training. **Assists in developing communication skills of Active-listening, I-messages, and problem-solving techniques to improve family relationships and promote a win-win environment.**

Information that appears in brackets has been added by the authors to clarify and enhance the use of nursing diagnoses.

Nursing Priority No. 3.

To promote optimal wellness:

· Involve all members of the family in learning. **The family system benefits from all members participating in learning new skills to enhance family relationships.**

· Encourage parents to identify positive outlets for meeting their own needs. **Activities, such as going out for dinner or dating, making time for their own interests and each other, promote general well-being and can enhance family relationships and improve family functioning.**

· Provide information, as indicated, including time management, stress-reduction techniques. **Learning about positive parenting skills, understanding growth and developmental expectations, and discovering ways to reduce stress and anxiety promote the individual's ability to deal with problems that may arise in the course of family relationships.**

· Discuss current "family rules," identifying areas of needed change. **Rules may be imposed by adults, rather than through a democratic process involving all family members, leading to conflict and angry confrontations. Setting positive family rules with all family members participating can promote an effective, functional family.**

· Discuss need for long-term planning and ways in which family can maintain desired positive relationships. **Each stage of life brings its own challenges and understanding and preparing for each stage enables family members to move through them in positive ways, promoting family unity and resolving inevitable conflicts with win-win solutions.**

Documentation Focus

Assessment/Reassessment

- Individual findings, including parenting skill level, parenting expectations, family makeup, and developmental stages.
- Availability and use of support systems and community resources.
- Motivation and expectations for change.

Planning

- Plan for enhancement, who is involved in planning.
- Teaching plan.

Implementation/Evaluation

- Family members' responses to interventions, teaching, and actions performed.

Information that appears in brackets has been added by the authors to clarify and enhance the use of nursing diagnoses.

- Attainment or progress toward desired outcome(s).
- Modifications to plan.

Discharge Planning
- Long-term needs and who is responsible for actions to be taken.
- Modification to plan.

Sample Nursing Outcomes & Interventions Classifications (NOC/NIC) NIC

NOC—Parenting Performance
NIC—Parent Education: Childrearing Family

---

risk for impaired Parenting

Taxonomy II: Role Relationships—Class 1 Caregiving Roles (00057)
[Diagnostic Division: Social Interaction]
Submitted 1978; Nursing Diagnosis Extension and Classification (NDEC) Revision 1998

Definition: Risk for inability of the primary caretaker to create, maintain, or regain an environment that promotes the optimum growth and development of the child

---

[NOTE: It is important to reaffirm that adjustment to parenting in general is a normal maturational process that elicits nursing behaviors to prevent potential problems and to promote a healthy relationship.]

Risk Factors

Infant or Child
Altered perceptual abilities; attention deficit-hyperactivity disorder
Difficult temperament; temperament conflicts with parental expectation
Premature birth; multiple births; not gender desired
Handicapping condition; developmental delay
Illness; prolonged separation from parent

Information that appears in brackets has been added by the authors to clarify and enhance the use of nursing diagnoses.

  Cultural Collaborative Community/Home Care

Knowledge

Unrealistic expectations of child; deficient knowledge about child development or health maintenance, or parenting skills

Low educational level or attainment; lack of cognitive readiness for parenthood; low cognitive functioning

Poor communication skills

Inability to respond to infant cues

Preference for physical punishment

Physiological

Physical illness

Psychological

Young parental age

Closely spaced pregnancies; high number of pregnancies; difficult birthing process

Sleep disruption or deprivation

Depression; history of mental illness or substance abuse

Disability

Social

Stress; job problems; unemployment; financial difficulties; poor home environment; relocation

Situational or chronic low self-esteem

Lack of family cohesiveness; marital conflict; change in family unit; inadequate childcare arrangements

Role strain; single parent; father or mother of child not involved; parent-child separation

Poor or lack of parental role model; lack of valuing of parenthood

Unplanned or unwanted pregnancy; late or lack of prenatal care

Low socioeconomic class; poverty; lack of resources or access to resources; lack of transportation

Poor problem-solving skills; maladaptive coping strategies

Lack of social support network; social isolation

History of being abused or being abusive; legal difficulties

> **NOTE:** A risk diagnosis is not evidenced by signs and symptoms, as the problem has not occurred; rather, nursing interventions are directed at prevention.

Information that appears in brackets has been added by the authors to clarify and enhance the use of nursing diagnoses.

Desired Outcomes/Evaluation Criteria—Parents Will:

- Verbalize awareness of individual risk factors.
- Identify own strengths, individual needs, and methods and resources to meet them.
- Demonstrate behavior and lifestyle changes to reduce potential for development of problem or reduce or eliminate effects of risk factors.
- Participate in activities, classes to promote growth.

Refer to NDs impaired Parenting; risk for impaired Attachment for interventions and documentation focus.

Sample Nursing Outcomes & Interventions Classifications (NOC/NIC) NIC

NOC—Parenting Performance
NIC—Parenting Promotion

---

ineffective peripheral tissue Perfusion

Taxonomy II: Activity/Rest—Class 4 Cardiovascular/Pulmonary Responses (00204)
[Diagnostic Division: Circulation]
Submitted 2008

Definition: Decrease in blood circulation to the periphery that may compromise health

---

Related Factors:

Deficient knowledge of aggravating factors (e.g., smoking, sedentary lifestyle, trauma, obesity, salt intake, immobility)
Deficient knowledge of disease process (e.g., diabetes, hyperlipidemia; [peripheral artery disease, chronic venous insufficiency])
Hypertension
Sedentary lifestyle
Smoking

Defining Characteristics

Subjective
Extremity pain; claudication
Paresthesia; [altered sensations]

Information that appears in brackets has been added by the authors to clarify and enhance the use of nursing diagnoses.

 Cultural   Collaborative   Community/Home Care

Objective

Diminished or absent pulses; [diminished arterial pulsations; bruits; blood pressure changes in extremities]

Altered skin characteristics (color, elasticity, hair, moisture, nails, sensation, temperature)

Skin color pale on elevation; color does not return to leg on lowering it; [skin erythema or dependent rubor with chronic dryness, scaling, flaking]

[Varicosities; spider veins]

Edema

Altered motor function

Delayed peripheral wound healing; [ulcerations]

Desired Outcomes/Evaluation Criteria—Client Will (include specific time frame):

- Demonstrate increased perfusion as individually appropriate (e.g., skin warm and dry, peripheral pulses present and strong, absence of edema, free of pain or discomfort).
- Verbalize understanding of condition, therapy regimen, side effects of medications, and when to contact healthcare provider.
- Demonstrate behaviors and lifestyle changes to improve circulation (e.g., engage in regular exercise, cessation of smoking, weight reduction, disease management).

Actions/Interventions

Nursing Priority No. 1.

To assess causative/contributing factors:

- Note current situation or presence of conditions that can affect perfusion to all body systems (e.g., congestive heart failure, lung disorders, major trauma, septic or hypovolemic shock, coagulopathies, sickle cell anemia) **affecting systemic circulation/perfusion.**
- Determine history of conditions associated with thrombus or emboli (e.g., problems with coronary or cerebral circulation, stroke; high-velocity trauma with fractures, abdominal or orthopedic surgery, long periods of immobility; inflammatory diseases; chronic lung disease; diabetes with coexisting peripheral vascular disease; estrogen therapy, cancer and cancer therapies, presence of central venous catheters) **to identify client at higher risk for venous stasis, vessel wall injury, and hypercoagulability.**

Information that appears in brackets has been added by the authors to clarify and enhance the use of nursing diagnoses.

- Identify presence of high-risk factors or conditions (e.g., smoking, uncontrolled hypertension, obesity, pregnancy, pelvic tumor, paralysis, hypercholesterolemia, varicose veins, arthritis, sepsis) that place client at greater risk for developing peripheral vascular disease (including arterial blockage and chronic venous insufficiency) with associated complications.
- Note location of restrictive clothing, pressure dressings, circular wraps, cast, or traction device **that may restrict circulation to limb.**
- Ascertain impact of condition on functioning and lifestyle.

Nursing Priority No. 2.
To evaluate degree of impairment:

- Compare skin temperature and color with other limb when assessing extremity circulation. **Helps differentiate type of problem (e.g., deep redness in both hands triggered by vibrating machinery is associated with Raynaud's; while edema, redness, swelling in calf of one leg is associated with localized thrombophlebitis).**
- Assess presence, location, and degree of swelling or edema formation. Measure circumference of extremities, noting differences in size. **Useful in identifying or quantifying edema in involved extremity.**
- Measure capillary refill **to determine adequacy of systemic circulation.**
- Note client's nutritional and fluid status. **Protein-energy malnutrition and weight loss make ischemic tissues more prone to breakdown. Dehydration reduces blood volume and compromises peripheral circulation.**
- Inspect lower extremities for skin texture (e.g., atrophic, shiny appearance, lack of hair; or dry/scaly, reddened skin), and skin breaks or ulcerations **that often accompany diminished peripheral circulation.**
- Palpate arterial pulses (bilateral femoral, popliteal, dorsalis pedis, and posterial tibial), using handheld Doppler if indicated **to determine level of circulatory blockage.**
- Note whether activity alters pulses (**e.g., client with intermittent claudication may have palpable pulses that disappear after ambulation**).
- Determine pulse equality, as well as intensity, (e.g., bounding, normal, diminished, or absent) and compare with unaffected extremity **to evaluate distribution and quality of blood flow, and success or failure of therapy.**

Information that appears in brackets has been added by the authors to clarify and enhance the use of nursing diagnoses.

- Evaluate extremity pain reports, noting associated symptoms (e.g., cramping or heaviness, discomfort with walking; progressive temperature or color changes; paresthesias).
- Determine time (day or night) that symptoms are worse, precipitating or aggravating events (e.g., walking), and relieving factors (e.g., rest, sitting down with legs in dependent position, oral analgesics) **to help isolate and differentiate problems such as intermittent chronic claudication versus loss of function and pain due to acute sustained ischemia related to loss of arterial blood flow.**
- Assess motor and sensory function. **Problems with ambulation; hypersensitivity; or loss of sensation, numbness and tingling are changes that can indicate neurovascular dysfunction or limb ischemia.**
- Check for calf tenderness or pain on dorsiflexion of foot (Homans' sign), swelling and redness. **Indicators of deep vein thrombosis (DVT), although DVT is often present without a positive Homans' sign.**
- Review laboratory studies such as clotting times, Hb/Hct, renal or cardiac function tests; and diagnostic studies (e.g., Doppler ultrasound, magnetic resonance angiography [MRA], venogram, contrast angiography; resting ankle-brachial index [ABI], leg segmental arterial pressure measurements).

Nursing Priority No. 3.

To maximize tissue perfusion:

- Collaborate in treatment of underlying conditions, such as diabetes, hypertension, cardiopulmonary conditions, blood disorders, traumatic injury, hypovolemia, hypoxemia **to maximize systemic circulation and organ perfusion.**
- Administer medications such as antiplatelet agents, thrombolytics, antibiotics **to improve tissue perfusion or organ function.**
- Administer fluids, electrolytes, nutrients, and oxygen as indicated **to promote optimal blood flow, organ perfusion, and function.**
- Assist with or prepare for medical procedures such as endovascular stent placement, surgical revascularization procedures, thrombectomy, **to improve peripheral circulation.**
- Assist with application of elasticized tubular support bandages, adhesive elastic or Velcro wraps (e.g., Circ-Aid), medication-impregnated layered bandage (e.g., Unna boot), multilayer bandage regimens, sequential pneumatic

---

Information that appears in brackets has been added by the authors to clarify and enhance the use of nursing diagnoses.

 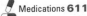

compression devices, and custom-fitted compression stockings, as indicated **to provide graduated compression of lower extremity in presence of venous stasis ulcer.**

- Refer to wound care specialist if arterial or venous ulcerations are present for in-depth wound care interventions.
- Provide interventions **to promote peripheral circulation and limit complications associated with poor perfusion and tissue injury:**

Encourage early ambulation when possible, and recommend regular exercise.

Recommend or provide foot and ankle exercises when client unable to ambulate freely.

Provide pressure-relieving devices for immobilized client (e.g., air mattress, foam or sheepskin padding, bed or foot cradle).

Apply intermittent compression devices and/or elastic compression stockings to lower extremities.

Assist or instruct client to change position at timed intervals, rather than using presence of pain as signal to change positions.

Elevate legs when sitting; avoid sharp angulation of the hips or knees.

Avoid massaging the leg in presence of thrombosis.

Avoid, or carefully monitor, use of heat or cold, such as hot water bottle, heating pad, or ice pack.

Refer to NDs risk for Peripheral Neurovascular Dysfunction, risk for impaired Skin Integrity, impaired Tissue Integrity, and disturbed Sensory Perception for additional interventions as appropriate.

Nursing Priority No. 4.

To promote wellness (Teaching/Discharge Considerations):

- Discuss relevant risk factors (e.g., family history, obesity, age, smoking, hypertension, diabetes, clotting disorders) and potential outcomes of atherosclerosis (e.g., systemic and peripheral vascular disease conditions). **Information necessary for client to make informed choices about remedial risk factors and commit to lifestyle changes.**
- Identify necessary changes in lifestyle and assist client to incorporate disease management into ADLs. **Promotes independence, enhances self-concept regarding ability to deal with change and manage own needs.**

Information that appears in brackets has been added by the authors to clarify and enhance the use of nursing diagnoses.

⊕ Cultural Ⓐ Collaborative 🏠 Community/Home Care

- Emphasize need for regular exercise program **to enhance circulation and promote general well-being.**
- Refer to dietitian for well-balanced, low-saturated-fat, low-cholesterol diet, or other modifications as indicated.
- Discuss care of dependent limbs, foot care as appropriate. **When circulation is impaired, changes in sensation place client at risk for development of lesions or ulcerations that are often slow to heal.**
- Discourage sitting or standing for extended periods of time, wearing constrictive clothing, or crossing legs when seated, **which restricts circulation and leads to venous stasis and edema.**
- Provide education about relationship between smoking and peripheral vascular circulation, as indicated. **Smoking contributes to development and progression of peripheral vascular disease, and is associated with higher rate of amputation in presence of Buerger's disease.**
- Educate client/SO in reportable symptoms, including any changes in pain level, difficulty walking, nonhealing wounds **to provide opportunity for timely evaluation and intervention.**
- Stress need for regular medical and laboratory follow-up **to evaluate disease progression and response to therapies.**
- Review medication regimen and possible harmful side effects with client/SO. **Client may be on various drugs (e.g., antiplatelet agents, blood-viscosity-reducing agents, vasodilators, anticoagulants, or cholesterol-lowering agents) for treatment of the particular vascular disorder. Many of these medications have harmful side effects and require client teaching and ongoing medical monitoring.**
- Emphasize importance of avoiding use of aspirin, some OTC drugs and supplements, or alcohol when taking anticoagulants.
- Refer to community resources such as smoking cessation assistance, weight control program, and exercise group **to provide support for lifestyle changes.**

Documentation Focus

Assessment/Reassessment
- Individual findings, noting nature, extent, and duration of problem, effect on independence and lifestyle.
- Characteristics of pain, precipitators, and what relieves pain.

Information that appears in brackets has been added by the authors to clarify and enhance the use of nursing diagnoses.

- Pulses and BP, including above and below suspected lesion as appropriate.

Planning
- Plan of care and who is involved in planning.
- Teaching plan.

Implementation/Evaluation
- Response to interventions, teaching, and actions performed.
- Attainment or progress toward desired outcome(s).
- Modifications to plan of care.

Discharge Planning
- Long-term needs and who is responsible for actions to be taken.
- Available resources, specific referrals made.

Sample Nursing Outcomes & Interventions Classifications (NOC/NIC) NIC

NOC—Tissue Perfusion: Peripheral
NIC—Circulatory Care: Arterial [or] Venous Insufficiency

risk for decreased cardiac tissue Perfusion

Taxonomy II: Activity/Rest—Class 4 Cardiovascular/
   Pulmonary Responses (00200)
[Diagnostic Division: Circulation]
Submitted 2008

Definition: At risk for decrease in cardiac (coronary) circulation

Risk Factors

Coronary artery spasm; cardiac surgery; cardiac tamponade
Lack of knowledge of modifiable risk factors (e.g., smoking, sedentary lifestyle, obesity); hypertension; hyperlipidemia
Birth control pills
Drug abuse
Elevated C-reactive protein; hypoxemia; hypoxia
Family history of coronary artery disease

Information that appears in brackets has been added by the authors to clarify and enhance the use of nursing diagnoses.

🌐 Cultural 🅐 Collaborative 🏠 Community/Home Care

> **NOTE:** A risk diagnosis is not evidenced by signs and symptoms, as the problem has not occurred; rather, nursing interventions are directed at prevention.

Desired Outcomes/Evaluation Criteria— Client Will:

- Demonstrate adequate coronary perfusion as individually appropriate (e.g., vital signs within client's normal range, free of chest pain or discomfort).
- Identify individual risk factors.
- Verbalize understanding of treatment regimen.
- Demonstrate behaviors and lifestyle changes to maintain or maximize circulation (e.g., cessation of smoking, relaxation techniques, exercise/dietary program).

Actions/Interventions

Nursing Priority No. 1.

To identify individual risk factors:

- Note presence of conditions such as congestive heart failure, major trauma with blood loss, recent coronary artery bypass graft (CABG) surgery or use of intra-aortic balloon pump, chronic anemia, sepsis, **which can affect systemic circulation, tissue oxygenation, and organ function.**
- Note client's age and gender when assessing risk for coronary artery spasm or myocardial infarction. **Risk for heart disorders increases with age. Although men are still considered at higher risk for myocardial infarction and experience them earlier in life, the rate of mortality among women with coronary artery disease is rising.**
- Identify lifestyle issues such as obesity, smoking, high cholesterol, excessive alcohol intake, use of drugs such as cocaine, and physical inactivity, **which can raise client's risk for coronary artery disease and impaired cardiac tissue perfusion.**
- Determine presence of breathing problems, such as obstructive sleep apnea with oxygen desaturation, **which can produce alveolar hypoventilation, respiratory acidosis and hypoxia, resulting in cardiac dysrhythmias and cardiac dysfunction.**
- Determine if client is experiencing usual degree or prolonged stress, or may have underlying psychiatric disorder (e.g., anxiety or panic).

Information that appears in brackets has been added by the authors to clarify and enhance the use of nursing diagnoses.

- Review client's medications **to note current use of vasoactive drugs such as nitroglycerin, calcium channel blockers, beta-adrenergic blockers that can exert undesirable side effects, increasing myocardial workload and oxygen consumption.**
- Review diagnostic studies (e.g., ECG, echocardiogram, angiography, Doppler ultrasound, chest radiography; pulse oximetry, oxygen saturation, capnometry,or ABGs; electrolytes, BUN/Cr, cardiac enzymes) **to identify conditions requiring treatment, and/or response to therapies.**

Nursing Priority No. 2.
To determine changes in cardiac status:

- Investigate reports of chest pain, noting changes in characteristics of pain **to evaluate for potential myocardial ischemia, or inadequate systemic oxygenation or perfusion of organs.**
- Monitor vital signs, especially noting blood pressure changes, including hypertension or hypotension.
- Assess heart sounds and pulses for dysrhythmias.
- Assess for restlessness, fatigue, changes in level of consciousness, decreased capillary refill time, diminished peripheral pulses, and pale, cool skin. **Signs and symptoms of inadequate systemic perfusion, which can affect cardiac function.**
- Inspect for pallor, mottling, cool or clammy skin, and diminished pulses **indicative of systemic vasoconstriction resulting from reduced cardiac output.**
- Investigate reports of difficulty breathing or respiratory rate outside acceptable parameters, **which can be indicative of oxygen exchange problems.**

Nursing Priority No. 3.
To maintain/maximize cardiac perfusion:

- Collaborate in treatment of underlying conditions.
- Provide supplemental oxygen as indicated **to improve or maintain cardiac and systemic tissue perfusion.**
- Administer fluids and electrolytes as indicated **to maintain systemic circulation and optimal cardiac function.**
- Administer medications (e.g., antihypertensive agents, analgesics, antidysrhythmics, bronchodilators, fibrinolytic agents).
- Provide periods of undisturbed rest and calming environment **to reduce myocardial workload.**

Information that appears in brackets has been added by the authors to clarify and enhance the use of nursing diagnoses.

🌐 Cultural   🅐 Collaborative   🏠 Community/Home Care

Nursing Priority No. 4.
To promote wellness (Teaching/Discharge Considerations):

- Discuss risk factors (e.g., family history, obesity, age, smoking, hypertension, diabetes, clotting disorders) and potential outcomes of atherosclerosis (e.g., systemic and cardiac disease conditions).
- Review modifiable risk factors **to assist client/SO in understanding those areas in which he or she can take action or make healthy-heart choices.**

  Recommend maintenance of normal weight, or weight loss if client obese. Review specific dietary concerns with client (e.g., reducing animal and dairy fats; increasing plant foods—fruits, vegetables, olive oil, nuts).

  Encourage smoking cessation, when indicated, offering information about smoking-cessation aids and programs.

  Encourage client to engage in regular exercise.

  Discuss cardiac effects of drug use, where indicated (including cocaine, methamphetamines, alcohol).

  Discuss coping and stress tolerance.

  Demonstrate and encourage use of relaxation and stress management techniques.

  Encourage client in high-risk categories (e.g., strong family history, diabetic, prior history of cardiac event) to have regular medical examinations.

- Review medications on regular basis **to manage those that affect cardiac function or those given to prevent blood pressure or thromboembolic problems.**
- Refer to educational/community resources, as indicated. **Client/SO may benefit from support to engage in healthier heart activities (e.g., weight loss, smoking cessation, exercise).**
- Instruct in blood pressure monitoring at home, if indicated; advise purchase of home monitoring equipment. **Facilitates management of hypertension, a major risk factor for damage to blood vessels, which contributes to coronary artery disease.**

Documentation Focus

Assessment/Reassessment
- Individual findings, noting specific risk factors.
- Vital signs, cardiac rhythm, presence of dysrhythmias.

Information that appears in brackets has been added by the authors to clarify and enhance the use of nursing diagnoses.

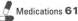

Planning
* Plan of care and who is involved in planning.
* Teaching plan.

Implementation/Evaluation
* Response to interventions, teaching, and actions performed.
* Attainment or progress toward desired outcome(s).
* Modifications to plan of care.

Discharge Planning
* Long-term needs and who is responsible for actions to be taken.
* Available resources, specific referrals made.

Sample Nursing Outcomes & Interventions Classifications (NOC/NIC) NIC

NOC—Tissue Perfusion: Cardiac
NIC—Cardiac Precautions

> ### risk for ineffective cerebral tissue **Perfusion**
>
> Taxonomy II: Activity/Rest—Class 4 Cardiovascular/
>   Pulmonary Responses (00201)
> [Diagnostic Division: Circulation]
> Submitted 2008
>
> **Definition:** At risk for a decrease in cerebral tissue circulation

Risk Factors:

Head trauma; cerebral aneurysm; brain tumor; neoplasm of the brain

Carotid stenosis; aortic atherosclerosis; arterial dissection

Atrial fibrillation; sick sinus syndrome; atrial myxoma; left atrial appendage thrombosis

Recent myocardial infarction; akinetic left ventricular segment; dilated cardiomyopathy; mitral stenosis; mechanical prosthetic valve; infective endocarditis; embolism

Coagulopathy (e.g., sickle cell anemia ; disseminated intravascular coagulation); abnormal partial thromboplastin time; abnormal prothrombin time

Hypertension; hypercholesterolemia

Information that appears in brackets has been added by the authors to clarify and enhance the use of nursing diagnoses.

Substance abuse

Treatment-related side effects (cardiopulmonary bypass, medications); thrombolytic therapy

> **NOTE:** A risk diagnosis is not evidenced by signs and symptoms, as the problem has not occurred; rather, nursing interventions are directed at prevention.

Desired Outcomes/Evaluation Criteria— Client Will

(Include Specific Time Frame):

- Display neurological signs within client's normal range.
- Verbalize understanding of condition, therapy regimen, side effects of medications, and when to contact healthcare provider.
- Demonstrate behaviors and lifestyle changes to improve circulation (e.g., cessation of smoking, relaxation techniques, exercise and dietary program).

Actions/Interventions

Nursing Priority No. 1.

To assess causative/contributing factors:

- Determine history of conditions associated with thrombus or emboli such as stroke, complicated pregnancy, sickle cell disease, fractures (especially long bones and pelvis) **to identify client at higher risk for decreased cerebral perfusion related to bleeding and/or coagulation problems.**
- Note current situation or presence of conditions (e.g., congestive heart failure, major trauma, sepsis, hypertension) **that can affect multiple body systems and systemic circulation/perfusion.**
- Ascertain potential for presence of acute neurological conditions, such as TBI, tumors, hemorrhage, anoxic brain injury associated with cardiac arrest, and toxic or viral encephalopathies. **These conditions alter the relationship between intracranial volume and pressure, potentially increasing intracranial pressure and decreasing cerebral perfusion.**
- Investigate client reports of headache, particularly when accompanied by a range of progressive neurological deficits. **May accompany cerebral perfusion deficits associated with conditions such as stroke, transient ischemic attack**

Information that appears in brackets has been added by the authors to clarify and enhance the use of nursing diagnoses.

(TIA), brain trauma, or cerebral arteriovenous malformations.

- Ascertain if client has history of cardiac problems (e.g., recent myocardial infarction, heart failure, heart valve dysfunction or replacement, chronic atrial fibrillation).
- Evaluate blood pressure. **Chronic or severe acute hypertension can precipitate cerebrovascular spasm and stroke. Low blood pressure or severe hypotension causes inadequate perfusion of brain.**
- Verify proper use of antihypertensive medications.
- Review medication regimen noting use of anticoagulants/ antiplatelet agents/other drugs **that could cause intracranial bleeding.**
- Review pulse oximetry or ABGs. **Hypoxia is associated with reduced cerebral perfusion.**
- Review laboratory studies **to identify disorders that increase risk of clotting or bleeding, or conditions contributing to decreased cerebral perfusion.**
- Review results of diagnostic studies (e.g., x-rays, cardiac output; ultrasound or other imaging scans such as echocardiography, CT, angiography).

Nursing Priority No. 2.
To maximize tissue perfusion:
- Collaborate in treatment of underlying conditions as indicated.
- Restore or maintain fluid balance **to maximize cardiac output and prevent decreased cerebral perfusion associated with hypovolemia.**
- Manage cardiac dysrhythmias via medication administration, pacemaker insertion.
- Restrict fluids, administer diuretics as indicated **to prevent decreased cerebral perfusion associated with hypertension and cerebral edema.**
- Maintain head of bed placement (e.g., 0, 15, 30 degrees) as indicated, **to promote optimal cerebral perfusion.**
- Administer vasoactive medications as indicated, **to increase cardiac output and/or adequate arterial blood pressure to maintain cerebral perfusion.**
- Administer other medications as indicated (**e.g., steroids may decrease edema, antihypertensives to manage high blood pressure, anticoagulants to prevent cerebral embolus**).
- Prepare client for surgery as indicated (e.g., carotid endarterectomy, evacuation of hematoma or space-occupying lesion) **to improve cerebral perfusion.**

Information that appears in brackets has been added by the authors to clarify and enhance the use of nursing diagnoses.

- Refer to NDs decreased Cardiac Output, decreased Intracranial Adaptive Capacity for additional interventions.

Nursing Priority No. 3.

To promote wellness (Teaching/Discharge Considerations):

 • Review modifiable risk factors, including hypertension, smoking, diet, physical activity, excessive alcohol intake, illicit drug use, as indicated. **Information necessary for client to make informed choices about remedial risk factors and commit to lifestyle changes as appropriate.**

• Discuss impact of unmodifiable risk factors such as family history, age, race. **Understanding effects and interrelationship of all risk factors may encourage client to address what can be changed to improve general well-being and reduce individual risk.**

• Assist client to incorporate disease management into ADLs. **Promotes independence; enhances self-concept regarding ability to deal with change and manage own needs.**

• Stress necessity of routine follow-up and laboratory monitoring as indicated **for effective disease management and possible changes in therapeutic regimen.**

• Refer to educational and community resources, as indicated. **Client/SO may benefit from instruction and support provided by agencies to engage in healthy activities (e.g., weight loss, smoking cessation, exercise).**

Documentation Focus ⎯⎯⎯⎯⎯⎯⎯⎯⎯⎯⎯⎯

Assessment/Reassessment

- Individual findings, noting specific risk factors.
- Vital signs, blood pressure, cardiac rhythm.
- Medication regimen.
- Diagnostic studies, laboratory results.

Planning

- Plan of care and who is involved in planning.
- Teaching plan.

Implementation/Evaluation

- Response to interventions, teaching, and actions performed.
- Attainment or progress toward desired outcome(s).
- Modifications to plan of care.

⎯⎯⎯⎯⎯⎯⎯⎯⎯⎯⎯⎯⎯⎯⎯⎯⎯⎯⎯⎯⎯⎯⎯⎯⎯⎯⎯⎯⎯

Information that appears in brackets has been added by the authors to clarify and enhance the use of nursing diagnoses.

Discharge Planning

- Long-term needs and who is responsible for actions to be taken.
- Available resources, specific referrals made.

Sample Nursing Outcomes & Interventions Classifications (NOC/NIC) NIC

NOC—Tissue Perfusion: Cerebral
NIC—Cerebral Perfusion Promotion

risk for ineffective gastrointestinal **Perfusion**

Taxonomy II: Activity/Rest Class 4: Cardiovascular/
  Pulmonary Responses (00197)
[Diagnostic Division: Circulation]
Submitted 2008

Definition: At risk for change in gastrointestinal circulation that may compromise health

Risk Factors

Acute gastrointestinal hemorrhage; [hypovolemia]

Trauma; abdominal compartment syndrome

Vascular disease (e.g., peripheral vascular disease, aortoiliac occlusive disease); abdominal aortic aneurysm

Poor left ventricular performance; hemodynamic instability

Coagulopathy (e.g., sickle cell anemia, disseminated intravascular coagulation), abnormal partial thromboplastin time, abnormal prothrombin time; [emboli]

Gastrointestinal disease (e.g., duodenal or gastric ulcer, ischemic colitis, ischemic pancreatitis); gastric paresis; gastroesphageal varices

Liver dysfunction; renal failure; diabetes mellitus; stroke

Smoking

Treatment-related side effects (e.g., cardiopulmonary bypass, medication, anesthesia, gastric surgery)

Age >60 years; female gender

NOTE: A risk diagnosis is not evidenced by signs and symptoms, as the problem has not occurred; rather, nursing interventions are directed at prevention.

Information that appears in brackets has been added by the authors to clarify and enhance the use of nursing diagnoses.

Cultural   Collaborative   Community/Home Care

Desired Outcomes/Evaluation Criteria: Client Will (Include Specific Time Frame)

- Demonstrate adequate tissue perfusion as evidenced by active bowel sounds; absence of abdominal pain, nausea, and vomiting
- Verbalize understanding of condition, therapy regimen, side effects of medication, and when to contact healthcare provider.
- Engage in behaviors and lifestyle changes to improve circulation.

Actions/Interventions

Nursing Priority No. 1.

To identify individual risk factors/needs:

- Note presence of conditions affecting systemic circulation and perfusion such as heart failure with left ventricular dysfunction, major trauma with blood loss and hypotension, septic shock, and so forth. **Blood loss and hypovolemic or hypotensive shock can result in GI hypoperfusion, and bowel ischemia.**
- Determine presence of disorders such as esophageal varices, pancreatitis; abdominal or chest trauma, increase of intra-abdominal pressure; prior history of bowel obstruction or strangulated hernia, **which could cause local or regional reduction in GI blood flow.**
- Identify client with history of bleeding or coagulation disorders, such as prior GI bleed, coagulopathies; cancer, **to identify risk for potential bleeding problems.**
- ∞ Note client's age and gender when assessing for impaired GI perfusion (**e.g., studies indicate that risk for GI bleeding increases with age in both sexes, but that risk for abdominal aortic aneurysm is higher in men than in women). Premature or low-birth-weight neonates are at risk for developing NEC.**
- Investigate reports of abdominal pain, noting location, intensity, and duration.
- Review routine medication regimen (e.g., NSAIDs, Coumadin, low-dose aspirin such as used for prophylaxsis in certain cardiovascular conditions, corticosteroids). **Likelihood of bleeding increases from use of these medications.**
- Note history of smoking, **which can potentiate vasoconstriction; or excessive alcohol use/abuse, which can cause**

Information that appears in brackets has been added by the authors to clarify and enhance the use of nursing diagnoses.

general inflammation of the stomach mucosa and potentiate risk of GI bleeding; or liver involvement and esophageal varices.

- Auscultate abdomen to evaluate peristaltic activity. **Hypoactive or absent bowel sounds may indicate intraperitoneal
injury, bowel perforation, and bleeding. Abdominal bruit
can indicate abdominal aortic injury or aneurysm.**
- Palpate abdomen for distention, masses, enlarged organs
(such as spleen, liver, or portions of colon); elicitation of pain
with touch; pulsation of aorta.
- Percuss abdomen for fixed or shifting dullness over regions
that normally contain air. **Can indicate accumulated blood
or fluid.**
- Measure and monitor progression of abdominal girth as indicated. **Can reflect bowel problems such as obstruction;
or organ failure (e.g., heart, liver, or kidney) or organ
injury with intra-abdominal fluid and gas accumulation.**
- Note reports of nausea or vomiting accompanied by problems
with bowel elimination.
- Assess client with severe or prolonged vomiting, or forceful
coughing, engaging in lifting or straining activities or childbirth, **which can result in a tear in the esophageal or stomach wall, resulting in hemorrhage.**
- Evaluate stool color and consistency. Test for occult blood,
as indicated.
- Test gastric suction contents for blood when tube is used to
decompress stomach and/or manage vomiting.
- Assess vital signs, noting sustained hypotension, **which can
result in hypoperfusion of abdominal organs.**
- Review laboratory and other diagnostic studies (e.g., CBC,
bilirubin, liver enzymes, electrolytes, stool guaiac; endoscopy, abdominal ultrasound or CT, aortic angiography, par-
acentesis) **to identify any conditions or disorders that may
affect GI perfusion and function.**

Nursing Priority No. 2.
To reduce or correct individual risk factors:

- Collaborate in treatment of underlying conditions **to correct
or treat disorders that could affect GI perfusion.**
- Administer fluids and electrolytes as indicated **to replace
losses and to maintain GI circulation and cellular function.**

Information that appears in brackets has been added by the authors to clarify
and enhance the use of nursing diagnoses.

- Administer prescribed prophylactic medications in at-risk clients during illness and hospitalization (e.g. anti-emetics, proton pump inhibitors, antihistamines, anticholinergics, antibiotics) **to reduce potential for stress-related GI complications.**
- Maintain gastric or intestinal decompression, when indicated; measure output periodically, and note characteristics of drainage.
- Provide small, easily digested food and fluids when oral intake tolerated.
- Encourage rest after meals **to maximize blood flow to digestive system.**
- Prepare client for surgery as indicated such as gastric resection, bypass graft, mesenteric endarterectomy.
- Refer to NDs dysfunctional gastrointestinal Motility, Nausea, imbalanced Nutrition: Less than body requirements, for additional interventions.

Nursing Priority No. 3.
To promote wellness (Teaching/Discharge Considerations):

- Discuss individual risk factors (e.g., family history, obesity, age, smoking, hypertension, diabetes, clotting disorders) and potential outcomes of atherosclerosis (e.g., systemic and peripheral vascular disease conditions), as appropriate. **Information necessary for client to make informed choices about remedial risk factors and commit to lifestyle changes.**
- Identify necessary changes in lifestyle and assist client to incorporate disease management into ADLs.
- Encourage client to quit smoking, join Smoke-out, other smoking-cessation programs.
- Establish regular exercise program **to enhance circulation and promote general well-being.**
- Stress necessity of routine follow-up and laboratory monitoring as indicated. **Important for effective disease management and possible changes in therapeutic regimen.**
- Emphasize importance of discussing with primary care provider current and new prescribed medications, and/or planned use of certain medications (e.g., anticoagulants, NSAIDs including aspirin; corticosteroids, some OTC drugs, herbals supplements), **which can be harmful to GI mucosa or cause bleeding.**

Information that appears in brackets has been added by the authors to clarify and enhance the use of nursing diagnoses.

Documentation Focus

Assessment/Reassessment
- Individual findings, noting specific risk factors.
- Vital signs, adequacy of circulation.
- Abdominal assessment, characteristics of emesis or gastric drainage and stools.

Planning
- Plan of care and who is involved in planning.
- Teaching plan.

Implementation/Evaluation
- Response to interventions, teaching, and actions performed.
- Attainment or progress toward desired outcome(s).
- Modifications to plan of care.

Discharge Planning
- Long-term needs and who is responsible for actions to be taken.
- Available resources, specific referrals made.

Sample Nursing Outcomes & Interventions Classifications (NOC/NIC) **NIC**

NOC—Tissue Perfusion: Abdominal Organs
NIC—Surveillance

risk for ineffective renal **Perfusion**

Taxonomy II: Activity/Rest—Class 4 Cardiovascular/
  Pulmonary Responses (00203)
[Diagnostic Division: Circulatory]
Submitted 2008

Definition: At risk for a decrease in blood circulation to the kidney that may compromise health

Risk Factors

Hypovolemia; [interuption of blood flow]; vascular embolism
  vasculitis
Hypertension; malignant hypertension; hyperlipidemia
Renal disease (polycystic kidney); polynephritis; exposure to
  toxins; bilateral cortical necrosis

Information that appears in brackets has been added by the authors to clarify
and enhance the use of nursing diagnoses.

🌐 Cultural ♻ Collaborative 🏠 Community/Home Care

Diabetes mellitus; malignancy

Cardiac surgery; cardiopulmonary bypass

Hypoxemia, hypoxia; metabolic acidosis

Multitrauma; abdominal compartment syndrome; burns; infection (e.g. sepsis, localized infection); systemic inflammatory response syndrome

Treatment-related side effects (e.g., medications)

Advanced age

> **NOTE:** A risk diagnosis is not evidenced by signs and symptoms, as the problem has not occurred; rather, nursing interventions are directed at prevention.

Desired Outcomes/Evaluation Criteria—Client Will:

- Demonstrate adequate renal perfusion as evidenced by urine output appropriate for individual, balanced intake and output, absence of edema formation or inappropriate weight gain.
- Verbalize understanding of condition, therapy regimen, side effects of medication, and when to contact healthcare provider.
- Engage in behaviors/lifestyle changes to improve circulation (e.g., smoking cessation, diabetic glucose control, medication management)

Actions/Interventions

Nursing Priority No. 1.

To assess causative/contributing factors:

- Determine history or presence of severe hypotension and hypoxemia, or shock (may be cardiogenic, hypovolemia, obstructive, or septic shock); blunt or penetrating trauma; surgery with excess bleeding or fluid loss, prolonged dehydration, poorly controlled diabetes, and so forth. **Conditions associated with decreased circulation and kidney ischemia.**
- Note history or presence of abrupt onset or severe hypertension, persistent hypertension (160/100) over time; or hypertension resistant to appropriately dosed antihypertensive therapy, **any of which places client at high risk for kidney damage associated with renovascular hypertension.**
- Assess hydration status. **Dehydration reduces glomerular filtration rate (GFR).**

Information that appears in brackets has been added by the authors to clarify and enhance the use of nursing diagnoses.

- Ascultate for bruit over each renal artery in abdomen at mid-clavicular line, **suggesting renal artery stenosis, which is associated with renal insufficiency.**
- Determine usual voiding pattern, and investigate reported deviations, such as low output or need for diuretics, **which may indicate problems with kidney perfusion.**
- Note urine color—pale (dilute), dark (concentrated)—and measure specific gravity, as indicated **to evaluate hydration status and kidney's ability to concentrate the urine.**
- Monitor fluid intake, urine output, and weight on a regular schedule **to provide noninvasive assessment of cardiovascular and renal function.**
- Note mentation and behavior. **Adverse changes may be the consequence of fluid shifts, accumulation of toxins, acid-base and/or electrolyte imbalances when kidney dysfunction is occurring.**
- Review laboratory studies (e.g., CBC, BUN/Cr levels, protein, specific gravity, 24-hour creatinine clearance, glucose, electrolytes) **to evaluate kidney function.**
- Review diagnostic studies, as indicated, including Doppler ultrasonography, CT, renogram, intravenous pyelogram (IVP); contrast or magnetic resonance angiography (MRA), **to evaluate kidney size, perfusion, and function.**
- Review medication regimen for medications **whose potential side or toxic effects may substantially alter kidney perfusion (e.g., ACE inhibitors, NSAIDs, radiocontrast agents, methotrexate).**

Nursing Priority No. 2.
To reduce or correct individual risk factors:

- Collaborate in treatment of underlying conditions (e.g., angioplasty with stent placement, surgical revascularization procedures, fluids, electrolytes, nutrients, antibiotics, thrombolytics, oxygen) **to improve tissue perfusion/organ function.**
- Administer medications (e.g., vasoactive medications, including antihypertensive agents, insulin) as indicated **to treat underlying condition and improve renal blood flow and function.**
- Exercise caution when administering nephrotoxic agents, particularly when dehydration is present, **to reduce risk for acute or chronic renal failure.**
- Provide for fluid and diet restrictions as indicated, while providing adequate calories and hydration **to meet the body's needs without overtaxing kidney function.**

Information that appears in brackets has been added by the authors to clarify and enhance the use of nursing diagnoses.

⊕ Cultural   ⊘ Collaborative   🏠 Community/Home Care

- Refer to NDs deficient [or] excess Fluid Volume, impaired Urinary Elimination for additional interventions.

Nursing Priority No. 3.
To promote wellness (Teaching/Discharge Considerations):

- Discuss individual risk factors (e.g., family history, obesity, age, smoking, hypertension, diabetes, clotting disorders) and potential outcomes of atherosclerosis such as systemic and peripheral vascular disease. **Information necessary for client to make informed choices about remedial risk factors and consider lifestyle changes to prevent onset of complications or manage symptoms when condition present.**

- Identify necessary changes in lifestyle and assist client to incorporate disease management into ADLs. **Promotes independence, enhances self-concept regarding ability to deal with change and manage own needs.**

- Emphasize need to manage blood pressure when client is hypertensive. Instruct about individual's antihypertensive medications (e.g., ACE inhibitors, diuretics, beta-adrenergic blockers), and necessity for taking them as prescribed and with physician follow-up **to reduce cardiovascular complications and slow progression of renal dysfunction.**

- Instruct in home blood pressure monitoring; advise purchase of appropriate equipment; refer to community resources as indicated. **Facilitates management of hypertension, which is a major risk factor for damage to blood vessels and organ function.**

- Encourage client to quit smoking, join Smoke-out or other smoking-cessation programs. **Smoking causes vasoconstriction, compromising renal perfusion.**

- Review specific fluid and dietary requirements with client/SO (e.g., reduction of cholesterol, carbohydrates, or sodium) as indicated by individual situation **to promote circulatory health and kidney function.**

- Establish regular exercise program **to enhance circulation and promote general well-being.**

- Encourage regular medical and laboratory follow-up **to provide monitoring and earlier intervention for underlying conditions, and to evaluate effectiveness of therapeutic interventions.**

- Refer to specific support groups, counseling as appropriate **to assist with problem solving, provide role model, enhance coping ability.**

Information that appears in brackets has been added by the authors to clarify and enhance the use of nursing diagnoses.

Documentation Focus

Assessment/Reassessment
- Individual physical findings; identified risk factors.
- Baseline kidney function.
- I&O and weight as indicated.

Planning
- Plan of care and who is involved in planning.
- Teaching plan.

Implementation/Evaluation
- Response to interventions, teaching, and actions performed.
- Attainment or progress toward desired outcome(s).
- Modifications to plan of care.

Discharge Planning
- Long-term needs and who is responsible for actions to be taken.
- Available resources, specific referrals made.

Sample Nursing Outcomes & Interventions Classifications (NOC/NIC) NIC

NOC—Kidney Function
NIC—Fluid/Electrolyte Management

> ### risk for Peripheral Neurovascular Dysfunction
>
> Taxonomy II: Safety/Protection—Class 2 Physical Injury (00086)
> [Diagnostic Division: Neurosensory]
> Submitted 1992
>
> **Definition:** At risk for disruption in circulation, sensation, or motion of an extremity

Risk Factors

Fractures; trauma; vascular obstruction
Mechanical compression (e.g., tourniquet, cane, cast, brace, dressing, restraint)

Information that appears in brackets has been added by the authors to clarify and enhance the use of nursing diagnoses.

🌐 Cultural   🅐 Collaborative   🏠 Community/Home Care

Orthopedic surgery; immobilization
Burns

Desired Outcomes/Evaluation Criteria— Client Will:

- Maintain function as evidenced by sensation and movement within normal range for the individual.
- Identify individual risk factors.
- Demonstrate and participate in behaviors and activities to prevent complications.
- Relate signs/symptoms that require medical reevaluation.

Actions/Interventions

Nursing Priority No. 1.
To determine significance/degree of potential for compromise:

- Assess for individual risk factors: (1) trauma to extremity(ies) that cause internal tissue damage (e.g., high-velocity and penetrating trauma); fractures (especially long-bone fractures) with hemorrhage, or external pressures from burn eschar; (2) immobility (e.g., long-term bedrest, tight dressings, splints, or casting); (3) presence of conditions affecting peripheral circulation, such as atherosclerosis, Raynaud's disease, or diabetes; and (4) smoking, obesity, and sedentary lifestyle, **which potentiate risk of circulation insufficiency and occlusion.**
- Assess presence, location, and degree of swelling or edema formation. Measure affected extremity and compare with unaffected extremity.
- Monitor for tissue bleeding and spread of hematoma formation, **which can compress blood vessels and raise compartment pressures.**
- Note position and location of casts, braces, traction apparatus **to ascertain potential for pressure on tissues.**
- Review recent and current drug regimen, noting use of anticoagulants and vasoactive agents.

Information that appears in brackets has been added by the authors to clarify and enhance the use of nursing diagnoses.

risk for PERIPHERAL NEUROVASCULAR DYSFUNCTION

Nursing Priority No. 2.

To prevent deterioration/maximize circulation of affected limb(s):

- Perform neurovascular assessment in person immobilized for any reason (e.g., surgery, diabetic neuropathy, fractures) or individuals with suspected neurovascular problems. **Provides baseline for future comparisons.**
- Evaluate for differences between affected extremity and unaffected extremity, noting pain, pulses, pallor, paresthesia, paralysis, changes in motor and sensory function.
- Ask client to localize pain or discomfort and to report numbness and tingling or presence of pain with exercise or rest (atherosclerotic changes). (Refer to ND ineffective peripheral tissue Perfusion, as appropriate.)
- Monitor presence and quality of peripheral pulse distal to injury or impairment via palpation or Doppler. **Occasionally a pulse may be palpated even though circulation is blocked by a soft clot through which pulsations may be felt; or perfusion through larger arteries may continue after increased compartment pressure has collapsed the arteriole/venule circulation in the muscle.**
- Assess capillary return, skin color, and warmth in the limb(s) at risk and compare with unaffected extremities. **Peripheral pulses, capillary refill, skin color, and sensation may be normal initially even in the presence of compartment syndrome because superficial circulation is usually not compromised.**
- Test sensation of peroneal nerve by pinch or pinprick in the dorsal web between first and second toe, and assess ability to dorsiflex toes if indicated (e.g., presence of leg fracture).
- Minimize edema formation and elevated tissue pressure:

  Remove jewelry from affected limb.

  Avoid or limit use of restraints. Pad limb, and evaluate status frequently if restraints are required.

  Observe position and location of supporting ring of orthopedic splints or sling. Readjust, as indicated.

  Maintain elevation of injured extremity(ies), unless contraindicated by confirmed presence of compartment syndrome. **In presence of increased compartment pressure, elevation of extremity actually impedes arterial flow, decreasing perfusion.**

  Apply ice bags around injury or fracture site, as indicated, for initial 24 to 48 hours.

Information that appears in brackets has been added by the authors to clarify and enhance the use of nursing diagnoses.

- Maximize circulation:

  Use techniques such as repositioning and padding **to relieve pressure.**

  Encourage client to routinely exercise digits or joints distal to injury.

  Encourage ambulation as soon as possible.

   Apply antiembolic hose or sequential pressure device, as indicated.

  Administer IV fluids, blood products, as needed, **to maintain circulating volume and tissue perfusion.**

  Administer anticoagulants or antithrombomic agents, as indicated, **to prevent deep vein thrombosis (DVT) or treat thrombotic vascular obstructions.**

  Split or bivalve cast, or reposition traction or restraints, as appropriate, **to quickly release pressure.**

  Prepare for surgical intervention (e.g., fibulectomy, fasciotomy), as indicated, **to relieve pressure and restore circulation.**

- Monitor for development of complications:

  Inspect tissues around cast edges for rough places, and pressure points. Investigate reports of "burning sensation" under cast.

  Evaluate for tenderness, swelling, pain on dorsiflexion of foot (positive Homans' sign).

  Monitor Hb/Hct, coagulation studies (e.g., prothrombin time).

  Investigate sudden signs of limb ischemia (e.g., decreased skin temperature, pallor, increased pain), reports of pain that are extreme for type of injury, increased pain on passive movement of extremity, development of paresthesia, muscle tension or tenderness with erythema, change in pulse quality distal to injury. Place limb in neutral position, avoiding elevation. Report symptoms to physician at once **to provide for timely intervention/limit severity of problem.**

  Assist with measurements of intracompartmental pressures, as indicated. **Provides for early intervention and evaluates effectiveness of therapy.**

Nursing Priority No. 3.
To promote wellness (Teaching/Discharge Considerations):

- Review proper body alignment, elevation of limbs, as appropriate.

Information that appears in brackets has been added by the authors to clarify and enhance the use of nursing diagnoses.

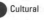 • Keep linens off affected extremity with bed cradle or cut-out box, as indicated.

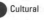 • Discuss necessity of avoiding constrictive clothing, sharp angulation of legs or crossing legs.

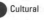 • Demonstrate proper application of antiembolic hose.

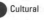 • Review safe use of heat or cold therapy, as indicated.

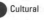 • Instruct client/SO(s) to check shoes and socks for proper fit and/or wrinkles.

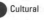 • Demonstrate and recommend continuation of exercises **to maintain function and circulation of limbs.**

Documentation Focus

Assessment/Reassessment
• Specific risk factors, nature of injury to limb.
• Assessment findings, including comparison of affected and unaffected limb, characteristics of pain in involved area.

Planning
• Plan of care and who is involved in the planning.
• Teaching plan.

Implementation/Evaluation
• Response to interventions, teaching, and actions performed.
• Attainment or progress toward desired outcome(s).
• Modification of plan of care.

Discharge Planning
• Long-term needs, referrals made, and who is responsible for actions to be taken.
• Specific referrals made.

Sample Nursing Outcomes & Interventions Classifications (NOC/NIC) (NIC)

NOC—Neurological Status: Peripheral
NIC—Peripheral Sensation Management

Information that appears in brackets has been added by the authors to clarify and enhance the use of nursing diagnoses.

🌐 Cultural   🅐 Collaborative   🏠 Community/Home Care

risk for **Poisoning**

Taxonomy II: Safety/Protection—Class 4 Environmental
Hazards (00037)
[Diagnostic Division: Safety]
Submitted 1980; Revised 2006

Definition: Accentuated risk of accidental exposure to, or
ingestion of, drugs or dangerous products in doses sufficient to cause poisoning [or the adverse effects of prescribed medication/drug use]

Risk Factors

Internal
Reduced vision
Lack of safety or drug education
Lack of proper precaution; [unsafe habits, disregard for safety
measures, lack of supervision]
Verbalization that occupational setting is without adequate safe-
guards
Cognitive or emotional difficulties
Age (e.g., young child, elderly person)
Chronic disease state, disability
Cultural or religious beliefs or practices

External
Large supplies of drugs in house
Medicines stored in unlocked cabinets accessible to children or
confused individuals
Availability of illicit drugs potentially contaminated by poison-
ous additives
Dangerous products placed within reach of children or confused
individuals
Therapeutic margin of safety of specific drugs (e.g., therapeutic
versus toxic level, half-life, method of uptake and degrada-
tion in body, adequacy of organ function)
Use of multiple herbal supplements or megadosing

> **NOTE:** A risk diagnosis is not evidenced by signs and
> symptoms, as the problem has not occurred; rather,
> nursing interventions are directed at prevention.

Information that appears in brackets has been added by the authors to clarify
and enhance the use of nursing diagnoses.

Desired Outcomes/Evaluation Criteria— Client Will:

- Verbalize understanding of dangers of poisoning.
- Identify hazards that could lead to accidental poisoning.
- Correct external hazards as identified.
- Demonstrate necessary actions/lifestyle changes to promote safe environment.
- Refer to NDs Contamination; risk for Contamination for additional interventions related to poisoning associated with environmental contaminants.

Actions/Interventions

Nursing Priority No. 1.

To assess causative/contributing factors:

- Identify internal and external risk factors in client's environment, including presence of infants, young children, or frail elderly **(who are at risk for accidental poisoning)** and teenagers or young adults **(who are at risk for medication experimentation);** confused or chronically ill person on multiple medications; person with potential for suicidal action; person who partakes in illicit drug use/dealing (e.g., marijuana, cocaine, heroin); person who manufactures drugs in home (e.g., methamphetamines).
- Note client's age, gender, socioeconomic status, developmental stage, decision-making ability, level of cognition and competence. **Affects client's ability to protect self/others and influences choice of interventions/teaching.**
- Assess mood, coping abilities, personality styles (e.g., temperament, impulsive behavior, level of self-esteem) **that may result in carelessness/increased risk-taking without consideration of consequences.**
- Assess client's knowledge of safe use of drugs/herbal supplements, safety hazards in the environment, and ability to respond to potential threat.
- Review results of laboratory tests and toxicology screening, as indicated.

Nursing Priority No. 2.

To assist in correcting factors that can lead to accidental poisoning:

- Discuss medication safety with client/SO(s) to:

Information that appears in brackets has been added by the authors to clarify and enhance the use of nursing diagnoses.

- Prevent accidental ingestion:
  Stress importance of supervising infant, child, frail elderly, or individuals with cognitive limitations.
  Keep medicines and vitamins out of sight or reach of children or cognitively impaired persons.
  Use child-resistant or tamper-resistant caps and lock medication cabinets.
  Recap medication containers immediately after obtaining current dosage.
  Code medicines for the visually impaired.
  Administer children's medications as drugs, not candy.
- Prevent duplication or possible overdose:
  Keep updated list of all medications (prescription, OTC, herbals, supplements) and review with healthcare providers when medications are changed, new ones added, or new healthcare providers are consulted.
  Keep prescription medication in original bottle with label. Do not mix with other medication/place in unmarked containers.
  Have responsible SO(s)/home health nurse supervise medication regimen/prepare medications for the cognitively or visually impaired, or obtain prefilled medication box from pharmacy.
  Take prescription medications, as prescribed on label.
  Do not adjust medication dosage.
  Retain and read safety information that accompanies prescriptions about expected effects, minor side effects, reportable or adverse affects that require medical intervention, and how to manage forgotten dose.
- Prevent taking medications that interact with one another or OTC, herbals, or other supplements in an undesired or dangerous manner:
  Keep list of medication allergies, including type of reaction to share with healthcare providers and pharmacist.
  Wear medical alert bracelet or necklace, as appropriate.
  Do not take outdated or expired medications. Do not save partial prescriptions to use another time.
  Encourage discarding outdated or unused drug safely (disposing in hazardous waste collection areas, not down drain or toilet).
  Do not take medications prescribed for another person.
  Coordinate care when multiple healthcare providers are involved to limit number of prescriptions and dosage levels.

Information that appears in brackets has been added by the authors to clarify and enhance the use of nursing diagnoses.

 Diagnostic Studies   Pediatric/Geriatric/Lifespan Medications **637**

Nursing Priority No. 3.

To promote wellness (Teaching/Discharge Considerations):

- Review drug side effects and potential interactions with client/SO(s). Discuss use of OTC drugs and herbal supplements and possibilities of misuse, drug interactions, and overdosing as with vitamin megadosing, and so forth.
- Obtain lab tests (e.g., prothrombin time/INR for Coumadin; drug levels for Dilantin, digoxin) at regular intervals **to ascertain that circulating blood levels are within therapeutic range.**
- Review periodic lab tests performed to monitor for adverse drug effect (e.g., liver function tests when lipid-lowering agents [statins] are prescribed, or renal or thyroid function and serum glucose levels for antimanics [lithium]).
- Discuss vitamins (especially those containing iron) that can be poisonous to children if taken in large doses.
- Review common analgesic safety (e.g., acetaminophen is an ingredient in many OTC medications, and unintentional overdose can occur).
- Ask healthcare provider or pharmacist about any considered medications if pregnant, nursing, or planning to become pregnant, **as some drugs are dangerous to fetus or nursing infant.**
- Provide list of emergency numbers (i.e., local/national poison control numbers, physician's office) to be placed by telephone **for use if poisoning occurs.**
- Encourage parent to place safety stickers on drugs/chemicals **to warn children of harmful contents.**
- Discuss use of ipecac syrup in home. **The use of ipecac is controversial, as it may delay appropriate medical treatment (e.g., reduce the effectiveness of activated charcoal or oral antidotes) or be used inappropriately with adverse effects. Therefore, use in the home without direct advice from poison control professionals is not recommended.**
- Refer substance abuser to detoxification programs, inpatient or outpatient rehabilitation, counseling, support groups, and psychotherapy.
- Encourage emergency measures, awareness, and education (e.g., CPR/first-aid class, community safety programs, ways to access emergency medical personnel).
- Institute community programs to assist individuals **to identify and correct risk factors in own environment.**

Information that appears in brackets has been added by the authors to clarify and enhance the use of nursing diagnoses.

Cultural Collaborative Community/Home Care

Documentation Focus

Assessment/Reassessment
- Identified risk factors noting internal and external concerns.
- Drug allergies or sensitivities.
- Current medications prescribed or available to individual, use of OTC medications, herbals or supplements, illicit drug use.

Planning
- Plan of care and who is involved in the planning.
- Teaching plan.

Implementation/Evaluation
- Response to interventions, teaching, and actions performed.
- Attainment or progress toward desired outcome(s).
- Modification to plan of care.

Discharge Planning
- Long-term needs and who is responsible for actions to be taken.
- Specific referrals made.

Sample Nursing Outcomes & Interventions Classifications (NOC/NIC) NIC

NOC—Safe Home Environment
NIC—Medication Management

Post-Trauma Syndrome [specify stage]

Taxonomy II: Coping/Stress Tolerance—Class 1 Post-Trauma Responses (00141)
[Diagnostic Division: Ego Integrity]
Submitted 1986; Nursing Diagnosis Extension and Classification (NDEC) Revision 1998

Definition: Sustained maladaptive response to a traumatic, overwhelming event

---

Related Factors

Events outside the range of usual human experience
Serious threat to self or loved ones

Information that appears in brackets has been added by the authors to clarify and enhance the use of nursing diagnoses.

Serious injury to self or loved ones; serious accidents (e.g., industrial, motor vehicle)

Abuse (physical and psychosocial); criminal victimization; rape

Witnessing mutilation or violent death; tragic occurrence involving multiple deaths

Disasters; sudden destruction of one's home or community; epidemics

Wars; being held prisoner of war; torture

Defining Characteristics

Subjective

Intrusive thoughts or dreams; nightmares; flashbacks; [excessive verbalization of the traumatic event]

Palpitations; headaches; [loss of interest in usual activities, loss of feeling of intimacy or sexuality]

Hopelessness; shame; guilt; [verbalization of survival guilt or guilt about behavior required for survival]

Anxiety; fear; grieving; depression

Reports feeling numb

Gastric irritability; [change in appetite; sleep disturbance/insomnia; chronic fatigue, easy fatigability]

Difficulty in concentrating

Objective

Hypervigilance; exaggerated startle response; irritability; neurosensory irritability

Anger; rage; aggression

Avoidance; repression; alienation; denial; detachment; psychogenic amnesia

Altered mood states; [poor impulse control/explosiveness]; panic attacks; horror

Substance abuse; compulsive behavior

Enuresis (in children)

[Difficulty with interpersonal relationships; dependence on others; work or school failure]

[**Stages:**

ACUTE: Begins within 6 months and does not last longer than 6 months.

CHRONIC: Lasts more than 6 months.

DELAYED ONSET: Period of latency of 6 months or more before onset of symptoms.]

Information that appears in brackets has been added by the authors to clarify and enhance the use of nursing diagnoses.

⊕ Cultural ⊛ Collaborative 🏠 Community/Home Care

Desired Outcomes/Evaluation Criteria— Client Will:

- Express own feelings or reactions, avoiding projection.
- Verbalize a positive self-image.
- Report reduced anxiety or fear when memories occur.
- Demonstrate ability to deal with emotional reactions in an individually appropriate manner.
- Demonstrate appropriate changes in behavior and lifestyle (e.g., share experiences with others, seek or get support from SO[s] as needed, change in job or residence).
- Report absence of physical manifestations (e.g., pain, chronic fatigue).
- Refer to ND Rape-Trauma Syndrome for additional outcomes when trauma is the result of rape.

Actions/Interventions

Nursing Priority No. 1.

To assess causative factor(s) and individual reaction:
Acute

- Observe for and elicit information about physical or psychological injury and note associated stress-related symptoms (e.g., "numbness," headache, tightness in chest, nausea, pounding heart).
- Identify psychological responses: anger, shock, acute anxiety, confusion, denial. Note laughter, crying, calm or agitated or excited (hysterical) behavior, expressions of disbelief, guilt or self-blame, labile emotions.
- Assess client's knowledge of and anxiety related to the situation. Note ongoing threat to self (e.g., contact with perpetrator and/or associates).
- Identify social aspects of trauma or incident (e.g., disfigurement, chronic conditions or permanent disabilities, loss of home or community).
 - Ascertain ethnic background and cultural or religious perceptions and beliefs about the occurrence (e.g., retribution from God).
- Determine degree of disorganization (e.g., task-oriented activity is not goal directed, organized, or effective; individual is overwhelmed by emotion most of the time).
- Identify whether incident has reactivated preexisting or co-existing situations (physical or psychological). **Affects how the client views the trauma.**

Information that appears in brackets has been added by the authors to clarify and enhance the use of nursing diagnoses.

- Determine disruptions in relationships (e.g., family, friends, coworkers, SOs). **Support persons may not know how to deal with client/situation (e.g., may be oversolicitous or withdraw).**
- Note withdrawn behavior, use of denial, and use of chemical substances or impulsive behaviors (e.g., chain smoking, overeating).
- Be aware of signs of increasing anxiety (e.g., silence, stuttering, inability to sit still). **Increasing anxiety may indicate risk for violence.**
- Note verbal and nonverbal expressions of guilt or self-blame when client has survived trauma in which others died. Validate congruency of observations with verbalizations.
- Assess signs and stage of grieving for self and others.
- Identify development of phobic reactions to ordinary articles (e.g., knives); situations (e.g., walking in groups of people, strangers ringing doorbell).

Chronic (In Addition to Above)

- Evaluate continued somatic complaints (e.g., gastric irritation, anorexia, insomnia, muscle tension, headache). Investigate reports of new or changes in symptoms.
- Note manifestations of chronic pain or pain symptoms in excess of degree of physical injury.
- Be aware of signs of severe or prolonged depression. Note presence of flashbacks, intrusive memories, nightmares; panic attacks; poor impulse control; problems with memory or concentration, thoughts and perceptions; and conflict, aggression or rage.
- Assess degree of dysfunctional coping (e.g., use or abuse of alcohol or other drugs; suicidal or homicidal ideation) and consequences.

Nursing Priority No. 2.

To assist client to deal with situation that exists:

Acute

- Provide a calm, safe environment. **Promotes sense of trust and safety.**
- Assist with documentation for police report, as indicated, and stay with the client.
- Listen to and investigate physical complaints, and take note of lack of physical complaints when injury may have occurred. **Emotional reactions may limit client's ability to recognize or verbalize physical injury.**

Information that appears in brackets has been added by the authors to clarify and enhance the use of nursing diagnoses.

🌐 Cultural 🔄 Collaborative 🏠 Community/Home Care

- Identify supportive persons for the individual (e.g., loved ones, counselor, spiritual advisor or pastor).
- Remain with client, listen as client recounts incident or concerns—possibly repeatedly. (If client does not want to talk, accept silence.) **Provides psychological support.**
- Provide environment in which client can talk freely about feelings and fears (including concerns about relationship with and response of SO), and trauma experiences and sensations (e.g., loss of control, "near-death experience").
• Help child express feelings about event using techniques appropriate to developmental level (e.g., play for young child, stories or puppets for preschooler, peer group for adolescent). **Children are more likely to express in play what they may not be able to verbalize directly. Adolescents may benefit from groups that help them gain knowledge, support, and a decreased sense of isolation.**
- Assist with practical realities (e.g., temporary housing, money, notifications of family members, or other needs).
- Be aware of and assist client to use ego strengths in a positive way by acknowledging ability to handle what is happening. **Enhances self-concept, supports self-esteem, and reduces sense of helplessness.**
- Allow client to work through own kind of adjustment. If the client is withdrawn or unwilling to talk, do not force the issue.
- Listen for expressions of fear of crowds and/or people.
- Administer anti-anxiety, sedative, or hypnotic medications with caution.

Chronic

- Continue listening to expressions of concern. **May need to continue to talk about the incident.**
- Permit free expression of feelings (may continue from the crisis phase). Avoid rushing client through expressions of feelings too quickly and refrain from providing reassurance inappropriately. **Client may believe pain and/or anguish is misunderstood and may be depressed. Statements such as "You don't understand" or "You weren't there" are a defense, a way of pushing others away.**
- Encourage client to talk out experience when ready, expressing feelings of fear, anger, loss, or grief. (Refer to ND complicated Grieving.)
• Ascertain and monitor sleep pattern of children as well as adults. **Sleep disturbances and/or nightmares may develop, delaying resolution, impairing coping abilities.**

Information that appears in brackets has been added by the authors to clarify and enhance the use of nursing diagnoses.

- Encourage client to become aware of and accept own feelings and reactions as being normal reactions in an abnormal situation.
- Acknowledge reality of loss of self that existed before the incident. Help client to move toward a state of acceptance as to the potential for growth that still exists within client.
- Continue to allow client to progress at own pace.
- Give "permission" to express and deal with anger at the assailant or situation in acceptable ways.
- Avoid prompting discussion of issues that cannot be resolved. Keep discussion on practical and emotional level rather than intellectualizing the experience, **which allows client to deal with reality while taking time to work out feelings.**
- Assist in dealing with practical concerns and effects of the incident, such as court appearances, altered relationships with SO(s), employment problems.
- Provide for sensitive, trained counselors/therapists and engage in therapies, such as psychotherapy, Implosive Therapy (flooding), hypnosis, relaxation, Rolfing, memory work, cognitive restructuring, Eye Movement Desensitization and Reprocessing (EMDR), physical and occupational therapies.
- Administer psychotropic medications, as indicated.

Nursing Priority No. 3.
To promote wellness (Teaching/Discharge Considerations):

- Assist client to identify and monitor feelings while therapy is occurring.
- Provide information about what reactions client may expect during each phase. Let client know these are common reactions. Be sure to phrase in neutral terms of "You may or you may not . . . ." **Helps reduce fear of the unknown.**
- Assist client to identify factors that may have created a vulnerable situation and that he or she may have power to change **to protect self in the future.**
- Avoid making value judgments.
- Discuss lifestyle changes client is contemplating and how they may contribute to recovery. **Helps client evaluate appropriateness of plans and identify shortcomings (e.g., moving away from effective support group).**
- Assist client to learn stress-management techniques.
- Discuss drug regimen, potential side effects of prescribed medications, and necessity of prompt reporting of untoward effects.

Information that appears in brackets has been added by the authors to clarify and enhance the use of nursing diagnoses.

• Discuss recognition of, and ways to manage, "anniversary reactions," reinforcing normalcy of recurrence of thoughts and feelings at this time.

• Suggest support group for SO(s) **to assist with understanding and ways to deal with client.**

• Encourage psychiatric consultation, especially if client is unable to maintain control, is violent, is inconsolable, or does not seem to be making an adjustment.

• Refer for long-term individual/family/marital counseling, if indicated.

• Refer to NDs Powerlessness; ineffective Coping; Grieving; complicated Grieving.

Documentation Focus

Assessment/Reassessment
• Individual findings, noting current dysfunction and behavioral and emotional responses to the incident.
• Specifics of traumatic event.
• Reactions of family/SO(s).
• Availability and use of resources.

Planning
• Plan of care and who is involved in the planning.
• Teaching plan.

Implementation/Evaluation
• Responses to interventions, teaching, and actions performed.
• Emotional changes.
• Attainment or progress toward desired outcome(s).
• Modifications to plan of care.

Discharge Planning
• Long-term needs and who is responsible for actions to be taken.
• Specific referrals mades.

Sample Nursing Outcomes & Interventions Classifications (NOC/NIC) NIC

NOC—Comfort Status: Psychospiritual
NIC—Crisis Intervention

Information that appears in brackets has been added by the authors to clarify and enhance the use of nursing diagnoses.

risk for **Post-Trauma Syndrome**

Taxonomy II: Coping/Stress Tolerance—Class 1 Post-
  Trauma Responses (00145)
[Diagnostic Division: Ego Integrity]
Submitted 1998; Nursing Diagnosis Extension and
  Classification (NDEC) Submission 1998

Definition: At risk for sustained maladaptive response to
a traumatic, overwhelming event

Risk Factors

Occupation (e.g., police, fire, rescue, corrections, emergency
  room staff, mental health worker, [and their family mem-
  bers])
Perception of event; exaggerated sense of responsibility; diminished ego strength
Survivor's role in the event
Inadequate social support; nonsupportive environment; displacement from home
Duration of the event

NOTE: A risk diagnosis is not evidenced by signs and
symptoms, as the problem has not occurred; rather,
nursing interventions are directed at prevention.

Desired Outcomes/Evaluation Criteria— Client Will:

• Verbalize absence of severe anxiety.
• Demonstrate ability to deal with emotional reactions in an
  individually appropriate manner.
• Report relief or absence of physical manifestations (pain,
  nightmares or flashbacks, fatigue) associated with event.

Actions/Interventions

Nursing Priority No. 1.
To assess contributing factors and individual reaction:

• Identify client who survived or witnessed traumatic event
  (e.g., airplane or motor vehicle crash, mass shooting, fire de-
  stroying home and lands, robbery at gunpoint, other violent

---

Information that appears in brackets has been added by the authors to clarify
and enhance the use of nursing diagnoses.

⊕ Cultural   ⊛ Collaborative   🏠 Community/Home Care

act) **to recognize individual at high risk for post-trauma syndrome.**

- Note occupation (e.g., police, fire, emergency services personnel or rescue workers, soldiers and support personnel in combat areas), as listed in Risk Factors. **Studies reveal a moderate to high percentage of post-traumatic stress disorders develop in these populations when they have been exposed to one or more traumatic incidents.**
- Assess client's knowledge of and anxiety related to potential for work-related trauma (e.g., shooting in line of duty, or viewing body of murdered child); and number, duration, and intensity of recurring situations (e.g., EMT personnel exposed to numerous on-the-job traumatic incidents; rescuers searching for victims of natural or man-made disasters).
- Identify how client's past experiences may affect current situation.
- Listen for comments of guilt, humiliation, shame, or taking on responsibility (e.g., "I should have been more careful/gone back to get her"; "Don't call me a hero, I couldn't save my partner"; "My kids are the same age as the ones that died").
- Evaluate for life factors or stressors currently or recently occurring, such as displacement from home due to catastrophic event (e.g., fire, flood, violent storm) happening to individual whose child is dying with cancer or who suffered abuse as a child. **This individual is at greater risk for developing traumatic symptoms (acute added to delayed-onset reactions).**
- Identify client's general health and coping mechanisms.
- Determine availability and effectiveness of client's support systems, family, social, community, and so forth. (*Note:* Family members can also be at risk.)

Nursing Priority No. 2.

To assist client to deal with situation that exists:

- Educate high-risk persons and families about signs/symptoms of post-trauma response, especially if it is likely to occur in their occupation/life.
- Identify and discuss client's strengths (e.g., very supportive family, usually copes well with stress) as well as vulnerabilities (e.g., client tends toward alcohol or other drugs for coping, client has witnessed a murder).
- Discuss how individual coping mechanisms have worked in past traumatic events. **Client/SO(s) may be able to employ previously successful strategies to deal with current incident.**

Information that appears in brackets has been added by the authors to clarify and enhance the use of nursing diagnoses.

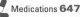

- Evaluate client's perceptions of events and personal significance (e.g., police officer—who is also a parent—investigating death of a child).
- Provide emotional and physical presence **to strengthen client's coping abilities.**
- Encourage expression of feelings and reinforce that feelings and reactions to trauma are common, and not indicators of weakness or failure. Note whether feelings expressed appear congruent with events the client experienced. **Incongruency may indicate deeper conflict and can impede resolution.**
- Observe for signs and symptoms of stress responses, such as nightmares, reliving an incident, poor appetite, irritability, numbness and crying, family or relationship disruption. **These responses are normal in the early postincident time frame. If prolonged and persistent, the client may be experiencing post-traumatic stress disorder.**

Nursing Priority No. 3.
To promote wellness (Teaching/Discharge Considerations):

- 🏠 Provide a calm, safe environment **in which client can deal with disruption of life.**
- 🏠 Encourage client to identify and monitor feelings on an ongoing basis. **Promotes awareness of changes in ability to deal with stressors.**
- 🏠 Encourage learning stress-management techniques **to help with resolution of situation.**
- 🏠 Recommend participation in debriefing sessions that may be provided following major events. **Dealing with the stressor promptly may facilitate recovery from event or prevent exacerbation, although issues about best timing of debriefing continue to be debated.**
- Ⓐ Explain that post-traumatic symptoms can emerge months or sometimes years after a traumatic experience and that help and support can be obtained when needed or desired if client begins to experience intrusive memories or other symptoms.
- Ⓐ Identify employment, community resource groups (e.g., Assistance Support and Self Help in Surviving Trauma [ASSIST], employee peer assistance programs, Red Cross or other survivor support services, Compassionate Friends). **Provides opportunity for ongoing support to deal with recurrent stressors.**
- Ⓐ Refer for individual or family counseling, as indicated.

Information that appears in brackets has been added by the authors to clarify and enhance the use of nursing diagnoses.

Documentation Focus

Assessment/Reassessment
- Identified risk factors noting internal and external concerns.
- Client's perception of event and personal significance.

Planning
- Plan of care and who is involved in the planning.
- Teaching plan.

Implementation/Evaluation
- Response to interventions, teaching, and actions performed.
- Attainment or progress toward desired outcome(s).

Discharge Planning
- Long-term needs and who is responsible for actions to be taken.
- Specific referrals made.

Sample Nursing Outcomes & Interventions Classifications (NOC/NIC) **NIC**

NOC—Comfort Status: Psychospiritual
NIC—Support System Enhancement

---

readiness for enhanced Power

Taxonomy II: Self-Perception—Class 1 Self-Concept (00187)
[Diagnostic Division: ego integrity]
Submitted 2006

Definition: A pattern of participating knowingly in change that is sufficient for well-being and can be strengthened

Related Factors

To be developed

Information that appears in brackets has been added by the authors to clarify and enhance the use of nursing diagnoses.

Defining Characteristics

Subjective

Expresses readiness to enhance power; knowledge for participation in change; awareness of possible changes to be made; identification of choices that can be made for change

Expresses readiness to enhance freedom; need to perform actions for change; involvement in creating change; participation in choices for daily living and health

> **NOTE:** Even though power (a response) and empowerment (an intervention approach) are different concepts, the literature related to both concepts supports the defining characteristics of this diagnosis.

Desired Outcomes/Evaluation Criteria— Client Will:

* Verbalize knowledge of what changes he or she wants to make.
* Express awareness of own ability to be in charge of changes to be made.
* Participate in classes or group activities to learn new skills.
* State readiness to take power over own life.

Actions/Interventions

Nursing Priority No. 1.

To determine need/motivation for improvement:

* Determine current situation and circumstances that client is experiencing leading to desire to improve life.
* Ascertain motivation and expectations for change.
* Identify emotional climate in which client and relationships live and work. **The emotional climate has a great impact between people. When a power differential exists in relationships, the atmosphere is largely determined by the person or people who have the power.**
* Identify client locus of control: internal (expressions of responsibility for self and ability to control outcomes) or external (expressions of lack of control over self and environment). **Understanding locus of control can help client work toward positive, internal control as he or she develops ability to freely recognize and choose own actions.**

Information that appears in brackets has been added by the authors to clarify and enhance the use of nursing diagnoses.

 Cultural Collaborative Community/Home Care

- Determine cultural factors/religious beliefs influencing client's self-view.
- Assess degree of mastery client has exhibited in his or her life. **Helps client understand how he or she has functioned in the past and what is needed to improve.**
- Note presence of family/SO(s) that can, or do, act as support systems for client.
- Determine whether client knows and/or uses assertiveness skills.

Nursing Priority No. 2.

To assist client to clarify needs relative to ability to improve feelings of power:

- Discuss needs and how client is meeting them at this time.
- Listen to, or Active-listen client's perceptions and beliefs about how power can be gained in his or her life.
- Identify strengths, assets, and past coping strategies that were successful and can be built on **to enhance feelings of control.**
- Discuss the importance of assuming personal responsibility for life and relationships. **This skill requires one to be open to new ideas and experiences and different values and beliefs and to be inquisitive.**
- Identify things client can and cannot control. **Avoids wasting time on things that are not in the control of the client.**
- Treat expressed desires and decisions with respect. Avoid critical parenting expressions.

Nursing Priority No. 3.

To promote optimum wellness, enhancing power (Teaching/Discharge Considerations):

- Assist client to set realistic goals for the future.
- Provide accurate verbal and written information about what is happening and discuss with client. **Reinforces learning and promotes self-paced review.**
- Assist client to learn and use assertive communication skills. **These techniques require practice, but as the client becomes more proficient they will help client to develop more effective relationships.**
- Use "I-messages" instead of "You-messages." **"I-messages" acknowledge ownership of what is said, while "You-messages" suggest that the other person is wrong or bad, fostering resentment and resistance instead of understanding and cooperation.**

Information that appears in brackets has been added by the authors to clarify and enhance the use of nursing diagnoses.

 Diagnostic Studies   ∞ Pediatric/Geriatric/Lifespan   Medications **651**

• Discuss importance of client paying attention to nonverbal communication. **Messages are often confusing or misinterpreted when verbal and nonverbal communications are not congruent.**

 • Help client learn to problem-solve differences. **Promotes win-win solutions.**

• Instruct and encourage use of stress-reduction techniques.

• Refer to support groups or classes, as indicated (e.g., assertiveness training, effectiveness for women, "Be your Best").

Documentation Focus

Assessment/Reassessment
• Individual findings, noting determination to improve sense of power, locus of control.
• Motivation and expectations for change.

Planning
• Plan of care, specific interventions, and who is involved in planning.
• Teaching plan.

Implementation/Evaluation
• Client's responses to interventions, teaching, and actions performed.
• Attainment or progress toward desired outcome(s).
• Modifications to plan of care.

Discharge Planning
• Long-term needs and who is responsible for actions to be taken.
• Specific referrals made.

Sample Nursing Outcomes & Interventions Classifications (NOC/NIC) NIC

NOC—Personal Autonomy
NIC—Self-Responsibility Facilitation

Information that appears in brackets has been added by the authors to clarify and enhance the use of nursing diagnoses.

⊕ Cultural 🅐 Collaborative 🏠 Community/Home Care

Powerlessness [specify level]

Taxonomy II: Self-Perception—Class 1 Self-Concept
(00125)
[Diagnostic Division: Ego Integrity]
Submitted 1982

Definition: Perception that one's own action will not significantly affect an outcome; a perceived lack of control over a current situation or immediate happening

Related Factors

Healthcare environment [e.g., loss of privacy, personal possessions, control over therapies]

Interpersonal interaction [e.g., misuse of power, force; abusive relationships]

Illness-related regimen [e.g., chronic/debilitating conditions]

Lifestyle of helplessness [e.g., repeated failures, dependency]

Defining Characteristics

Subjective

Low

Expressions of uncertainty about fluctuating energy levels

Moderate

Expressions of dissatisfaction or frustration over inability to perform previous tasks or activities

Expressions of doubt regarding role performance

Fear of alienation from caregivers

Reluctance to express true feelings; resentment; anger; guilt

Severe

Verbal expressions of having no control (e.g., over self-care, situation, outcome)

Depression over physical deterioration

Objective

Low

Passivity

Moderate

Dependence on others that may result in irritability

Inability to seek information regarding care

Information that appears in brackets has been added by the authors to clarify and enhance the use of nursing diagnoses.

 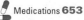

Passivity

Nonparticipation in care or decision making when opportunities are provided; does not monitor progress

Does not defend self-care practices when challenged

Severe

Apathy [withdrawal, resignation, crying]

Desired Outcomes/Evaluation Criteria— Client Will:

- Express sense of control over the present situation and future outcome.
- Make choices related to and be involved in care.
- Identify areas over which individual has control.
- Acknowledge reality that some areas are beyond individual's control.

Actions/Interventions

Nursing Priority No. 1.

To assess causative/contributing factors:

- Identify situational circumstances (e.g., unfamiliar environment, immobility, diagnosis of terminal or chronic illness, lack of support system, lack of knowledge about situation).
- Determine client's perception and knowledge of condition and treatment plan.
- Ascertain client response to treatment regimen. Does client see reason(s) and understand regimen is in the client's best interest, or is client compliant and helpless?
- Identify client locus of control: internal (expressions of responsibility for self and ability to control outcomes— "I didn't quit smoking") or external (expressions of lack of control over self and environment—"Nothing ever works out"; "What bad luck to get lung cancer").
- Note cultural factors or religious beliefs that may contribute to how client is handling the situation.
- Assess degree of mastery client has exhibited in life. **Passive individual may have more difficulty being assertive and standing up for rights.**
- Determine if there has been a change in relationships with SO(s). **Conflict in the family, loss of a family member, or divorce can contribute to feelings of powerlessness and lack of ability to manage situation.**
- Note availability and use of resources.

Information that appears in brackets has been added by the authors to clarify and enhance the use of nursing diagnoses.

 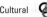 Cultural · Collaborative · Community/Home Care

• Investigate caregiver practices. Do they support client control or responsibility?

Nursing Priority No. 2.
To assess degree of powerlessness experienced by client:

• Listen to statements client makes: "They don't care"; "It won't make any difference"; "Are you kidding?"
• Note expressions that indicate "giving up," such as "It won't do any good."
• Note behavioral responses (verbal and nonverbal) including expressions of fear, interest or apathy, agitation, withdrawal.
• Note lack of communication, flat affect, and lack of eye contact.
• Identify the use of manipulative behavior and reactions of client and caregivers. **Manipulation is used for management of powerlessness because of distrust of others, fear of intimacy, search for approval, and validation of sexuality.**

Nursing Priority No. 3.
To assist client to clarify needs relative to ability to meet them:

• Show concern for client as a person.
• Make time to listen to client's perceptions and concerns and encourage questions.
• Accept expressions of feelings, including anger and hopelessness.
• Avoid arguing or using logic with hopeless client. **Client will not believe it can make a difference.**
• Deal with manipulative behavior by being straightforward and honest with your communication and letting client know that this is a better way to get needs met.
• Express hope for the client. **(There is always hope of something.)**
• Identify strengths and assets, and past coping strategies that were successful. **Helps client to recognize own ability to deal with difficult situation.**
• Assist client to identify what he or she can do for self. Identify things the client can and cannot control.
• Encourage client to maintain a sense of perspective about the situation.

Nursing Priority No. 4.
To promote independence:

• Use client's locus of control to develop individual plan of care (e.g., for client with internal control, encourage client to take

---

Information that appears in brackets has been added by the authors to clarify and enhance the use of nursing diagnoses.

POWERLESSNESS [specify level]

control of own care; for those with external control, begin with small tasks and add, as tolerated).

- Develop contract with client specifying goals agreed on. **Enhances commitment to plan, optimizing outcomes.**
- Treat expressed decisions and desires with respect. Avoid critical parenting behaviors and communications.
- Provide client opportunities to control as many events as energy and restrictions of care permit.
- Discuss needs openly with client and set up agreed-on routines for meeting identified needs. **Minimizes use of manipulation.**
- Minimize rules and limit continuous observation to the degree that safety permits **to provide sense of control for the client.**
- Support client efforts to develop realistic steps to put plan into action, reach goals, and maintain expectations.
- Provide positive reinforcement for desired behaviors.
- Direct client's thoughts beyond present state to future when appropriate.
- Schedule frequent brief visits to check on client, deal with client needs, and let client know someone is available.
- Involve SO(s) in client care as appropriate.

Nursing Priority No. 5.
To promote wellness (Teaching/Discharge Considerations):

- Instruct in and encourage use of anxiety and stress-reduction techniques.
- Provide accurate verbal and written information about what is happening and discuss with client/SO(s). Repeat as often as necessary.
- Assist client to set realistic goals for the future.
- Assist client to learn and use assertive communication skills. **Use of I-messages, Active-listening, and problem solving encourages client to be more in control of own life.**
- Refer to occupational therapist or vocational counselor, as indicated. **Facilitates return to a productive role in whatever capacity possible for the individual.**
- Encourage client to think productively and positively and take responsibility for choosing own thoughts.
- Model problem-solving process with client/SO(s). **Outcome is more likely to be accepted when arrived at by all parties involved, and participating in win-win solutions promotes sense of self-worth.**
- Suggest periodic review of own needs and goals.
- Refer to support groups, counseling or therapy, and so forth, as indicated.

Information that appears in brackets has been added by the authors to clarify and enhance the use of nursing diagnoses.

Cultural Collaborative Community/Home Care

Documentation Focus

Assessment/Reassessment
- Individual findings, noting degree of powerlessness, locus of control, individual's perception of the situation.
- Specific culteral or religious factors.
- Availability and use of support system and resources.

Planning
- Plan of care and who is involved in the planning.
- Teaching plan.

Implementation/Evaluation
- Responses to interventions, teaching, and actions performed.
- Specific goals and expectations.
- Attainment or progress toward desired outcome(s).
- Modifications to plan of care.

Discharge Planning
- Long-term needs and who is responsible for actions to be taken.
- Specific referrals made.

Sample Nursing Outcomes & Interventions Classifications (NOC/NIC) (NIC)

NOC—Personal Resiliency
NIC—Self-Responsibility Facilitation

> ### risk for **Powerlessness**
>
> Taxonomy II: Self-Perception—Class 1 Self-Concept (00125)
> [Diagnostic Division: Ego Integrity]
> Submitted 2000
>
> **Definition:** At risk for perceived lack of control over a situation and/or one's ability to significantly affect an outcome

Risk Factors

Physiological
Illness [hospitalization, intubation, ventilator, suctioning]; dying

---

Information that appears in brackets has been added by the authors to clarify and enhance the use of nursing diagnoses.

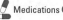

Acute injury; progressive debilitating disease process (e.g., spinal cord injury, multiple sclerosis)

Aging [e.g., decreased physical strength, decreased mobility]

Psychosocial

Deficient knowledge (e.g., of illness or healthcare system)

Lifestyle of dependency

Inadequate coping patterns

Absence of integrality (e.g., essence of power)

Situational or chronic low self-esteem; disturbed body image

> **NOTE:** A risk diagnosis is not evidenced by signs and symptoms, as the problem has not occurred; rather, nursing interventions are directed at prevention.

Desired Outcomes/Evaluation Criteria—Client Will:

- Express sense of control over the present situation and hopefulness about future outcomes.
- Verbalize positive self-appraisal in current situation.
- Make choices related to and be involved in care.
- Identify areas over which individual has control.
- Acknowledge reality that some areas are beyond individual's control.

Actions/Interventions

Nursing Priority No. 1.

To assess causative/contributing factors:

- Identify situational circumstances (e.g., acute illness, sudden hospitalization; diagnosis of terminal or debilitating, chronic illness; very young or aged individual with decreased physical strength and mobility; lack of knowledge about illness or healthcare system).
- Determine client's perception and knowledge of condition and proposed treatment plan.
- Identify client's locus of control: internal (expressions of responsibility for self and environment) or external (expressions of lack of control over self and environment). **May affect willingness to accept responsibility to manage situation.**
- Assess client's self-esteem and degree of mastery client has exhibited in life situations. **Passive individual may have more difficulty being assertive and standing up for rights.**

Information that appears in brackets has been added by the authors to clarify and enhance the use of nursing diagnoses.

⊕ Cultural ⟨A⟩ Collaborative 🏠 Community/Home Care

- Determine cultural values or religious beliefs impacting self-view.
- Note availability and use of resources.
- Listen to statements client makes (e.g., "They can't really help"; "It probably won't make a difference"). **Suggests concerns regarding own power and ability to control situation.**
- Determine congruency of responses (verbal and nonverbal) and note expressions of fear, disinterest or apathy, or withdrawal.
- Be alert for signs of manipulative behavior and note reactions of client and caregivers. **Manipulation may be used for management of powerlessness because of fear and distrust.**

Nursing Priority No. 2.
To assist client to clarify needs and ability to meet them:

- Make time to listen to client's perceptions of the situation. **Shows concern for client as a person.**
- Encourage questions.
- Accept expressions of feelings, including anger and reluctance, to try to work things out. **Being able to express feelings freely enables client sort out what is happening and come to a positive and realistic conclusion.**
- Express hope for client and encourage review of past experiences with successful strategies.
- Assist client to identify what he or she can do to help self, and what situations can and cannot be controlled.

Nursing Priority No. 3.
To promote wellness (Teaching/Discharge Considerations):

- Encourage client to think productively and positively, and to take responsibility for choosing own thoughts and reactions. **Can enhance feelings of power and sense of positive self-esteem.**
- Provide accurate verbal and written instructions about what is happening and what realistically might happen. **Reinforces learning and promotes self-paced review.**
- Involve client/SO(s) in planning process and problem-solve, using client's locus of control (e.g., for client with internal control, encourage client to take control of own care; for those with external control, begin with small tasks and add, as tolerated).
- Support client efforts to develop realistic steps to put plan into action, reach goals, and maintain expectations.

Information that appears in brackets has been added by the authors to clarify and enhance the use of nursing diagnoses.

Diagnostic Studies   ∞ Pediatric/Geriatric/Lifespan   Medications **659**

- Identify resource books or classes for assertiveness training and stress reduction, as appropriate.
- Encourage client to be active in long-term healthcare management and to engage in periodic review of own needs and goals.
- Refer to support groups for chronic conditions or disability (e.g., MS Society, Easter Seals, Alzheimer's Association, Al-Anon) or counseling or therapy, as appropriate.

Documentation Focus

Assessment/Reassessment
- Individual findings, noting potential for powerlessness, locus of control, individual's perception of the situation.
- Cultural values or religious beliefs.
- Availability and use of resources.

Planning
- Plan of care and who is involved in the planning.
- Teaching plan.

Implementation/Evaluation
- Responses to interventions, teaching, and actions performed.
- Specific goals and expectations.
- Modifications to plan of care.

Discharge Planning
- Long-term needs and who is responsible for actions to be taken.
- Specific referrals made.

Sample Nursing Outcomes & Interventions Classifications (NOC/NIC) NIC

NOC—Personal Autonomy
NIC—Self-Responsibility Facilitation

---

ineffective Protection

Taxonomy II: Safety/Protection—Class 2 Physical Injury (00043)
[Diagnostic Division: Safety]
Submitted 1990

Definition: Decrease in the ability to guard self from internal or external threats such as illness or injury

---

Information that appears in brackets has been added by the authors to clarify and enhance the use of nursing diagnoses.

Related Factors

Extremes of age
Inadequate nutrition
Alcohol abuse
Abnormal blood profiles (e.g., leukopenia, thrombocytopenia, anemia, coagulation)
Drug therapies (e.g., antineoplastic, corticosteroid, immune, anticoagulant, thrombolytic)
Treatments (e.g., surgery, radiation)
Cancer; immune disorders

Defining Characteristics

Subjective
Neurosensory alterations
Chilling
Itching
Insomnia; fatigue; weakness
Anorexia

Objective
Deficient immunity
Impaired healing; altered clotting
Maladaptive stress response
Perspiring [inappropriately]
Dyspnea; cough
Restlessness; immobility
Disorientation
Pressure sores

NOTE: The purpose of this diagnosis seems to combine multiple NDs under a single heading for ease of planning care when a number of variables may be present. Outcomes/evaluation criteria and interventions are specifically tied to individual related factors that are present, such as:

Extremes of age: Concerns may include Body Temperature or Thermoregulation; Memory, Thought Process or Sensory-Perceptual alterations, as well as impaired Mobility, risk for Falls, sedentary Lifestyle, Self-Care deficits; risk for Trauma, Suffocation, or Poisoning; risk for Skin/Tissue Integrity; and Fluid Volume imbalances.

Information that appears in brackets has been added by the authors to clarify and enhance the use of nursing diagnoses.

Inadequate nutrition: Brings up issues of Nutrition: less than body requirements, risk for unstable Blood Glucose Levels; risk for Infection, delayed Surgical Recovery; impaired Swallowing; disturbed Thought Processes, impaired Skin/Tissue Integrity; Trauma, ineffective Coping, and interrupted Family Processes.

Alcohol [other drug] abuse: May be situational or chronic, with problems ranging from ineffective Breathing Pattern, decreased Cardiac Output, impaired Liver Function, and Fluid Volume deficits, to nutritional concerns, Infection, Trauma, disturbed Thought Processes, and Coping or Family Process difficulties.

Abnormal blood profile: Suggests possibility of Fluid Volume deficits, decreased tissue Perfusion, impaired Gas Exchange, Activity Intolerance, or risk for Infection or Injury.

Drug therapies, treatments, and disease concerns: Would include ineffective tissue Perfusion, Activity Intolerance; cardiovascular, respiratory, and elimination concerns; risk for Infection, Fluid Volume imbalances, impaired Skin/Tissue Integrity, impaired Liver Function; Pain, nutritional problems, Fatigue or Sleep Deprivation, ineffective self Health Management; and emotional responses (e.g., Anxiety, Sorrow, Grieving, Coping difficulties).

It is suggested that the user refer to specific NDs based on identified related factors and individual concerns for this client to find appropriate outcomes and interventions, and Documentation Focus.

Sample Nursing Outcomes & Interventions Classifications (NOC/NIC) NIC

NOC/NICs also depend on the specifics of the client's situation such as:

NOC—Blood Coagulation; Immune Status; Neurological Status: Consciousness

NIC—Bleeding Precautions; Infection Protection; Postanesthesia Care

---

Information that appears in brackets has been added by the authors to clarify and enhance the use of nursing diagnoses.

⊕ Cultural 🔣 Collaborative 🏠 Community/Home Care

Rape-Trauma Syndrome (specify)

Taxonomy II: Coping/Stress Tolerance—Class 1 Post-
   Trauma Responses (see A, [B], [C], following)
[Diagnostic Division: Ego Integrity]
Submitted 1980; Nursing Diagnosis Extension and Clas-
   sification (NDEC) Revision 1998

Definition: Sustained maladaptive response to a forced,
violent sexual penetration against the victim's will and
consent [Rape is not a sexual crime, but a crime of violence and identified as sexual assault. Although attacks
are most often directed toward women, men also may
be victims.]

NOTE: This syndrome includes the following three
subcomponents: [A] Rape-Trauma; [B] Compound
Reaction; and (C) Silent Reaction.

[A] Rape-Trauma—(00142)

Related Factors

Rape [actual or attempted forced sexual penetration]

Defining Characteristics

Subjective

Embarrassment; humiliation; shame; guilt; self-blame
Loss of self-esteem; helplessness; powerlessness
Shock; fear; anxiety; anger; revenge
Nightmares; sleep disturbances
Change in relationships; sexual dysfunction

Objective

Physical trauma [e.g., bruising, tissue irritation]; muscle tension
   or spasms
Confusion; disorganization; impaired decision making
Agitation; hyperalertness; aggression
Mood swings; vulnerability; dependence; depression
Substance abuse; suicide attempts
Denial; phobias; paranoia; dissociative disorders

Information that appears in brackets has been added by the authors to clarify
and enhance the use of nursing diagnoses.

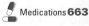

[B] Compound Reaction—(00143) Retired from Taxonomy 2009

Definition: Forced violent sexual penetration against the victim's will and consent. The trauma syndrome that develops from this attack or attempted attack includes an acute phase of disorganization of the victim's lifestyle and a long-term process of reorganization of lifestyle.

Related Factors

To be developed

Defining Characteristics

Subjective

Acute Phase
Emotional reactions (e.g., anger, embarrassment, fear of physical violence and death, humiliation, self-blame, revenge)

Multiple physical symptoms (e.g., GI irritability, genitourinary discomfort, muscle tension, sleep pattern disturbance)

Reactivated symptoms of previous conditions (e.g., physical or psychiatric illness); substance abuse

Long-Term Phase
Changes in lifestyle (e.g., changes in residence, dealing with repetitive nightmares and phobias, seeking family or social network support)

[C] Silent Reaction—(00141) Retired from Taxonomy 2009

Definition: Forced violent sexual penetration against the victim's will and consent. The trauma syndrome that develops from this attack or attempted attack includes an acute phase of disorganization of the victim's lifestyle and a long-term process of reorganization of lifestyle.

Related Factors

To be developed

Information that appears in brackets has been added by the authors to clarify and enhance the use of nursing diagnoses.

🌐 Cultural   🔧 Collaborative   🏠 Community/Home Care

Defining Characteristics

Subjective
Increase in nightmares
Abrupt changes in relationships with men
Pronounced changes in sexual behavior

Objective
Increasing anxiety during interview (e.g., blocking of associations, long periods of silence, minor stuttering, physical distress)
No verbalization of the occurrence of rape
Sudden onset of phobic reactions

Desired Outcomes/Evaluation Criteria—Client Will:

- Deal appropriately with emotional reactions as evidenced by behavior and expression of feelings.
- Report absence of physical complications, pain, and discomfort.
- Verbalize a positive self-image.
- Verbalize recognition that incident was not of own doing.
- Identify behaviors or situations within own control that may enhance sense of safety, reduce risk of recurrence.
- Deal with practical aspects (e.g., court appearances).
- Demonstrate appropriate changes in lifestyle (e.g., change in job, residence) as necessary and seek or obtain support from SO(s) as needed.
- Interact with individuals and groups in desired and acceptable manner.

Actions/Interventions

Nursing Priority No. 1.
To assess trauma and individual reaction, noting length of time since occurrence of event:

- Observe for and elicit information about physical injury and assess stress-related symptoms, such as numbness, headache, tightness in chest, nausea, and pounding heart.
- Identify psychological responses: anger, shock, acute anxiety, confusion, denial. Note laughter, crying, calm or agitated state, excited (hysterical) behavior, expressions of disbelief, and/or self-blame.

Information that appears in brackets has been added by the authors to clarify and enhance the use of nursing diagnoses.

- Note signs of increasing anxiety (e.g., silence, stuttering, inability to sit still). **Indicates need for immediate interventions to prevent panic reaction.**
- Determine degree of disorganization. **(May need help to manage ADLs and other aspects of life.)**
- Identify whether incident has reactivated preexisting or co-existing situations (physical/psychological). **Can affect how the client views the trauma, and reactive preexisting problems.**

- Ascertain cultural values or religious beliefs that may affect how client views incident, self, and expectations of SO/family reaction.
- Determine disruptions in relationships with men and with others (e.g., family, friends, coworkers, SO[s]).
- Identify development of phobic reactions to ordinary articles (e.g., knives, buildings) and situations (e.g., walking in groups of people, strangers ringing doorbell).
- Note degree of intrusive repetitive thoughts, sleep disturbances.
- Assess degree of dysfunctional coping (e.g., use of alcohol, other drugs, suicidal/homicidal ideation, marked change in sexual behavior).

Nursing Priority No. 2.
To assist client to deal with situation that exists:

- Explore own feelings (nurse/caregiver) regarding rape or incest issue prior to interacting with the client. **Need to recognize own biases to prevent imposing them on the client.**

Acute Phase

- Stay with the client, do not leave child unattended. **Provides reassurance and sense of safety.**
- Involve rape response team where available. Provide same-sex examiner when appropriate.
- Evaluate infant, child, or adolescent as dictated by age, sex, and developmental level.
- Assist with documentation of incident for police or child-protective services reports, maintain sequencing and collection of evidence (chain of evidence), label each specimen, and store and package properly. **Protecting evidence is important to the judicial process when offender goes to trial.**
- Provide environment in which client can talk freely about feelings and fears, including concerns about relationship with and response of SO(s), pregnancy, sexually transmitted diseases.

Information that appears in brackets has been added by the authors to clarify and enhance the use of nursing diagnoses.

Cultural   Collaborative   Community/Home Care

- Provide psychological support by listening and remaining with client. If client does not want to talk, accept silence. **May indicate Silent Reaction.**
- Listen to and investigate physical complaints. Assist with medical treatments, as indicated. **Emotional reactions may limit client's ability to recognize physical injury.**
- Assist with practical realities (e.g., safe temporary housing, money, or other needs).
- Determine client's ego strengths and assist client to use them in a positive way by acknowledging client's ability to handle what is happening.
- Identify support persons for this individual. **The client's partner can be important to her or his recovery by being patient and comforting. When partners talk through the incident, the relationship can be strengthened.**

Postacute Phase

- Allow the client to work through own kind of adjustment (may be withdrawn or unwilling to talk); do not force the issue, but be available, if needed.
- Listen for expressions of fear of crowds, men, being alone in home, and so forth. **May reveal developing phobias.**
- Discuss specific concerns and fears. Identify appropriate actions (e.g., diagnostic testing for pregnancy, sexually transmitted diseases) and provide information, as indicated.
- Include written instructions that are concise and clear regarding medical treatments, crisis support services, and so forth. **Reinforces teaching, provides opportunity to deal with information at own pace.**

Long-Term Phase

- Continue listening to expressions of concern. May need to continue to talk about the assault. Note persistence of somatic complaints (e.g., nausea, anorexia, insomnia, muscle tension, headache).
- Permit free expression of feelings (may continue from the crisis phase). Refrain from rushing client through expressions of feelings and avoid reassuring inappropriately. **Client may believe pain and/or anguish is misunderstood and depression may limit responses.**
- Acknowledge reality of loss of self that existed before the incident. Assist client to move toward an acceptance of the potential for growth that exists within individual.
- Continue to allow client to progress at own pace.

Information that appears in brackets has been added by the authors to clarify and enhance the use of nursing diagnoses.

- Give "permission" to express/deal with anger at the perpetrator and situation in acceptable ways. Set limits on destructive behaviors. **Facilitates resolution of feelings without diminishing self-concept.**
- Keep discussion on practical and emotional level rather than intellectualizing the experience, **which allows client to avoid dealing with feelings.**
- Assist in dealing with ongoing concerns about and effects of the incident, such as court appearance, pregnancy, sexually transmitted disease, and relationship with SO(s).
- Provide for sensitive, trained counselors, considering individual needs. **(Male or female counselors may be best determined on an individual basis as counselor's gender may be an issue for some clients, affecting ability to disclose.)**

Nursing Priority No. 3.

To promote wellness (Teaching/Discharge Considerations):

- Provide information about what reactions client may expect during each phase. Let client know these are common reactions and phrase in neutral terms of "You may or may not . . . ." (Be aware that, although male rape perpetrators are usually heterosexual, the male victim may be concerned about his own sexuality and may exhibit a homophobic response.)
- Assist client to identify factors that may have created a vulnerable situation and that she or he may have power to change **to protect self in the future.**
- Avoid making value judgments.
- Discuss lifestyle changes client is contemplating and how they will contribute to recovery. **Helps client evaluate appropriateness of plans and make decisions that will be helpful to eventual recovery.**
- Encourage psychiatric consultation if client is violent, inconsolable, or does not seem to be making an adjustment. **Participation in a group may be helpful.**
- Refer to family/marital counseling, as indicated.
- Refer to NDs Powerlessness; ineffective Coping; Grieving; complicated Grieving; Anxiety; Fear.

Documentation Focus

Assessment/Reassessment

- Individual findings, including nature of incident, individual reactions and fears, degree of trauma (physical and emotional), effects on lifestyle.

Information that appears in brackets has been added by the authors to clarify and enhance the use of nursing diagnoses.

⊕ Cultural 🐾 Collaborative 🏠 Community/Home Care

- Cultural or religious factors.
- Reactions of family/SO(s).
- Samples gathered for evidence, disposition, and storage (chain of evidence).

Planning
- Plan of action and who is involved in planning.
- Teaching plan.

Implementation/Evaluation
- Responses to interventions, teaching, and actions performed.
- Attainment or progress toward desired outcome(s).
- Modifications to plan of care.

Discharge Planning
- Long-term needs and who is responsible for actions to be taken.
- Specific referrals made.

Sample Nursing Outcomes & Interventions Classifications (NOC/NIC) (NIC)

NOC—Abuse Recovery: Sexual
NIC—Rape Trauma Treatment

Compound Reaction
NOC—Coping
NIC—Crises Intervention

Silent Reaction
NOC—Abuse Recovery: Emotional
NIC—Counseling

---

readiness for enhanced **Relationship**

Taxonomy II: Role Relationships—Class 3 Role
  Performance (00207)
[Diagnostic Division: Ego Integrity]
Submitted 2008

Definition: A pattern of mutual partnership that is sufficient to provide each other's needs and can be strengthened

---

Information that appears in brackets has been added by the authors to clarify and enhance the use of nursing diagnoses.

 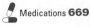

Related Factors

To be developed

Defining Characteristics

Subjective
Expresses:
Desire to enhance communication between partners
Satisfaction with sharing of information and ideas between partners
Satisfaction with fulfilling physical and emotional needs by one's partner
Satisfaction with complementary relation between partners
Identifies each other as a key person

Objective
Demonstrates:
Mutual respect between partners
Well-balanced autonomy and collaboration between partners
Mutual support in daily activities between partners
Understanding of partner's insufficient (physical, social, psychological) function
Meets developmental goals appropriate for family life cycle stage

Sample Clinical Applications

Chronic conditions (e.g., MS, spinal cord injury, gastric bypass surgery, mental health problems, depression, anxiety, bipolar disorder, substance abuse)

Desired Outcomes/Evaluation Criteria: Client Will (Include Specific Time Frames)

- Verbalize a desire to learn more effective communication skills.
- Verbalize understanding of current relationship with partner.
- Seek information to improve emotional and physical needs of both partners.
- Talk with partner about circumstances that can be improved.
- Develop realistic plans to strengthen relationship.

Actions/Interventions

Nursing Priority No. 1.
To assess current situation and determine needs:

- Determine makeup of family (e.g., includes couple only, parents and children, older and younger members). **Life changes,**

Information that appears in brackets has been added by the authors to clarify and enhance the use of nursing diagnoses.

🌐 Cultural 🔘 Collaborative 🏠 Community/Home Care

such as developmental, situational, health-illness, can affect relationship between partners and require readjustment and thinking of ways to enhance situation.

- Discuss client's perception of needs and how partner sees desire to improve relationship.
- Identify use of effective communication skills. **May need to improve understanding of words partners use in discussion of sensitive subjects.**
- Help client identify thoughts and feelings when starting a discussion with partner. **A system of thinking (referred to as a paradigm) forms the basis for how we look at and experience life and determines how we perceive our world, forms the basis for our reality, and exists below our level of conscience.**
- Ask partners how they deal with conflict.
- Ascertain client's view of sexual aspects of relationship. **Changes that occur with aging or medical conditions, such as hysterectomy, erectile dysfunction, can affect the relationship and need specific interventions to resolve.**
- Identify cultural factors relating to individual's view of role in relationship.
- Discuss how family as a whole functions. **Interrelationships with members of the family, personal and family history, and situational dynamics can improve the functioning of the whole family.**

Nursing Priority No. 2.
To assist the client to enhance existing situation:

- Maintain positive attitude toward client. **Promotes safe relationship in which client can feel free to speak openly and plan for a positive future.**
- Have couple discuss paradigms that they have become aware of in own thinking that interfere with relationship.
- Determine how each person views themselves as a positive or negative person. One's self-image influences behavior and how they relate to others. When emotional needs are met individuals relate to others in positive ways, while unmet needs result in low self-image and insecurity.
- Discuss the skills of emotional intelligence that are important for maintaining positive relationships. **This is the ability to recognize and effectively control our own emotions and to recognize the emotions of others.**
- Help couple to recognize that surface symptoms of dysfunctional relationships are not the problems that need to be dealt

---

Information that appears in brackets has been added by the authors to clarify and enhance the use of nursing diagnoses.

with. **Underlying emotions influence our behaviors and individuals often are not aware of them and continue to deal with the superficial conflicts.**

- Explore individual's emotional needs. **Relationships are often motivated by unconscious desires to gain acceptance, recognition, sense of being cared about or valued.**
- Note client's awareness of nonverbal communications. **Body language, tone of voice, a roll of the eyes or subtle movements convey strong messages, positive or negative, that need to be discussed and clarified.**
- Discuss effective conflict resolution skills.
- Encourage client to remain calm and focused regardless of circumstances. **Maintaining a calm demeanor helps individual to be able to think more clearly and be more rational in dealing with situation.**
- Recommend cross-checking or verifying what listener believes speaker said. **Clarifies communication and allows speaker to respond or correct perception of listener as needed.**
- Help partners to learn win-win method of conflict resolution.
- Role-play ways to defuse arguments and repair injured feelings. **Provides a realistic situation where each person can identify own and partner's view and practice new ways of interacting.**
- Provide open environment for partners to discuss sexual concerns and questions.
- Discuss nonblameful self-disclosure when having a dialogue. **Partners take turns talking about own needs and feelings without blaming the other, resulting in being able to find a solution in a climate of mutual consideration and respect.**

Nursing Priority No. 3.

To promote optimal functioning (Teaching/Discharge Considerations):

- Provide information for partners, using bibliotherapy, appropriate Web sites.
- Encourage couple to use humor and playfulness in their relationship. **Sharing laughter and enjoying life helps weather difficult times.**
- Discuss the importance of being an empathic, understanding, and nonjudgmental listener when either partner has a problem.

Information that appears in brackets has been added by the authors to clarify and enhance the use of nursing diagnoses.

⊕ Cultural   ⊗ Collaborative   🏠 Community/Home Care

- Help individuals to learn to use the skill of Active-listening. **This avoids giving advice and helps other person to find own solution, enhancing self-esteem.**
• Refer to support groups, classes on assertiveness, parenting, as indicated by individual needs.
- Include family members in discussions as needed.
• Refer for care as indicated by psychological or physical concerns of either individual.

Documentation Focus

Assessment/Reassessment
- Baseline information, individuals' perception of situation and self.
- Reasons for desire to improve relationship.
- Motivation and expectations for change.

Planning
- Plan of care and who is involved in planning.
- Teaching Plan.

Implementation/Evaluation
- Response of partners to plan, interventions, and actions performed.
- Attainment or progress toward desired outcomes(s).

Discharge Planning
- Long-range plan and who is responsible for actions to be taken.

Sample Nursing Outcomes & Interventions Classifications (NOC/NIC) NIC

NOC—Role Enhancement
NIC—Social Interaction Skills

---

impaired Religiosity

Taxonomy II: Life Principles—Class 3 Value/Belief/Action Conguence (00169)
[Diagnostic Division: Ego Integrity]
Submitted 2004

Definition: Impaired ability to exercise reliance on beliefs and/or participate in rituals of a particular faith tradition

---

Information that appears in brackets has been added by the authors to clarify and enhance the use of nursing diagnoses.

NOTE: NANDA recognizes that the term "religiosity" may be culture specific; however, the term is useful in the United States and is well supported in the U.S. literature.

Related Factors

Developmental and Situational
Life transitions; aging; end-stage life crises

Physical
Illness; pain

Psychological Factors
Ineffective support or coping
Anxiety; fear of death
Personal crisis/[/disaster], lack of security
Use of religion to manipulate

Sociocultural
Cultural or environmental barriers to practicing religion
Lack of social integration; lack of sociocultural interaction

Spiritual
Spiritual crises; suffering

Defining Characteristics

Subjective
Expresses emotional distress because of separation from faith community
Expresses a need to reconnect with previous belief patterns/customs
Questions religious belief patterns/customs
Difficulty adhering to prescribed religious beliefs and rituals (e.g., religious ceremonies, dietary regulations, clothing, prayer, worship/religious services, private religious behaviors/reading religious materials/media, holiday observances, meetings with religious leaders)

Desired Outcomes/Evaluation Criteria—Client Will:

• Express ability to once again participate in beliefs and rituals of desired religion.

Information that appears in brackets has been added by the authors to clarify and enhance the use of nursing diagnoses.

Cultural   Collaborative   Community/Home Care

- Discuss beliefs and values about spiritual or religious issues.
- Attend religious or worship services of choice as desired.
- Verbalize concerns about end-of-life issues and fear of death.

Actions/Interventions

Nursing Priority No. 1.
To assess causative/contributing factors:

- Determine client's usual religious or spiritual beliefs, values, past spiritual commitment. **Provides a baseline for understanding current problem or need.**
- Note client's/SO's reports and expressions of anger, alienation from God, sense of guilt or retribution. **Perception of guilt may cause spiritual crisis and suffering resulting in rejection of religious symbols.**
- Determine sense of futility, feelings of hopelessness, lack of motivation to help self. **Indicators that client may see no, or only limited, options, alternatives or personal choices.**
- Assess extent of depression client may be experiencing. **Some studies suggest that a focus on religion may protect against depression.**
- Note recent changes in behavior (e.g., withdrawal from others or religious activities; dependence on alcohol or medications). **Lack of connectedness with self/others impairs ability to trust others or feel worthy of trust from others or God.**

Nursing Priority No. 2.
To assist client/SO(s) to deal with feelings/situation:

- Use therapeutic communication skills of reflection and active-listening. **Communicates acceptance and enables client to find own solutions to concerns.**
- Encourage expression of feelings about illness, condition, death.
- Suggest use of journaling and reminiscence. **Promotes life review and can assist in clarifying values and ideas, recognizing and resolving feelings or situation.**
- Discuss differences between grief and guilt, and help client to identify and deal with each. Point out consequences of actions based on guilt.
- Encourage client to identify individuals (e.g., spiritual advisor, parish nurse) who can provide needed support.
- Review client's religious affiliation, associated rituals, and beliefs. **Helps client examine what has been important in the past.**

Information that appears in brackets has been added by the authors to clarify and enhance the use of nursing diagnoses.

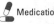

- Provide opportunity for nonjudgmental discussion of philosophical issues related to religious belief patterns and customs. **Open communication can assist client to check reality of perceptions and identify personal options and willingness to resume desired activities.**
- Discuss desire to continue or reconnect with previous belief patterns and customs and current barriers.
- Involve client in refining healthcare goals and therapeutic regimen, as appropriate. **Identifies role illness is playing in current concerns about ability to participate or appropriateness of participating in desired religious activities.**

Nursing Priority No. 3.

To promote spiritual wellness (Teaching/Discharge Considerations):

• Assist client to identify spiritual resources that could be helpful (e.g., contacting spiritual advisor who has qualifications and experience in dealing with specific problems individual is concerned about). **Provides answers to spiritual questions, assists in the journey of self-discovery, and can help client learn to accept and forgive self.**
- Provide privacy for meditation, prayer, or performance of rituals, as appropriate.
- Explore alternatives or modifications of ritual based on setting and individual needs and limitations.

Documentation Focus

Assessment/Reassessment
- Individual findings, including nature of spiritual conflict, effects of participation in treatment regimen.
- Physical and emotional responses to conflict.

Planning
- Plan of care and who is involved in planning.
- Teaching plan.

Implementation/Evaluation
- Responses to interventions, teaching, and actions performed.
- Attainment or progress toward desired outcome(s).
- Modifications to plan of care.

Information that appears in brackets has been added by the authors to clarify and enhance the use of nursing diagnoses.

Discharge Planning

- Long-term needs and who is responsible for actions to be taken.
- Available resources, specific referrals made.

Sample Nursing Outcomes & Interventions Classifications (NOC/NIC) NIC

NOC—Spiritual Health
NIC—Religious Ritual Enhancement

---

readiness for enhanced **Religiosity**

Taxonomy II: Life Principles—Class 3 Value/Belief/Action Conguence (00171)
[Diagnostic Division: Ego Integrity]
Submitted 2004

Definition: Ability to increase reliance on religious beliefs and/or participate in rituals of a particular faith tradition

---

NOTE: NANDA recognizes that the term "religiosity" may be culture specific; however, the term is useful in the United States and is well supported in the U.S. literature.

Related Factors

To be developed

Defining Characteristics

Subjective

Expresses desire to strengthen religious belief patterns or customs that had provided comfort or religion in the past

Request for assistance to increase participation in prescribed religious beliefs (e.g., religious ceremonies, dietary regulations/rituals, clothing, prayer, worship/religious services, private religious behaviors, reading religious materials/media, holiday observances)

Requests assistance expanding religious options/religious materials/experiences

---

Information that appears in brackets has been added by the authors to clarify and enhance the use of nursing diagnoses.

 Diagnostic Studies   Pediatric/Geriatric/Lifespan Medications **677**

Requests meeting with religious leaders/facilitators
Requests forgiveness, reconciliation
Questions or rejects belief patterns or customs that are harmful

Desired Outcomes/Evaluation Criteria— Client Will:

- Acknowledge need to strengthen religious affiliations and continue or resume previously comforting rituals.
- Verbalize willingness to seek help to enhance desired religious beliefs.
- Become involved in spiritually based programs of own choice.
- Recognize the difference between belief patterns and customs that are helpful and those that may be harmful.

Actions/Interventions

Nursing Priority No. 1.

To determine spiritual state/motivation for growth:

- Determine client's current thinking about desire to learn more about religious beliefs and actions.
- Ascertain religious beliefs of family of origin and climate in which client grew up. **Early religious training deeply affects children and is carried on into adulthood. Conflict between family's beliefs and client's current learning may need to be addressed.**
- Discuss client's spiritual commitment, beliefs, and values. **Enables examination of these issues and helps client learn more about self and what he or she desires/believes.**
- Explore how spirituality and religious practices have affected client's life.
- Ascertain motivation and expectations for change.

Nursing Priority No. 2.

To assist client to integrate values and beliefs to strengthen sense of wholeness and achieve optimum balance in daily living:

- Establish nurse-client relationship in which dialogue can occur. **Client can feel safe to say anything and know it will be accepted.**
- Identify barriers and beliefs that might hinder growth and/or self-discovery. **Previous practices and beliefs may need to**

Information that appears in brackets has been added by the authors to clarify and enhance the use of nursing diagnoses.

   Cultural   Collaborative   Community/Home Care

be considered and accepted or discarded in new search for religious beliefs.

• Discuss cultural beliefs of family of origin and how they have influenced client's religious practices. **As client expands options for learning new or other religious beliefs and practices, these influences will provide information for comparing and contrasting new information.**

• Explore connection of desire to strengthen belief patterns and customs to daily life. **Becoming aware of how these issues affect the individual's daily life can enhance ability to incorporate them into everything he or she does.**

• Identify ways in which individual can develop a sense of harmony with self and others.

Nursing Priority No. 3.
To enhance optimum spiritual wellness:

• Encourage client to seek out and experience different religious beliefs, services, and ceremonies. **Trying out different religions will give client more information to contrast and compare what will fit his or her belief system.**

• Provide bibliotherapy or reading materials pertaining to spiritual issues client is interested in learning about.

• Help client learn about stress-reducing activities (e.g., meditation, relaxation exercises, mindfulness). **Promotes general well-being and sense of control over self and ability to choose religious activities desired. Mindfulness is a method of being in the moment.**

• Encourage participation in religious activities, worship or religious services, reading religious materials or reviewing multimedia sources, study groups, volunteering in choir, or undertaking other needed duties.

• Refer to community resources (e.g., parish nurse, religion classes, other support groups).

Documentation Focus

Assessment/Reassessment
• Assessment findings, including client's religious beliefs and practices, perception of need.
• Motivation and expectations for growth or enhancement.

Planning
• Plan for growth and who is involved in planning.

Information that appears in brackets has been added by the authors to clarify and enhance the use of nursing diagnoses.

Implementation/Evaluation
- Response to activities, learning, and actions performed.
- Attainment or progress toward desired outcome(s).
- Modifications to plan.

Discharge Planning
- Long-term needs/expectations and plan of action.
- Specific referrals made.

Sample Nursing Outcomes & Interventions Classifications (NOC/NIC) NIC

NOC—Spiritual Health
NIC—Spiritual Growth Facilitation

risk for impaired Religiosity

Taxonomy II: Life Principles—Class 3 Value/Belief/Action Conguence (00170)
[Diagnostic Division: Ego Integrity]
Submitted 2004

Definition: At risk for an impaired ability to exercise reliance on religious beliefs and/or participate in rituals of a particular faith tradition

NOTE: NANDA recognizes that the term "religiosity" may be culture specific; however, the term is useful in the United States and is well supported in the U.S. literature.

Risk Factors

Developmental
Life transitions

Environmental
Lack of transportation
Barriers to practicing religion

Physical
Illness; hospitalization; pain

Information that appears in brackets has been added by the authors to clarify and enhance the use of nursing diagnoses.

Psychological
Ineffective support, coping, or caregiving
Depression
Lack of security

Sociocultural
Lack of social interaction; social isolation
Cultural barrier to practicing religion

Spiritual
Suffering

> **NOTE:** A risk diagnosis is not evidenced by signs and symptoms, as the problem has not occurred; rather, nursing interventions are directed at prevention.

Desired Outcomes/Evaluation Criteria—Client Will:

- Express understanding of relation of situation/health status to thoughts and feelings of concern about ability to participate in desired religious activities.
- Seek solutions to individual factors that may interfere with reliance on religious beliefs/participation in religious rituals.
- Identify and use resources appropriately.

Actions/Interventions

Nursing Priority No. 1.
To assess causative/contributing factors:

- Ascertain current situation (e.g., illness, hospitalization, prognosis of death, depression, lack of support systems, financial concerns). **Identifies problems client is dealing with in the moment that may be affecting desire to be involved with religious activities.**
- Note client's concerns or expressions of anger, belief that illness or situation is result of lack of faith. **Individual may blame himself or herself for what has happened and could reject religious beliefs and/or God.**
- Determine client's usual religious or spiritual beliefs, past or current involvement in specific church activities.
- Identify cultural values and expectations regarding religious beliefs and/or practices.

Information that appears in brackets has been added by the authors to clarify and enhance the use of nursing diagnoses.

- Note quality of relationships with significant others and friends. **Individual may withdraw from others in relation to the stress of illness, pain, and suffering. Others may be encouraging client to rely on religious beliefs at a time when individual is questioning own beliefs in the current situation.**
- Assess for barriers (e.g., lack of transportation, lack of family involvement) to participation in desired religious activities.
- Ascertain substance use or abuse. **Individuals often turn to use of various substances in distress, and this can affect the ability to deal with problems in a positive manner.**

Nursing Priority No. 2.

To assist client to deal with feelings/situation:

- Develop nurse-client relationship. **Individual can express feelings and concerns freely when he or she feels safe to do so.**
- Use therapeutic communications skills of Active-listening, reflection, and I-messages. **Helps client find own solutions to problems and concerns and promotes sense of control.**
- Have client identify and prioritize current or immediate needs. **Dealing with current needs is easier than trying to predict the future.**
- Provide time for nonjudgmental discussion of individual's spiritual beliefs and fears about impact of current illness and/or treatment regimen. **Helps clarify thoughts and promote ability to deal with stresses of what is happening.**
- Review with client past difficulties in life and coping skills that were used at those times.
- Encourage client to discuss feelings about death and end-of-life issues when illness or prognosis is grave.

Nursing Priority No. 3.

To promote spiritual wellness (Teaching/Discharge Considerations):

- Have client identify support systems available.
- Help client learn relaxation techniques, meditation, guided imagery, and mindfulness/living in the moment and enjoying it.
- Take the lead from the client in initiating participation in religious activities, prayer, other activities. **Client may be vulnerable in current situation and must be allowed to decide own participation in these actions.**

Information that appears in brackets has been added by the authors to clarify and enhance the use of nursing diagnoses.

⊕ Cultural ⊛ Collaborative 🏠 Community/Home Care

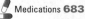

• Refer to appropriate resources (e.g., crisis counselor, governmental agencies, spiritual advisor) who has qualifications or experience dealing with specific problems, such as death/dying, relationship problems, substance abuse, suicide, hospice, psychotherapy, Alcoholics or Narcotics Anonymous.

Documentation Focus

Assessment/Reassessment
• Individual findings, including risk factors, nature of current distress.
• Physical and emotional response to distress.
• Availability and use of resources.

Planning
• Plan of care and who is involved in planning.
• Teaching plan.

Implementation/Evaluation
• Responses to interventions, teaching, and actions performed.
• Attainment or progress toward desired outcome(s).
• Modifications to plan of care.

Discharge Planning
• Long-term needs and who is responsible for actions to be taken.
• Available resources, specific referrals made.

Sample Nursing Outcomes & Interventions Classifications (NOC/NIC) NIC

NOC—Spiritual Health
NIC—Spiritual Support

Relocation Stress Syndrome

Taxonomy II: Coping/Stress Tolerance—Class 1 Post-Trauma Responses (00114)
[Diagnostic Division: Ego Integrity]
Submitted 1992; Revised 2000

Definition: Physiological and/or psychosocial disturbance following transfer from one environment to another

---

Information that appears in brackets has been added by the authors to clarify and enhance the use of nursing diagnoses.

Related Factors

Losses; feeling of powerlessness

Lack of adequate support system; lack of predeparture counseling; unpredictability of experience

Isolation; language barrier

Impaired psychosocial health; passive coping

Decreased health status

Defining Characteristics

Subjective

Anxiety (e.g., separation); anger

Insecurity; worry; fear

Loneliness; depression

Unwillingness to move; concern over relocation

Sleep disturbance

Objective

Move from one environment to another

Increased [frequency of] verbalization of needs

Pessimism; frustration

Increased physical symptoms or illness

Withdrawal; aloneness; alienation; [hostile behavior or outbursts]

Loss of identity, self-worth, or self-esteem; dependency

Increased confusion or cognitive impairment

Desired Outcomes/Evaluation Criteria— Client Will:

- Verbalize understanding of reason(s) for change.
- Demonstrate appropriate range of feelings and lessened fear.
- Participate in routine and special or social events as able.
- Verbalize acceptance of situation.
- Experience no catastrophic event.

Actions/Interventions

Nursing Priority No. 1.

To assess degree of stress as perceived/experienced by client and determine issues of safety:

- Determine situation or cause for relocation (e.g., planned move for new job; loss of home or community due to natural

---

Information that appears in brackets has been added by the authors to clarify and enhance the use of nursing diagnoses.

   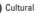 Cultural   Collaborative   Community/Home Care

or man-made disaster such as fire, earthquake, flood, war or act of terror; older adult unable to care for self, caregiver burnout; change in marital or health status). **Influences needs and choice of interventions.**

- Ascertain if client participated in the decision to relocate and perceptions about change(s) and expectations for the future. **Decision may have been made without client's input or understanding of event or consequences, which can impact adjustment.**

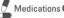• Note client's age, developmental level, role in family. **Child can be traumatized by transfer to new school or loss of peers; elderly persons may be affected by loss of long-term home, neighborhood setting, and support persons.**

- Determine presence of cultural and/or religious concerns or conflicts.

- Monitor behavior, noting presence of anxiety, suspiciousness or paranoia, irritability, defensiveness. Compare with SO's/ staff's description of customary responses. **Move may temporarily exacerbate mental deterioration (cognitive inaccessibility) and impair communication (social inaccessibility).**

- Note signs of increased stress (e.g., irritability, withdrawal, crying, moodiness, problems sleeping, increased use of alcohol or other drugs), reports of "new" physical discomfort or pain (e.g., stomach aches, headaches, back pain); change in appetite; greater susceptiblilty to colds, fatigue.

- Determine involvement of family/SO(s). Note availability and use of support systems and resources.

- Identify issues of safety that may be involved.

Nursing Priority No. 2.

To assist client to deal with situation/changes:

- Encourage visit to new community, surroundings, school prior to transfer when possible. **Provides opportunity to "get acquainted" with new situation, reducing fear of unknown.**

- Encourage free expression of feelings about reason for relocation, including venting of anger; grief; loss of personal space, belongings, or friends; financial strains; powerlessness; and so forth. Acknowledge reality of situation and maintain hopeful attitude regarding move/change. Refer to NDs relating to client's particular situation (e.g., Grieving; ineffective Coping) for additional interventions.

Information that appears in brackets has been added by the authors to clarify and enhance the use of nursing diagnoses.

- Identify strengths and successful coping behaviors the individual has used previously. **Incorporating these into problem solving builds on past successes.**
- Orient to surroundings and schedules. Introduce to neighbors, staff members, roommate or residents. Provide clear, honest information about actions and events.
- Encourage individual/family to personalize area with pictures, own belongings, as possible and appropriate. **Enhances sense of belonging and creates personal space.**
- Determine client's usual schedule of activities and incorporate into routine as possible. **Reinforces sense of importance of individual.**
- Introduce planned diversional activities, such as movies, meals with new acquaintances, art therapy, music, religious activities. **Involvement increases opportunity to interact with others, decreasing isolation.**
- Place in private facility room, if appropriate, and include SO(s)/family into care activities, mealtime and so forth.
- Encourage hugging and use of touch unless client is paranoid or agitated at the moment. **Human connection reaffirms acceptance of individual.**
- Deal with aggressive behavior by imposing calm, firm limits. Control environment and protect others from client's disruptive behavior. **Promotes safety for client and others.**
- Remain calm, place in a quiet environment, providing time-out, as indicated, **to prevent escalation into panic state and violent behavior.**
- Collaborate in treatment of underlying conditions (e.g., chronic confusional states/brain injury, post-trauma rehabilitation) and physical stress symptoms **that are potentially exacerbating relocation stress.**
- Refer to social worker, financial resources, mental healthcare provider, minister/spiritual advisor for additional assessment and interventions, as indicated. **May be needed if client has special needs and/or persistent problems with adaptation.**

Nursing Priority No. 3.
To promote wellness (Teaching/Discharge Considerations):
- Involve client in formulating goals and plan of care when possible. **Supports independence and commitment to achieving outcomes.**
- Discuss benefits of adequate nutrition, rest, and exercise **to maintain physical well-being.**

Information that appears in brackets has been added by the authors to clarify and enhance the use of nursing diagnoses.

Cultural   Collaborative   Community/Home Care

• Involve in anxiety- and stress-reduction activities (e.g., meditation, progressive muscle relaxation, group socialization), as able, to enhance psychological well-being.

 • Encourage participation in activities, hobbies, and personal interactions as appropriate. **Promotes creative endeavors, stimulating the mind.**

 • Identify community supports, cultural or ethnic groups client can access.

 • Support self-responsibility and coping strategies. Foster sense of control and self-worth.

Documentation Focus

Assessment/Reassessment
- Assessment findings, individual's perception of the situation and changes, sense of loss, specific behaviors.
- Cultural or religious concerns.
- Safety issues.

Planning
- Note plan of care, who is involved in planning, and who is responsible for proposed actions.
- Teaching plan.

Implementation/Evaluation
- Response to interventions (especially time out or seclusion), teaching, and actions performed.
- Sentinel events.
- Attainment or progress toward desired outcome(s).
- Modifications to plan of care.

Discharge Planning
- Long-term needs and who is responsible for actions to be taken.
- Specific referrals made.

Sample Nursing Outcomes & Interventions Classifications (NOC/NIC) NIC

NOC—Psychosocial Adjustment: Life Change
NIC—Relocation Stress Reduction

Information that appears in brackets has been added by the authors to clarify and enhance the use of nursing diagnoses.

risk for Relocation Stress Syndrome

Taxonomy II: Coping/Stress Tolerance—Class 1 Post-
Trauma Responses (00149)
[Diagnostic Division: Ego Integrity]
Submitted 2000

Definition: At risk for physiological and/or psychosocial
disturbance following transfer from one environment to
another

Risk Factors

Move from one environment to another
Moderate to high degree of environmental change [e.g., physi-
cal, ethnic, cultural]
Lack of adequate support system or group; lack of predeparture
counseling
Passive coping; feelings of powerlessness; losses
Moderate mental competence
Unpredictability of experiences
Decreased health status

NOTE: A risk diagnosis is not evidenced by signs and
symptoms, as the problem has not occurred; rather,
nursing interventions are directed at prevention.

Desired Outcomes/Evaluation Criteria—
Client Will:

- Verbalize understanding of reason(s) for change.
- Express feelings and concerns openly and appropriately.
- Experience no catastrophic event.

Actions/Interventions

Nursing Priority No. 1.
To assess causative/contributing factors:

- Determine situation or cause for relocation (e.g., planned
move for new job; loss of home or community due to natural
or man-made disaster such as fire, earthquake, war; older adult
unable to care for self, caregiver burnout; change in marital

Information that appears in brackets has been added by the authors to clarify
and enhance the use of nursing diagnoses.

🌐 Cultural   Ⓐ Collaborative   🏠 Community/Home Care

or health status). **Influences needs and choice of interventions.**

 • Determine presence of cultural and/or religious concerns or conflicts.

• Ascertain if client participated in decision to relocate and perceptions about change(s) and expectations for the future. **Decision can be made without client's input or understanding of event or consequences, which can impact adjustment and sense of control over life.**

∞ • Note client's age, developmental level, role in family. **Child can be traumatized by transfer to new school/loss of peers; elderly persons may be affected by loss of long-term home, neighborhood setting, and support persons.**

• Determine physical and emotional health status. **Stress associated with move, even if desired, can exacerbate health problems.**

• Note whether relocation will be temporary (e.g., extended care for rehabilitation therapies, moving in with family while house is being repaired after fire) or long term or permanent (e.g., move from home of many years; placement in retirement center or long-term care facility). **Client may be willing to relocate on temporary basis, seeing it as step to health and independence, but may view long-term placement as unbearable loss.**

• Evaluate client/caregiver's resources and coping abilities. Determine family's/SO's degree of involvement and willingness to be involved.

• Identify issues of safety that may be involved.

Nursing Priority No. 2.

To prevent/minimize adverse response to change:

• Involve client in formulating goals and plan of care when possible. **Supports independence and commitment to achieving outcomes.**

• Encourage client/SO(s) to accept that relocation is an adjustment and that it takes time to adapt to new circumstances and environment.

• Allow as much time as possible for move preparation and provide information and support in planning.

• Support self-responsibility and coping strategies **to foster sense of control and self-worth.**

🏠 • Encourage visit to new community or surroundings prior to transfer when possible. **Provides opportunity to "get**

Information that appears in brackets has been added by the authors to clarify and enhance the use of nursing diagnoses.

acquainted" with new situation, thus reducing fear of unknown.

Refer to ND Relocation Stress Syndrome for additional Actions/Interventions and Documentation Focus.

---

impaired individual **Resilience**

Taxonomy II: Coping/Stress Tolerance—Class 2 Coping Responses (00210)
[Diagnostic Division: Ego Integrity]
Submitted 2008

Definition: Decreased ability to sustain a pattern of positive responses to an adverse situation or crisis

---

Related Factors

Demographics that increase chance of maladjustment; large family size; minority status; poverty; gender

Vulnerability factors which encompass indices that exacerbate the negative effects of the risk condition; drug use; poor impulse control; violence in neighborhood

Low intelligence; low maternal education

Inconsistent parenting; parental mental illness

Psychological disorders; violence

Defining Characteristics

Subjective

Depression; guilt; isolation or social isolation; low self-esteem; shame

Lower perceived health status

Renewed elevation of distress

Decreased interest in academic activities; vocational activities

Objective

Using maladaptive coping skills (i.e., drug use, violence, etc.)

Desired Outcomes/Evaluation Criteria Client Will (Include Specific Time Frame)

• Acknowledge reality of current situation or crisis.
• Express positive feelings about self and situation.

Information that appears in brackets has been added by the authors to clarify and enhance the use of nursing diagnoses.

⊕ Cultural ✇ Collaborative 🏠 Community/Home Care

- Seek appropriate resources to change circumstances that affect adaptation and resilience.
- Be involved in programs to address problems presenting in life (e.g., substance abuse, low self-esteem, poverty).

Actions/Interventions

Nursing Priority No. 1.
To assess causative/contributing factors:

- Determine individuals involved, family, children; and ages and current circumstances. **Understanding the family makeup provides information that will guide choice of interventions.**
- Note underlying stressors, health concerns, debilitating conditions, mental health or behavioral issues such as unemployment, poverty, diabetes, obesity, COPD, Alzheimer's disease, parental mental illness.
- Identify locus of control. **Individuals with external locus of control are less likely to feel in control or to rely on their own abilities or judgment to manage a situation.**
- Determine client's education level, family dynamics, and parenting styles if relevant. **Drug use, violence, and poor impulse control affect individual's ability to develop resilience in adverse situations or crisis. Individual may see self as a victim rather than a survivor.**
- Note communication patterns within the family. **Skills learned within the family can determine whether the individual develops low self-esteem or positive feelings about self.**
- Identify maladaptive coping skills used by individual and in the family. **Focusing on negative in situations impairs one's ability to adjust positively and learn attributes of resiliency.**
- Note parental status including age and maturity. **Young parents may lack ability to deal with family responsibilities, financial concerns, factors associated with low socioeconomic status.**
- Ascertain stability of relationship, presence of separation or divorce. **Family members are vulnerable to breakup of the family unit and may see it as causing long-term harm.**
- Determine availability and use of resources, family, support groups, financial aid.

Information that appears in brackets has been added by the authors to clarify and enhance the use of nursing diagnoses.

- Note cultural factors and religious beliefs that may affect interpretation of, or response to, situation. **Helps determine individual needs and possible options.**

Nursing Priority No. 2.

To assist client to improve skills to deal with adverse situations or crises:

- Encourage free expressions of feelings, including feelings of anger and hostility, setting limits on unacceptable behavior. **Unacceptable behavior leads to feelings of shame and guilt if not controlled.**
- Listen to client's concerns and acknowledge difficulty of adversity and making changes in situation. **Being listened to provides opportunity for client to feel valued, capable, and like a survivor rather than a victim.**
- Help client assume responsibility for own life, look at situation as a challenge rather than an obstacle, and refrain from viewing crisis as insurmountable. **People learn and develop resilience as they deal with adversities of life.**
- Provide information at client's level of comprehension, being honest in explanations. **Provides data to assist in decision-making process.**
- Have client paraphrase information provided during teaching session to **assure understanding and to provide opportunity to correct misunderstandings.**
- Promote parent involvement in developing a positive mindset for fostering resilience in their children.
- Facilitate communication skills between client and family. **Sometimes, individuals who find themselves in difficult situations withdraw because they do not know what to do or say.**
- Focus on strengths of the individual as the problems are being assessed and diagnosed.
- Teach client/parents to practice empathy with family members.
- Discuss individual issues, such as obesity, substance use, poor impulse control, violent behavior; providing information about the risks and helping client/parent understand how they can help family members develop habits that will promote physical and mental well-being.

Nursing Priority No. 3.

To promote wellness (Teaching/Discharge Considerations):

- Reinforce that client is responsible for self, for choices made, and actions taken. **The road to resilience is developed by**

Information that appears in brackets has been added by the authors to clarify and enhance the use of nursing diagnoses.

Cultural   Collaborative   Community/Home Care

the individual accepting that change is a part of living, and then beginning to live life more fully.

 • Provide or identify learning opportunities specific to individual needs. **Activities such as assertiveness, regular exercise, parenting classes can enhance knowledge and help develop a resilient mind-set.**

• Discuss use of the problem-solving method to set mutually agreed on goals.

• Provide anticipatory guidance relevant to current situation and long-term expectations. **Client may have many issues to resolve, and planning ahead can help individuals make changes, have hope for the future, and have a sense of control over their lives.**

• Encourage client/parents to take time for themselves. **Provides opportunity for personal growth; respite allows individuals to pursue own interests and return to tasks of life/parenting with renewed vigor.**

 • Refer to community resources as appropriate, such as social services, financial, domestic violence/elder abuse program, family therapy, divorce counseling, special-needs support services.

Documentation Focus

Assessment/Reassessment
• Findings, including specifics of individual situations, parental concerns, perceptions, expectations.
• Locus of control and cultural beliefs.

Planning
• Plan of care and who is involved in the planning.
• Teaching plan.

Implementation/Evaluation
• Response to interventions, teaching, and actions performed.
• Attainment or progress toward desired outcome(s).
• Modifications to plan of care.

Discharge Planning
• Long-term needs and who is responsible for actions to be taken.
• Specific referrals made.

Information that appears in brackets has been added by the authors to clarify and enhance the use of nursing diagnoses.

Sample Nursing Outcomes & Interventions Classifications (NOC/NIC) NIC

NOC—Personal Resiliency
NIC—Resiliency Promotion

readiness for enhanced Resilience

Taxonomy II: Coping/Stress Tolerance—Class 2 Coping Responses (00212)
[Diagnostic Division: Ego Integrity]
Submitted 2008

Definition: A pattern of positive responses to an adverse situation or crisis that can be strengthened to optimize human potential

Related Factors

Demographics that increase chance of maladjustment; large family size; minority status; poverty; gender
Vulnerability factors, which encompass indices that exacerbate the negative effects of the risk condition; drug use; poor impulse control
Low intelligence; low maternal education
Inconsistent parenting; parental mental illness
Psychological disorders; violence

Defining Characteristics

Subjective
Presence of a crisis
Verbalizes an enhanced sense of control/self-esteem; takes responsibilities for actions
Expressed desire to enhance resilience
Sets goals; makes progress toward goals
Identifies available resources or support systems
Involvement in activities

Objective
Demonstrates positive outlook
Enhances personal coping; use of effective communication skills; effective use of conflict management strategies
Increases positive relationships with others
Access to resources

Information that appears in brackets has been added by the authors to clarify and enhance the use of nursing diagnoses.

⊕ Cultural ⊛ Collaborative 🏠 Community/Home Care

Desired Outcomes/Evaluation Criteria—Client Will (Include Specific Time Frames):

- Describe current situation accurately.
- Identify positive responses currently being used.
- Verbalize feelings congruent with behavior.
- Express desire to strengthen ability to deal with current situation or crisis.

Actions/Interventions

Nursing Priority No. 1.
To determine needs and desires for improvement:

- Evaluate client's perception and ability to provide a realistic view of the situation. **Provides information about how client views the situation and specific expectations to aid in formulating plan of care.**
- Determine client's coping abilities in current situation and expectations for change. **Motivation to improve and high expectations can encourage client to make changes that will improve his or her life. However, unrealistic expectations may hamper efforts.**
- Note client's verbal expressions indicating belief that he or she owns the responsibility for how to deal with adverse situation. **When client has internal locus of control, he or she accepts that life has its adversities and one needs to deal with them.**
- Discuss religious and cultural beliefs held by the individual.
- Identify support systems available to client.

Nursing Priority No. 2.
To assist client to enhance resilience to adverse situation:

- Active-listen and identify client's concerns about situation. **Reflecting client's statements helps to clarify what he or she is thinking and promotes accurate interpretation of reality.**
- Determine previous methods of dealing with adversity. **Helps client to remember successful skills used in the past, and see what might be helpful in current situation.**
- Discuss desire to improve ability to handle adverse situations that arise throughout life. **Willingness to be open to change requires a curiosity, listening to others ideas and beliefs, looking at new ways to do things.**

Information that appears in brackets has been added by the authors to clarify and enhance the use of nursing diagnoses.

Diagnostic Studies   ∞ Pediatric/Geriatric/Lifespan   Medications **695**

- Discuss concept of what can be changed versus what cannot be changed.
- Determine how client is dealing with activities of daily living (ADLs). **While client may have some transient problems with sleeping or managing daily affairs, most people have the ability to function in a healthy manner over time.**
- Help client to learn how to empathize with others. **Understanding own emotions as well as feelings of others enhances one's resiliency during stressful times.**

Nursing Priority No. 3.
To promote optimum growth and resiliency:

- Provide factual information and anticipatory guidance relevant to current situation and long-term expectations. **Planning ahead allows for problem solving and review of options in a relaxed atmosphere, reinforcing sense of control and hope for the future.**
- Review factors that might impact individual's response to stress.
- Encourage client to maintain or establish good relationships with family and friends.
- Help client avoid seeing situation as insurmountable. **While one cannot change the fact of the circumstances, how individual interprets and responds is within one's control.**
- Recommend setting realistic goals and doing something regularly, even if it is small.
- Encourage client to maintain a hopeful outlook, nurture a positive view of self, and take care of self. **Keeping a long-term perspective and paying attention to own needs helps maintain and build resilience.**
- Refer to classes and/or reading materials as appropriate.

Documentation Focus

Assessment/Reassessment
- Baseline information, including client's perception of situation, view of own ability to be resilient, and support systems available.
- Ways of dealing with previous life problems.
- Motivation and expectations for change.
- Cultural or religious influences.

Information that appears in brackets has been added by the authors to clarify and enhance the use of nursing diagnoses.

Planning
- Plan of care and who is involved in planning.
- Educational plan.

Implementation/Evaluation
- Responses to interventions, teaching, and actions performed.
- Attainment or progress toward desired outcomes(s).
- Modifications to plan.

Discharge Planning
- Long-term needs and who is responsible for actions to be taken.
- Specific referrals made.

Sample Nursing Outcomes & Interventions Classifications (NOC/NIC) NIC

NOC—Personal Resiliency
NIC—Resiliency Promotion

---

risk for compromised **Resilience**

Taxonomy II: Coping/Stress Tolerance—Class 2 Coping Responses (00211)
[Diagnostic Division: Ego Integrity]
Submitted 2008

Definition: At risk for decreased ability to sustain a pattern of positive responses to an adverse situation or crisis

---

Risk Factors

Chronicity of existing crises

Multiple coexisting adverse situations

Presence of an additional new crisis (e.g., unplanned pregnancy, death of a spouse or family member, loss of job, illness, loss of housing)

NOTE: A risk diagnosis is not evidenced by signs and symptoms, as the problem has not occurred; rather, nursing interventions are directed at prevention.

Information that appears in brackets has been added by the authors to clarify and enhance the use of nursing diagnoses.

Desired Outcomes/Evaluation Criteria—Client Will (Include Specific Time Frame):

- Acknowledge reality of individual situation or crisis.
- Verbalize feelings associated with chronic situation.
- Verbalize awareness of own ability to deal with problems.
- Identify resources for assisting with chronic and new adverse occurrence.

Actions/Interventions

Nursing Priority No. 1.
To determine individual stressors/potential challenges:

- Note underlying stressors, health concerns, debilitating conditions, mental health or behavioral issues such as unemployment, pregnancy, diabetes, Alzheimer's disease, anxiety disorder.
- Determine alcohol or other drug use, smoking, sleeping and eating habits, **which can affect ability to cope with added stress of crises effectively and in a healthy manner.**
- Assess functional capacity and how it affects client's ability to manage daily needs.
- Evaluate client's ability to verbalize and understand current situation and impact of new crisis. **Informed choice cannot be made without a good understanding of reality of situation.**
- Note speech and communication patterns. **Provides information about level of education, ability to understand situation and to relate problems to caregiver(s).**
- Determine locus of control. **Individuals with external locus of control are less likely to feel in control or to rely on their own abilities or judgment to manage a situation.**
- Evaluate client's current decision-making ability. **Crises affect individual's ability to think clearly and trust own ability to deal with situation.**
- Ascertain stability of relationship, presence of separation or divorce, deteriorating health, or recent death of family member. **Family members are vulnerable to breakup of the family unit and may see it as causing long-term liability.**

Nursing Priority No. 2.
To assess coping skills and degree of resilience:

- Active-listen and identify client's perceptions of what has occurred, as well as previous concerns.

Information that appears in brackets has been added by the authors to clarify and enhance the use of nursing diagnoses.

- Determine how adverse situation is affecting client's ability to deal with what is happening now. **When an unplanned situation occurs in addition to existing problems, it often results in decreased ability to maintain optimism.**
- Determine how individual has dealt with problems in the past. **Having client remember these skills helps in thinking about what can be used to enhance current response or address future challenges.**
- Note cultural factors and religious beliefs that may affect interpretation of, or response to, situation. **Helps determine individual needs and possible options.**
- Determine availability and use of resources, family, support groups, financial aid. **Appropriate use can help the individual continue to manage problems in their lives and plan for future needs.**

Nursing Priority No. 3.
To assist client to deal with current/future situation:

- Ask client what name he or she prefers. **Acknowledging how the individual wants to be addressed provides sense of self, promoting esteem.**
- Encourage free expressions of feelings, including feelings of anger and hostility, setting limits on unacceptable behavior. **Unacceptable behavior leads to feeling of shame and guilt if not controlled.**
- Allow client to react in own way without judgment by caregivers. Provide support and diversion as indicated. **Unconditional positive regard and support promote acceptance and help client to realize own ability to deal with situation.**
- Listen to client's concerns and acknowledge difficulty of adversity and possible need to make changes. **Often individuals who are feeling that life is being difficulty begin to doubt their ability to deal with circumstances. Being listened to provides opportunity for client to feel valued, capable, and like a survivor rather than a victim.**
- Encourage communication with caregivers and significant other(s).
- Provide reality orientation when necessary. **Depending on nature of crisis, client may be disoriented by change in environment, serious diagnosis or treatment regimen, loss of family member.**
- Provide client with factual information and expected course of situation or crisis if known. **Knowledge helps to allay anxiety, enabling client to manage more effectively and to**

Information that appears in brackets has been added by the authors to clarify and enhance the use of nursing diagnoses.

begin to consider possible resolution of the current situation.

- Focus on strengths of the individual as problems are being assessed and diagnosed. Improving future for client is based on strengthening the capacity to deal successfully with obstacles one meets in life.

Nursing Priority No. 4.

To promote wellness (Teaching/Discharge Considerations):

- Provide or identify learning opportunities specific to individual needs. **Activities such as assertiveness, regular exercise, parenting classes, can enhance knowledge and help develop a resilient mind-set.**
- Encourage an attitude of realistic hope. **Client can accept that change is a part of living and, while some plans cannot be obtained because of crisis or new circumstances, new goals can be developed and life can move forward.**
- Support client in evaluating current lifestyle and changes that need to be made.
- Provide anticipatory guidance relevant to current situation and long-term expectations.
- Determine need or desire for religious or spiritual counselor and make arrangements for visit. **Providing client an opportunity to discuss concerns about what has happened helps to build resilience to face future stressors.**
- Reinforce importance of client/SO taking time for self. **Provides opportunity for personal growth; respite allows individuals to pursue own interests and return to tasks of life with renewed vigor.**
- Refer to community resources as appropriate. **May need professional counseling, assistance with financial concerns, special-needs support services, child or parenting care to move forward.**

Documentation Focus

Assessment/Reassessment

- Assessment findings, including details of this client's situation or crisis, expectations.
- Client's degree of resiliency.

Planning

- Plan of care, and who is involved in planning.
- Teaching plan.

Information that appears in brackets has been added by the authors to clarify and enhance the use of nursing diagnoses.

⊕ Cultural   ⚲ Collaborative   🏠 Community/Home Care

Implementation/Evaluation

- Response to interventions, teaching, and actions performed.
- Attainment or progress toward desired outcome(s).
- Modifications to plan of care.

Discharge Planning

- Long-term needs and who is responsible for actions to be taken.
- Support systems available, specific referrals made.

Sample Nursing Outcomes & Interventions Classifications (NOC/NIC) NIC

NOC—Personal Resiliency
NIC—Resiliency Promotion

---

ineffective **Role Performance**

Taxonomy II: Role Relationships—Class 3 Role Performance (00055)
[Diagnostic Division: Social Interaction]
Submitted 1978; Revised 1996, 1998

Definition: Patterns of behavior and self-expression that do not match the environmental context, norms, and expectations

---

[**NOTE:** There is a typology of roles: sociopersonal (friendship, family, marital, parenting, community); home management; intimacy (sexuality, relationship building); leisure, exercise, or recreation; self-management; socialization (developmental transitions), community contributor; and religious.]

Related Factors

Knowledge
Inadequate or lack of role model
Inadequate role preparation (e.g., role transition, skill rehearsal, validation)
Lack of education
Developmental transitions
Unrealistic role expectations

Information that appears in brackets has been added by the authors to clarify and enhance the use of nursing diagnoses.

Physiological
Body image alteration; cognitive deficits; neurological deficits; physical illness; mental illness; depression; low self-esteem
Fatigue; pain; substance abuse

Social
Inadequate role socialization [e.g., role model, expectations, responsibilities]
Young age, developmental level
Lack of resources; low socioeconomic status
Stress; conflict; job schedule demands
[Family conflict]; domestic violence
Inadequate support system; lack of rewards
Inappropriate linkage with the healthcare system

Defining Characteristics

Subjective
Altered role perceptions; change in self-/other's perception of role
Change in usual patterns of responsibility or capacity to resume role
Inadequate opportunities for role enactment
Role dissatisfaction, overload, or denial
Discrimination [by others]; powerlessness

Objective
Deficient knowledge; inadequate role competency or skills
Inadequate adaptation to change; inappropriate developmental expectations
Inadequate confidence, motivation, self-management, or coping
Inadequate external support for role enactment
Role strain, conflict, confusion, or ambivalence; [failure to assume role]
Uncertainty; anxiety; depression; pessimism
Domestic violence; harassment; system conflict

Desired Outcomes/Evaluation Criteria—
Client Will:

- Verbalize understanding of role expectations and obligations.
- Verbalize realistic perception and acceptance of self in changed role.
- Talk with family/SO(s) about situation and changes that have occurred and limitations imposed.

Information that appears in brackets has been added by the authors to clarify and enhance the use of nursing diagnoses.

⊕ Cultural   Ⓐ Collaborative   🏠 Community/Home Care

• Develop realistic plans for adapting to new role or role changes.

Actions/Interventions

Nursing Priority No. 1.

To assess causative/contributing factors:

• Identify type of role dysfunction: for example, developmental (adolescent to adult); situational (husband to father, gender identity); transitions from health to illness.
• Determine client role in family constellation.
• Identify how client sees self as a man or woman in usual lifestyle or role functioning.
• Ascertain client's view of sexual functioning (e.g., loss of childbearing ability following hysterectomy).
• Identify cultural factors relating to individual's sexual roles. **Cultures define male and female roles differently (e.g., Muslim culture demands that the woman adopt a subservient role, whereas the man is seen as the powerful one in the relationship).**
• Determine client's perceptions or concerns about current situation. **May believe current role is more appropriate for the opposite sex (e.g., passive role of the patient may be somewhat less threatening for women).**
• Interview SO(s) regarding their perceptions and expectations. **Influences client's view of self.**

Nursing Priority No. 2.

To assist client to deal with existing situation:

• Discuss perceptions and significance of the situation as seen by client.
• Maintain positive attitude toward the client.
• Provide opportunities for client to exercise control over as many decisions as possible. **Enhances self-concept and promotes commitment to goals.**
• Offer realistic assessment of situation while communicating sense of hope.
• Discuss and assist client/SO(s) to develop strategies for dealing with changes in role related to past transitions, cultural expectations, and value or belief challenges. **Helps those involved deal with differences between individuals (e.g., adolescent task of separation in which parents clash with child's choices; individual's decision to change religious affiliation).**

Information that appears in brackets has been added by the authors to clarify and enhance the use of nursing diagnoses.

- Acknowledge reality of situation related to role change and help client express feelings of anger, sadness, and grief. Encourage celebration of positive aspects of change and expressions of feelings.
- Provide open environment for client to discuss concerns about sexuality. **Embarrassment can block discussion of sensitive subject.** (Refer to NDs Sexual Dysfunction; ineffective Sexuality Pattern.)
- Identify role model for client. Educate about role expectations using written and audiovisual materials.
- Use the techniques of role rehearsal to help client develop new skills **to cope with changes.**

Nursing Priority No. 3.

To promote wellness (Teaching/Discharge Considerations):

- Make information available for client to learn about role expectations or demands that may occur. **Provides opportunity to be proactive in dealing with changes.**
- Accept client in changed role. Encourage and give positive feedback for changes and goals achieved. **Provides reinforcement and facilitates continuation of efforts.**
- Refer to support groups, employment counselors, parent effectiveness classes, counseling/psychotherapy, as indicated by individual need(s). **Provides ongoing support to sustain progress.**
- Refer to NDs Self-Esteem [specify] and the Parenting diagnoses.

Documentation Focus

Assessment/Reassessment
- Individual findings, including specifics of predisposing crises or situation, perception of role change.
- Expectations of SO(s).

Planning
- Plan of care and who is involved in planning.
- Teaching plan.

Implementation/Evaulation
- Responses to interventions, teaching, and actions performed.
- Attainment or progress toward desired outcome(s).
- Modifications plan of care.

Information that appears in brackets has been added by the authors to clarify and enhance the use of nursing diagnoses.

Cultural   Collaborative   Community/Home Care

Discharge Planning
- Long-term needs and who is responsible for actions to be taken.
- Specific referrals made.

Sample Nursing Outcomes & Interventions Classifications (NOC/NIC) **NIC**

NOC—Role Performance
NIC—Role Enhancement

---

readiness for enhanced Self-Care

Taxonomy II: Activity/Rest—Class 5 Self-Care (00182)
[Diagnostic Division: teaching/learning]
Submitted 2006

Definition: A pattern of performing activities for oneself that helps to meet health-related goals and can be strengthened

---

Related Factors

To be developed

Defining Characteristics

Subjective
Expresses desire to enhance independence in maintaining: life, health, personal development, or well-being
Expresses desire to enhance self-care, knowledge for strategies for self-care, or responsibility for self-care

[NOTE: Based on the definition and defining characteristics of this ND, the focus appears to be broader than simply meeting routine basic ADLs and addresses independence in maintaining overall health, personal development, and general well-being.]

Desired Outcomes/Evaluation Criteria— Client Will:

- Maintain responsibility for planning and achieving self-care goals and general well-being.

Information that appears in brackets has been added by the authors to clarify and enhance the use of nursing diagnoses.

 Diagnostic Studies ∞ Pediatric/Geriatric/Lifespan Medications **705**

- Demonstrate proactive management of chronic conditions, potential complications or changes in capabilities.
- Identify and use resources appropriately.
- Remain free of preventable complications.

Actions/Interventions

Nursing Priority No. 1.

To determine current self-care status and motivation for growth:

- Determine individual strengths and skills of the client. **Establishes comparative baseline for potential growth and/or modifications in current stratagies.**
- Ascertain motivation and expectations for change.
- Note availability and use of resources, supportive person(s), assistive devices.
- ∞ Determine age and developmental issues, presence of medical conditions **that could impact potential for growth or interrupt client's ability to meet own needs.**
- Assess for potential barriers to enhanced participation in self-care (e.g., lack of information, insufficient time for discussion, sudden or progressive change in health status, catastrophic events).

Nursing Priority No. 2.

To assist client's/SO's plan to meet individual needs:

- Discuss client's understanding of situation.
- Provide accurate and relevant information regarding current and future needs **so that client can incorporate into self-care plans, while minimizing problems associated with change.**
- Promote client's/SO's participation in problem identification and decision making. **Optimizes outcomes and supports health promotion.**
- Active-listen client's/SO's concerns **to exhibit regard for client's values and beliefs, to support positive responses, and to address questions or concerns.**
- Encourage communication among those who are involved in the client's health promotion. **Periodic review allows for clarification of issues, reinforcement of successful interventions, and possibility for early intervention (where needed) to manage chronic conditions.**

Information that appears in brackets has been added by the authors to clarify and enhance the use of nursing diagnoses.

Nursing Priority No. 3.

To promote optimum functioning (Teaching/Discharge Considerations):

• Assist client to set realistic goals for the future.

• Support client in making health-related decisions and pursuit of self-care practices that promote health **to foster self-esteem and support positive self-concept.**

• Identify reliable reference sources regarding individual needs and strategies for self-care. **Reinforces learning and promotes self-paced review.**

• Provide for ongoing evaluation of self-care program **to identify progress and needed changes for continuation of health, adaptation in management of limiting conditions.**

• Review safety concerns and modification of medical therapies or activities and environment, as needed, **to prevent injury and enhance successful functioning.**

• Refer to home care provider, social services, physical or occupational therapy, rehabilitation, and counseling resources, as indicated or requested, **for education, assistance, adaptive devices, and modifications that may be desired.**

• Identify additional community resources (e.g., senior services, handicap transportation van for appointments, accessible and safe locations for social or sports activities, Meals on Wheels).

Documentation Focus

Assessment/Reassessment
• Individual findings including strengths, health status, and any limitation(s).
• Availability and use of community resources, support person(s), assistive devices.
• Motivation and expectations for change.

Planning
• Plan of care, specific interventions, and who is involved in planning.
• Teaching plan.

Implementation/Evaluation
• Client's responses to interventions, teaching, and actions performed.
• Attainment or progress toward desired outcome(s).
• Modifications to plan.

Information that appears in brackets has been added by the authors to clarify and enhance the use of nursing diagnoses.

Discharge Planning

- Long-term needs and who is responsible for actions to be taken.
- Type of and source for assistive devices.
- Specific referrals made.

Sample Nursing Outcomes & Interventions Classifications (NOC/NIC) NIC

NOC—Self-Care Status
NIC—Self-Modification Assistance

Self-Care Deficit: bathing, dressing, feeding, toileting

Taxonomy II: Activity/Rest—Class 5 Self-Care (Bathing 00108, Dressing 00109, Feeding 00102, Toileting 00110) [Diagnostic Division: Hygiene]
Submitted 1980; Nursing Diagnosis Extension and Classification (NDEC) Revision 1998

Definition: Impaired ability to perform or complete feeding, bathing/hygiene, dressing and grooming, or toileting activities for oneself

---

[NOTE: Self-care also may be expanded to include the practices used by the client to promote health, the individual responsibility for self, a way of thinking. Refer to NDs impaired Home Maintenance; ineffective Health Maintenance.]

Related Factors

Weakness; fatigue; decreased motivation
Neuromuscular or musculoskeletal impairment
Environmental barriers
Severe anxiety
Pain; discomfort
Perceptual or cognitive impairment
Inability to perceive body part or spatial relationship [bathing]
Impaired transfer ability [self-toileting]

Information that appears in brackets has been added by the authors to clarify and enhance the use of nursing diagnoses.

Cultural Collaborative Community/Home Care

Impaired mobility status [self-toileting]
Mechanical restrictions such as cast, splint, traction, ventilator

Defining Characteristics

feeding Self-Care Deficit

Inability to:
Prepare food for ingestion; open containers
Handle utensils; get food onto utensil; bring food from a receptacle to the mouth
Ingest food safely; manipulate food in mouth; chew or swallow food
Pick up cup or glass
Use assistive device
Ingest sufficient food; complete a meal
Ingest food in a socially acceptable manner

bathing Self-Care Deficit

Inability to:
Get bath supplies
Wash body
Obtain water source; regulate bath water
Access bathroom [tub]
Dry body

dressing Self-Care Deficit

Inability to:
Choose clothing; pick up clothing
Put clothing on upper or lower body; put on socks or shoes; remove clothing
Use zippers or assistive devices
Maintain appearance at a satisfactory level
Impaired ability to obtain clothing; put on or take off necessary items of clothing; fasten clothing

toileting Self-Care Deficit

Inability to:
Get to toilet or commode
Manipulate clothing for toileting
Sit on or rise from toilet or commode

Information that appears in brackets has been added by the authors to clarify and enhance the use of nursing diagnoses.

Carry out proper toilet hygiene

Flush toilet or [empty] commode

Desired Outcomes/Evaluation Criteria— Client Will:

- Identify individual areas of weakness or needs.
- Verbalize knowledge of healthcare practices.
- Demonstrate techniques and lifestyle changes to meet self-care needs.
- Perform self-care activities within level of own ability.
- Identify personal and community resources that can provide assistance.

Actions/Interventions

Nursing Priority No. 1.

To identify causative/contributing factors:

- Determine age and developmental issues **affecting ability of individual to participate in own care.**
- Note concomitant medical problems or existing conditions that may be factors for care (e.g., recent trauma or surgery, heart disease, renal failure, spinal cord injury, CVA, MS, malnutrition, pain, Alzheimer's disease).
- Review medication regimen for possible effects on alertness/mentation, energy level, balance, perception.
- Note other etiological factors present, including language barriers, speech impairment, visual acuity or hearing problem, emotional stability/ability. (Refer to NDs impaired verbal Communication; impaired Environmental Interpretation; risk for unilateral Neglect; disturbed Sensory Perception [specify] for related interventions.)
- Assess barriers to participation in regimen (e.g., lack of information, insufficient time for discussion; psychological and/or intimate family problems that may be difficult to share; fear of appearing stupid or ignorant; social, economic, work or home environment problems).

Nursing Priority No. 2.

To assess degree of disability:

- Identify degree of individual impairment and functional level according to scale (as listed in ND impaired physical Mobility).

Information that appears in brackets has been added by the authors to clarify and enhance the use of nursing diagnoses.

  Cultural   Collaborative   Community/Home Care

- Assess memory and intellectual functioning. Note developmental level to which client has regressed or progressed.
- Determine individual strengths and skills of the client.
- Note whether deficit is temporary or permanent, should decrease or increase with time.

Nursing Priority No. 3.

To assist in correcting/dealing with situation:

- Perform or assist with meeting client's needs when he or she is unable to meet own needs (e.g., personal care assistance is part of nursing care and should not be neglected while self-care independence is promoted and integrated).
- Promote client's/SO's participation in problem identification and desired goals and decision making. **Enhances commitment to plan, optimizing outcomes, and supporting recovery and/or health promotion.**
- Develop plan of care appropriate to individual situation, scheduling activities to conform to client's usual or desired schedule.
- Plan time for listening to the client's/SO's feelings and concerns **to discover barriers to participation in regimen and to work on problem solutions.**
- Practice and promote short-term goal setting and achievement **to recognize that today's success is as important as any long-term goal, accepting ability to do one thing at a time, and conceptualization of self-care in a broader sense.**
- Provide for communication among those who are involved in caring for or assisting the client. **Enhances coordination and continuity of care.**
- Establish remotivation or resocialization programs when indicated.
- Establish "contractual" partnership with client/SO(s) **if appropriate for motivation or behavioral modification.**
- Refer to and assist with rehabilitation program **to enhance client's capabilities and promote independence.**
- Provide privacy and equipment within easy reach during personal care activities.
- Allow sufficient time for client to accomplish tasks to fullest extent of ability. Avoid unnecessary conversation or interruptions.
- Assist with necessary adaptations to accomplish ADLs. Begin with familiar, easily accomplished tasks **to encourage client and build on successes.**

Information that appears in brackets has been added by the authors to clarify and enhance the use of nursing diagnoses.

- Collaborate with rehabilitation professionals to identify and obtain assistive devices, mobility aids, and home modification as necessary (e.g., adequate lighting, visual aids; bedside commode; raised toilet seat and grab bars for bathroom; modified clothing; modified eating utensils).
- Identify energy-saving behaviors (e.g., sitting instead of standing when possible). (Refer to NDs Activity Intolerance; Fatigue for additional interventions.)
- Implement bowel or bladder training program, as indicated. (Refer to NDs Constipation; Bowel Incontinence; impaired Urinary Elimination for appropriate interventions.)
- Encourage food and fluid choices reflecting individual likes and abilities that meet nutritional needs. Provide assistive devices or alternate feeding methods, as appropriate. (Refer to ND impaired Swallowing for related interventions.)
- Assist with medication regimen as necessary, encouraging timely use of medications (e.g., taking diuretics in morning when client is more awake and able to manage toileting, use of pain relievers prior to activity to facilitate movement, postponing intake of medications that cause sedation until self-care activities completed).
- Make home visit, as indicated **to assess environmental and discharge needs.**

Nursing Priority No. 4.
To promote wellness (Teaching/Discharge Considerations):

- Assist the client to become aware of rights and responsibilities in health and healthcare and to assess own health strengths—physical, emotional, and intellectual.
- Support client in making health-related decisions and assist in developing self-care practices and goals that promote health.
- Provide for ongoing evaluation of self-care program, identifying progress and needed changes.
- Review and modify program periodically to accommodate changes in client's abilities. **Assists client to adhere to plan of care to fullest extent.**
- Encourage keeping a journal of progress and practicing of independent living skills **to foster self-care and self-determination.**
- Review safety concerns. Modify activities or environment **to reduce risk of injury and promote successful community functioning.**

Information that appears in brackets has been added by the authors to clarify and enhance the use of nursing diagnoses.

• Refer to home care provider, social services, physical or occupational therapy, rehabilitation, and counseling resources, as indicated.

• Identify additional community resources (e.g., senior services, Meals on Wheels).

• Review instructions from other members of the healthcare team and provide written copy. **Provides clarification, reinforcement; allows periodic review by client/caregivers.**

• Give family information about respite or other care options. **Allows them free time away from the care situation to renew themselves.** (Refer to ND Caregiver Role Strain for additional interventions.)

• Assist and support family with alternative placements as necessary. **Enhances likelihood of finding individually appropriate situation to meet client's needs.**

• Be available for discussion of feelings about situation (e.g., grieving, anger).

• Refer to NDs risk for Falls; risk for Injury; ineffective Coping; compromised family Coping; risk for Disuse Syndrome; situational low Self-Esteem; impaired physical Mobility; Powerlessness, as appropriate.

Documentation Focus

Assessment/Reassessment
• Individual findings, functional level, and specifics of limitation(s).
• Needed resources and adaptive devices.
• Availability and use of community resources.
• Who is involved in care or provides assistance.

Planning
• Plan of care and who is involved in planning.
• Teaching plan.

Implementation/Evaluation
• Response to interventions, teaching, and actions performed.
• Attainment or progress toward desired outcome(s).
• Modifications of plan of care.

Discharge Planning
• Long-term needs and who is responsible for actions to be taken.

Information that appears in brackets has been added by the authors to clarify and enhance the use of nursing diagnoses.

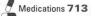

- Type of and source for assistive devices.
- Specific referrals made.

Sample Nursing Outcomes & Interventions Classifications (NOC/NIC) NIC

Bathing Deficit
NOC—Self-Care: Bathing
NIC—Self-Care Assistance: Bathing/Hygiene

Dressing Deficit
NOC—Self-Care: Dressing
NIC—Self-Care Assistance: Dressing/Grooming

Feeding Deficit
NOC—Self-Care: Eating
NIC—Self-Care Assistance: Feeding

Toileting Deficit
NOC—Self-Care: Toileting
NIC—Self-Care Assistance: Toileting

---

readiness for enhanced Self-Concept

Taxonomy II: Self-Perception—Class 1 Self-Concept (00167)
[Diagnostic Division: ego integrity]
Submitted 2002

Definition: A pattern of perceptions or ideas about the self that is sufficient for well-being and can be strengthened

---

Related Factors

To be developed

Defining Characteristics

Subjective
Expresses willingness to enhance self-concept
Accepts strengths, limitations
Expresses confidence in abilities

Information that appears in brackets has been added by the authors to clarify and enhance the use of nursing diagnoses.

 Cultural   Collaborative   Community/Home Care

Expresses satisfaction with thoughts about self, sense of wor-
thiness

Expresses satisfaction with body image, personal identity, role
performance

Objective
Actions are congruent with expressed feelings and thoughts

Desired Outcomes/Evaluation Criteria— Client Will:

- Verbalize understanding of own sense of self-concept.
- Participate in programs and activities to enhance self-esteem.
- Demonstrate behaviors and lifestyle changes to promote pos-
itive self-esteem.
- Participate in family, group, or community activities to en-
hance self-concept.

Actions/Interventions

Nursing Priority No. 1.
To assess current situation and desire for improvement:

- Determine current status of individual's belief about self.
**Self-concept consists of the physical self (body image), the
personal self (identity), and self-esteem. Information
about client's current thinking about self provides a beginning for making changes to improve self.**
- Determine availability and quality of family/SO(s) support.
**Presence of supportive people who reflect positive atti-
tudes regarding the individual promotes a positive sense
of self.**
- Identify family dynamics—present and past. **Self-esteem begins in early childhood and is influenced by perceptions
of how the individual is viewed by SOs. Provides information about family functioning that will help to develop
plan of care for enhancing client's self-concept.**
- Note willingness to seek assistance and motivation for
change. **Individuals who have a sense of their own self-
image and are willing to look at themselves realistically
will be able to progress in the desire to improve.**
- Determine client's concept of self in relation to cultural or
religious ideals and beliefs. **Cultural characteristics are
learned in the family of origin and shape how the individual views self.**

Information that appears in brackets has been added by the authors to clarify
and enhance the use of nursing diagnoses.

- Observe nonverbal behaviors and note congruence with verbal expressions. Discuss cultural meanings of nonverbal communication. **Incongruencies between verbal and nonverbal communication require clarification. Interpretation of nonverbal expressions is culturally determined and needs to be clarified to avoid misinterpretation.**

Nursing Priority No. 2.

To facilitate personal growth:

- Develop therapeutic relationship. Be attentive, maintain open communication, use skills of Active-listening and I-messages. **Promotes trusting situation in which client is free to be open and honest with self and others.**
- Validate client's communication, provide encouragement for efforts.
- Accept client's perceptions or view of current status. **Provides opportunity for client to develop realistic plan for improving self-concept, while feeling safe in existing self view.**
- Be aware that people are not programmed to be rational. **Individuals must seek information—choosing to learn; to think rather than merely to accept or react, in order to have respect for self, facts, and honesty, and to develop positive self-esteem.**
- Discuss client perception of self, confronting misconceptions and identifying negative self-talk. Address distortions in thinking, such as self-referencing (beliefs that others are focusing on individual's weaknesses or limitations); filtering (focusing on negative and ignoring positive); catastrophizing (expecting the worst outcomes). **Addressing these issues openly allows client to identify things that may negatively affect self-esteem, and provides opportunity for change.**
- Have client list current and past successes and strengths. **Emphasizes fact that client is and has been successful in many actions taken.**
- Use positive I-messages rather than praise. **Praise is a form of external control, coming from outside sources, whereas I-messages allow the client to develop internal sense of self-esteem.**
- Discuss what behavior does for client (positive intention). Ask what options are available to the client/SO(s). **Encourages thinking about what inner motivations are and what actions can be taken to enhance self-esteem.**

Information that appears in brackets has been added by the authors to clarify and enhance the use of nursing diagnoses.

- Give reinforcement for progress noted. **Positive words of encouragement support development of effective coping behaviors.**
- Encourage client to progress at own rate. **Adaptation to a change in self-concept depends on its significance to the individual and disruption to lifestyle.**
- Involve in activities or exercise program of choice, promote socialization. **Enhances sense of well-being and can help to energize client.**

Nursing Priority No. 3.
To promote optimum sense of self-worth and happiness:

- Assist client to identify goals that are personally achievable. Provide positive feedback for verbal and behavioral indications of improved self-view. **Increases likelihood of success and commitment to change.**
- Refer to vocational or employment counselor, educational resources, as appropriate. **Assists with improving development of social or vocational skills.**
- Encourage participation in classes, activities, or hobbies that client enjoys or would like to experience. **Provides opportunity for learning new information and skills that can enhance feelings of success, improving self-esteem.**
- Reinforce that current decision to improve self-concept is ongoing. **Continued work and support are necessary to sustain behavior changes and personal growth.**
- Discuss ways to develop optimism. **Optimism is a key ingredient in happiness and can be learned.**
- Suggest assertiveness training classes. **Enhances ability to interact with others and develop more effective relationships, enhancing one's self-concept.**
- Emphasize importance of grooming and personal hygiene and assist in developing skills to improve appearance and dress for success as needed. **Looking one's best improves sense of self-esteem and presenting a positive appearance enhances how others see one.**

Documentation Focus

Assessment/Reassessment
- Individual findings, including evaluations of self and others, current and past successes.

Information that appears in brackets has been added by the authors to clarify and enhance the use of nursing diagnoses.

- Interactions with others, lifestyle.
- Motivation for and willingness to change.

Planning
- Plan of care and who is involved in planning.
- Educational plan.

Implementation/Evaluation
- Responses to interventions, teaching, and actions performed.
- Attainment or progress toward desired outcome(s).
- Modifications to plan of care.

Discharge Planning
- Long-term needs and who is responsible for actions to be taken.
- Specific referrals made.

Sample Nursing Outcomes & Interventions Classifications (NOC/NIC) NIC

NOC—Self-Esteem
NIC—Self-Modification Assistance

chronic low Self-Esteem

Taxonomy II: Self-Perception—Class 2 Self-Esteem (00119)
[Diagnostic Division: Ego Integrity]
Submitted 1988; Revised 1996

Definition: Long-standing negative self-evaluation/feelings about self or self-capabilities

Related Factors

Repeated negative reinforcement, failures
Lack of affection, approval, or membership in group
Perceived lack of belonging or respect from others
Perceived discrepancy between self and cultural or spiritual norms
Traumatic event or situation
Ineffective adaptation to loss
Psychiatric disorders; fixation in earlier level of development
Personal vulnerability

Information that appears in brackets has been added by the authors to clarify and enhance the use of nursing diagnoses.

Cultural   Collaborative   Community/Home Care

Defining Characteristics

Subjective

Self-negating verbalization
Expressions of shame or guilt
Evaluates self as unable to deal with events
Rejects positive or exaggerates negative feedback about self

Objective

Hesitant to try new things or situations
Frequent lack of success in work or in life events
Overly conforming; dependent on others' opinions
Lack of eye contact
Nonassertive; passive; indecisive
Excessively seeks reassurance

Desired Outcomes/Evaluation Criteria—Client Will:

- Verbalize understanding of negative evaluation of self and reasons for this problem.
- Participate in treatment program to promote change in self-evaluation.
- Demonstrate behaviors and lifestyle changes to promote positive self-image.
- Verbalize increased sense of self-worth in relation to current situation.
- Participate in family, group, or community activities to enhance change.

Actions/Interventions

Nursing Priority No. 1.

To assess causative/contributing factors:

- Determine factors of low self-esteem related to current situation (e.g., family crises, physical disfigurement, social isolation), noting age and developmental level of individual. **Current crises may exacerbate long-standing feelings and perception of self-evaluation as not being worthwhile.**
- Assess content of negative self-talk. Note client's perceptions of how others view him or her.
- Determine availability and quality of family/SO(s) support.
- Identify family dynamics—present and past—and cultural influences. **Family may engage in "put-downs" or "teasing"**

Information that appears in brackets has been added by the authors to clarify and enhance the use of nursing diagnoses.

 Diagnostic Studies ∞ Pediatric/Geriatric/Lifespan 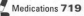 Medications **719** in ways that give client the message that he or she is worthless.

• Be alert to client's concept of self in relation to cultural/religious ideal(s).
- Note nonverbal behavior (e.g., nervous movements, lack of eye contact). **Incongruencies between verbal/nonverbal communication require clarification.**
- Determine degree of participation and cooperation with therapeutic regimen (e.g., maintaining scheduled medications such as antidepressants/antipsychotics).
- Note willingness to seek assistance, motivation for change.

Nursing Priority No. 2.
To promote client sense of self-esteem in dealing with current situation:

- Develop therapeutic relationship. Be attentive, validate client's communication, provide encouragement for efforts, maintain open communication, use skills of Active-listening and I-messages. **Promotes trusting situation in which client is free to be open and honest with self and therapist.**
- Address presenting medical/safety issues.
- Accept client's perceptions or view of situation. Avoid threatening existing self-esteem.
- Be aware that people are not programmed to be rational. **To have respect for self, facts, honesty, and to develop positive self-esteem, one must seek information—choosing to learn; to think rather than merely accepting/reacting.**
- Discuss client perceptions of self related to what is happening; confront misconceptions and negative self-talk. Address distortions in thinking, such as self-referencing (belief that others are focusing on individual's weaknesses/limitations), filtering (focusing on negative and ignoring positive), catastrophizing (expecting the worst outcomes). **Addressing these issues openly provides opportunity for change.**
- Emphasize need to avoid comparing self with others. Encourage client to focus on aspects of self that can be valued.
- Have client review past successes and strengths. **May help client see that he or she can develop an internal locus of control (a belief that one's successes and failures are the result of one's efforts).**
- Use positive I-messages rather than praise. **Assists client to develop internal sense of self-esteem.**
- Discuss what a given behavior does for client (positive intention). What options are available to the client/SO(s)?

Information that appears in brackets has been added by the authors to clarify and enhance the use of nursing diagnoses.

 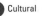 Cultural   Collaborative   Community/Home Care

- Assist client to deal with sense of powerlessness. (Refer to ND Powerlessness.)
- Set limits on aggressive or problem behaviors such as acting out, suicide preoccupation, or rumination. Put self in client's place (empathy not sympathy). **These negative behaviors diminish sense of self-concept.**
- Give reinforcement for progress noted. **Positive words of encouragement promote continuation of efforts, supporting development of coping behaviors.**
- Encourage client to progress at own rate. **Adaptation to a change in self-concept depends on its significance to individual, disruption to lifestyle, and length of illness/debilitation.**
- Assist client to recognize and cope with events, alterations, and sense of loss of control by incorporating changes accurately into self-concept.
- Involve in activities or exercise program, promote socialization. **Enhances sense of well-being/can help energize client.**

Nursing Priority No. 3.
To promote wellness (Teaching/Discharge Considerations):

- Discuss inaccuracies in self-perception with client/SO(s).
- Model behaviors being taught, involving client in goal setting and decision making. **Facilitates client's developing trust in own unique strengths.**
- Prepare client for events/changes that are expected, when possible **to provide opportunity for client to prepare self, or reduce negative reactions associated with the unknown.**
- Provide structure in daily routine/care activities.
- Emphasize importance of grooming and personal hygiene. Assist in developing skills as indicated (e.g., makeup classes, dressing for success). **People feel better about themselves when they present a positive outer appearance.**
- Assist client to identify goals that are personally achievable. Provide positive feedback for verbal and behavioral indications of improved self-view. **Increases likelihood of success and commitment to change.**
- Refer to vocational or employment counselor, educational resources, as appropriate. **Assists with development of social or vocational skills, enhancing sense of self-concept and inner locus of control.**
- Encourage participation in classes, activities, or hobbies that client enjoys or would like to experience.

Information that appears in brackets has been added by the authors to clarify and enhance the use of nursing diagnoses.

🏠 • Reinforce that this therapy is a brief encounter in overall life of the client/SO(s), with continued work and ongoing support being necessary **to sustain behavior changes and personal growth.**

🤝 • Refer to classes (e.g., assertiveness training, positive self-image, communication skills) **to assist with learning new skills to promote self-esteem.**

🤝 • Refer to counseling, therapy, mental health, or special-needs support groups, as indicated.

Documentation Focus

Assessment/Reassessment
• Individual findings, including early memories of negative evaluations (self and others), subsequent or precipitating failure events.
• Effects on interactions with others, lifestyle.
• Specific medical and safety issues.
• Motivation for and willingness to change.

Planning
• Plan of care and who is involved in planning.
• Teaching plan.

Implementation/Evaluation
• Responses to interventions, teaching, and actions performed.
• Attainment or progress toward desired outcome(s).
• Modifications to plan of care.

Discharge Planning
• Long-term needs and who is responsible for actions to be taken.
• Specific referrals made.

Sample Nursing Outcomes & Interventions Classifications (NOC/NIC) NIC

NOC—Self-Esteem
NIC—Self-Esteem Enhancement

Information that appears in brackets has been added by the authors to clarify and enhance the use of nursing diagnoses.

⊕ Cultural 🤝 Collaborative 🏠 Community/Home Care

situational low Self-Esteem

Taxonomy II: Self-Perception—Class 2 Self-Esteem
(00120)
[Diagnostic Division: Ego Integrity]
Submitted 1988; Revised 1996, 2000

Definition: Development of a negative perception of self-worth in response to a current situation (specify)

Related Factors

Developmental changes [e.g., maturational transitions, adolescence, aging]
Functional impairment; disturbed body image
Loss [e.g., loss of health status, body part, independent functioning; memory deficit, cognitive impairment]
Social role changes
Failures; rejections; lack of recognition[or rewards; feelings of abandonment by SO]
Behavior inconsistent with values

Defining Characteristics

Subjective
Verbally reports current situational challenge to self-worth
Expressions of helplessness or uselessness
Evaluation of self as unable to deal with situations or events

Objective
Self-negating verbalizations
Indecisive or nonassertive behavior

Desired Outcomes/Evaluation Criteria— Client Will:

- Verbalize understanding of individual factors that precipitated current situation.
- Identify feelings and underlying dynamics for negative perception of self.
- Express positive self-appraisal.
- Demonstrate behaviors to restore positive self-esteem.
- Participate in treatment regimen or activities to correct factors that precipitated crisis.

Information that appears in brackets has been added by the authors to clarify and enhance the use of nursing diagnoses.

Actions/Interventions

Nursing Priority No. 1.

To assess causative/contributing factors:

- Determine individual situation (e.g., family crisis, termination of a relationship, loss of employment, physical disfigurement) related to low self-esteem in the present circumstances.
- Identify client's basic sense of self-esteem and image client has of self: existential, physical, psychological.
- Assess degree of threat and perception of client in regard to crisis. **One individual views a serious situation as manageable, while another individual may be overly concerned about a minor problem.**
- Ascertain sense of control client has (or perceives self to have) over self and situation. Note client's locus of control (internal or external). **Locus of control is important in determining whether the client believes he or she has control over the situation, or whether one is at the mercy of fate or luck.**
- Determine client's awareness of own responsibility for dealing with situation, personal growth, and so forth. **When client is aware of and accepts own responsibility, may indicate internal locus of control.**
- Verify client's concept of self in relation to cultural/religious ideals. **May provide client with support or reinforce negative self-evaluation.**
- Review past coping skills in relation to current episode.
- Assess negative attitudes and/or self-talk.
- Note nonverbal body language. **Incongruencies between verbal and nonverbal communication require clarification.**
- Assess for self-destructive or suicidal behavior. (Refer to ND risk for Suicide, as appropriate.)
- Identify previous adaptations to illness or disruptive events in life. **May be predictive of current outcome.**
- Assess family/SO(s) dynamics and support of client.
- Note availability and use of resources.

Nursing Priority No. 2.

To assist client to deal with loss/change and recapture sense of positive self-esteem:

- Assist with treatment of underlying condition when possible. **For example, cognitive restructuring and improved**

Information that appears in brackets has been added by the authors to clarify and enhance the use of nursing diagnoses.

 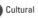

concentration in mild brain injury often result in restoration of positive self-esteem.

- Encourage expression of feelings, anxieties. **Facilitates grieving the loss.**
- Active-listen client's concerns and negative verbalizations without comment or judgment.
- Identify individual strengths and assets, and aspects of self that remain intact and can be valued. Reinforce positive traits, abilities, self-view.
- Help client identify own responsibility and control or lack of control in situation. **When able to acknowledge what is out of his or her control, client can focus attention on area of own responsibility.**
- Assist client to problem-solve situation, developing plan of action and setting goals to achieve desired outcome. **Enhances commitment to plan, optimizing outcomes.**
- Convey confidence in client's ability to cope with current situation.
- Mobilize support systems.
- Provide opportunity for client to practice alternative coping strategies, including progressive socialization opportunities.
- Encourage use of visualization, guided imagery, and relaxation **to promote positive sense of self.**
- Provide feedback of client's self-negating remarks or behavior, using I-messages, **to allow the client to experience a different view.**
- Encourage involvement in decisions about care when possible.

Nursing Priority No. 3.
To promote wellness (Teaching/Discharge Considerations):

- Encourage client to set long-range goals for achieving necessary lifestyle changes. **Supports view that this is an ongoing process.**
- Support independence in ADLs or mastery of therapeutic regimen. **Confident individual is more secure and positive in self-appraisal.**
- Promote attendance in therapy or support group, as indicated.
- Involve extended family/SO(s) in treatment plan. **Increases likelihood they will provide appropriate support to client.**
- Provide information to assist client in making desired changes. **Appropriate books, DVDs, or other resources allow client to learn at own pace.**

Information that appears in brackets has been added by the authors to clarify and enhance the use of nursing diagnoses.

🏠 • Suggest participation in group or community activities (e.g., assertiveness classes, volunteer work, support groups).

Documentation Focus

Assessment/Reassessment
- Individual findings, noting precipitating crisis, client's perceptions, effects on desired lifestyle/interaction with others.
- Cultural values or religious beliefs, locus of control.
- Family support, availability and use of resources.

Planning
- Plan of care and who is involved in planning.
- Teaching plan.

Implementation/Evaluation
- Responses to interventions, teaching, actions performed, and changes that may be indicated.
- Attainment or progress toward desired outcome(s).
- Modifications to plan of care.

Discharge Planning
- Long-term needs and goals and who is responsible for actions to be taken.
- Specific referrals made.

Sample Nursing Outcomes & Interventions Classifications (NOC/NIC) (NIC)

NOC—Self-Esteem
NIC—Self-Esteem Enhancement

---

risk for situational low Self-Esteem

Taxonomy II: Self-Perception—Class 2 Self-Esteem (00153)
[Diagnostic Division: Ego Integrity]
Submitted 2000

Definition: At risk for developing negative perception of self-worth in response to a current situation (specify)

Information that appears in brackets has been added by the authors to clarify and enhance the use of nursing diagnoses.

🌐 Cultural 🐾 Collaborative 🏠 Community/Home Care

Risk Factors

Developmental changes
Disturbed body image; functional impairment
Loss [e.g., loss of health status, body part, independent functioning; memory deficit, cognitive impairment]
Social role changes
Unrealistic self-expectations; history of learned helplessness
History of neglect, abuse, or abandonment
Behavior inconsistent with values
Lack of recognition; failures; rejections
Decreased control over environment
Physical illness

> **NOTE:** A risk diagnosis is not evidenced by signs and symptoms, as the problem has not occurred; rather, nursing interventions are directed at prevention.

Desired Outcomes/Evaluation Criteria—Client Will:

- Acknowledge factors that lead to possibility of feelings of low self-esteem.
- Verbalize view of self as a worthwhile, important person who functions well both interpersonally and occupationally.
- Demonstrate self-confidence by setting realistic goals and actively participating in life situation.

Actions/Interventions

Nursing Priority No. 1.

To assess causative/contributing factors:

- Determine individual factors that could contribute to diminished self-esteem.
- Identify client's basic sense of self-worth and image client has of self: existential, physical, psychological.
- Note client's perception of threat to self in current situation.
- Ascertain sense of control client has (or perceives to have) over self and situation.
- Determine client awareness of own responsibility for dealing with situation, personal growth, and so forth.
- Verify client's concept of self in relation to cultural or religious ideals. **Conflict between current situation and these ideals may contribute to risk of low self-esteem.**

Information that appears in brackets has been added by the authors to clarify and enhance the use of nursing diagnoses.

- Assess negative attitudes and/or self-talk. **Contributes to view of situation as hopeless, difficult.**
- Note nonverbal body language. **Incongruencies between verbal and nonverbal communication require clarification.**
- Listen for self-destructive/suicidal verbalizations, noting behaviors that indicate these thoughts. **Necessitates intervention to prevent client following through on thoughts.**
- Identify previous adaptations to illness/disruptive events in life. **May be predictive of current outcome.**
- Assess family/SO(s) dynamics and support of client.
- Note availability and use of resources.
- Refer to NDs situational low Self-Esteem; chronic low Self-Esteem, as appropriate, for additional nursing priorities and interventions.

Documentation Focus

Assessment/Reassessment
- Individual findings, including individual expressions of lack of self-esteem, effects on interactions with others or lifestyle.
- Underlying dynamics and duration (situational or situational exacerbating chronic).
- Cultural values or religious beliefs, locus of control.
- Family support, availability and use of resources.

Planning
- Plan of care and who is involved in planning.
- Teaching plan.

Implementation/Evaluation
- Responses to interventions, teaching, actions performed, and changes that may be indicated.
- Attainment or progress toward desired outcome(s).
- Modifications to plan of care.

Discharge Planning
- Long-term needs, goals, and who is responsible for actions to be taken.
- Specific referrals made.

Information that appears in brackets has been added by the authors to clarify and enhance the use of nursing diagnoses.

Sample Nursing Outcomes & Interventions Classifications (NOC/NIC) (NIC)

NOC—Self-Esteem
NIC—Self-Esteem Enhancement

Self-Mutilation

Taxonomy II: Safety/Protection—Class 3 Violence (00151)
[Diagnostic Division: Safety]
Submitted 2000

Definition: Deliberate self-injurious behavior causing tissue damage with the intent of causing nonfatal injury to attain relief of tension

Related Factors

Adolescence; peers who self-mutilate; isolation from peers

Dissociation; depersonalization; psychotic state (e.g., command hallucinations); character disorder; borderline personality disorders; emotionally disturbed; developmentally delayed; autistic individual

History of: self-injurious behavior, inability to plan solutions, inability to see long-term consequences

Childhood illness, surgery, or sexual abuse; battered child

Disturbed body image; eating disorders

Ineffective coping; perfectionism

Negative feelings (e.g., depression, rejection, self-hatred, separation anxiety, guilt, depersonalization); low self-esteem; unstable self-esteem/body image

Poor communication between parent and adolescent; lack of family confidant

Feels threatened with loss of significant relationship [loss of parent/parental relationship]

Disturbed interpersonal relationships; use of manipulation to obtain nurturing relationship with others

Family alcoholism, divorce; violence between parental figures; family history of self-destructive behaviors

Living in nontraditional settings (e.g., foster, group, or institutional care); incarceration

Inability to express tension verbally; mounting tension that is intolerable; needs quick reduction of stress

---

Information that appears in brackets has been added by the authors to clarify and enhance the use of nursing diagnoses.

Irresistible urge to cut or damage self; impulsivity; labile behavior
Sexual identity crisis
Substance abuse

Defining Characteristics

Subjective
Self-inflicted burns [e.g., eraser, cigarette]
Ingestion or inhalation of harmful substances

Objective
Cuts or scratches on body
Picking at wounds
Biting; abrading; severing
Insertion of object into body orifice
Hitting
Constricting a body part

Desired Outcomes/Evaluation Criteria— Client Will:

- Verbalize understanding of reasons for occurrence of behavior.
- Identify precipitating factors or awareness of arousal state that occurs prior to incident.
- Express increased self-concept or self-esteem.
- Seek help when feeling anxious and having thoughts of harming self.

Actions/Interventions

Nursing Priority No. 1.
To assess causative/contributing factors:

- Determine underlying dynamics of individual situation as listed in Related Factors. Note presence of inflexible, maladaptive personality traits that reflect personality or character disorder (e.g., impulsive, unpredictable, inappropriate behaviors, intense anger, or lack of control of anger).
- Evaluate history of mental illness (e.g., borderline personality, identity disorder, bipolar disorder).
- Identify previous episodes of self-mutilation behavior. *Note:* **Some body piercing (e.g., ears) is generally accepted as decorative; piercing of multiple sites often is an attempt**

Information that appears in brackets has been added by the authors to clarify and enhance the use of nursing diagnoses.

Cultural Collaborative Community/Home Care

to establish individuality, addressing issues of separation and belonging, but is not considered as self-injury behavior.
- Determine relationship of previous self-mutilating behavior to stressful events. **Self-injury is considered to be an attempt to alter a mood state.**
- Note use or abuse of addicting substances.
- Review laboratory findings (e.g., blood alcohol, polydrug screen, glucose, and electrolyte levels). **Drug use may affect self-injury behavior.**

Nursing Priority No. 2.
To structure environment to maintain client safety:
- Assist client to identify feelings leading up to desire for self-mutilation. **Early recognition of recurring feelings provides opportunity to seek and learn other ways of coping.**
- Provide external controls/limit setting. **May decrease the opportunity to self-mutilate.**
- Include client in development of plan of care. **Commitment to plan increases likelihood of adherence.**
- Encourage appropriate expression of feelings. **Identifies feelings and promotes understanding of what leads to development of tension.**
- Note feelings of healthcare providers and family, such as frustration, anger, defensiveness, need to rescue. **Client may be manipulative, evoking defensiveness and conflict. These feelings need to be identified, recognized, and dealt with openly with staff/family and client.**
- Provide care for client's wounds, when self-mutilation occurs, in a matter-of-fact manner **that conveys empathy and concern.** Refrain from offering sympathy or additional attention **that could provide reinforcement for maladaptive behavior and may encourage its repetition.**

Nursing Priority No. 3.
To promote movement toward positive changes:
- Involve client in developing goals for stopping behavior. **Enhances commitment, optimizing outcomes.**
- Develop a contract between client and counselor **to enable the client to stay physically safe, such as "I will not cut or harm myself for the next 24 hours."** Renew contract on a regular basis and have both parties sign and date each contract.

Information that appears in brackets has been added by the authors to clarify and enhance the use of nursing diagnoses.

- Provide avenues of communication **for times when client needs to talk to avoid cutting or damaging self.**
- Assist client to learn assertive behavior. Include the use of effective communication skills, focusing on developing self-esteem by replacing negative self-talk with positive comments.
- Use interventions that help the client to reclaim power in own life (e.g., experiential and cognitive).

Nursing Priority No. 4.
To promote wellness (Teaching/Discharge Considerations):

🏠 • Discuss commitment to safety and ways in which client will deal with precursors to undesired behavior. **Provides opportunity for client to assume responsibility for self.**

🏠 • Promote the use of healthy behaviors, identifying consequences and outcomes of current actions.

🏠 • Identify support systems.

🏠 • Discuss living arrangements when client is discharged/relocated. **May need assistance with transition to changes required to avoid recurrence of self-mutilating behaviors.**

🕸 • Involve family/SO(s) in planning for discharge and in group therapies, as appropriate. **Promotes coordination and continuation of plan, commitment to goals.**

🏠 • Discuss information about the role neurotransmitters play in predisposing an individual to beginning this behavior. **It is believed that problems in the serotonin system may make the person more aggressive and impulsive, especially when combined with an environment where he or she learned that feelings are bad or wrong, leading client to turn aggression on self.**

💊 • Provide information and discuss the use of medication, as appropriate. **Antidepressant medications may be useful, but they need to be weighed against the potential for overdosing.**

- Refer to NDs Anxiety; impaired Social Interaction; Self-Esteem (specify).

Documentation Focus

Assessment/Reassessment
- Individual findings, including risk factors present, underlying dynamics, prior episodes.
- Cultural or religious practices.
- Laboratory test results.
- Substance use or abuse.

Information that appears in brackets has been added by the authors to clarify and enhance the use of nursing diagnoses.

Planning
- Plan of care and who is involved in planning.
- Teaching plan.

Implementation/Evaluation
- Response to interventions, teaching, and actions performed.
- Attainment or progress toward desired outcome(s).
- Modifications to plan of care.

Discharge Planning
- Long-term needs and who is responsible for actions to be taken.
- Community resources, referrals made.

Sample Nursing Outcomes & Interventions Classifications (NOC/NIC) NIC

NOC—Self-Mutilation Restraint
NIC—Behavior Management: Self-Harm

---

risk for Self-Mutilation

Taxonomy II: Safety/Protection—Class 3 Violence (00139)
[Diagnostic Division: Safety]
Submitted 1992; Revised 2000

Definition: At risk for deliberate self-injurious behavior causing tissue damage with the intent of causing nonfatal injury to attain relief of tension

---

Risk Factors

Adolescence; peers who self-mutilate; isolation from peers
Dissociation; depersonalization; psychotic state (e.g., command hallucinations); character disorders; borderline personality disorders; emotionally disturbed child; developmentally delayed, autistic individuals
History of: self-injurious behavior, inability to plan solutions, inability to see long-term consequences
Childhood illness, surgery, or sexual abuse; battered child
Disturbed body image; eating disorders
Ineffective coping; loss of control over problem-solving situations; perfectionism

---

Information that appears in brackets has been added by the authors to clarify and enhance the use of nursing diagnoses.

 Diagnostic Studies Pediatric/Geriatric/Lifespan ✎ Medications

Negative feelings (e.g., depression, rejection, self-hatred, separation anxiety, guilt); low or unstable self-esteem

Feels threatened with loss of significant relationship; loss of significant relationship; lack of family confidant

Disturbed interpersonal relationships; use of manipulation to obtain nurturing relationship with others

Family alcoholism, divorce; violence between parental figures; family history of self-destructive behaviors

Living in nontraditional settings (e.g., foster, group, or institutional care); incarceration

Inability to express tension verbally; mounting tension that is intolerable; needs quick reduction of stress; irresistable urge to damage self; impulsivity

Sexual identity crisis

Substance abuse

> **NOTE:** A risk diagnosis is not evidenced by signs and symptoms, as the problem has not occurred; rather, nursing interventions are directed at prevention.

Desired Outcomes/Evaluation Criteria— Client Will:

- Verbalize understanding of reasons for wanting to cut or harm self.
- Identify precipitating factors or awareness of arousal state that occurs prior to incident.
- Express increased self-concept or self-esteem.
- Demonstrate self-control as evidenced by lessened (or absence of) episodes of self-injury.
- Engage in use of alternative methods for managing feelings and individuality.

Actions/Interventions

Nursing Priority No. 1.

To assess causative/contributing factors:

- Determine underlying dynamics of individual situation as listed in Risk Factors. Note presence of inflexible, maladaptive personality traits (e.g., impulsive, unpredictable, inappropriate behaviors; intense anger or lack of control of anger) **reflecting personality or character disorder or mental illness (e.g., bipolar disorder)** or conditions that may interfere

---

Information that appears in brackets has been added by the authors to clarify and enhance the use of nursing diagnoses.

🌐 Cultural   🅰 Collaborative   🏠 Community/Home Care

with ability to control own behavior (e.g., psychotic state, mental retardation, autism).

- Identify previous episodes of self-mutilating behavior (e.g., cutting, scratching, bruising). *Note:* **Some body piercing (e.g., ears) is generally accepted as decorative; piercing of multiple sites often is an attempt to establish individuality, addressing issues of separation and belonging, but is not considered as self-injury behavior.**
- Note beliefs, cultural and religious practices that may be involved in choice of behavior. **Growing up in a family that did not allow feelings to be expressed, individuals learn that feelings are bad or wrong. Family dynamics may come out of religious or cultural expectations that believe in strict punishment for transgressions.**
- Determine use or abuse of addictive substances. **May be trying to resist impulse to self-injure by turning to drugs.**
- Review laboratory findings (e.g., blood alcohol, polydrug screen, glucose, electrolyte levels).
- Note degree of impairment in social and occupational functioning. **May dictate treatment setting (e.g., specific outpatient program, short-stay inpatient).**

Nursing Priority No. 2.

To structure environment to maintain client safety:

- Assist client to identify feelings and behaviors that precede desire for mutilation. **Early recognition of recurring feelings provides client opportunity to seek other ways of coping.**
- Provide external controls and limit setting **to decrease the need to mutilate self.**
- Include client in development of plan of care. **Being involved in own decisions can help reestablish ego boundaries and strengthen commitment to goals and participation in therapy.**
- Encourage client to recognize and appropriately express feelings verbally.
- Keep client in continuous staff view and provide special observation checks during inpatient therapy **to promote safety.**
- Structure inpatient milieu to maintain positive, clear, open communication among staff and clients, with an understanding that "secrets are not tolerated" and failure to maintain openness will be confronted.
- Develop schedule of alternative, healthy, success-oriented activities, including involvement in such groups as Overeaters

---

Information that appears in brackets has been added by the authors to clarify and enhance the use of nursing diagnoses.

Anonymous (OA) or similar 12-step program based on individual needs; self-esteem activities include positive affirmations, visiting with friends, and exercise.
- Note feelings of healthcare providers and family, such as frustration, anger, defensiveness, distraction, despair and powerlessness, and need to rescue. **Client may be manipulative, evoking defensiveness and conflict. These feelings need to be identified, recognized, and dealt with openly with staff, family, and client.**

Nursing Priority No. 3.
To promote movement toward positive actions:
- Involve client in developing goals for preventing undesired behavior. **Enhances commitment, optimizing outcomes.**
- Assist client to learn assertive behavior. Include the use of effective communication skills, focusing on developing self-esteem by replacing negative self-talk with positive comments.
- Develop a contract between client and counselor **to enable the client to stay physically safe, such as "I will not cut or harm myself for the next 24 hours."** Renew contract on a regular basis and have both parties sign and date each contract. Make contingency arrangements **so client can talk to counselor, as needed.**
- ∞ Discuss with client/family normalcy of adolescent task of separation and ways of achieving.
- Promote the use of healthy behaviors, identifying the consequences and outcomes of current actions: "Does this get you what you want?" "How does this behavior help you achieve your goals?" **Dialectical Behavior Therapy is an effective therapy in reducing self-injurious behavior along with appropriate medication.**
- Provide reinforcement for use of assertive behavior rather than nonassertive or aggressive behavior.
- Use interventions that help the client to reclaim power in own life (e.g., experiential and cognitive).
- Involve client/family in group therapies as appropriate.

Nursing Priority No. 4.
To promote wellness (Teaching/Discharge Considerations):
- Discuss commitment to safety and ways in which client will deal with precursors to undesired behavior.
- Mobilize support systems.

Information that appears in brackets has been added by the authors to clarify and enhance the use of nursing diagnoses.

🌐 Cultural   🔄 Collaborative   🏠 Community/Home Care

• Involve family/SO(s) in planning for discharge, as appropriate. **Promotes coordination and continuation of plan, commitment to goals.**

• Identify living circumstances client will be going to once discharged/relocated. **May need assistance with transition to changes required to reduce risk or avoid recurrence of self-mutilating behaviors.**

• Arrange for continued involvement in group therapy(ies).

• Discuss and provide information about the use of medication, as appropriate. **Antidepressant medications may be useful, but use needs to be weighed against potential for overdosing or adverse side effects (e.g., the antidepressant Effexor can cause hostility, suicidal ideas, and self-harm). Medications that stabilize moods, ease depression, and calm anxiety may be tried to reduce the urge to self-harm.**

• Refer to NDs Anxiety; impaired Social Interaction; Self-Esteem (specify).

Documentation Focus

Assessment/Reassessment
• Individual findings, including risk factors present, underlying dynamics, prior episodes.
• Cultural or religious practices.
• Laboratory test results.
• Substance use or abuse.

Planning
• Plan of care and who is involved in planning.
• Teaching plan.

Implementation/Evaluation
• Response to interventions, teaching, and actions performed.
• Attainment or progress toward desired outcome(s).
• Modifications to plan of care.

Discharge Planning
• Long-term needs and who is responsible for actions to be taken.
• Community resources, referrals made.

Information that appears in brackets has been added by the authors to clarify and enhance the use of nursing diagnoses.

Sample Nursing Outcomes & Interventions Classifications (NOC/NIC) [NIC]

NOC—Self-Mutilation Restraint
NIC—Behavior Management: Self-Harm

---

disturbed Sensory Perception (specify: visual, auditory, kinesthetic, gustatory, tactile, olfactory)

Taxonomy II: Perception/Cognition—Class 3 Sensation/Perception (00122)
[Diagnostic Division: Neurosensory]
Submitted 1978; Revised 1980, 1998 (by small group work 1996)

Definition: Change in the amount or patterning of incoming stimuli accompanied by a diminished, exaggerated, distorted, or impaired response to such stimuli

---

Related Factors

Insufficient environmental stimuli [therapeutically restricted environments (e.g., isolation, intensive care, bedrest, traction, confining illnesses, incubator); socially restricted environment (e.g., institutionalization, homebound, aging, chronic or terminal illness, infant deprivation); stigmatized (e.g., mentally ill, developmentally delayed, handicapped)]

Excessive environmental stimuli [excessive noise level, such as work environment, client's immediate environment (ICU with support machinery, etc.)]

Altered sensory reception, transmission, or integration [neurological disease, trauma, or deficit; altered status of sense organs]

Biochemical imbalances [e.g., elevated BUN, elevated ammonia, hypoxia]; electrolyte imbalance; [drugs, e.g., stimulants or depressants, mind-altering drugs]

Psychological stress; [sleep deprivation]

Defining Characteristics

Subjective

[Reported] change in sensory acuity [e.g., photosensitivity, hypoesthesias or hyperesthesias, diminished or altered sense of taste, inability to tell position of body parts (proprioception)]
Sensory distortions

Information that appears in brackets has been added by the authors to clarify and enhance the use of nursing diagnoses.

Cultural   Collaborative   Community/Home Care

Objective

[Measured] change in sensory acuity

Change in usual response to stimuli [e.g., rapid mood swings, exaggerated emotional responses, anxiety, panic state]

Change in behavior pattern; restlessness; irritability

Change in problem-solving abilities; poor concentration

Disorientation; hallucinations; [illusions]; [bizarre thinking]

Impaired communication

Motor incoordination, altered sense of balance/falls (e.g., Ménière's syndrome)

Desired Outcomes/Evaluation Criteria—Client Will:

- Regain or maintain usual level of cognition.
- Recognize and correct or compensate for sensory impairments.
- Verbalize awareness of sensory needs and presence of overload and/or deprivation.
- Identify and modify external factors that contribute to alterations in sensory or perceptual abilities.
- Use resources effectively and appropriately.
- Be free of injury.

Actions/Interventions

Nursing Priority No. 1.

To assess causative/contributing factors and degree of impairment:

- Identify client with condition that can affect sensing, interpreting, and communicating stimuli (e.g., stroke, brain injury, cognitive impairment, dementia; pain, surgery, or trauma involving sensory organs; central nervous system disorders [e.g., spinal cord injury, cerebral palsy, Parkinson's disease]; peripheral neuropathies).
- Review results of laboratory tests (e.g., serum electrolytes, chemical profile, ABGs, serum drug levels).
- Assist with and review diagnostic studies and sensory/motor neurological testing.
- Monitor drug regimen **to identify medications with effects or drug interactions that may cause or exacerbate sensory or perceptual problems.**
- Assess ability to speak, hear, interpret, and respond to simple commands **to obtain an overview of client's mental and cognitive status and ability to interpret stimuli.**

Information that appears in brackets has been added by the authors to clarify and enhance the use of nursing diagnoses.

- Evaluate sensory awareness: stimulus of hot and cold, dull or sharp; smell, taste, visual acuity, and hearing; gait, mobility; location and function of body parts.
- Determine response to painful stimuli **to note whether response is appropriate to stimulus, immediate, or delayed.**
- Observe for behavioral responses (e.g., illusions, hallucinations, delusions, withdrawal, hostility, crying, inappropriate affect, confusion or disorientation).
- Ascertain client's/SO's perception of problem/changes in activities of daily living. Listen to and respect client's expressions of deprivation and take these into consideration in planning care.

Nursing Priority No. 2.

To promote normalization of response to stimuli:

- Provide means of communication, as indicated.
- Encourage use of listening devices (e.g., hearing aid, audiovisual amplifier, closed-caption TV, signing interpreter) **to assist in managing auditory impairment.**
- Avoid isolation of client, physically or emotionally, **to prevent sensory deprivation/limit confusion.**
- Promote a stable environment with continuity of care by same personnel as much as possible.
- Interpret stimuli and offer feedback **to assist client to separate reality from fantasy or altered perception.**
- Reorient to person, place, time, and events, as necessary.
- Explain procedures and activities, expected sensations, and outcomes.
- Limit and carefully monitor use of sedation, especially in older population.
- Minimize discussion of negatives (e.g., client and personnel problems) within client's hearing. **Client may misinterpret and believe references are to himself or herself.**
- Eliminate extraneous noise and stimuli, including nonessential equipment, alarms or audible monitor signals when possible.
- Provide undisturbed rest and sleep periods.
- Speak to visually impaired or unresponsive client during care **to provide auditory stimulation and prevent startle reflex.**
- Provide tactile stimulation as care is given. **Touching is an important part of caring and a deep psychological need communicating presence and connection with another human being.**

Information that appears in brackets has been added by the authors to clarify and enhance the use of nursing diagnoses.

Cultural · Collaborative · Community/Home Care

- Encourage SO(s) to bring in familiar objects, talk to, and touch the client frequently.
- Provide sensory stimulation, including familiar smells and sounds, tactile stimulation with a variety of objects, changing of light intensity and other cues (e.g., clocks, calendars).
- Provide diversional activities, as able (e.g., TV, radio, conversation, large-print or talking books). (Refer to ND deficient Diversional Activity.)
- Promote meaningful socialization. (Refer to ND Social Isolation.)
 - Collaborate with other health-team members in providing rehabilitative therapies and stimulating modalities (e.g., music therapy, sensory training, remotivation therapy) **to achieve maximal gains in function and psychosocial well-being.**
- Identify and encourage use of resources and prosthetic devices (e.g., hearing aids, computerized visual aid, glasses with a level plumbline for balance). **Useful for augmenting senses.**

Nursing Priority No. 3.
To prevent injury/complications:
- Record perceptual deficit on chart **so that caregivers are aware.**
- Place call bell or other communication device within reach and be sure client knows where it is and how to use it.
- Provide safety measures, as needed (e.g., siderails, bed in low position, adequate lighting; assistance with walking; use of vision or hearing devices).
- Review basic and specific safety information (e.g., "I am on your right side"; "This water is hot"; "Swallow now"; "Stand up"; "You cannot drive").
- Position doors and furniture so they are out of travel path for client with impaired vision, or strategically place items or grab bars **to aid in maintaining balance.**
- Ambulate with assistance and devices **to enhance balance.**
- Describe where affected areas of body are when moving client.
- Monitor use of heating pads or ice packs; use thermometer to measure temperature of bath water **to protect from thermal injury.**
- Refer to NDs risk for Injury; risk for Trauma; risk for Falls.

Nursing Priority No. 4.
To promote wellness (Teaching/Discharge Considerations):

Information that appears in brackets has been added by the authors to clarify and enhance the use of nursing diagnoses.

🏠 • Assist client/SO(s) to learn effective ways of coping with and managing sensory disturbances, anticipating safety needs according to client's sensory deficits and developmental level.

🏠 • Identify alternative ways of dealing with perceptual deficits (e.g., vision and hearing aids; augmentative communication devices; computer technologies; specific deficit-compensation techniques).

🏠 • Provide explanations of and plan care with client, involving SO(s) as much as possible. **Enhances commitment to and continuation of plan, optimizing outcomes.**

🏠 • Review home safety measures pertinent to deficits.

💊 • Discuss drug regimen, noting possible toxic side effects of both prescription and OTC drugs. **Prompt recognition of side effects allows for timely intervention/change in drug regimen.**

• Demonstrate use and care of sensory prosthetic devices (e.g., assistive vision or listening devices, etc.).

🏠 • Identify resources and community programs for acquiring and maintaining assistive devices.

🏠 • Discuss with client/SO ways to prevent or limit exposure to conditions affecting sensory functions (e.g., how exposure to loud noise and toxic side effects of some drugs can impair hearing; early childhood screening for speech and language disorders; vaccines to prevent measles, mumps, meningitis [**once known to be major causes of hearing loss**]).

🌐 • Refer to appropriate helping resources, such as Society for the Blind, Self-Help for the Hard of Hearing (SHHH), or local support groups, screening programs, and so forth.

Documentation Focus

Assessment/Reassessment
• Individual findings, noting specific deficit and associated symptoms, perceptions of client/SO(s).
• Assistive device needs.

Planning
• Plan of care, including who is involved in planning.
• Teaching plan.

Implementation/Evaluation
• Responses to interventions, teaching, and actions performed.
• Attainment or progress toward desired outcome(s).
• Modifications to plan of care.

Information that appears in brackets has been added by the authors to clarify and enhance the use of nursing diagnoses.

Discharge Planning
- Long-term needs and who is responsible for actions to be taken.
- Available resources; specific referrals made.

Sample Nursing Outcomes & Interventions Classifications (NOC/NIC) NIC

Auditory
NOC—Hearing Compensation Behavior
NIC—Communication Enhancement: Hearing Deficit

Visual
NOC—Vision Compensation Behavior
NIC—Communication Enhancement: Visual Deficit

Gustatory/Olfactory
NOC—Sensory Function: Taste & Smell
NIC—Nutrition Management

Kinesthetic
NOC—Sensory Function: Proprioception
NIC—Body Mechanics Promotion

Tactile
NOC—Sensory Function: Cutaneous
NIC—Peripheral Sensation Management

Sexual Dysfunction

Taxonomy II: Sexuality—Class 2 Sexual Function (00059)
[Diagnostic Division: Sexuality]
Submitted 1980; Revised 2006

Definition: The state in which an individual experiences a change in sexual function during the sexual response phases of desire, excitation, and/or orgasm, which is viewed as unsatisfying, unrewarding, or inadequate

Related Factors

Ineffectual or absent role models; lack of SO
Lack of privacy
Misinformation or lack of knowledge

Information that appears in brackets has been added by the authors to clarify and enhance the use of nursing diagnoses.

Vulnerability

Physical abuse; psychosocial abuse (e.g., harmful relationships)

Altered body function or structure (e.g., pregnancy, recent childbirth, drugs, surgery, anomalies, disease process, trauma, radiation, [effects of aging])

Biopsychosocial alteration of sexuality

Values conflict

Defining Characteristics

Subjective

Verbalization of problem [e.g., loss of sexual desire, disruption of sexual response patterns such as premature ejaculation, dyspareunia, vaginismus]; alterations in achieving perceived sex role

Actual or perceived limitations imposed by disease or therapy

Alterations in achieving sexual satisfaction; inability to achieve desired satisfaction

Perceived deficiency of sexual desire or alteration in sexual excitation

Seeking confirmation of desirability [concern about body image]

Change of interest in self/others; [alteration in relationship with SO]

Desired Outcomes/Evaluation Criteria— Client Will:

- Verbalize understanding of sexual anatomy and function, and alterations that may affect function.
- Verbalize understanding of individual reasons for sexual problems.
- Identify stressors in lifestyle that may contribute to the dysfunction.
- Identify satisfying and acceptable sexual practices and alternative ways of dealing with sexual expression.
- Discuss concerns about body image, sex role, desirability as a sexual partner with partner/SO.

Actions/Interventions

Nursing Priority No. 1.

To assess causative/contributing factors:

- Do a complete history and physical, including a sexual history, which would include usual pattern of functioning and

---

Information that appears in brackets has been added by the authors to clarify and enhance the use of nursing diagnoses.

⊕ Cultural 🄲 Collaborative 🏠 Community/Home Care

level of desire. Note vocabulary used by the individual to maximize communication/understanding.

- Have client describe problem in own words.
- Determine importance of sex to individual/partner and client's motivation for change. **Interpersonal problems (marital and relationship), lack of trust and open communication between partners can contribute to client's concern.**
- Be alert to comments of client, **as sexual concerns are often disguised as humor, sarcasm, and/or offhand remarks.**
- Assess knowledge of client/SO regarding sexual anatomy and function, and effects of current situation or condition. **Individuals are often ignorant of anatomy of sexual system and how it works, impacting client's understanding of situation and expectations.**
- Determine preexisting problems that may be factors in current situation (e.g., marital or job stress, role conflicts).
- Identify current stress factors in individual situation. **These factors may be producing enough anxiety to cause depression or other psychological reaction(s) leading to physiological symptoms.**

- Discuss cultural values, religious beliefs or conflicts present. **Client may have anxiety and guilt as a result of family beliefs about sex and genital area of the body because of how sexuality was communicated to the client as he or she was growing up.**
- Determine pathophysiology, illness, surgery, or trauma involved, and impact on (perception of) individual/SO. **The client may be more concerned about these issues when the sexual parts of the body are involved (e.g., mastectomy, hysterectomy, prostatectomy).**

- Review medication regimen and drug use (prescriptions, OTC, illegal, alcohol) and cigarette use. **Antihypertensives may cause erectile dysfunction; monoamine oxidase inhibitors and tricyclics can cause erection or ejaculation problems and anorgasmia in women; narcotics and alcohol can produce impotence and inhibit orgasm; smoking creates vasoconstriction and may be a factor in erectile dysfunction.**
- Observe behavior and stage of grieving when related to body changes or loss of a body part (e.g., pregnancy, obesity, amputation, mastectomy).
- Discuss client's view of body, concern about penis size, failure with performance.

- Assist with diagnostic studies to determine cause of erectile dysfunction. **More than half of the cases have a physical**

Information that appears in brackets has been added by the authors to clarify and enhance the use of nursing diagnoses.

cause such as diabetes, vascular problems. Monitor penile tumescence during REM sleep **to assist in determining physical ability.**

* Explore with client the meaning of client's behavior. **(Masturbation, for instance, may have many meanings or purposes, such as for relief of anxiety, sexual deprivation, pleasure, a nonverbal expression of need to talk, way of alienating.)** (*Note:* Nurse needs to be aware of and be in control of own feelings and response to client expressions or self-revelation.)
* Avoid making value judgments, **as they do not help the client to cope with the situation.**

Nursing Priority No. 2.

To assist client/SO to deal with individual situation:

* Establish therapeutic nurse-client relationship **to promote treatment and facilitate sharing of sensitive information and feelings.**
* Assist with treatment of underlying medical conditions, including changes in medication regimen, weight management, and cessation of smoking.
* Provide factual information about individual condition involved. **Promotes informed decision making.**
* Determine what client wants to know **to tailor information to client needs.** *Note:* Information affecting client safety or consequences of actions may need to be reviewed and reinforced.
* Encourage and accept expressions of concern, anger, grief, fear. **Client needs to talk about these feelings to begin resolution.**
* Assist client to be aware of and deal with stages of grieving for loss or change.
* Encourage client to share thoughts and concerns with partner, and to clarify values and impact of condition on relationship.
* Provide for or identify ways to obtain privacy **to allow for sexual expression for individual and/or between partners without embarrassment and/or objections of others.**
* Assist client/SO to problem-solve alternative ways of sexual expression. **When client is unable to perform in usual manner, there are many ways the couple can learn to satisfy sexual needs.**
* Provide information about availability of corrective measures such as medication (e.g., papaverine or sildenafil [Viagra] for

---

Information that appears in brackets has been added by the authors to clarify and enhance the use of nursing diagnoses.

    Cultural   Collaborative   Community/Home Care

erectile dysfunction) or reconstructive surgery (e.g., penile/breast implants) when indicated.

• Refer to appropriate resources as need indicates (e.g., health-care coworker with greater comfort level and/or knowledge-able clinical nurse specialist or professional sex therapist, family counseling).

Nursing Priority No. 3.

To promote wellness (Teaching/Discharge Considerations):

• Provide sex education, explanation of normal sexual functioning when necessary.

• Provide written material appropriate to individual needs (include list of books related to client's concerns) **for reinforcement at client's leisure and readiness to deal with sensitive materials.**

• Encourage ongoing dialogue and take advantage of teachable moments that occur. **Nurse needs to become comfortable with talking about sexual issue so he or she can recognize these moments and be willing to discuss the client's concerns.**

• Demonstrate and assist client to learn relaxation and/or visualization techniques.

• Encourage client to engage in regular self-examination, as indicated (e.g., breast/testicular examinations).

• Identify community resources for further assistance (e.g., Reach for Recovery, CanSurmount, Ostomy Association, family or sex therapist).

• Refer for further professional assistance concerning relationship difficulties, low sexual desire, and other sexual concerns (e.g., premature ejaculation, vaginismus, painful intercourse).

• Identify resources for assistive devices or sexual "aids."

Documentation Focus

Assessment/Reassessment

• Individual findings including nature of dysfunction, predisposing factors, perceived effect on sexuality and relationships.
• Cultural or religious factors, conflicts.
• Response of SO.
• Motivation for change.

Planning

• Plan of care and who is involved in planning.
• Teaching plan.

Information that appears in brackets has been added by the authors to clarify and enhance the use of nursing diagnoses.

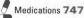

Implementation/Evaluation
- Response to interventions, teaching, and actions performed.
- Attainment or progress toward desired outcome(s).
- Modifications to plan of care.

Discharge Planning
- Long-term needs, referrals made, and who is responsible for actions to be taken.
- Community resources, specific referrals made.

Sample Nursing Outcomes & Interventions Classifications (NOC/NIC) NIC

NOC—Sexual Functioning
NIC—Sexual Counseling

ineffective Sexuality Pattern

Taxonomy II: Sexuality—Class 2 Sexual Function (00065)
[Diagnostic Division: Sexuality]
Submitted 1986; Revised 2006

Definition: Expressions of concern regarding own sexuality

Related Factors

Knowledge or skill deficit about alternative responses to health-related transitions, altered body function or structure, illness, or medical treatment
Lack of privacy
Impaired relationship with a SO; lack of SO
Ineffective or absent role models
Conflicts with sexual orientation or variant preferences
Fear of pregnancy or acquiring a sexually transmitted disease

Defining Characteristics

Subjective
Reported difficulties, limitations, or changes in sexual behaviors or activities
Alteration in relationship with SO
Alterations in achieving perceived sex role

Information that appears in brackets has been added by the authors to clarify and enhance the use of nursing diagnoses.

    Cultural   Collaborative   Community/Home Care

Conflicts involving values
Expressions of feeling alienated, lonely, loss, powerless, angry

Desired Outcomes/Evaluation Criteria— Client Will:

- Verbalize understanding of sexual anatomy and function.
- Verbalize knowledge and understanding of sexual limitations, difficulties, or changes that have occurred.
- Verbalize acceptance of self in current (altered) condition.
- Demonstrate improved communication and relationship skills.
- Identify individually appropriate method of contraception.

Actions/Interventions

Nursing Priority No. 1.
To assess causative/contributing factors:

- Obtain complete physical and sexual history, as indicated, including perception of normal function. **Sexuality is multifaceted, beginning with one's body, biological sex, and gender (biological, social, and legal status as girls or boys, women or men).**
- Note use of vocabulary (assessing basic knowledge) and comments or concerns about sexual identity. **Components of sexual identity include one's gender identity (how one feels about his or her gender) as well as one's sexual orientation (straight, lesbian, gay, bisexual, transgendered).**
- Determine importance of sex and a description of the problem in the client's own words. Be alert to comments of client/SO (e.g., discounting overt or covert sexual expressions such as "He's just a dirty old man"). **Sexual concerns are often disguised as sarcasm, humor, or in offhand remarks.**
- Elicit impact of perceived problem on SO/family. **One's values about life, love, and the people in one's life are also components of one's sexuality.**
- Note cultural values or religious beliefs and conflicts that may exist. **Individuals are enculturated as they grow up and, depending on particular family views and taboos, may harbor feelings of shame and guilt about their sexual feelings.**
- Assess stress factors in client's environment that might cause anxiety or psychological reactions (e.g., power issues involving SO, adult children, aging, employment, loss of prowess).

Information that appears in brackets has been added by the authors to clarify and enhance the use of nursing diagnoses.

 Diagnostic Studies ∞ Pediatric/Geriatric/Lifespan Medications **749**

- Explore knowledge of effects of altered body function/ limitations precipitated by illness (e.g., MS, arthritis, mutilating cancer surgery) or medical treatment of alternative sexual responses and expressions (e.g., undescended testicle in young male, gender change or reassignment procedure).
- Review history of substance use (prescription medications, OTC drugs, alcohol, and illicit drugs). **May be used by client to handle underlying feelings or anxiety.**
- Explore issues and fears associated with sex (pregnancy, sexually transmitted diseases, trust and control issues, inflexible beliefs, preference confusion, altered performance).
- Determine client's interpretation of the altered sexual activity or behavior (e.g., a way of controlling, relief of anxiety, pleasure, lack of partner). **These behaviors (when related to body changes, including pregnancy, weight loss or gain, or loss of body part) may reflect a stage of grieving.**
- Assess life cycle issues, such as adolescence, young adulthood, menopause, aging. **All people are sexual beings from birth to death. Each transition has its own concerns and needs specific education to help the client deal with it in a healthy manner.**

Nursing Priority No. 2.

To assist client/SO to deal with individual situation:

- Provide atmosphere in which discussion of sexual problems is encouraged and permitted. **Sense of trust or comfort enhances ability to discuss sensitive matters.**
- Avoid value judgments—**they do not help the client cope with the situation.**
- Provide information about individual situation, determining client needs and desires.
- Encourage discussion of individual situation, with opportunity for expression of feelings without judgment. **Sexuality also includes feelings, attitudes, relationships, self-image, ideals, and behaviors, and influences how one experiences the world.** (*Note:* Nurse needs to be aware of and in control of own feelings and responses to the client's expressions and/ or concerns.)
- Provide specific information and suggestions about interventions directed toward the identified problems.
- Identify alternative forms of sexual expression that might be acceptable to both partners. **When illness or trauma (e.g., rheumatoid arthritis, paraplegia, long-term chronic condition) interferes with usual sexual expression, there are**

Information that appears in brackets has been added by the authors to clarify and enhance the use of nursing diagnoses.

Cultural   Collaborative   Community/Home Care

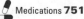

many different methods that can be used to obtain sexual satisfaction.

- Discuss ways to manage individual devices or appliances (e.g., ostomy bag, breast prostheses, urinary collection device) **when change in body image or medical condition is involved.**
- Provide anticipatory guidance about losses that are to be expected (e.g., loss of known self when transsexual surgery is planned).
- Introduce client to individuals who have successfully managed a similar problem. **Provides positive role model and support for problem solving.**

Nursing Priority No. 3.

To promote wellness (Teaching/Discharge Considerations):

- Provide factual information about problem(s), as identified by the client.
- Engage in ongoing dialogue with the client and SO(s), as situation permits.
- Discuss methods, effectiveness and side effects of contraceptives, if indicated. **Assists individual/couple to make an informed decision on a method that meets own values or religious beliefs.**
- Refer to community resources (e.g., Planned Parenthood; gender-identity clinic; social services; Parents, Families and Friends of Lesbians and Gays [PFLAG]), as indicated.
- Refer for intensive individual or group psychotherapy, which may be combined with couple or family and/or sex therapy, as appropriate.
- Refer to NDs Sexual Dysfunction; disturbed Body Image; Self-Esteem [specify].

Documentation Focus

Assessment/Reassessment

- Individual findings, including nature of concern, perceived difficulties, limitations or changes, specific needs and desires.
- Cultural or religious beliefs, conflicts.
- Response of SO(s).

Planning

- Plan of care and who is involved in the planning.
- Teaching plan.

Information that appears in brackets has been added by the authors to clarify and enhance the use of nursing diagnoses.

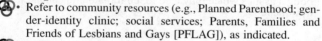

Implementation/Evaluation
- Response to interventions, teaching, and actions performed.
- Attainment or progress toward desired outcome(s).
- Modifications to plan of care.

Discharge Planning
- Long-term needs, teaching, and referrals made, and who is responsible for actions to be taken.
- Community resources, specific referrals made.

Sample Nursing Outcomes & Interventions Classifications (NOC/NIC) **NIC**

NOC—Sexual Identity
NIC—Teaching: Sexuality

---

risk for **Shock**

Taxonomy II: Activity/Rest—Class 4 Cardiovascular/
Pulmonary Responses (00205)
[Diagnostic Division: Circulation]
Submitted 2008

Definition: At risk for an inadequate blood flow to the body's tissues which may lead to life-threatening cellular dysfunction

---

Risk Factors

Hypotension
Hypovolemia
Hypoxemia, hypoxia
Infection, sepsis; systemic inflammatory response syndrome

NOTE: A risk diagnosis is not evidenced by signs and symptoms, as the problem has not occurred; rather, nursing interventions are directed at prevention.

Desired Outcomes/Evaluation Criteria—Client Will:

- Display hemodynamic stability as evidenced by vital signs within normal range for client; prompt capillary refill; adequate urinary output with normal specific gravity; usual level of mentation.

Information that appears in brackets has been added by the authors to clarify and enhance the use of nursing diagnoses.

Cultural   Collaborative   Community/Home Care

- Be afebrile and free of other signs of infection, achieve timely wound healing.
- Verbalize understanding of disease process, risk factors, and treatment plan.

Actions/Interventions

Nursing Priority No. 1.

To assess causative/contributing factors:

- Note possible medical diagnoses or disease processes that can result in one or more types of shock, such as major trauma with heavy internal or external bleeding; heart failure; head or spinal cord injury; allergic reactions; pregnancy-related complications; intra-abdomimal infections, open wounds, or other conditions associated with sepsis.
- Assess for history or presence of conditions leading to hypovolemic shock, such as trauma, surgery, inadequate clotting, anticoagulant therapy; gastrointestinal or other organ hemorrhage; prolonged vomiting and diarrhea; diabetes insipidus; overuse or misuse of diuretics resulting in dehydration. **These conditions deplete the body's circulating blood volume and ability to maintain organ perfusion and function.**
- Assess for conditions associated with *cardiogenic shock,* including myocardial infarction, cardiac arrest, lethal ventricular dysrhythmias, severe valvular dysfunction, cardiomyopathies, malignant hypertension. **These conditions directly impair the heart muscle and ability to pump.**
- Assess for conditions associated with *obstructive shock,* including pulmonary embolus, aortic stenosis, cardiac tamponade, tension pneumothorax. **In these conditions the heart itself may be healthy but cannot pump because of conditions outside the heart that prevent normal filling or adequate outflow.**
- Assess for conditions associated with *distributive shock—neural-induced* including pain, anesthesia, spinal cord or head injury; or *chemical-induced* including peritonitis, sepsis, burns, anaphylaxis, hyperglycemia. **These situations result in loss of sympathetic tone, blood vessel dilation, pooling of venous blood and increased capillary permeability with shifting of fluids.**
- Monitor for persistent or heavy fluid loss, including wounds, drains, vomiting, gastrointestinal tube, chest tube. Check all secretions and excretions for occult blood. Refer to NDs, risk

Information that appears in brackets has been added by the authors to clarify and enhance the use of nursing diagnoses.

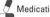 Diagnostic Studies ∞ Pediatric/Geriatric/Lifespan Medications **753**

for Bleeding; risk for imbalanced Fluid Volume for additional interventions.

- Inspect skin, noting presence of traumatic or surgical wounds, erythema, edema, tenderness, petechiae; rashes or hives **for evidence of hemorrhage, localized infections, or hypersensitivity reaction.**
- Investigate reports of increased or sudden pain in wounds or body parts, **which could indicate ischemia or infection.**
- Be aware of invasive devices such as urinary and intravascular cathethers, ET tube, implanted prosthetic devices **that potentiate risk for localized and systemic infections.**
- Assess vital signs and tissue and organ perfusion **for changes associated with shock states:**

Heart rate and rhythm—noting progressive changes in heart rate **(reflecting an attempt to increase cardiac output)** and development of dysrhythmias **suggesting electrolyte imbalances, hypoxia.**

Respirations—noting rapid, shallow breathing, use of accessory muscles **(in an attempt to increase vital capacity and compensate for metabolic acidosis associated with poor tissue perfusion and anaerobic metabolism),** which can progress to respiratory failure.

Blood pressure—noting hypotension, postural hypotension, and narrowed pulse pressure.

Pulses and neck veins—noting rapid, weak, thready peripheral pulses; and congested or flat neck veins. **Signs associated with changes in circulating volume, cardiac ouput, and progressive changes in vascular tone and/or capillary permeability.**

Temperature—higher than 100.4°F (38°C) or lower than 96.8°F (36°C) may indicate infectious process. **Temperature changes in presence of elevated heart and respiratory rate, along with mildly elevated white blood cell (WBC) count in absence of documented infection, is suggestive of systemic inflammatory response syndrome (SIRS).**

State of consciousness and mentation—noting anxiety, restlessness, confusion, lethargy, or unresponsiveness. **Can occur because of changes in oxygenation, acid-base imbalances, and toxins associated with hypoperfusion.**

Skin color and moisture—noting overall flushing or pallor; bluish lips and fingernails, slow capillary refill; or cool, clammy skin.

Information that appears in brackets has been added by the authors to clarify and enhance the use of nursing diagnoses.

⊕ Cultural   Ⓐ Collaborative   🏠 Community/Home Care

Urine output—noting decreased ouput. **One of the most sensitive indicators of change in circulating volume or poor perfusion.**

Urine characteristics—noting color and odor **suggestive of infection source.**

Bowel sounds—noting diminished or absent bowel sounds, or other changes in gastrointestinal function such as vomiting; or change in color, amount or frequency of stools, **reflecting hypoperfusion of gastrointestinal tract.**

- Measure invasive hemodynamic parameters when available—CVP, MAP, cardiac output—**to determine if intravascular fluid deficit or cardiac dysfunction exists.**
- Obtain specimens of wounds, drains, central lines, blood for culture and sensitivity.
- Review laboratory data such as CBC with WBCs and differential; platelet numbers and function; other coagulation factors; tests for cardiac, renal, and hepatic function; pulse oximetry/ABGs; blood urine cultures **to identify potential sources of shock and degree of organ involvement.**
- Review diagnostic studies such as x-rays, ECG; echocardiogram, angiography with ejection fraction; CT or MRI scans, ultrasound **to determine presence of injuries or disorders that could cause or lead to shock conditions.**
- Refer to NDs, ineffective peripheral tissue Perfusion, risk for decreased cardiac tissue Perfusion, risk for ineffective cerebral tissue Perfusion, risk for ineffective gastrointestinal Perfusion, risk for ineffective renal Perfusion for additional interventions and rationales.

Nursing Priority No. 2.

To prevent/correct potential causes of shock:

- Collaborate in prompt treatment of underlying conditions such as trauma, heart failure, infections; and prepare for, assist with medical and surgical interventions **to maximize systemic circulation and tissue and organ perfusion.**
- Administer oxygen by appropriate route (e.g., nasal prongs, mask, ventilator) **to maximize oxygenation of tissues.**
- Administer fluids, electrolytes, colloids, blood or blood products, as indicated **to rapidly restore or sustain circulating volume, electrolyte balance, and prevent shock state.**
- Administer medications as indicated (e.g., vasoactive drugs, cardiac glycosides, thrombolytics, anticoagulants, antimicrobials, analgesics).

Information that appears in brackets has been added by the authors to clarify and enhance the use of nursing diagnoses.

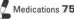

- Provide client care with infection-prevention interventions, such as diligent attention to hand hygiene between clients, aseptic wound care or dressing changes, isolation precautions, early intervention in potential infectious condition.
- Provide nutrition by best means—oral, enteral, or parenteral feeding. Refer to nutritionist or dietitian **to provide foods rich in nutrients, vitamins, and minerals needed to promote healing and support immune system health.**

Nursing Priority No. 3.
Promote wellness (Teaching/Discharge Considerations):

- Instruct client/SO in ways to prevent and/or manage underlying conditions that cause shock, including heart disease, injuries, dehydration, and infection.
- Identify reportable signs and symptoms, including unrelieved pain, unresolved bleeding, excessive fluid loss, persistent fever and chills, change in skin color accompanied by chest pain **for timely evaluation and intervention.**
- Stress need for recognition of substances that cause hypersensitivity or allergic reactions (e.g., insects, medicines, foods, latex).
- Teach client purpose, dosage, schedule, precautions, and potential side effects of medications given to treat underlying conditions. **Enhances compliance with drug regimen, reducing individual risk.**
- Instruct in wound and skin care as indicated **to prevent infection and promote healing.**
- Teach client/caregivers importance of good hand hygiene, clean environment, and avoiding crowds when ill, especially if client is immunocompromised.
- Reinforce importance of immunization against infections such as influenza and pneumonia, especially in client with chronic conditions.
- Encourage consumption of healthy diet, participation in regular exercise, and adequate rest **for healing and immune system support.**
- Recommend that client at risk for hypersensitivity reactions wear Medic-Alert bracelet, maintain readily accessible emergency medication (e.g., Benadryl and/or Epi-pen).

Documentation Focus

Assessment/Reassessment
- Individual risk factors such as blood loss, presence of infection.

Information that appears in brackets has been added by the authors to clarify and enhance the use of nursing diagnoses.

- Assessment findings, including respiratory rate, character of breath sounds; heart rate and rhythm; temperature; frequency, amount, and appearance of secretions; presence of cyanosis; and mentation level.
- Results of laboratory tests and diagnostic studies.

Planning
- Plan of care, specific interventions, and who is involved in the planning.
- Teaching plan.

Implementation/Evaluation
- Clients responses to treatment, teaching, and actions performed.
- Attainment or progress toward desired outcome(s).
- Modifications to plan of care.

Discharge Planning
- Long-term needs, identifying who is responsible for actions to be taken.
- Community resources for equipment and supplies postdischarge.
- Specific referrals made.

Sample Nursing Outcomes & Interventions Classifications (NOC/NIC) NIC

NOC—Circulation Status
NIC—Shock Management

---

impaired Skin Integrity

Taxonomy II: Safety/Protection—Class 2 Physical Injury (00046)
[Diagnostic Division: Safety]
Submitted 1975; Revised 1998 (by small group work 1996)

Definition: Altered epidermis and/or dermis

Related Factors

External
Hyperthermia; hypothermia
Chemical substance; radiation; medications

Information that appears in brackets has been added by the authors to clarify and enhance the use of nursing diagnoses.

Physical immobilization

Humidity; moisture; [excretions or secretions]

Mechanical factors (e.g., shearing forces, pressure, restraint); [trauma: injury, surgery]

Extremes in age

Internal

Imbalanced nutritional state (e.g., obesity, emaciation); impaired metabolic state; changes in fluid status

Skeletal prominence; changes in turgor; [presence of edema]

Impaired circulation or sensation; changes in pigmentation

Developmental factors

Immunological deficit

Psychogenetic factors

Defining Characteristics

Subjective

Reports of itching, pain, numbness of affected or surrounding area

Objective

Disruption of skin surface [epidermis]

Destruction of skin layers [dermis]

Invasion of body structures

Desired Outcomes/Evaluation Criteria—Client Will:

- Display timely healing of skin lesions, wounds, or pressure sores without complication.
- Maintain optimal nutrition and physical well-being.
- Participate in prevention measures and treatment program.
- Verbalize feelings of increased self-esteem and ability to manage situation.

Actions/Interventions

Nursing Priority No. 1.

To assess causative/contributing factors:

- Identify underlying condition or pathology involved (e.g., skin and other cancers, burns, scleroderma, lupus, psoriasis, acne, allergic reaction, diabetes, occupational hazards, familial

---

Information that appears in brackets has been added by the authors to clarify and enhance the use of nursing diagnoses.

Cultural   Collaborative   Community/Home Care

history, trauma, surgical incision or amputation, communicable diseases).

- Note general debilitation, reduced mobility, changes in skin and muscle mass associated with aging or chronic disease, presence of incontinence, or problems with self-care.
- Assess blood supply and sensation (nerve damage) of affected area. Calculate ankle-brachial index (ABI) **to evaluate actual/potential for impairment of circulation to lower extremities.** *Note:* **Result less than 0.9 indicates need for close monitoring or more aggressive intervention (e.g., tighter blood glucose and weight control in diabetic client).**
- Determine nutritional status and potential for delayed healing or tissue injury exacerbated by malnutrition (e.g., pressure points on emaciated and/or elderly client).
- Review medication and therapy regimen (e.g., steroid use, chemotherapy, radiation).
- Evaluate client with impaired cognition, developmental delay, need for or use of restraints, long-term immobility **to identify risk for injury and safety requirements.**
- Review laboratory results pertinent to causative factors (e.g., studies such as Hb/Hct, blood glucose, infectious agents [viral, bacterial, fungal], albumin and protein). (*Note:* Albumin less than 3.5 correlates to decreased wound healing and increased frequency of pressure ulcers.)
- Obtain specimen from draining wounds when appropriate for culture and sensitivities, or Gram's stain **to determine appropriate therapy.**

Nursing Priority No. 2.

To assess extent of involvement/injury:

- Obtain a history of condition, including age at onset, date of first episode, original site/characteristics of lesions, duration of problem, and changes that have occurred over time.
- Note skin color, texture, and turgor. Assess areas of least pigmentation for color changes (e.g., sclera, conjunctiva, nailbeds, buccal mucosa, tongue, palms, and soles of feet).
- Palpate skin lesions for size, shape, consistency, texture, temperature, and hydration.
- Determine degree and depth of injury or damage to integumentary system (i.e., involves epidermis, dermis, and/or underlying tissues).
- Measure length, width, depth of ulcer or wound. Note extent of tunneling or undermining, if present.

Information that appears in brackets has been added by the authors to clarify and enhance the use of nursing diagnoses.

- Inspect surrounding skin for erythema, induration, maceration.
- Photograph lesion(s)/burns, as appropriate, **to document status and provide visual baseline for future comparisons.**
- Note odors emitted from the skin, lesion, or wound.
- Classify ulcer using tool such as Wagner Ulcer Classification System. **Provides consistent terminology for documentation.**

Nursing Priority No. 3.
To determine impact of condition:

- Ascertain attitudes of individual/SO(s) about condition (e.g., cultural values, stigma). Note misconceptions. **Identifies areas to be addressed in teaching plan and potential referral needs.**
- Determine impact on life (e.g., work, leisure, increased caregiver requirements).
- Obtain psychological assessment of client's emotional status, as indicated, noting potential for sexual problems arising from presence of condition.
- Note presence of compromised vision, hearing, or speech. **Skin is a particularly important avenue of communication for this population and, when compromised, may affect responses.**

Nursing Priority No. 4.
To assist client with correcting/minimizing condition and promote optimal healing:

- Inspect skin on a daily basis, describing wound or lesion characteristics and changes observed.
- Periodically remeasure and photograph wound, and observe for complications (e.g., infection, dehiscence) **to monitor progress of wound healing.**
- Keep the area clean and dry, carefully dress wounds, support incision (e.g., use of Steri-Strips, splinting when coughing), prevent infection, manage incontinence, and stimulate circulation to surrounding areas **to assist body's natural process of repair.**
- Assist with débridement or enzymatic therapy, as indicated (e.g., burns, severe pressure sores), **to remove nonviable, contaminated, or infected tissue.**
- Use appropriate barrier dressings, wound coverings, drainage appliances, vacuum-assisted closure device (wound vac), and

---

Information that appears in brackets has been added by the authors to clarify and enhance the use of nursing diagnoses.

 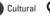

skin-protective agents for open, draining wounds and stomas **to protect the wound and/or surrounding tissues.**

- Apply appropriate dressing (e.g., adhesive or nonadhesive film, hydrofiber or gel, acrylics, hydropolymers) **for wound healing and to best meet needs of client and caregiver or care setting.**
- Maintain appropriate moisture environment for particular wound (e.g., expose lesion or ulcer to air and light if excess moisture is impeding healing, or use occlusive dressings to maintain a moist environment for autolytic débridement of wound), as indicated.
- Avoid or limit use of plastic material (e.g., plastic-backed linen savers). Remove wet and wrinkled linens promptly. **Moisture potentiates skin breakdown.**
- Use paper tape or nonadherent dressing on frail skin and remove gently. Use stockinette, gauze wrap, or any other similar type of wrap instead of tape to secure dressings and drains.
- Reposition client on regular schedule, involving client in reasons for and decisions about times and positions **to enhance understanding and cooperation.**
- Use appropriate padding devices (e.g., air or water mattress, gel pad, waffle boots), when indicated, **to reduce pressure on, and enhance circulation to, compromised tissues.** Avoid use of sheepskin, **which may retain heat and moisture.**
- Encourage early ambulation or mobilization. **Promotes circulation and reduces risks associated with immobility.**
- Provide optimum nutrition, including vitamins (e.g., A, C, D, E) and increased protein intake, **to provide a positive nitrogen balance to aid in skin and tissue healing and to maintain general good health.**
- Monitor periodic laboratory studies relative to general well-being and status of specific problem.
- Consult with wound or stoma specialist, as indicated, **to assist with developing plan of care for problematic or potentially serious wounds.**

Nursing Priority No. 5.
To promote wellness (Teaching/Discharge Considerations):

- Review importance of health, intact skin, as well as measures to maintain proper skin functioning. **The integumentary system is the largest multifunctional organ of the body.**
- Discuss importance of early detection of skin changes and/or complications.

Information that appears in brackets has been added by the authors to clarify and enhance the use of nursing diagnoses.

🏠 • Assist the client/SO(s) in understanding and following medical regimen and developing program of preventive care and daily maintenance. **Enhances commitment to plan, optimizing outcomes.**

🏠 • Review measures to avoid spread of communicable disease or reinfection.

🏠 • Emphasize importance of proper fit of clothing and shoes, use of specially lined shock-absorbing socks or pressure-reducing insoles for shoes **in presence of reduced sensation/ circulation.**

🏠 • Identify safety factors for use of equipment or appliances (e.g., heating pad, ostomy appliances, padding straps of braces).

🏠 • Encourage client to verbalize feelings and discuss how or if condition affects self-concept or self-esteem. (Refer to NDs disturbed Body Image; situational low Self-Esteem.)

🏠 • Assist client to work through stages of grief and feelings associated with individual condition.

🏠 • Lend psychological support and acceptance of client, using touch, facial expressions, and tone of voice.

🏠 • Assist client to learn stress-reduction and alternate therapy techniques **to control feelings of helplessness and deal with situation.**

🔗 • Refer to dietitian or certified diabetes educator, as appropriate, **to enhance healing, reduce risk of recurrence of diabetic ulcers.**

Documentation Focus

Assessment/Reassessment
• Characteristics of lesion(s) or condition, ulcer classification.
• Causative and contributing factors.
• Impact of condition on personal image and lifestyle.

Planning
• Plan of care and who is involved in planning.
• Teaching plan.

Implementation/Evaluation
• Responses to interventions, teaching, and actions performed.
• Attainment or progress toward desired outcome(s).
• Modifications to plan of care.

Information that appears in brackets has been added by the authors to clarify and enhance the use of nursing diagnoses.

Discharge Planning

- Long-term needs and who is responsible for actions to be taken.
- Specific referrals made.

Sample Nursing Outcomes & Interventions Classifications (NOC/NIC) NIC

NOC—Tissue Integrity: Skin & Mucous Membranes
NIC—Pressure Ulcer Care

---

risk for impaired Skin Integrity

Taxonomy II: Safety/Protection—Class 2 Physical Injury (00047)
[Diagnostic Division: Safety]
Submitted 1975; Revised 1998 (by small group work 1996)

Definition: At risk for skin being adversely altered

NOTE: Risk should be determined by use of a standardized risk assessment tool [e.g., Braden Scale].

Risk Factors

External

Chemical substance; radiation
Hypothermia; hyperthermia
Physical immobilization
Excretions; secretions; humidity; moisture
Mechanical factors (e.g., shearing forces, pressure, restraint)
Extremes of age

Internal

Medications
Imbalanced nutritional state (e.g., obesity, emaciation); impaired metabolic state; [fluid status]
Skeletal prominence; changes in skin turgor; [presence of edema]
Impaired circulation or sensation; changes in pigmentation

Information that appears in brackets has been added by the authors to clarify and enhance the use of nursing diagnoses.

Developmental factors
Psychogenetic factors
Immunological factors

> **NOTE:** A risk diagnosis is not evidenced by signs and symptoms as the problem has not occurred; rather, nursing interventions are directed at prevention.

Desired Outcomes/Evaluation Criteria—Client Will:

- Identify individual risk factors.
- Verbalize understanding of treatment/therapy regimen.
- Demonstrate behaviors and techniques to prevent skin breakdown.

Actions/Interventions

Nursing Priority No. 1.
To assess causative/contributing factors:

- Assess skin routinely, noting moisture, color, and elasticity. Review with client/SO history of past skin problems (e.g., allergic reactions, rashes, easy bruising or skin tears) **that may indicate particular vulnerability.**
- Note presence of conditions or situations (e.g., age-related changes in skin and muscle mass, general debilitation, impaired mobility, poor nutritional status, presence of chronic conditions/immunosuppression, incontinence, problems of self-care, side or adverse effects of medication or therapy) **that may impair skin integrity.**
- Assess for diminished circulation in lower extremities. Calculate ABI, as appropriate (diabetic clients or others with impaired circulation to lower extremities). **Result less than 0.9 indicates need for more aggressive preventive interventions (e.g., stricter blood glucose and weight control).**
- Review pertinent laboratory results (e.g., studies such as Hb/Hct, blood glucose, infectious agents [viral, bacterial, fungal], albumin and protein). (*Note:* Albumin less than 3.5 correlates with decreased wound healing and increased frequency of pressure ulcers.)

Nursing Priority No. 2.
To maintain skin integrity at optimal level:

Information that appears in brackets has been added by the authors to clarify and enhance the use of nursing diagnoses.

  Cultural   Collaborative   Community/Home Care

• Handle client gently (particularly infant, young child, elderly). **Epidermis of infants and very young children is thin and lacks subcutaneous depth that will develop with age. Skin of the older client is also thin, less elastic, and prone to injury, such as bruising and skin tears.**

• Inspect skin surfaces and pressure points routinely, especially in mobility-impaired client.

• Observe for reddened or blanched areas or skin rashes, and institute treatment immediately. **Reduces likelihood of progression to skin breakdown.**

• Maintain meticulous skin hygiene, using mild nondetergent soap, drying gently and thoroughly, and lubricating with lotion or emollient, as indicated.

• Massage bony prominences and use proper positioning, turning, lifting, and transferring techniques when moving client **to prevent friction or shear injury.**

• Change position in bed or chair on a regular schedule. Encourage client participation in early ambulation, active and assistive range-of-motion exercises.

• Provide adequate clothing or covers; protect from drafts **to prevent vasoconstriction.**

• Keep bedclothes dry and wrinkle-free; use nonirritating linens.

• Provide protection by use of pads, pillows, foam mattress, water bed, and so forth, **to increase circulation and limit or eliminate excessive tissue pressure.**

• Use paper tape or a nonadherent dressing on frail skin and remove it gently. Or use stockinette, gauze wrap, or any other similar type of wrap instead of tape to secure dressings and drains.

• Provide for safety measures during ambulation and other therapies that might cause dermal injury (e.g., use of properly fitting hose and footwear, safe use of heating pads or lamps, restraints).

• Provide preventive skin care to incontinent client: Change continence pads or diapers frequently; cleanse perineal skin daily, and after each incontinence episode apply skin protectant ointment **to minimize contact with irritants (urine, stool, excessive moisture).**

Nursing Priority No. 3.
To promote wellness (Teaching/Discharge Considerations):

• Provide information to client/SO(s) about the importance of regular observation and effective skin care in preventing problems.

Information that appears in brackets has been added by the authors to clarify and enhance the use of nursing diagnoses.

🏠 • Emphasize importance of adequate nutritional and fluid intake **to maintain general good health and skin turgor.**

🏠 • Encourage continuation of regular exercise program (active or assistive) **to enhance circulation.**

🏠 • Recommend elevation of lower extremities when sitting **to enhance venous return and reduce edema formation.**

🏠 • Encourage abstinence from or restriction of tobacco, **which can cause vasoconstriction.**

🏠 • Suggest use of ice, colloidal bath, lotions **to decrease irritable itching.**

🏠 • Recommend keeping nails short or wearing gloves **to reduce risk of dermal injury when severe itching is present.**

🏠 • Discuss importance of avoiding exposure to sunlight in specific conditions (e.g., systemic lupus, tetracycline or psychotropic drug use, radiation therapy) as well as potential for development of skin cancer.

• Advise regular use of sunscreen, particularly on young child, client with fair skin (prone to burn), or client using multiple medications, and so forth, **to limit skin damage (immediate and over time) associated with sun exposure.**

🏠 • Counsel diabetic and neurologically impaired clients about importance of skin care, especially of lower extremities.

🏠 • Perform periodic assessment using a tool such as the Braden Scale **to determine changes in risk status and need for alterations in the plan of care.**

🔬 • Refer to dietitian or certified diabetes educator, as appropriate, **to identify nutritional needs/maintain proper diabetic control.**

Documentation Focus

Assessment/Reassessment
• Individual findings, including individual risk factors.

Planning
• Plan of care and who is involved in planning.
• Teaching plan.

Implementation/Evaluation
• Responses to interventions, teaching, and actions performed.
• Attainment or progress toward desired outcome(s).
• Modifications to plan of care.

Information that appears in brackets has been added by the authors to clarify and enhance the use of nursing diagnoses.

🌐 Cultural   🔬 Collaborative   🏠 Community/Home Care

Discharge Planning

- Long-term needs and who is responsible for actions to be taken.

Sample Nursing Outcomes & Interventions Classifications (NOC/NIC) NIC

NOC—Risk Control
NIC—Skin Surveillance

readiness for enhanced Sleep

Taxonomy II: Activity/Rest—Class 1 Sleep/Rest (00165)
[Diagnostic Division: Activity/Rest]
Submitted 2002

Definition: A pattern of natural, periodic suspension of consciousness that provides adequate rest, sustains a desired lifestyle, and can be strengthened

Related Factors

To be developed

Defining Characteristics

Subjective
Expresses willingness to enhance sleep
Expresses a feeling of being rested after sleep
Follows sleep routines that promote sleep habits

Objective
Amount of sleep is congruent with developmental needs
Occasional use of medications to induce sleep

Desired Outcomes/Evaluation Criteria— Client Will:

- Identify individually appropriate interventions to promote sleep.
- Verbalize feeling rested after sleep.
- Adjust lifestyle to accommodate routines that promote sleep.

Information that appears in brackets has been added by the authors to clarify and enhance the use of nursing diagnoses.

Actions/Interventions ─────────────────

readiness for enhanced SLEEP

Nursing Priority No. 1.
To determine motivation for continued growth:

- Listen to client's reports of sleep quantity and quality. Determine client's/SO's perception of adequate sleep. **Reveals client's experience and expectations. Provides opportunity to address misconceptions or unrealistic expectations and plan for interventions.**
- Observe and/or obtain feedback from client/SO(s) regarding usual bedtime, desired rituals and routines, number of hours of sleep, time of arising, and environmental needs **to determine usual sleep pattern and provide comparative baseline for improvements.**
- Ascertain motivation and expectation for change.
- Note client report of potential for alteration of habitual sleep time (e.g., change of work pattern, rotating shifts) or change in normal bedtime (e.g., hospitalization). **Helps identify circumstances that are known to interrupt sleep patterns and that could disrupt the person's biological rhythms.**

Nursing Priority No. 2.
To assist client to enhance sleep/rest:

- Recommend limiting intake of chocolate and caffeine or alcoholic beverages (especially prior to bedtime), **which are substances known to impair falling or staying asleep.** *Note:* **Use of alcohol at bedtime may help individual initially fall asleep, but ensuing sleep is then fragmented.**
- Limit fluid intake in evening if nocturia or bedwetting is a problem, **to reduce need for nighttime elimination.**
- Recommend appropriate changes to usual bedtime rituals:

  Provide quiet environment and comfort measures (e.g., back rub, washing hands and face, cleaning and straightening sheets). **Promotes relaxation and readiness for sleep.**

  Explore use of warm bath, comfortable room temperature, use of soothing music, favorite calming TV show. **Nonpharmaceutical aids may enhance falling asleep.**

  ∞ Implement effective age-appropriate bedtime rituals for infant/child (e.g., soothing bath, rocking, story reading, cuddling, favorite blanket or toy). **Rituals can enhance ability to fall asleep, reinforce that bed is a place to sleep, and promote sense of security for child.**

───────────────

Information that appears in brackets has been added by the authors to clarify and enhance the use of nursing diagnoses.

768   ⊕ Cultural   ⊛ Collaborative   🏠 Community/Home Care

- Assist client in use of necessary equipment, instructing as necessary. **Client may use oxygen or CPAP system to improve sleep/rest if hypoxia or sleep apnea diagnosed.**
- Investigate use of sleep mask, darkening shades or curtains, earplugs, low-level background (white) noise. **Aids in blocking out light and disturbing noise.**
- Arrange care **to provide for uninterrupted periods for rest.** Explain necessity of disturbances for monitoring vital signs and/or other care when client is hospitalized. Do as much care as possible without waking client during night. **Allows for longer periods of uninterrupted sleep, especially during night.**

Nursing Priority No. 3.
To promote optimum wellness:

- Assure client that occasional sleeplessness should not threaten health. **Knowledge that occasional insomnia is universal and usually not harmful may promote relaxation and relief from worry.**
- Encourage regular exercise during the day **to aid in stress control and release of energy.** *Note:* **Exercise at bedtime may stimulate rather than relax client and actually interfere with sleep.**
- Advise using barbiturates and/or other sleeping medications sparingly. **These medications, while useful for promoting sleep in the short term, can interfere with REM sleep.**

Documentation Focus

Assessment/Reassessment
- Assessment findings, including specifics of current and past sleep pattern, and effects on lifestyle and level of functioning.
- Medications, interventions, and previous therapies used.
- Motivation and expectations for change.

Planning
- Plan of care and who is involved in planning.
- Teaching plan.

Implementation/Evaluation
- Client's response to interventions, teaching, and actions performed.

Information that appears in brackets has been added by the authors to clarify and enhance the use of nursing diagnoses.

- Attainment or progress toward desired outcome(s).
- Modifications to plan of care.

Discharge Planning
- Long-term needs and who is responsible for actions to be taken.
- Specific referrals made.

Sample Nursing Outcomes & Interventions Classifications (NOC/NIC) **NIC**

NOC—Sleep
NIC—Sleep Enhancement

Sleep Deprivation

Taxonomy II: Activity/Rest—Class 1 Sleep/Rest (00096)
[Diagnostic Division: Activity/Rest]
Nursing Diagnosis Extension and Classification (NDEC)
   Submission Date 1998

Definition: Prolonged periods of time without sleep (sustained natural, periodic suspension of relative consciousness)

Related Factors

Sustained environmental stimulation or uncomfortable sleep environment

Inadequate daytime activity; sustained circadian asynchrony; aging-related sleep stage shifts; non–sleep-inducing parenting practices

Sustained inadequate sleep hygiene; prolonged use of pharmacological or dietary antisoporifics

Prolonged discomfort (e.g., physical, psychological); periodic limb movement (e.g., restless leg syndrome, nocturnal myoclonus); sleep-related enuresis/painful erections

Nightmares; sleepwalking; sleep terror

Sleep apnea

Sundowner's syndrome; dementia

Idiopathic CNS hypersomnolence; narcolepsy; familial sleep paralysis

---

Information that appears in brackets has been added by the authors to clarify and enhance the use of nursing diagnoses.

Cultural   Collaborative   Community/Home Care

Defining Characteristics

Subjective

Daytime drowsiness; decreased ability to function

Malaise; lethargy; fatigue

Anxiety

Perceptual disorders (e.g., disturbed body sensation, delusions, feeling afloat); heightened sensitivity to pain

Objective

Restlessness; irritability

Inability to concentrate; slowed reaction

Listlessness; apathy

Fleeting nystagmus; hand tremors

Acute confusion; transient paranoia; agitation; combativeness; hallucinations

Desired Outcomes/Evaluation Criteria— Client Will:

- Identify individually appropriate interventions to promote sleep.
- Verbalize understanding of sleep disorder.
- Adjust lifestyle to accommodate chronobiological rhythms.
- Report improvement in sleep and rest pattern.

Family Will:

- Deal appropriately with parasomnias.

Actions/Interventions

Nursing Priority No. 1.

To assess causative/contributing factors:

- Determine presence of physical or psychological stressors, including night-shift working hours or rotating shifts, pain, advanced age, current or recent illness, death of a spouse.
- Note medical diagnoses that affect sleep (e.g., dementia, encephalitis, brain injury, narcolepsy, depression, asthma, sleep-induced respiratory disorders or obstructive sleep apnea, nocturnal myoclonus [jerking of legs causing repeated awakening]).

Information that appears in brackets has been added by the authors to clarify and enhance the use of nursing diagnoses.

- Evaluate for use of medications and/or other drugs affecting sleep (e.g., diet pills, antidepressives, antihypertensives, stimulants, sedatives, diuretics, opioids, alcohol).
- Note environmental factors affecting sleep (e.g., unfamiliar or uncomfortable sleep environment, excessive noise and light, uncomfortable temperature, roommate actions—e.g., snoring, watching TV late at night).
- Determine presence of parasomnias: nightmares, terrors, or somnambulism (e.g., sitting, sleepwalking, or other complex behavior during sleep).
- Note reports of terror, brief periods of paralysis, sense of body being disconnected from the brain. **Occurrence of sleep paralysis (although not widely recognized in the United States, has been well documented elsewhere) may result in feelings of fear and reluctance to go to sleep.**

Nursing Priority No. 2.
To assess degree of impairment:

- Determine client's usual sleep pattern and expectations. **Provides comparative baseline.**
- Ascertain duration of current problem and effect on life and functional ability.
- Listen to client's/SO's subjective reports of client's sleep quality and family concerns.
- Observe for physical signs of fatigue (e.g., frequent yawning, restlessness, irritability; inability to tolerate stress; disorientation; problems with concentration or memory; behavioral, learning, or social problems).
- Determine interventions client has tried in the past. **Helps identify appropriate options.**
- Distinguish client's beneficial bedtime habits from detrimental ones (e.g., drinking late-evening milk versus drinking late-evening coffee).
- Instruct client and/or bed partner to keep a sleep-wake log **to document symptoms and identify factors that are interfering with sleep.**
- Do a chronological chart **to determine peak performance rhythms.**

Nursing Priority No. 3.
To assist client to establish optimal sleep pattern:

- Encourage client to restrict late afternoon or evening intake of caffeine, alcohol, and other stimulating substances and to

---

Information that appears in brackets has been added by the authors to clarify and enhance the use of nursing diagnoses.

🌐 Cultural 🅐 Collaborative 🏠 Community/Home Care

avoid eating large evening or late-night meals. **These factors are known to disrupt sleep patterns.**

• Recommend light bedtime snack (protein, simple carbohydrate, and low fat) for young children 15 to 30 minutes before retiring. **Sense of fullness and satiety promotes sleep and reduces likelihood of gastric upset.**

• Promote adequate physical exercise activity during day. **Enhances expenditure of energy and release of tension so that client feels ready for sleep or rest.**

• Review current medications and their effect on sleep, suggesting modifications in regimen **if medications are found to be interfering.**

• Suggest abstaining from daytime naps **because they may impair ability to sleep at night.**

• Investigate anxious feelings **to help determine basis and appropriate anxiety-reduction techniques.**

• Recommend quiet activities, such as reading or listening to soothing music in the evening, **to reduce stimulation so client can relax.**

• Instruct in relaxation techniques, music therapy, meditation, and so forth, **to decrease tension, prepare for rest or sleep.**

• Limit evening fluid intake if nocturia is present **to reduce need for nighttime elimination.**

• Discuss and implement effective age-appropriate bedtime rituals (e.g., going to bed at same time each night, drinking warm milk, soothing bath, rocking, story reading, cuddling, favorite blanket or toy) **to enhance client's ability to fall asleep; reinforce that bed is a place to sleep, and promote sense of security for child.**

• Provide calm, quiet environment and manage controllable sleep-disrupting factors (e.g., noise, light, room temperature).

• Administer sedatives or other sleep medications, when indicated, noting client's response. Time pain medications for peak effect and duration **to reduce need for redosing during prime sleep hours.**

• Instruct client to get out of bed, leave bedroom, engage in relaxing activities if unable to fall asleep, and not return to bed until feeling sleepy.

• Review with client the physician's recommendations for medications or surgery (alteration of facial structures, tracheotomy) and/or apneic oxygenation therapy—continuous positive airway pressure (CPAP) such as Respironics—**when sleep apnea is the cause for sleep disturbance, as documented by sleep disorder studies.**

Information that appears in brackets has been added by the authors to clarify and enhance the use of nursing diagnoses.

Nursing Priority No. 4.

To promote wellness (Teaching/Discharge Considerations):

- Review possibility of next-day drowsiness or "rebound" insomnia and temporary memory loss **that may be associated with prescription sleep medications.**
- Discuss use and appropriateness of OTC sleep medications or herbal supplements. Note possible side effects and drug interactions.
- Refer to support group or counselor **to help deal with psychological stressors (e.g., grief, sorrow).** (Refer to NDs Grieving; chronic Sorrow.)
- Encourage family counseling **to help deal with concerns arising from parasomnias.**
- Refer to sleep specialist or sleep laboratory **when problem is unresponsive to interventions.**

Documentation Focus

Assessment/Reassessment

- Assessment findings, including specifics of current and past sleep pattern and effects on lifestyle and level of functioning.
- Medications, interventions tried, previous therapies.
- Family history of similar problem.

Planning

- Plan of care and who is involved in planning.
- Teaching plan.

Implementation/Evaluation

- Client's response to interventions, teaching, and actions performed.
- Attainment or progress toward desired outcome(s).
- Modifications to plan of care.

Discharge Planning

- Long-term needs and who is responsible for actions to be taken.
- Specific referrals made.

Sample Nursing Outcomes & Interventions Classifications (NOC/NIC) (NIC)

NOC—Sleep
NIC—Sleep Enhancement

Information that appears in brackets has been added by the authors to clarify and enhance the use of nursing diagnoses.

 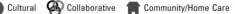 Cultural   Collaborative   Community/Home Care

disturbed Sleep Pattern

Domain 4: Activity/Rest– Class 1 Sleep/Rest (00198)
[Diagnostic Division: Activity/Rest]
Resubmitted 2006

Definition: Time-limited interruptions of sleep amount and quality due to external factors

Related Factors

Ambient temperature, humidity; lighting; noise; noxious odors; physical restraint
Change in daylight-darkness exposure
Caregiving responsibilities
Lack of sleep privacy or control; sleep partner
Unfamiliar sleep surroundings
Interruptions (e.g., for therapeutics, monitoring, lab tests)

Defining Characteristics

Subjective
Reports no difficulty falling asleep; reports being awakened
Verbal complaints of not feeling well rested; dissatisfaction with sleep

Objective
Change in normal sleep pattern
Decreased ability to function

Desired Outcomes/Evaluation Criteria—Client Will (Include Specific Time Frame):

Report improved sleep.
Report increased sense of well-being and feeling rested.
Identify individually appropriate interventions to promote sleep.

Actions/Interventions

Nursing Priority No. 1.
To assess causative/contributing factors:

• Identify presence of factors known to interfere with sleep, including current illness, hospitalization; new baby or sick

---

Information that appears in brackets has been added by the authors to clarify and enhance the use of nursing diagnoses.

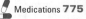

family member in home. **Sleep problems can arise from internal and external factors, and may require assessment over time to differentiate specific cause(s).**

- Ascertain presence of short-term alteration in sleep patterns, such as can occur with travel (jet-lag), sharing bed with new sleep partner, fighting with family member, crisis at work, loss of job, death in family. **Helps identify circumstances that are known to interrupt sleep acutely, but not necessarily long term.**
- Note environmental factors, such as unfamiliar or uncomfortable room; excessive noise and light, uncomfortable temperature; frequent medical and monitoring interventions; and roommate actions—snoring, watching television late at night, wanting to talk. **These factors can reduce client's ability to rest and sleep at a time when more rest is needed.** *Note:* **Clients in critical care units are known to experience lack of sleep or frequent disruptions, often compounding their illness.**

Nursing Priority No. 2.

To evaluate sleep and degree of dysfunction:

- Assess client's usual sleep patterns, and compare with current sleep disturbance, relying on client/SO report of problem **to ascertain intensity and duration of problems.**
- Listen to reports of sleep quality (e.g., "short, interrupted") and response from lack of good sleep (feeling foggy, sleepy, and woozy; fighting sleep; fatigue). **Helps clarify client's perception of sleep quantity and quality and response to inadequate sleep**.
- Determine client's sleep expectations. **Individual may have faulty beliefs or attitudes about sleep, and/or unrealistic sleep expectations (e.g., "I must get 8 hours of sleep every night or I can't accomplish anything").**
- Observe for physical signs of fatigue (e.g., restlessness, hand tremors, thick speech, drooping eyes, inattention, lack of interest in activities).
- Incorporate screening information into in-depth sleep diary or testing if needed **to evaluate the type and etiology of sleep disturbance and to identify useful treatment options.**

Nursing Priority No. 3.

To assist client to establish optimal sleep/rest patterns:

- Manage environment for hospitalized client:
  Adjust ambient lighting **to maintain daytime light and nighttime dark.**

Information that appears in brackets has been added by the authors to clarify and enhance the use of nursing diagnoses.

   Cultural   Collaborative   Community/Home Care

Request visitors to leave, close room door, post "Quiet, patient sleeping" sign as indicated **to provide privacy.**

Encourage usual bedtime routines such as washing face and hands, and brushing teeth.

Provide bedtime care such as straightening bed sheets, changing damp linens or gown, back massage **to promote physical comfort.**

Turn on soft music, calm TV program, or quiet environment, as client prefers **to enhance relaxation.**

Minimize sleep-disrupting factors (e.g., shut room door, adjust room temperature as needed, reduce talking and other disturbing noises such as phones, beepers, alarms) **to promote readiness for sleep, and improve sleep duration and quality.**

Perform monitoring and care activities without waking client whenever possible. **Allows for longer periods of uninterrupted sleep, especially during night.**

Avoid or limit use of physical restraints in accordance with client's needs and facility policy.

- Refer to physician or sleep specialist as indicated **for specific interventions and/or therapies, including medications, biofeedback.**
- Refer to NDs Insomnia and Sleep Deprivation for related interventions and rationale.

Nursing Priority No. 4.

To promote wellness (Teaching/Discharge Considerations):

- Assure client that occasional sleeplessness should not threaten health, and that resolving time-limited situation can restore healthful sleep. **Knowledge that occasional insomnia is universal and usually not harmful may promote relaxation and relief from worry, which can perpetuate the problem.**
- Problem-solve immediate needs. **Short-term solutions (e.g., sleeping in different rooms if partner's illness is keeping client awake, acquiring a fan if sleeping quarters too warm or lacks ventilation) may be needed until client adjusts to situation or crisis is resolved, with resulting return to more usual sleep pattern.**
- Encourage appropriate indoor light settings during day and night, avoidance of daytime napping as appropriate for age and situation, being active during day and more passive in evening. **Helps in promotion of normal sleep-wake patterns.**
- Investigate use of aids to block out light and sound, such as sleep mask, room-darkening shades, earplugs, "white noise."

Information that appears in brackets has been added by the authors to clarify and enhance the use of nursing diagnoses.

 Diagnostic Studies ∞ Pediatric/Geriatric/Lifespan 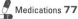 Medications **777**

🏠 • Discuss use and appropriateness of OTC sleep medications or herbal supplements **to provide assistance in falling and staying asleep.**

Documentation Focus

Assessment/Reassessment

- Assessment findings, including specifics of current and past sleep pattern, and effects on lifestyle and level of functioning.
- Specific interventions, medications, or previously tried therapies.

Planning

- Plan of care and who is involved in planning.
- Teaching plan.

Implementation/Evaluation

- Response to interventions, teaching, and actions performed.
- Attainment or progress toward desired outcome(s).
- Modifications to plan of care.

Discharge Planning

- Long-term needs and who is responsible for actions to be taken.
- Available resources, specific referrals made.

Sample Nursing Outcomes & Interventions Classifications (NOC/NIC) NIC

NOC—Sleep
NIC—Sleep Enhancement

---

impaired Social Interaction

Taxonomy II: Role Relationship—Class 3 Role Performance (00052)
[Diagnostic Division: Social Interaction]
Submitted 1986

Definition: Insufficient or excessive quantity or ineffective quality of social exchange

---

Related Factors

Deficit about ways to enhance mutuality (e.g., knowledge, skills)

Information that appears in brackets has been added by the authors to clarify and enhance the use of nursing diagnoses.

⊕ Cultural   ⊛ Collaborative   🏠 Community/Home Care

Communication barriers [including head injury, stroke, other neurological conditions affecting ability to communicate]
Self-concept disturbance
Absence of SOs
Limited physical mobility [e.g., neuromuscular disease]
Therapeutic isolation
Sociocultural dissonance
Environmental barriers
Disturbed thought processes

Defining Characteristics

Subjective
Discomfort in social situations
Inability to communicate/receive a satisfying sense of social engagement (e.g., belonging, caring, interest, or shared history)
Family report of changes in interaction (e.g., style, pattern)

Objective
Use of unsuccessful social interaction behaviors
Dysfunctional interaction with others

Desired Outcomes/Evaluation Criteria— Client Will:

- Verbalize awareness of factors causing or promoting impaired social interactions.
- Identify feelings that lead to poor social interactions.
- Express desire for, and be involved in, achieving positive changes in social behaviors and interpersonal relationships.
- Give self positive reinforcement for changes that are achieved.
- Develop effective social support system; use available resources appropriately.

Actions/Interventions

Nursing Priority No. 1.
To assess causative/contributing factors:
- Review social history with client/SO(s) going back far enough in time to note when changes in social behavior or patterns of relating occurred or began: for example, loss or long-term illness of loved one; failed relationships; loss of occupation, financial, or social or political (power) position; change in

---

Information that appears in brackets has been added by the authors to clarify and enhance the use of nursing diagnoses.

status in family hierarchy (job loss, aging, illness); poor coping or adjustment to developmental stage of life, as with marriage, birth or adoption of child, or children leaving home.

- Ascertain ethnic, cultural, or religious implications for the client **because these impact choice of behaviors and may even script interactions with others.**
- Review medical history, noting stressors of physical or long-term illness (e.g., stroke, cancer, MS, head injury, Alzheimer's disease); mental illness (e.g., schizophrenia); medications or drugs, debilitating accidents, learning disabilities (e.g., sensory integration difficulties, Asperger's disorder/autism spectrum disorder); and emotional disabilities.
- Determine family patterns of relating and social behaviors. Explore possible family scripting of behavioral expectations in the children and how the client was affected. **May result in conforming or rebellious behaviors. Parents are important in teaching their children social skills (e.g., sharing, taking turns, and allowing others to talk without interrupting).**
- Observe client while relating to family/SO(s) **to note prevalent interaction patterns.**
- Encourage client to verbalize feeling of discomfort about social situations. Identify causative factors, if any, recurring precipitating patterns, and barriers to using support systems.

Nursing Priority No. 2.
To assess degree of impairment:

- Encourage client to verbalize perceptions of problem and causes. Active-listen, noting indications of hopelessness, powerlessness, fear, anxiety, grief, anger, feeling unloved or unlovable, problems with sexual identity, hate (directed or not).
- Observe and describe social and interpersonal behaviors in objective terms, noting speech patterns, body language—in the therapeutic setting and in normal areas of daily functioning (if possible)—such as in family, job, social or entertainment settings. **Helps identify the kinds and extent of problems client is exhibiting.**
- Determine client's use of coping skills and defense mechanisms. **Affects ability to be involved in social situations.**
- Evaluate possibility of client being the victim of or using destructive behaviors against self or others. (Refer to NDs risk for other-/self-directed Violence.) **Problems with communication lead to frustration and anger, leaving the individual**

Information that appears in brackets has been added by the authors to clarify and enhance the use of nursing diagnoses.

🌐 Cultural   🅰 Collaborative   🏠 Community/Home Care

with few coping skills, and may result in destructive behaviors.

- Interview family, SO(s), friends, spiritual leaders, coworkers, as appropriate, **to obtain observations of client's behavioral changes and effect on others.**

- Note effects of changes on socioeconomic level, ethnic and religious practices.

Nursing Priority No. 3.

To assist client/SO(s) to recognize/make positive changes in impaired social and interpersonal interactions:

- Establish therapeutic relationship using positive regard for the client, Active-listening, and providing safe environment for self-disclosure.
- Have client list behaviors that cause discomfort. **Once recognized, client can choose to change as he or she learns to listen and communicate in socially acceptable ways.**
- Have family/SO(s) list client's behaviors that are causing discomfort for them. **Family needs to understand that the client is unable to use social skills that have not been learned.**
- Review/list negative behaviors observed previously by caregivers, coworkers, and so forth.
- Compare lists and validate reality of perceptions. Help client prioritize those behaviors needing change.
- Explore with client and role-play means of making agreed upon changes in social interactions and behaviors.
- Role-play random social situations in therapeutically controlled environment with "safe" therapy group. Have group note behaviors, both positive and negative, and discuss these and any changes needed.
- Role-play changes and discuss impact. Include family/SO(s), as indicated. **Enhances comfort with new behaviors.**
- Provide positive reinforcement for improvement in social behaviors and interactions. **Encourages continuation of desired behaviors and efforts for change.**
- Participate in multidisciplinary client-centered conferences to evaluate progress. Involve everyone associated with client's care, family members, SO(s), and therapy group.
- Work with client to alleviate underlying negative self-concepts **because they often impede positive social interactions. Attempts at trying to connect with another can become devastating to self-esteem and emotional well-being.**
- Involve neurologically impaired client in individual and/or group interactions or special classes, as situation allows.

Information that appears in brackets has been added by the authors to clarify and enhance the use of nursing diagnoses.

- Refer for family therapy, as indicated, **because social behaviors and interpersonal relationships involve more than the individual.**

Nursing Priority No. 4.
To promote wellness (Teaching/Discharge Considerations):

- Encourage client to keep a daily journal in which social interactions of each day can be reviewed and the comfort/discomfort experienced noted with possible causes or precipitating factors. **Helps client identify responsibility for own behavior(s) and learn new skills that can be used to enhance social interactions.**
- Assist the client to develop positive social skills through practice of skills in real social situations accompanied by a support person. Provide positive feedback during interactions with client.
- Seek community programs for client involvement that promote positive behaviors the client is striving to achieve.
- Encourage classes, reading materials, community support groups, and lectures for self-help in alleviating negative self-concepts that lead to impaired social interactions.
- Involve client in a music-based program, if available (e.g., The Listening Program). **There is a direct correlation between the musical portion of the brain and the language area, and the use of these programs may result in better communication skills.**
- Encourage ongoing family or individual therapy as long as it is promoting growth and positive change. (However, be alert to possibility of therapy being used as a crutch.)
- Provide for occasional follow-up, as appropriate, **for reinforcement of positive behaviors after professional relationship has ended.**
- Refer to psychiatric clinical nurse specialist for additional assistance when indicated.

Documentation Focus

Assessment/Reassessment
- Individual findings, including factors affecting interactions, nature of social exchanges, specifics of individual behaviors, type of learning disability present.
- Cultural or religious beliefs and expectations.
- Perceptions and response of others.

Information that appears in brackets has been added by the authors to clarify and enhance the use of nursing diagnoses.

⊕ Cultural Collaborative Community/Home Care

Planning

- Plan of care and who is involved in the planning.
- Teaching plan.

Implementation/Evaluation

- Responses to interventions, teaching, and actions performed.
- Attainment or progress toward desired outcome(s).
- Modifications to plan of care.

Discharge Planning

- Long-term needs and who is responsible for actions to be taken.
- Community resources, specific referrals made.

Sample Nursing Outcomes & Interventions Classifications (NOC/NIC) NIC

NOC—Social Interaction Skills
NIC—Socialization Enhancement

Social Isolation

Taxonomy II: Comfort—Class 3 Social Comfort (00053)
[Diagnostic Division: Social Interaction]
Submitted 1982

Definition: Aloneness experienced by the individual and perceived as imposed by others and as a negative or threatened state

---

Related Factors

Factors contributing to the absence of satisfying personal relationships (e.g., delay in accomplishing developmental tasks); immature interests
Alterations in physical appearance or mental status
Altered state of wellness
Unaccepted social behavior or values
Inadequate personal resources
Inability to engage in satisfying personal relationships
Traumatic incidents or events causing physical and/or emotional pain

---

Information that appears in brackets has been added by the authors to clarify and enhance the use of nursing diagnoses.

Diagnostic Studies   ∞ Pediatric/Geriatric/Lifespan   Medications **783**

Defining Characteristics

Subjective

Expresses feelings of aloneness imposed by others, differences from others, rejection

Expresses values unacceptable to the dominant cultural group

Inability to meet expectations of others

Inadequate purpose in life

Developmentally inappropriate interests

Insecurity in public

Objective

Absence of supportive SO(s)—[family, friends, group]

Sad or dull affect

Developmentally inappropriate behaviors

Projects hostility

Evidence of handicap (e.g., physical/mental); illness

Uncommunicative; withdrawn; no eye contact

Preoccupation with own thoughts; repetitive or meaningless actions

Seeks to be alone; exists in a subculture

Shows behavior unaccepted by dominant cultural group

Desired Outcomes/Evaluation Criteria— Client Will:

- Identify causes and actions to correct isolation.
- Verbalize willingness to be involved with others.
- Participate in activities or programs at level of ability and desire.
- Express increased sense of self-worth.

Actions/Interventions

Nursing Priority No. 1.

To assess causative/contributing factors:

- Determine presence of factors as listed in Related Factors and other concerns (e.g., elderly, female, adolescent, ethnic or racial minority, economically/educationally disadvantaged).
- Note onset of physical or mental illness and whether recovery is anticipated or condition is chronic or progressive. **May affect client's desire to isolate self.**
- Do physical exam, paying particular attention to any illnesses that are identified. **Individuals who are isolated appear to**

Information that appears in brackets has been added by the authors to clarify and enhance the use of nursing diagnoses.

  Cultural Collaborative Community/Home Care

be susceptible to health problems, especially coronary heart disease, although little is understood about why this is true.

- Identify blocks to social contacts (e.g., physical immobility, sensory deficits, housebound, incontinence). **Client may be unable to go out, embarrassed to be with others, and reluctant to solve these problems.**

 • Ascertain implications of cultural values or religious beliefs for the client **because these impact choice of behaviors and may even script interactions with others.**

- Assess factors in client's life that may contribute to sense of helplessness (e.g., loss of spouse/parent). **Client may withdraw and fail to seek out friends who may have been in his or her life previously.**

- Ascertain client's perception regarding sense of isolation. Differentiate isolation from solitude and loneliness, **which may be acceptable or by choice.**

- Assess client's feelings about self, sense of ability to control situation, sense of hope.

- Note use and effectiveness of coping skills.

- Identify support systems available to the client, including presence of and relationship with extended family.

- Determine drug use (legal and illicit). **Possibility of a relationship between unhealthy behaviors and social isolation or the influence others have on the individual.**

- Identify behavior response of isolation (e.g., excessive sleeping or daydreaming, substance use), **which also may potentiate isolation.**

- Review history and elicit information about traumatic events that may have occurred. (Refer to ND Post-Trauma Syndrome.)

Nursing Priority No. 2.
To alleviate conditions contributing to client's sense of isolation:

- Establish therapeutic nurse-client relationship. **Promotes trust, allowing client to feel free to discuss sensitive matters.**

- Spend time visiting with client, and identify other resources available (e.g., volunteer, social worker, chaplain).

- Develop plan of action with client: Look at available resources, support risk-taking behaviors to engage in social interactions, management of personal resources, appropriate medical care or self-care, and so forth. **Learning to manage**

Information that appears in brackets has been added by the authors to clarify and enhance the use of nursing diagnoses.

issues of daily living can increase self-confidence and promote comfort in social settings.

- Introduce client to those with similar or shared interests and other supportive people. **Provides role models, encourages problem solving, and possibly making friends that will relieve client's sense of isolation.**
- Provide positive reinforcement when client makes move(s) toward others. **Encourages continuation of efforts.**
- Provide for placement in sheltered community when necessary.
- Assist client to problem-solve solutions to short-term or imposed isolation (e.g., communicable disease measures, including compromised host).
- Encourage open visitation when possible and/or telephone contacts **to maintain involvement with others.**
- Provide environmental stimuli (e.g., open curtains, pictures, TV, and radio).
- Promote participation in recreational or special interest activities in setting that client views as safe.
- Identify foreign-language resources, such as interpreter, newspaper, radio programming, as appropriate.

Nursing Priority No. 3.
To promote wellness (Teaching/Discharge Considerations):

- Assist client to learn or enhance skills (e.g., problem solving, communication, social skills, self-esteem, ADLs).
- Encourage or assist client to enroll in classes, as desired (e.g., assertiveness, vocational, sex education).
- Involve children and adolescents in age appropriate programs and activities **to promote socialization skills and peer contact.**
- Help client differentiate between isolation and loneliness or aloneness and about ways to prevent slipping into an undesired state.
- Involve client in programs directed at correction and prevention of identified causes of problem (e.g., senior citizen services, daily telephone contact, house sharing, pets, day-care centers, religious or spiritual resources). **Social isolation seems to be growing and may be related to time stressors, watching TV, prolonged Internet use, or fatigue, resulting in individuals finding they don't have a close friend they can share intimate thoughts with.**

Information that appears in brackets has been added by the authors to clarify and enhance the use of nursing diagnoses.

⊕ Cultural Ⓐ Collaborative 🏠 Community/Home Care

· Refer to therapists, as appropriate, **to facilitate grief work, relationship building, and so forth.**

Documentation Focus

Assessment/Reassessment
* Individual findings, including precipitating factors, effect on lifestyle and relationships, and functioning.
* Client's perception of situation.
* Cultural or religious factors.
* Availability and use of resources and support systems.

Planning
* Plan of care and who is involved in planning.
* Teaching plan.

Implementation/Evaluation
* Responses to interventions, teaching, and actions performed.
* Attainment or progress toward desired outcome(s).
* Modifications to plan of care.

Discharge Planning
* Long-term needs, referrals made, and who is responsible for actions to be taken.
* Available resources, specific referrals made.

Sample Nursing Outcomes & Interventions Classifications (NOC/NIC) NIC

NOC—Social Involvement
NIC—Social Enhancement

---

chronic Sorrow

Taxonomy II: Coping/Stress Tolerance—Class 2 Coping Responses (00137)
[Diagnostic Division: Ego Integrity]
Submitted 1998

Definition: Cyclical, recurring, and potentially progressive pattern of pervasive sadness experienced (by a parent, caregiver, individual with chronic illness or disability) in response to continual loss, throughout the trajectory of an illness or disability

---

Information that appears in brackets has been added by the authors to clarify and enhance the use of nursing diagnoses.

 Diagnostic Studies   Pediatric/Geriatric/Lifespan   Medications **787**

Related Factors

Death of a loved one
Experiences chronic illness or disability (e.g., physical or mental); crises in management of the illness
Crises related to developmental stages; missed opportunities or milestones
Unending caregiving

Defining Characteristics

Subjective

Expresses negative feelings (e.g., anger, being misunderstood, confusion, depression, disappointment, emptiness, fear, frustration, guilt, self-blame, helplessness, hopelessness, loneliness, low self-esteem, recurring loss, overwhelmed)
Expresses feelings of sadness (e.g., periodic, recurrent)
Expresses feelings that interfere with ability to reach highest level of personal or social well-being

Desired Outcomes/Evaluation Criteria— Client Will:

- Acknowledge presence and impact of sorrow.
- Demonstrate progress in dealing with grief.
- Participate in work and/or self-care ADLs as able.
- Verbalize a sense of progress toward resolution of sorrow and hope for the future.

Actions/Interventions

Nursing Priority No. 1.

To assess causative/contributing factors:

- Determine current and recent events or conditions contributing to client's state of mind, as listed in Related Factors (e.g., death of loved one, chronic physical or mental illness, disability).
- Look for cues of sadness (e.g., sighing, faraway look, unkempt appearance, inattention to conversation, refusing food). **Chronic sorrow has a cyclical effect, ranging from times of deepening sorrow to times of feeling somewhat better.**
- Determine level of functioning, ability to care for self.
- Note avoidance behaviors (e.g., anger, withdrawal, denial).
- Identify cultural factors or religious conflicts. **Family may experience conflict between the feelings of sorrow and**

Information that appears in brackets has been added by the authors to clarify and enhance the use of nursing diagnoses.

anger because of change in expectation that has occurred (e.g., newborn with a disability when the expectation was for a perfect child, while religious belief is that all children are gifts from God and that the individual/parent is never "given" more than he or she can handle).

- Ascertain response of family/SO(s) to client's situation. Assess needs of family/SO. **Family may have difficulty dealing with child/ill person because of their own feelings of sorrow and loss, and will do better when their needs are met.**
- Refer to complicated Grieving; Caregiver Role Strain; ineffective Coping, as appropriate.

Nursing Priority No. 2.
To assist client to move through sorrow:

- Encourage verbalization about situation (**helpful in beginning resolution and acceptance**). Active-listen feelings and be available for support/assistance.
- Encourage expression of anger, fear, and anxiety. Refer to appropriate NDs.
- Acknowledge reality of feelings of guilt/blame, including hostility toward spiritual power. (Refer to ND Spiritual Distress.) **When feelings are validated, client is free to take steps toward acceptance.**
- Provide comfort and availability as well as caring for physical needs.
- Discuss ways individual has dealt with previous losses. Reinforce use of previously effective coping skills.
- Instruct in, and encourage use of, visualization and relaxation skills.
- Discuss use of medication when depression is interfering with ability to manage life. **Client may benefit from the short-term use of an antidepressant medication to help with dealing with situation.**
- Assist SO to cope with client response. **Family/SO may not be dysfunctional but may be intolerant.**
- Include family/SO in setting realistic goals for meeting individual needs.

Nursing Priority No. 3.
To promote wellness (Teaching/Discharge Considerations):

- Discuss healthy ways of dealing with difficult situations.
- Have client identify familial, religious, and cultural factors that have meaning for him or her. **May help bring loss or**

Information that appears in brackets has been added by the authors to clarify and enhance the use of nursing diagnoses.

distressing situation into perspective and facilitate resolution of grief and sorrow.

🏠 • Encourage involvement in usual activities, exercise, and socialization within limits of physical and psychological state. **Maintaining usual activities may keep individuals from deepening sorrow and depression.**

🏠 • Introduce concept of mindfulness (living in the moment). **Promotes feelings of capability and belief that this moment can be dealt with.**

⊗ • Refer to other resources (e.g., pastoral care, counseling, psychotherapy, respite-care providers, support groups). **Provides additional help when needed to resolve situation, continue grief work.**

Documentation Focus

Assessment/Reassessment
• Physical and emotional response to conflict, expressions of sadness.
• Cultural issues or religious conflicts.
• Reactions of family/SO.

Planning
• Plan of care and who is involved in planning.
• Teaching plan.

Implementation/Evaluation
• Response to interventions, teaching, and actions performed.
• Attainment or progress toward desired outcome(s).
• Modifications to plan of care.

Discharge Planning
• Long-term needs and who is responsible for actions to be taken.
• Available resources, specific referrals made.

Sample Nursing Outcomes & Interventions Classifications (NOC/NIC) NIC

NOC—Depression Level
NIC—Hope Inspiration

Information that appears in brackets has been added by the authors to clarify and enhance the use of nursing diagnoses.

🌐 Cultural ⊗ Collaborative 🏠 Community/Home Care

Spiritual Distress

Taxonomy II: Life Principles—Class 3 Value/Belief/Action
  Congruence (00066)
[Diagnostic Division: Ego Integrity]
Submitted 1978; Revised 2002

Definition: Impaired ability to experience and integrate
meaning and purpose in life through connectedness with
self, others, art, music, literature, nature, and/or a power
greater than oneself

Related Factors

Active dying
Loneliness; social alienation; self-alienation; sociocultural dep-
  rivation
Anxiety; pain
Life change
Chronic illness [of self or others]; death
Challenged belief or value system (e.g., moral or ethical impli-
  cations of therapy)

Defining Characteristics

Subjective

Connections to Self
Expresses lack of: hope, meaning or purpose in life, serenity
  (e.g., peace), love, acceptance, forgiveness of self, courage
Expresses anger; guilt

Connections With Others
Refuses interactions with SO(s) or spiritual leaders
Verbalizes being separated from support system
Expresses alienation

**Connections With Art, Music,
Literature, Nature**
Inability to express previous state of creativity (e.g., singing/
  listening to music, writing)
Disinterested in nature or reading spiritual literature

Connections With Power Greater Than Self
Sudden changes in spiritual practices
Inability to pray or participate in religious activities, or to ex-
  perience the transcendent

Information that appears in brackets has been added by the authors to clarify
and enhance the use of nursing diagnoses.

Diagnostic Studies   Pediatric/Geriatric/Lifespan   Medications **791**

Expresses hopelessness, suffering, or having anger toward God
Expresses being abandoned
Request to see a religious leader

Objective

Connections to Self
Poor coping

Connections With Power Greater Than Self
Inability to be introspective

Desired Outcomes/Evaluation Criteria— Client Will:

- Verbalize increased sense of connectedness and hope for future.
- Demonstrate ability to help self and participate in care.
- Participate in activities with others, actively seek relationships.
- Discuss beliefs and values about spiritual issues.
- Verbalize acceptance of self as not deserving illness or situation; "no one is to blame."

Actions/Interventions

Nursing Priority No. 1.
To assess causative/contributing factors:

- Determine client's religious or spiritual orientation, current involvement, presence of conflicts. **Individual spiritual practices or restrictions may affect client care or create conflict between spiritual beliefs and treatment.**
- Listen to client's/SO's reports or expressions of concern, anger, alienation from God, belief that illness or situation is a punishment for wrongdoing, and so forth. **Suggests need for spiritual advisor to address client's belief system, if desired.**
- Determine sense of futility, feelings of hopelessness and helplessness, lack of motivation to help self. **Indicators that client may see no, or only limited, options, alternatives, or personal choices available and lacks energy to deal with situation.**
- Note expressions of inability to find meaning in life, reason for living. Evaluate suicidal ideation. **Crisis of the spirit or**

Information that appears in brackets has been added by the authors to clarify and enhance the use of nursing diagnoses.

 Cultural Collaborative Community/Home Care

loss of will-to-live places client at increased risk for inattention to personal well-being or harm to self.

- Note recent changes in behavior (e.g., withdrawal from others and creative or religious activities, dependence on alcohol or medications). **Helpful in determining severity and duration of situation and possible need for additional referrals, such as substance withdrawal.**
- Assess sense of self-concept, worth, ability to enter into loving relationships. **Lack of connectedness with self and others impairs client's ability to trust others or feel worthy of trust from others.**
- Observe behavior indicative of poor relationships with others (e.g., manipulative, nontrusting, demanding). **Manipulation is used for management of client's sense of powerlessness because of distrust of others.**
- Determine support systems available to client/SO(s) and how they are used. **Provides insight to client's willingness to pursue outside resources.**
- Be aware of influence of care provider's belief system. **(It is still possible to be helpful to client while remaining neutral and refraining from promoting own beliefs.)**

Nursing Priority No. 2.
To assist client/SO(s) to deal with feelings/situation:
- Develop therapeutic nurse-client relationship. Ascertain client's views as to how care provider(s) can be most helpful. Convey acceptance of client's spiritual beliefs and concerns. **Promotes trust and comfort, encouraging client to be open about sensitive matters.**
- Establish environment that promotes free expression of feelings and concerns.
- Suggest use of journaling. **Can assist in clarifying values and ideas, or recognizing and resolving feelings or situation.**
- Encourage client/family to ask questions. **Demonstrates support for individual's willingness to learn.**
- Identify inappropriate coping behaviors currently being used and associated consequences. **Recognizing negative consequences of actions may enhance desire to change.**
- Ascertain past coping behaviors **to determine approaches used previously that may be more effective in dealing with current situation.**
- Problem-solve solutions and identify areas for compromise **that may be useful in resolving possible conflicts.**

Information that appears in brackets has been added by the authors to clarify and enhance the use of nursing diagnoses.

- Provide calm, peaceful setting when possible. **Promotes relaxation and enhances opportunity for reflection on situation, discussions with others, meditation.**
- Set limits on acting-out behavior that is inappropriate or destructive. **Promotes safety for client/others and helps prevent loss of self-esteem.**
- Make time for nonjudgmental discussion of philosophical issues or questions about spiritual impact of illness or situation and/or treatment regimen. **Open communication can assist client in reality checks of perceptions and identifying personal options.**

Nursing Priority No. 3.

To facilitate setting goals and moving forward:

- Involve client in refining healthcare goals and therapeutic regimen, as appropriate. **Enhances commitment to plan, optimizing outcomes.**
- Discuss difference between grief and guilt and help client to identify and deal with each. Point out consequences of actions based on guilt. **Aids client in assuming responsibility for own actions and avoiding acting out of false guilt.**
- Use therapeutic communication skills of reflection and active-listening. **Helps client find own solutions to concerns.**
- Identify role models (e.g., nurse, individual experiencing similar situation). **Provides opportunities for sharing of experiences, finding hope, and identifying options to deal with situation.**
- Assist client to learn use of meditation, prayer and forgiveness **to heal past hurts.**
- Provide information that anger with God is a normal part of the grieving process. **Realizing these feelings are not unusual can reduce sense of guilt, encourage open expression, and facilitate resolution of conflict.**
- Provide time and privacy to engage in spiritual growth and religious activities (e.g., prayer, meditation, scripture reading, listening to music). **Allows client to focus on self and seek connectedness.**
- Encourage and facilitate outings to neighborhood park, nature walks, or similar outings when able. **Sunshine, fresh air, and activity can stimulate release of endorphins, promoting sense of well-being.**
- ∞ Provide play therapy for child that encompasses spiritual data. **Interactive pleasurable activity promotes open discussion**

Information that appears in brackets has been added by the authors to clarify and enhance the use of nursing diagnoses.

⊕ Cultural ⊛ Collaborative 🏠 Community/Home Care

and enhances retention of information. Also provides opportunity for child to practice what has been learned.
- Abide by parents' wishes in discussing and implementing child's spiritual support. **Limits confusion for child and prevents conflict of values or beliefs.**
- Refer to appropriate resources (e.g., pastoral or parish nurse, religious counselor, crisis counselor, hospice; psychotherapy; Alcoholics or Narcotics Anonymous). **Useful in dealing with immediate situation and identifying long-term resources for support to help foster sense of connectedness.**
- Refer to NDs ineffective Coping; Powerlessness; Self-Esteem [specify]; Social Isolation; risk for Suicide.

Nursing Priority No. 4.
To promote wellness (Teaching/Discharge Considerations):
- Assist client to develop goals for dealing with life/illness situation. **Enhances commitment to goal, optimizing outcomes.**
- Encourage life-review by client. Help client find a reason for living. **Promotes sense of hope and willingness to continue efforts to improve situation.**
- Assist in developing coping skills **to deal with stressors of illness or necessary changes in lifestyle.**
- Assist client to identify SO(s) and people who could provide support as needed. **Ongoing support is required to enhance sense of connectedness and continue progress toward goals.**
- Encourage family to provide a quiet, calm atmosphere. Be willing to just "be" there and not have a need to "do" something. **Helps client to think about self in the context of current situation.**
- Assist client to identify spiritual resources that could be helpful (e.g., contact spiritual advisor who has qualifications or experience in dealing with specific problems, such as death and dying, relationship problems, substance abuse, suicide). **Provides answers to spiritual questions, assists in the journey of self-discovery, and can help client learn to accept and forgive self.**

Documentation Focus

Assessment/Reassessment
- Individual findings, including nature of spiritual conflict, effects of participation in treatment regimen.
- Physical and emotional responses to conflict.

Planning
- Plan of care and who is involved in planning.
- Teaching plan.

Implementation/Evaluation
- Responses to interventions, teaching, and actions performed.
- Attainment or progress toward desired outcome(s).
- Modifications to plan of care.

Discharge Planning
- Long-term needs and who is responsible for actions to be taken.
- Available resources, specific referrals made.

Sample Nursing Outcomes & Interventions Classifications (NOC/NIC) (NIC)

NOC—Spiritual Health
NIC—Spiritual Support

risk for Spiritual Distress

Taxonomy II: Life Principles—Class 3 Value/Belief/Action Congruence (00067)
[Diagnostic Division: Ego Integrity]
Nursing Diagnosis Extension and Classification (NDEC) Submission 1998; Revised 2004

Definition: At risk for an impaired ability to experience and integrate meaning and purpose in life through connectedness with self, others, art, music, literature, nature, and/or a power greater than oneself

Risk Factors

Physical
Physical or chronic illness, substance abuse

Psychosocial
Stress; anxiety; depression
Low self-esteem; poor relationships; blocks to experiencing love; inability to forgive; loss; separated from support systems; racial or cultural conflict
Change in religious rituals or spiritual practices

Information that appears in brackets has been added by the authors to clarify and enhance the use of nursing diagnoses.

Developmental
Life changes

Environmental
Environmental changes; natural disasters

> **NOTE:** A risk diagnosis is not evidenced by signs and symptoms, as the problem has not occurred; rather, nursing interventions are directed at prevention.

Desired Outcomes/Evaluation Criteria— Client Will:

- Identify meaning and purpose in own life that reinforces hope, peace, and contentment.
- Verbalize acceptance of self as being worthy, not deserving of illness or situation, and so forth.
- Identify and use resources appropriately.

Actions/Interventions

Nursing Priority No. 1.
To assess causative/contributing factors:

- Ascertain current situation (e.g., natural disaster, death of a spouse, personal injustice).
- Listen to client's/SO's expressions of anger or concern, belief that illness or situation is a punishment for wrongdoing, and so forth. **May indicate possibility of becoming distressed about spiritual and religious beliefs.**
- Note client's reason for living and whether it is directly related to situation (e.g., home and business washed away in a flood, parent whose only child is terminally ill). **Questioning meaning or purpose of life may indicate inner conflict about religious beliefs.**
- Determine client's religious or spiritual orientation, current involvement, presence of conflicts, especially in current circumstances.
- Assess sense of self-concept, worth, ability to enter into loving relationships. **Feelings of abandonment may accompany sense of "not being good enough" in face of illness, disaster.**
- Observe behavior indicative of poor relationships with others (e.g., manipulative, nontrusting, demanding).

Information that appears in brackets has been added by the authors to clarify and enhance the use of nursing diagnoses.

 Diagnostic Studies ∞ Pediatric/Geriatric/Lifespan 💊 Medications **797**

- Determine support systems available to and used by client/SO(s).
- Ascertain substance use or abuse. **Affects ability to deal with problems in a positive manner.**

Nursing Priority No. 2.
To assist client/SO(s) to deal with feelings/situation:

- Establish environment that promotes free expression of feelings and concerns. **Listening, and a quiet demeanor can convey acceptance to the client.**
- Have client identify and prioritize current or immediate needs. **Helps client focus on what needs to be done and identify manageable steps to take.**
- Make time for nonjudgmental discussion of philosophical issues or questions about spiritual impact of illness or situation and/or treatment regimen. **Client may believe that illness is the result of being sinful, bad, or that God has abandoned him or her.**
- Discuss difference between grief and guilt and help client to identify and deal with each, assuming responsibility for own actions, expressing awareness of the consequences of acting out of false guilt. **Client needs to decide whether guilt is deserved or not. Cultural and religious beliefs may lead client to feel guilty when in fact nothing has been done to feel guilty about.**
- Use therapeutic communication skills of reflection and Active-listening. **Helps client find own solutions to concerns.**
- Review coping skills used and their effectiveness in current situation. **Identifies strengths to incorporate into plan and techniques needing revision.**
- Provide role model (e.g., nurse, individual experiencing similar situation or disease). **Sharing of experiences and hope assists client to deal with reality.**
- Suggest use of journaling. **Can assist in clarifying values and ideas, recognizing and resolving feelings or situation.**
- Discuss client's interest in the arts, music, literature. **Provides insight into meaning of these issues and how they are integrated into the individual's life.**
- Refer to appropriate resources for help (e.g., crisis counselor, governmental agencies; pastoral or parish nurse, or spiritual advisor who has qualifications or experience dealing with specific problems [e.g., death and dying, relationships, substance

---

Information that appears in brackets has been added by the authors to clarify and enhance the use of nursing diagnoses.

Cultural Collaborative Community/Home Care

abuse, suicide]; hospice, psychotherapy, Alcoholics or Narcotics Anonymous).

Nursing Priority No. 3.
To promote wellness (Teaching/Discharge Considerations):

- Role-play new coping techniques **to enhance integration of new skills or necessary changes in lifestyle.**
- Encourage individual to become involved in cultural activities of his or her choosing. **Art, music, plays, and other cultural activities provide a means of connecting with self and others.**
- Discuss possibilities of taking classes, being involved in discussion groups or community programs.
- Assist client to identify SO(s) and individuals or support groups that could provide ongoing support **because this is a daily need, requiring lifelong commitment.**
- Abide by parents' wishes in discussing and implementing child's spiritual support.
- Discuss benefit of family counseling, as appropriate. **Issues of this nature (e.g., situational losses, natural disasters, difficult relationships) affect family dynamics.**

Documentation Focus

Assessment/Reassessment
- Individual findings, including risk factors, nature of current distress.
- Physical and emotional responses to distress.
- Access to and use of resources.

Planning
- Plan of care and who is involved in planning.
- Teaching plan.

Implementation/Evaluation
- Responses to interventions, teaching, and actions performed.
- Attainment or progress toward desired outcome(s).
- Modifications to plan of care.

Discharge Planning
- Long-term needs and who is responsible for actions to be taken.
- Available resources, specific referrals made.

Information that appears in brackets has been added by the authors to clarify and enhance the use of nursing diagnoses.

 Diagnostic Studies   ∞ Pediatric/Geriatric/Lifespan   Medications **799**

Sample Nursing Outcomes & Interventions
Classifications (NOC/NIC) NIC

NOC—Spiritual Health
NIC—Spiritual Support

readiness for enhanced **Spiritual Well-Being**

Taxonomy II: Life Principles—Class 2 Beliefs (00068)
[Diagnostic Division: Ego Integrity]
Submitted 1994; Revised 2002

Definition: Ability to experience and integrate meaning and purpose in life through connectedness with self, others, art, music, literature, nature, and/or a power greater than oneself that can be strengthened

Defining Characteristics

Subjective

Connections to Self
Expresses desire for enhanced acceptance; coping; courage; forgiveness of self; hope; joy; love; meaning or purpose in life; satisfying philosophy of life; surrender
Expresses lack of serenity (e.g., peace)
Meditation

Connections With Others
Requests interactions with significant others or spiritual leaders
Requests forgiveness of others

Connections With Powers Greater Than Self
Participates in religious activities; prays
Expresses reverence or awe; reports mystical experiences

Objective

Connections With Others
Provides service to others

Connections With Art, Music, Literature, Nature
Displays creative energy (e.g., writing poetry, singing); listens to music; reads spiritual literature; spends time outdoors

Information that appears in brackets has been added by the authors to clarify and enhance the use of nursing diagnoses.

 Cultural Collaborative Community/Home Care

Desired Outcomes/Evaluation Criteria— Client Will:

- Acknowledge the stabilizing and strengthening forces in own life needed for balance and well-being of the whole person.
- Identify meaning and purpose in own life that reinforces hope, peace, and contentment.
- Verbalize a sense of peace or contentment and comfort of spirit.
- Demonstrate behavior congruent with verbalizations that lend support and strength for daily living.

Actions/Interventions

Nursing Priority No. 1.

To determine spiritual state/motivation for growth:

- Ascertain client's perception of current state and degree of connectedness and expectations. **Provides insight into where client is currently and what his or her hopes for the future may be.**
- Identify motivation and expectations for change.
- Review spiritual and religious history, activities, rituals, and frequency of participation. **Provides basis to build on for growth or change.**
- Determine relational values of support systems to one's spiritual centeredness. **The client's family of origin may have differing beliefs from those espoused by the individual that may be a source of conflict for the client. Comfort can be gained when family and friends share client's beliefs and support search for spiritual knowledge.**
- Explore meaning or interpretation and relationship of spirituality, life, death, and illness to life's journey. **Identifying the meaning of these issues is helpful for the client to use the information in forming a belief system that will enable him or her to move forward and live life to the fullest.**
- Clarify the meaning of one's spiritual beliefs or religious practice and rituals to daily living. **Discussing these issues allows client to explore spiritual needs and decide what fits own view of the world to enhance life.**
- Explore ways that spirituality or religious practices have affected one's life and given meaning and value to daily living. Note consequences as well as benefits. **Understanding that there is a difference between spirituality and religion and how each can be useful will help client begin to view the information in a new way.**

Information that appears in brackets has been added by the authors to clarify and enhance the use of nursing diagnoses.

- Discuss life's or God's plan for the individual, if client desires. **Helpful in determining individual goals and choosing specific options.**

Nursing Priority No. 2.

To assist client to integrate values and beliefs to achieve a sense of wholeness and optimum balance in daily living:

- Explore ways beliefs give meaning and value to daily living. **As client develops understanding of these issues, the beliefs will provide support for dealing with current and future concerns.**
- Clarify reality and appropriateness of client's self-perceptions and expectations. **Necessary to provide firm foundation for growth.**
- Determine influence of cultural beliefs and values. **Most individuals are strongly influenced by the spiritual or religious orientation of their family of origin, which can be a very strong determinant for client's choice of activities and receptiveness to various options.**
- Discuss the importance and value of connections to one's daily life. **The contact that one has with others maintains a feeling of belonging and connection and promotes feelings of wholeness and well-being.**
- Identify ways to achieve connectedness or harmony with self, others, nature, higher power (e.g., meditation, prayer, talking or sharing oneself with others; being out in nature, gardening, walking; attending religious activities). **This is a highly individual and personal decision, and no action is too trivial to be considered.**

Nursing Priority No. 3.

To enhance optimum wellness:

- Encourage client to take time to be introspective in the search for peace and harmony. **Finding peace within oneself will carry over to relationships with others and own outlook on life.**
- Discuss use of relaxation or meditative activities (e.g., yoga, tai chi, prayer). **Helpful in promoting general well-being and sense of connectedness with self, nature or spiritual power.**
- Suggest attendance or involvement in dream-sharing group **to develop and enhance learning of the characteristics of spiritual awareness and facilitate the individual's growth.**

Information that appears in brackets has been added by the authors to clarify and enhance the use of nursing diagnoses.

🌐 Cultural   🔵 Collaborative   🏠 Community/Home Care

- 🏠 • Identify ways for spiritual or religious expression. **There are multiple options for enhancing spirituality through connectedness with self/others (e.g., volunteering time to community projects, mentoring, singing in the choir, painting, or spiritual writings).**
- 🏠 • Encourage participation in desired religious activities, contact with minister or spiritual advisor. **Validating own beliefs in an external way can provide support and strengthen the inner self.**
- 🏠 • Discuss and role-play, as necessary, ways to deal with alternative view or conflict that may occur with family/SO(s), society or cultural group. **Provides opportunity to try out different behaviors in a safe environment and be prepared for potential eventualities.**
- 🏠 • Provide bibliotherapy, list of relevant resources (e.g., study groups, parish nurse, poetry society), and possible Web sites **for later reference or self-paced learning and ongoing support.**

Documentation Focus

Assessment/Reassessment
- Assessment findings, including client perception of needs and desire for growth or enhancement.
- Motivation and expectations for change.

Planning
- Plan for growth and who is involved in planning.

Implementation/Evaluation
- Response to activities, learning, and actions performed.
- Attainment or progress toward desired outcome(s).
- Modifications to plan.

Discharge Planning
- Long-term needs, expectations, and plan of action.
- Specific referrals made.

Sample Nursing Outcomes & Interventions Classifications (NOC/NIC) NIC

NOC—Spiritual Health
NIC—Spiritual Growth Facilitation

Information that appears in brackets has been added by the authors to clarify and enhance the use of nursing diagnoses.

Stress Overload

Taxonomy II: Coping/Stress Tolerance—Class 2 Coping Responses (00177)
[Diagnostic Division: Ego Intregrity]
Submitted 2006

Definition: Excessive amounts and types of demands that require action

Related Factors

Inadequate resources (e.g., financial, social, education/knowledge level)
Intense, repeated stressors (e.g., family violence, chronic illness, terminal illness)
Multiple coexisting stressors (e.g., environmental threats/demands; physical threats/demands; social threats/demands)

Defining Characteristics

Subjective
Expresses difficulty in functioning or problems with decision making
Expresses a feeling of pressure, tension, increased feelings of impatience, or anger
Reports negative impact from stress (e.g., physical symptoms, psychological distress, feeling of being sick or of going to get sick)
Reports situational stress as excessive (e.g., rates stress level as a 7 or above on a 10-point scale)

Objective
Demonstrates increased feelings of impatience/anger

Desired Outcomes/Evaluation Criteria— Client Will:

- Assess current situation accurately.
- Identify ineffective stress-management behaviors and consequences.
- Meet psychological needs as evidenced by appropriate expression of feelings, identification of options, and use of resources.
- Verbalize or demonstrate reduced stress reaction.

Information that appears in brackets has been added by the authors to clarify and enhance the use of nursing diagnoses.

Actions/Interventions

Nursing Priority No. 1.

To identify causative/precipitating factors and degree of impairment:

- Ascertain what events have occurred (e.g., family violence, death of loved one, chronic or terminal illness, workplace stress or loss of job, catastrophic natural or man-made event) over remote and recent past **to assist in determining number, duration, and intensity of events causing perception of overwhelming stress.**

- Determine client's/SO's understanding of events, noting differences in viewpoints.

• Note client's gender, age, and developmental level of functioning. **Women, children, young adults, and divorced and separated persons tend to have higher stress levels. Multiple stressors can weaken the immune system and tax physical and emotional coping mechanisms in persons of any age, but particularly the elderly.**

• Note cultural values or religious beliefs that may affect client's expectation for self in dealing with situation and expectations placed on client by SO(s)/family. **For example, in dealing with Navajo parents, it is important to look at how they define family (can be nuclear, extended, or clan), who are the primary caregivers, and what are their social goals.**

- Identify client locus of control: internal (expressions of responsibility for self and ability to control outcomes: "I didn't quit smoking") or external (expressions of lack of control over self and environment: "Nothing ever works out"). **Knowing client's locus of control will help in developing a plan of care reflecting client's ability to realistically make changes that will help to manage stress better.**

- Assess emotional responses and coping mechanisms being used.

- Determine stress feelings and self-talk client is engaging in. **Negative self-talk, all or nothing or pessimistic thinking, exaggeration, or unrealistic expectations all contribute to stress overload.**

- Assess degree of mastery client has exhibited in life. **Passive individual may have more difficulty being assertive and standing up for rights.**

- Determine presence or absence and nature of resources (e.g., whether family/SO(s) are supportive, lack of money, problems with relationship or social functioning).

Information that appears in brackets has been added by the authors to clarify and enhance the use of nursing diagnoses.

- Note change in relationships with SO(s). **Conflict in the family, loss of a family member, divorce can result in a change in support client is accustomed to and impair ability to manage situation.**
- Evaluate stress level, using appropriate tool (e.g., Stress & Depression, Self-Assessment Tool) to help identify areas of most distress. **While most stress seems to come from disastrous events in individual's life, positive events can also be stressful.**

Nursing Priority No. 2.
To assist client to deal with current situation:

- Active-listen concerns and provide empathetic presence, using talk and silence as needed.
- Provide for or encourage restful environment where possible.
- Discuss situation or condition in simple, concise manner. Devote time for listening. **May help client express emotions, grasp situation, and feel more in control.**
- Deal with the immediate issues first (e.g., treatment of acute physical or psychological illness, meet safety needs, removal from traumatic or violent environment).
- Assist client in determining whether he or she can change stressor or response. **May help client to sort out things over which he or she has control, and/or determine responses that can be modified.**
- Allow client to react in own way without judgment. Provide support and diversion as indicated.
- Help client set limits on acting-out behaviors and learn ways to express emotions in an acceptable manner. **Promotes internal locus of control, enabling client to maintain self-concept and feel more positive about self.**
- Address use of ineffective or dangerous coping mechanisms (e.g., substance use or abuse, self or other-directed violence) and refer for counseling as indicated.
- Collaborate in treatment of underlying conditions (e.g., physical injury, depression, anger management).

Nursing Priority No. 3.
To promote wellness (Teaching/Discharge Considerations):

- Use client's locus of control to develop individual plan of care **(e.g., for client with internal control, encourage client to take control of own care; for those with external control, begin with small tasks and add as tolerated).**

Information that appears in brackets has been added by the authors to clarify and enhance the use of nursing diagnoses.

Cultural   Collaborative   Community/Home Care

- Incorporate strengths, assets, and past coping strategies that were successful for client. **Reinforces that client is able to deal with difficult situations.**
- Provide information about stress and exhaustion phase, which occurs when person is experiencing chronic or unresolved stress. **Release of cortisol can contribute to reduction in immune function, resulting in physical illness, mental disability, and life dysfunction.**
- Review stress management and coping skills that client can use:

  Practice behaviors that may help reduce negative consequences—change thinking by focusing on positives, reframing thoughts, changing lifestyle.

  Take a step back, simplify life; learn to say "no" **to reduce sense of being overwhelmed.**

  Learn to control and redirect anger.

  Develop and practice positive self-esteem skills.

  Rest, sleep, and exercise **to recuperate and rejuvenate self.**

  Participate in self-help actions (e.g., deep breathing, find time to be alone, get involved in recreation or desired activity, plan something fun, develop humor) **to actively relax.**

  Eat right; avoid junk food, excessive caffeine, alcohol, and nicotine **to support general health.**

  Develop spiritual self (e.g., meditate or pray; block negative thoughts; learn to give and take, speak and listen, forgive and move on).

  Interact socially, reach out, nurture self and others **to reduce loneliness or sense of isolation.**

- Review proper medication use to manage exacerbating conditions (e.g., depression, mood disorders).
- Identify community resources (e.g., vocational counseling, educational programs, child/elder care, WIC or food stamps, home or respite care) **that can help client manage lifestyle and environmental stress.**
- Refer for therapy as indicated (e.g., medical treatment, psychological counseling, hypnosis, massage, biofeedback).

Documentation Focus

Assessment/Reassessment

- Individual findings, noting specific stressors, individual's perception of the situation, locus of control.
- Specific cultural or religious factors.
- Availability and use of support systems and resources.

Information that appears in brackets has been added by the authors to clarify and enhance the use of nursing diagnoses.

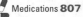

Diagnostic Studies   ∞ Pediatric/Geriatric/Lifespan   Medications **807**

Planning
* Plan of care and who is involved in planning.
* Teaching plan.

Implementation/Evaluation
* Responses to interventions, teaching, and actions performed.
* Attainment or progress toward desired outcome(s).
* Modifications to plan of care.

Discharge Planning
* Long-term needs and who is responsible for actions to be taken.
* Specific referrals made.

Sample Nursing Outcomes & Interventions Classifications (NOC/NIC) NIC

NOC—Stress Level
NIC—Coping Enhancement

---

risk for Suffocation

Taxonomy II: Safety/Protection—Class 2 Physical Injury (00036)
[Diagnostic Division: Safety]
Submitted 1980

Definition: Accentuated risk of accidental suffocation (inadequate air available for inhalation)

Risk Factors

Internal
Reduced olfactory sensation
Reduced motor abilities
Lack of safety education or precautions
Cognitive or emotional difficulties [e.g., altered consciousness/ mentation]
Disease or injury process

External
Pillow or propped bottle placed in an infant's crib
Hanging a pacifier around infant's neck
Playing with plastic bags; inserting small objects into airway

---

Information that appears in brackets has been added by the authors to clarify and enhance the use of nursing diagnoses.

 Cultural 🐾 Collaborative 🏠 Community/Home Care

Leaving children unattended in water

Discarded refrigerators without removed doors

Vehicle warming in closed garage [or faulty exhaust system];
use of fuel-burning heaters not vented to outside

Household gas leaks; smoking in bed

Low-strung clothesline

Eating large mouthfuls [or pieces] of food

> **NOTE:** A risk diagnosis is not evidenced by signs and symptoms, as the problem has not occurred; rather, nursing interventions are directed at prevention.

Desired Outcomes/Evaluation Criteria—
Client/Caregiver Will:

- Verbalize knowledge of hazards in the environment.
- Identify interventions appropriate to situation.
- Correct hazardous situations to prevent or reduce risk of suffocation.
- Demonstrate CPR skills and how to access emergency assistance.

Actions/Interventions

Nursing Priority No. 1.
To assess causative/contributing factors:

∞ • Note presence of internal and external factors in individual situation (e.g., seizure activity; asthma; frail elderly; impaired cognition or consiousness; risky teen behavior, such as playing suffocation game, sniffing inhalants; hazards in or around home [e.g., abandoned large appliances, swimming pool]; inadequate supervision of infants/small children).
- Determine client's/SO's knowledge of safety factors or hazards present in the environment.
- Identify level of concern or awareness and motivation of client/SO(s) to correct safety hazards and improve individual situation.
- Assess neurological status and note factors that have potential to compromise airway or affect ability to swallow (e.g., stroke, cerebral palsy, MS, ALS).
- Determine use of antiepileptics and how well epilepsy is controlled.
- Note reports of sleep disturbance and fatigue; **may be indicative of sleep apnea (airway obstruction).**

Information that appears in brackets has been added by the authors to clarify and enhance the use of nursing diagnoses.

 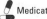

- Assess for allergies (e.g., medications, foods, environmental) **to which individual could have severe/anaphylactic reaction resulting in respiratory arrest.**

Nursing Priority No. 2.
To reverse/correct contributing factors:

- Identify and encourage relevant safety measures (e.g., seizure precautions; close supervision of toddler; avoiding smoking in bed, propping baby bottle, or running automobile in closed garage) **to prevent or minimize risk of injury.**
- Recommend storing small toys, coins, cords or drawstrings, and plastic bags out of reach of infants and young children. Avoid use of plastic mattress or crib covers, comforter, or fluffy pillows in cribs **to reduce risk of accidental suffocation.**
- Use proper positioning, suctioning; use airway adjuncts, as indicated, for comatose individual or client with swallowing impairment or obstructive sleep apnea **to protect and maintain airway.**
- Provide diet modifications as indicated by specific needs (e.g., developmental level, presence and degree of swallowing disability, impaired cognition) **to reduce risk of aspiration.**
- Monitor medication regimen (e.g., anticonvulsants, analgesics, sedatives), noting potential for oversedation.
- Discuss with client/SO(s) identified environmental or work-related safety hazards and problem-solve methods for resolution.
- Emphasize importance of periodic evaluation and repair of gas appliances, furnace, automobile exhaust system **to prevent exposure to carbon monoxide.**

Nursing Priority No. 3.
To promote wellness (Teaching/Discharge Considerations):

- Review safety factors identified in individual situation and methods for remediation.
- Develop plan with client/caregiver for long-range management of situation to avoid injuries. **Enhances commitment to plan, optimizing outcomes.**
- Review importance of chewing carefully, taking small amounts of food, using caution when talking or drinking while eating. Discuss possibility of choking **because of throat muscle relaxation and impaired judgment when drinking alcohol and eating.**

Information that appears in brackets has been added by the authors to clarify and enhance the use of nursing diagnoses.

🌐 Cultural ♨ Collaborative 🏠 Community/Home Care

- Emphasize the importance of getting help when beginning to choke; instead of leaving table, remain calm and make gesture across throat, making sure someone recognizes the emergency.
- Promote public education in techniques for clearing blocked airways, backblows, Heimlich maneuver, CPR.
- Collaborate in community public health education regarding hazards for children (e.g., appropriate toy size for young child) discussing dangers of "huffing" [inhalants] and playing choking or hanging games with preteens; fire safety drills; bathtub rules; how to spot potential for depression and risk of suicidagestures in adolescent **to reduce potential for accidental or intentional suffocation.**
- Assist individuals to learn to read package labels and identify safety hazards.
- Promote pool safety, use of approved flotation devices, proper fencing enclosure or alarm system for home pools.
- Discuss safety measures regarding use of heaters, household gas appliances, old or discarded appliances.
- Refer to NDs ineffective Airway Clearance; risk for Aspiration; ineffective Breathing Pattern; impaired Parenting.

Documentation Focus

Assessment/Reassessment
- Individual risk factors, including individual's cognitive status and level of knowledge.
- Level of concern and motivation for change.
- Equipment or airway adjunct needs.

Planning
- Plan of care and who is involved in planning.
- Teaching plan.

Implementation/Evaluation
- Responses to interventions, teaching, and actions performed.
- Attainment or progress toward desired outcome(s).
- Modifications to plan of care.

Discharge Planning
- Long-term needs, appropriate preventive measures, and who is responsible for actions to be taken.
- Specific referrals made.

Information that appears in brackets has been added by the authors to clarify and enhance the use of nursing diagnoses.

 Diagnostic Studies Pediatric/Geriatric/Lifespan Medications **811**

Sample Nursing Outcomes & Interventions Classifications (NOC/NIC) NIC

NOC—Risk Control
NIC—Airway Management

risk for Suicide

Taxonomy II: Safety/Protection—Class 3 Violence (00150)
[Diagnostic Division: Safety]
Submitted 2000

Definition: At risk for self-inflicted, life-threatening injury

Risk Factors/[Indicators]

Behavioral
History of prior suicide attempt
Buying a gun; stockpiling medicines
Making or changing a will; giving away possessions
Sudden euphoric recovery from major depression
Impulsiveness; marked changes in behavior, attitude, or school performance

Verbal
Threats of killing oneself; states desire to die [or end it all]

Situational
Living alone; retired; economic instability; relocation; institutionalization
Loss of autonomy or independence
Presence of gun in home
Adolescents living in nontraditional settings (e.g., juvenile detention center, prison, half-way house, group home)

Psychological
Family history of suicide; childhood abuse
Substance abuse
Psychiatric illness or disorder (e.g., depression, schizophrenia, bipolar disorder)
Guilt
Gay or lesbian youth

Information that appears in brackets has been added by the authors to clarify and enhance the use of nursing diagnoses.

 Cultural Collaborative Community/Home Care

Demographic
Age (e.g., elderly, young adult males, adolescents)
Race (e.g., Caucasian, Native American)
Male gender
Divorced; widowed

Physical
Physical or terminal illness; chronic pain

Social
Loss of important relationship; disrupted family life; poor support systems; social isolation
Grief; loneliness
Hopelessness; helplessness
Legal or disciplinary problem
Cluster suicides

> **NOTE:** A risk diagnosis is not evidenced by signs and symptoms, as the problem has not occurred; rather, nursing interventions are directed at prevention.

Desired Outcomes/Evaluation Criteria— Client Will:

- Acknowledge difficulties perceived in current situation.
- Identify current factors that can be dealt with.
- Be involved in planning course of action to correct existing problems.
- Make decision that suicide is not the answer to the perceived problems.

Actions/Interventions

Nursing Priority No. 1.
To assess causative/contributing factors:

- Identify degree of risk or potential for suicide and seriousness of threat. Use a scale of 1 to 10 and prioritize according to severity of threat, availability of means.
- Note behaviors indicative of intent (e.g., gestures; presence of means, such as guns; threats; giving away possessions; previous attempts; and presence of hallucinations or delusions). **Many people signal their intent, particularly to healthcare providers.**

Information that appears in brackets has been added by the authors to clarify and enhance the use of nursing diagnoses.

 Diagnostic Studies ∞ Pediatric/Geriatric/Lifespan 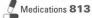 Medications **813**

- Ask directly if person is thinking of acting on thoughts or feelings. **Determines intent. Most people will answer honestly because they actually want help.**
- Note age and gender. **Risk of suicide is greater in males, teens, and the elderly, but there is a rising awareness of risk in early childhood.**
- Review family history for suicidal behavior. **Individual risk is increased, especially when the person who commited suicide was close to the client.**
- Identify conditions, such as acute or chronic brain syndrome, panic state, hormonal imbalance (e.g., premenstrual syndrome [PMS], postpartum psychosis, drug-induced) **that may interfere with ability to control own behavior and will require specific interventions to promote safety.**
- Review laboratory findings (e.g., blood alcohol, blood glucose, ABGs, electrolytes, renal function tests), **to identify factors that may affect reasoning ability.**
- Note withdrawal from usual activities, lack of social interactions.
- Assess physical complaints (e.g., sleeping difficulties, lack of appetite).
- Determine drug use or "self" medication.
- Note history of disciplinary problems or involvement with judicial system.
- Assess coping behaviors presently used. *Note:* Client may believe there is no alternative except suicide.
- Determine presence of SO(s)/friends who are available for support.

Nursing Priority No. 2.

To assist clients to accept responsibility for own behavior and prevent suicide:

- Develop therapeutic nurse-client relationship, providing consistent caregiver. **Promotes sense of trust, allowing individual to discuss feelings openly.**
- Maintain straightforward communication **to avoid reinforcing manipulative behavior.**
- Explain concern for safety and willingness to help client stay safe.
- Encourage expression of feelings and make time to listen to concerns. **Acknowledges reality of feelings and that they are okay. Helps individual sort out thinking and begin to develop understanding of situation and look at other alternatives.**

Information that appears in brackets has been added by the authors to clarify and enhance the use of nursing diagnoses.

🌐 Cultural   🐝 Collaborative   🏠 Community/Home Care

- Give permission to express angry feelings in acceptable ways and let client know someone will be available to assist in maintaining control. **Promotes acceptance and sense of safety.**
- Acknowledge reality of suicide as an option. Discuss consequences of actions if they follow through on intent. Ask how it will help individual to resolve problems. **Helps to focus on consequences of actions and possibility of other options.**
- Maintain observation of client and check environment for hazards that could be used to commit suicide **to increase client safety or reduce risk of impulsive behavior.**
- Help client identify more appropriate solutions/behaviors (e.g., motor activities/exercise) **to lessen sense of anxiety and associated physical manifestations.**
- Provide directions for actions client can take, avoiding negative statements, such as "do nots." **Promotes a positive attitude.**
- Discuss use of psychotropic medication, positive and negative aspects. **There has been concern about the increased risk of suicide from these drugs, and research is ongoing to determine whether they help or harm.**
- Reevaluate potential for suicide periodically at key times (e.g., mood changes, increasing withdrawal), as well as when client is feeling better and discharge planning becomes active. **The highest risk exists when the client has both suicidal ideation and sufficient energy with which to act.**

Nursing Priority No. 3.
To assist client to plan course of action to correct/deal with existing situation:

- Gear interventions to individual involved (e.g., age, relationship, current situation).
- Negotiate contract with client regarding willingness not to do anything lethal for a stated period of time. Specify what caregiver will be responsible for and what client responsibilities are.
- Specify alternative actions necessary if client is unwilling to negotiate contract. **May need hospitalization to provide safety.**
- Discuss losses client has experienced and meaning of those losses. **Unresolved issues may be contributing to thoughts of hopelessness.**

Information that appears in brackets has been added by the authors to clarify and enhance the use of nursing diagnoses.

Diagnostic Studies   ∞ Pediatric/Geriatric/Lifespan   Medications **815**

Nursing Priority No. 4.

To promote wellness (Teaching/Discharge Considerations):

- Promote development of internal control by helping client look at new ways to deal with problems.
- Assist with learning problem solving, assertiveness training, and social skills.
- Engage in physical activity programs. Releases endorphins **promoting feelings of self-worth and improving sense of well-being.**
- Determine nutritional needs and help client to plan for meeting them.
- Involve family/SO(s) in planning **to improve understanding and support.**
- Refer to formal resources as indicated (e.g., individual/group/marital psychotherapy, substance abuse treatment program, and social services).

Documentation Focus

Assessment/Reassessment
- Individual findings, including nature of concern (e.g., suicidal/behavioral risk factors and level of impulse control, plan of action and means to carry out plan).
- Client's perception of situation, motivation for change.

Planning
- Plan of care and who is involved in the planning.
- Details of contract regarding suicidal ideation or plans.
- Teaching plan.

Implementation/Evaluation
- Actions taken to promote safety.
- Response to interventions, teaching, and actions performed.
- Attainment or progress toward desired outcome(s).
- Modifications to plan of care.

Discharge Planning
- Long-term needs and who is responsible for actions to be taken.
- Available resources, specific referrals made.

Information that appears in brackets has been added by the authors to clarify and enhance the use of nursing diagnoses.

  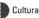 Cultural Collaborative Community/Home Care

Sample Nursing Outcomes & Interventions Classifications (NOC/NIC) NIC

NOC—Suicide Self-Restraint
NIC—Suicide Prevention

delayed Surgical Recovery

Taxonomy II: Activity/Rest—Class 2 Activity/Exercise (00100)
[Diagnostic Division: Safety]
Submitted 1998; Revised 2006

Definition: Extension of the number of postoperative days required to initiate and perform activities that maintain life, health, and well-being

Related Factors

Extensive or prolonged surgical procedure
Pain
Obesity
Preoperative expectations
Postoperative surgical site infection

Defining Characteristics

Subjective
Perception that more time is needed to recover
Report of pain or discomfort; fatigue
Loss of appetite with or without nausea
Postpones resumption of work or employment activities

Objective
Evidence of interrupted healing of surgical area (e.g., red, indurated, draining, immobilized)
Difficulty in moving about; requires help to complete self-care

Desired Outcomes/Evaluation Criteria—Client Will:

• Display complete healing of surgical area.
• Be able to perform desired self-care activities.

Information that appears in brackets has been added by the authors to clarify and enhance the use of nursing diagnoses.

• Report increased energy, able to participate in usual (work or employment) activities.

Actions/Interventions

Nursing Priority No. 1.
To assess causative/contributing factors:

• Identify vulnerable client (e.g., low socioeconomic status, lack of resources, challenges related to poverty, lack of insurance or transportation, severe trauma or prolonged hospitalization with multiple complicating factors) **who is at higher risk for adverse outcomes.**

• Determine extent of surgical involvement of organs or tissues, noting age and developmental level, and general state of health **to provide anticipatory guidance in postoperative care.**

• Identify underlying condition/pathology (e.g., cancers, burns, diabetes, multiple trauma, infections, cardiopulmonary disorders, debilitating illness), **which may affect healing and recovery.**

• Note other factors that may impede recovery (e.g., obesity, cigarette smoking, sedentary lifestyle, steroid use, prolonged preoperative hospital stay, radiation therapy).

• Ascertain presence and severity of perioperative complications (e.g., lengthy time under anesthesia; trauma or other conditions requiring multiple surgeries) and development of postoperative complications (e.g., surgical site infection, ventilator-associated pneumonia, deep vein thrombosis) **that can prolong recovery.**

• Assess nutritional status and current intake **to determine if nutrition is adequate to support healing.**

• Review current medication regimen and determine dosages and use of multiple drugs with potential for adverse side effects and interactions **affecting cognition, organ function, and tissue healing.**

• Perform pain assessment **to ascertain whether pain management is adequate to meet client's needs during recovery.**

• Evaluate client's cognitive and emotional state, noting presence of postoperative changes, including confusion, depression, apathy, expressions of helplessness **to determine possible psychological interferences.**

• Review results of laboratory tests (e.g., CBC, blood or wound cultures, glucose) **to assess for presence and type of**

Information that appears in brackets has been added by the authors to clarify and enhance the use of nursing diagnoses.

Cultural Collaborative Community/Home Care

infections, metabolic or endocrine dysfunction, or other conditions affecting body's ability to heal.

 • Determine cultural expectations regarding recovery process and participation of client/others (e.g., client is expected to be inactive and cared for by others).

Nursing Priority No. 2.

To determine impact of delayed recovery:

• Note length of hospitalization and progress in recovery to date and compare with expectations for procedure and situation.
• Determine client's/SO's expectations for recovery and specific stressors related to delay (e.g., return to work or school, home responsibilities, child care, financial difficulties, limited support system).
• Determine energy level and current participation in ADLs. Compare with usual level of function.
• Ascertain whether client usually requires assistance in home setting and who provides it, current availability, and capability.
• Obtain psychological assessment of client's emotional status, noting potential problems arising from current situation.

Nursing Priority No. 3.

To promote optimal recovery:

• Inspect incisions or wounds routinely, describing changes (e.g., deepening or healing, wound measurements, presence and type of drainage, development of necrosis).
• Collaborate in treatment of complications (e.g., infection, dehiscence).
• Assist with wound care as indicated (e.g., débridement, barrier dressings, wound coverings, skin-protective agents for open or draining wounds).
• Include wound care specialist or stoma therapist as appropriate **to problem-solve healing difficulties.**
• Avoid or limit use of plastics or latex materials. **Client may be sensitive.**
• Provide optimal nutrition and adequate protein intake **to provide a positive nitrogen balance, aiding in healing, and achieving good health.**
• Encourage early ambulation, regular exercise **to promote circulation, improve strength, and reduce risks associated with immobility.**
• Recommend alternating activity with adequate rest periods **to reduce fatigue.**

Information that appears in brackets has been added by the authors to clarify and enhance the use of nursing diagnoses.

- Administer medications as indicated (e.g., client may be experiencing stubborn infection requiring IV antibiotics or management of chronic pain).
- Instruct client/SO(s) in necessary self-care of incisions and specific symptom management. **With short hospital stays, client/SO(s) usually provide a great deal of postoperative care and monitoring at home.**
- Encourage client to adhere to medical regimen and follow-up care **to monitor healing process and provide for timely intervention as needed.**
- Refer for outpatient or follow-up care as indicated (e.g., telephone monitoring, home visit, wound care clinic, pain management program).

Nursing Priority No. 4.
To promote wellness (Teaching/Discharge Considerations):

- Demonstrate self-care skills, provide client/SO(s) with health-related information and psychosocial support **to manage symptoms and pain, enhancing well-being.**
- Discuss reality of recovery process in comparison with client's/SO's expectations. **Individuals are often unrealistic regarding energy and time required for healing and own abilities and responsibilities to facilitate process.**
- Involve client/SO(s) in setting incremental goals. **Enhances commitment to plan and reduces likelihood of frustration blocking progress.**
- Refer to physical or occupational therapists, as indicated, **to identify assistive devices to facilitate independence in ADLs.**
- Identify suppliers for dressings or wound care items and assistive devices as needed.
- Consult dietitian for individual dietary plan **to meet increased nutritional needs that reflect personal situation and resources.**
- Evaluate home situation (e.g., lives alone, bedroom or bathroom on second floor, availability of assistance). **Identifies necessary adjustments, such as moving bedroom to first floor, arranging for commode during recovery, obtaining a Lifeline emergency call system.**
- Discuss alternative placement (e.g., convalescent or rehabilitation center, as appropriate).
- Identify community resources, as indicated (e.g., visiting nurse, home healthcare agency, Meals on Wheels, respite care). **Facilitates adjustment to home setting.**

Information that appears in brackets has been added by the authors to clarify and enhance the use of nursing diagnoses.

Cultural   Collaborative   Community/Home Care

• Recommend support group or self-help program for smoking cessation.

• Refer for counseling or support. **May need additional help to overcome feelings of discouragement, deal with changes in life.**

Documentation Focus

Assessment/Reassessment
• Assessment findings, including individual concerns, family involvement, and support factors and availability of resources.
• Cultural expectations.
• Assistive device use or need.

Planning
• Plan of care and who is involved in planning.
• Teaching plan.

Implementation/Evaluation
• Responses of client/SO(s) to plan, interventions, teaching, and actions performed.
• Attainment or progress toward desired outcome(s).
• Modifications to plan of care.

Discharge Planning
• Long-range needs and who is responsible for actions to be taken.
• Specific referrals made.

Sample Nursing Outcomes & Interventions Classifications (NOC/NIC) NIC

NOC—Self-Care: Activities of Daily Living (ADLs)
NIC—Self-Care Assistance

---

impaired Swallowing

Taxonomy II: Nutrition—Class 1 Ingestion (00103)
[Diagnostic Division: Food/Fluid]
Submitted 1986; Nursing Diagnosis Extension and
  Classification (NDEC) Revision 1998

Definition: Abnormal functioning of the swallowing mechanism associated with deficits in oral, pharyngeal, or esophageal structure or function

---

Information that appears in brackets has been added by the authors to clarify and enhance the use of nursing diagnoses.

Related Factors

Congenital Deficits

Upper airway anomalies; mechanical obstruction (e.g., edema, tracheostomy tube, tumor); history of tube feeding

Neuromuscular impairment (e.g., decreased or absent gag reflex, decreased strength or excursion of muscles involved in mastication, perceptual impairment, facial paralysis); conditions with significant hypotonia

Respiratory disorders; congenital heart disease

Behavioral feeding problems; self-injurious behavior

Failure to thrive; protein energy malnutrition

Neurological Problems

Nasal or nasopharyngeal cavity defects; oropharynx, upper airway, or laryngeal anomalies; tracheal, laryngeal, or esophageal defects

Gastroesophageal reflux disease; achalasia

Traumas; acquired anatomical defects; cranial nerve involvement; traumatic head injury; developmental delay; cerebral palsy

Prematurity

Defining Characteristics

Subjective

Esophageal Phase Impairment

Complaints [reports] of "something stuck"; odynophagia

Food refusal; volume limiting

Heartburn; epigastric pain

Nighttime coughing or awakening

Objective

Oral Phase Impairment

Weak suck, resulting in inefficient nippling

Slow bolus formation; lack of tongue action to form bolus; premature entry of bolus

Incomplete lip closure; food pushed out of or falls from mouth

Lack of chewing

Coughing, choking, or gagging before a swallow

Piecemeal deglutition; abnormality in oral phase of swallow study

---

Information that appears in brackets has been added by the authors to clarify and enhance the use of nursing diagnoses.

🌐 Cultural   Ⓐ Collaborative   🏠 Community/Home Care

Inability to clear oral cavity; pooling in lateral sulci; nasal reflux; sialorrhea; drooling
Long meals with little consumption

Pharyngeal Phase Impairment
Food refusal
Altered head positions; delayed or multiple swallows
Inadequate laryngeal elevation; abnormality in pharyngeal
phase by swallow study
Choking; coughing; gagging; nasal reflux; gurgly voice quality
Unexplained fevers; recurrent pulmonary infections

Esophageal Phase Impairment
Observed evidence of difficulty in swallowing (e.g., stasis of
food in oral cavity, coughing/choking); abnormality in esoph-
ageal phase by swallow study
Hyperextension of head (e.g., arching during or after meals)
Repetitive swallowing; bruxism
Unexplained irritability surrounding mealtime
Acidic smelling breath; regurgitation of gastric contents (wet
burps); vomitus on pillow; vomiting; hematemesis

Desired Outcomes/Evaluation Criteria—
Client Will:

- Pass food and fluid from mouth to stomach safely.
- Maintain adequate hydration as evidenced by good skin turgor, moist mucous membranes, and individually appropriate
urine output.
- Achieve and/or maintain desired body weight.

Client/Caregiver Will:

- Verbalize understanding of causative or contributing factors.
- Identify individually appropriate interventions or actions to
promote intake and prevent aspiration.
- Demonstrate feeding methods appropriate to the individual
situation.
- Demonstrate emergency measures in the event of choking.

Actions/Interventions

Nursing Priority No. 1.
To assess causative/contributing factors and degree of impairment:

Information that appears in brackets has been added by the authors to clarify
and enhance the use of nursing diagnoses.

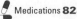

Diagnostic Studies   Pediatric/Geriatric/Lifespan   Medications **823**

- Assess sensory-perceptual status (sensory awareness, orientation, concentration, motor coordination).
- Note symmetry of facial structures and muscle tone.
- Assess strength and excursion of muscles involved in mastication and swallowing.
- Inspect oropharyngeal cavity for edema, inflammation, altered integrity of oral mucosa, adequacy of oral hygiene.
- Verify proper fit of dentures if present.
- Ascertain presence and strength of cough and gag reflex.
- Evaluate ability to swallow using small sips of water.
- Determine ability to initiate and sustain effective suck. **Weak suck results in inefficient nippling, suggesting ineffective movement of tongue and mouth muscles, impairing ability to swallow.**
- Note hyperextension of head or arching of neck during or after meals, or repetitive swallowing **suggesting inability to complete swallowing process.**
- Auscultate breath sounds **to evaluate the presence of aspiration.**
- Record current weight and recent changes.
- Prepare for and assist with diagnostic testing of swallowing activity.

Nursing Priority No. 2.
To prevent aspiration and maintain airway patency:
- Identify individual factors that can precipitate aspiration or compromise airway.
- Move client to chair for meals, snacks, and drinks when possible; if client must be in bed, raise head of bed as upright as possible with head in anatomical alignment and slightly flexed forward during feeding. Keep head of bed elevated for 30 to 45 minutes after feeding, if possible, **to reduce risk of regurgitation or aspiration.**
- Suction oral cavity prn. Teach client self-suction when appropriate. **Promotes airway safety and independence, and sense of control with managing secretions.**

Nursing Priority No. 3.
To enhance swallowing ability to meet fluid and caloric body requirements:
- Refer to gastroenterologist or neurologist as indicated **for treatment (e.g., reconstructive facial surgery, esophageal dilatation) that may result in improved swallowing.**

Information that appears in brackets has been added by the authors to clarify and enhance the use of nursing diagnoses.

  Cultural 🐊 Collaborative 🏠 Community/Home Care

- Refer to speech therapist **to identify specific techniques to enhance client efforts and safety measures.**
- Encourage a rest period before meals **to minimize fatigue.**
- Provide analgesics prior to feeding, as indicated, **to enhance comfort, being cautious to avoid decreasing awareness or sensory perception.**
- Focus client's attention on feeding and swallowing activity. Decrease environmental stimuli and talking, **which may be distracting or promote choking during feeding.**
- Determine food preferences of client **to incorporate as possible, enhancing intake.** Present foods in an appealing, attractive manner.
- Ensure temperature (hot or cold vs. tepid) of foods and fluid, **which will stimulate sensory receptors.**
- Provide a consistency of food and fluid that is most easily swallowed. **Risk of choking or aspiration is reduced when food can be formed into a bolus before swallowing, such as gelatin desserts prepared with less water than usual; pudding and custard or liquids are thickened (addition of thickening agent, or yogurt, cream soups prepared with less water); thinned purees (hot cereal with added water); thick drinks, such as nectars; fruit juices that have been frozen into "slush" consistency (thin fluids are most difficult to control); medium-soft boiled or scrambled eggs; canned fruit; soft-cooked vegetables.**
- Avoid milk products and chocolate, **which may thicken oral secretions.**
- Feed one consistency and/or texture of food at a time.
- Place food in unaffected side of client's mouth **(when one side of the mouth is affected by condition, e.g., hemiplegia),** and have client use tongue to assist with moving food bolus to swallowing postion.
- Manage size of bites **(e.g., small bites of 1/2 tsp or less are usually easier to swallow).** Use a teaspoon or small spoon **to encourage smaller bites.** Cut all solid foods into small pieces.
- Place food midway in oral cavity; provide medium-sized bites (about 15 mL) **to adequately trigger the swallowing reflex.**
- Provide cognitive cues (e.g., remind client to chew and swallow as indicated) **to enhance concentration and performance of swallowing sequence.**
- Instruct to chew food on unaffected side as appropriate.
- Massage the laryngopharyngeal musculature (sides of trachea and neck) gently **to stimulate swallowing.**

Information that appears in brackets has been added by the authors to clarify and enhance the use of nursing diagnoses.

- Observe oral cavity after each bite and have client check around cheeks with tongue for remaining food. Remove food if unable to swallow.
- Incorporate client's eating style and pace when feeding **to avoid fatigue and frustration with process.**
- Allow ample time for eating (feeding).
- Remain with client during meal to reduce anxiety and offer assistance.
- Use a glass with a nose cutout **to avoid posterior head tilting while drinking.** Refrain from pouring liquid into the mouth or "washing food down" with liquid. *Note:* Some people find drinking from a straw easier than sipping from a cup (if a straw is easier, consider using a flexible one-way straw; if a cup is easier, consider using a "nosey" cup that is double handled and made of durable plastic).
- Monitor intake, output, and body weight to evaluate adequacy of fluid and caloric intake.
- Provide positive feedback for client's efforts.
- Provide oral hygiene following each feeding.
- Consider tube feedings or parenteral solutions, as indicated, **for the client unable to achieve adequate nutritional intake.**
- Consult with dysphagia specialist or rehabilitation team, as indicated.
- Refer to lactation counselor or support group (e.g., La Leche League) **for breastfeeding guidance.**
- Refer to NDs ineffective Breastfeeding; ineffective Infant Feeding Pattern for additional interventions for infants.

Nursing Priority No. 4.
To promote wellness (Teaching/Discharge Considerations):

- Consult with dietitian **to establish optimum dietary plan.**
- Place medication in gelatin, jelly, or puddings. Consult with pharmacist **to determine if pills may be crushed or if liquids or capsules are available.**
- Assist client and/or SO(s) in learning specific feeding techniques and swallowing exercises.
- Encourage continuation of facial exercise program **to maintain or improve muscle strength.**
- Instruct client and/or SO(s) in emergency measures in event of choking.
- Establish routine schedule for monitoring weight.
- Refer to ND risk for imbalanced Nutrition: less than body requirements.

Information that appears in brackets has been added by the authors to clarify and enhance the use of nursing diagnoses.

 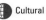 Cultural · Collaborative · Community/Home Care

Documentation Focus

Assessment/Reassessment

- Individual findings, including degree and characteristics of impairment, current weight and recent changes.
- Nutritional status.
- Effects on lifestyle and socialization.

Planning

- Plan of care and who is involved in planning.
- Teaching plan.

Implementation/Evaluation

- Response to interventions, teaching, and actions performed.
- Attainment or progress toward desired outcome(s).
- Modifications to plan of care.

Discharge Planning

- Long-term needs and who is responsible for actions to be taken.
- Available resources and specific referrals made.

Sample Nursing Outcomes & Interventions Classifications (NOC/NIC) `NIC`

NOC—Swallowing Status
NIC—Swallowing Therapy

[effective Therapeutic Regimen Management]

Taxonomy II: Health Promotion—Class 2 Health Management (00082)
[Diagnostic Division: Teaching/Learning]
Submitted 1994/Retired from Taxonomy 2009

Definition: Pattern of regulating and integrating into daily living a program for treatment of illness and its sequelae that is satisfactory for meeting specific health goals

---

Related Factors

To be developed
[Complexity of healthcare management; therapeutic regimen]

Information that appears in brackets has been added by the authors to clarify and enhance the use of nursing diagnoses.

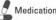

[Added demands made on individual or family]
[Adequate social supports]

Defining Characteristics

Subjective
Verbalizes desire to manage the treatment of illness or prevention of sequelae
Verbalizes intent to reduce risk factors for progression of illness and sequelae

Objective
Appropriate choices of daily activities for meeting the goals of a treatment/prevention program
Illness symptoms within a normal range of expectation

Desired Outcomes/Evaluation Criteria— Individual Will:

- Develop plan to address individual risk factors for progression of illness/sequelae.
- Demonstrate effective problem-solving in integration changes of therapeutic regimen into lifestyle.
- Identify and use available resources.
- Remain free of preventable complications or progression of illness and sequelae.

Actions/Interventions

Nursing Priority No. 1.
To assess situation and individual needs:
- Ascertain client's knowledge and understanding of condition and treatment needs. Note specific health goals.
- Identify individual's perceptions of adaptation to treatment and anticipated changes.
- Note treatments added to present regimen and client's/SO's associated learning needs.
- Discuss present resources used by client **to note whether changes need to be arranged (e.g., increased hours of home care assistance; access to case manager to support complex or long-term program).**

Nursing Priority No. 2.
To assist client/SO(s) in developing strategies to meet increased demands of therapeutic regimen:

Information that appears in brackets has been added by the authors to clarify and enhance the use of nursing diagnoses.

- Identify steps necessary to reach desired health goal(s).
- Accept client's evaluation of own strengths and limitations while working together to improve abilities. **Promotes sense of self-esteem and confidence to continue efforts.**
- Provide information about individual healthcare needs, using client's/SO's preferred learning style (e.g., pictures, words, video, Internet) **to help client understand own situation and enhance interest/involvement in own health.** *Note:* When referencing the Internet, nontraditional, or unproven resources, the individual must exercise some restraint and determine the reliability of the source and information provided before acting on it.
- Acknowledge individual efforts and capabilities **to reinforce movement toward attainment of desired outcomes.**

Nursing Priority No. 3.
To promote wellness (Teaching/Discharge Considerations):

- Promote client/caregiver choices and involvement in planning and implementing added tasks/responsibilities.
- Provide for follow-up contact or home visit, as appropriate.
- Assist in implementing strategies for monitoring progress/responses to therapeutic regimen. **Promotes proactive problem solving.**
- Refer to family and community support systems, as indicated, **for assistance with lifestyle or relationship issues, finances, housing, or legal concerns (e.g., advance directives, healthcare choices).**

Documentation Focus

Assessment/Reassessment
- Findings, including dynamics of individual situation.
- Individual strengths and additional needs.

Planning
- Plan of care and who is involved in planning.
- Teaching plan.

Implementation/Evaluation
- Response to interventions, teaching, and actions performed.
- Attainment or progress toward desired outcome(s).
- Modifications to plan of care.

Information that appears in brackets has been added by the authors to clarify and enhance the use of nursing diagnoses.

Discharge Planning
- Short- and long-term needs and who is responsible for actions.
- Available resources, specific referrals made.

Sample Nursing Outcomes & Interventions Classifications (NOC/NIC) NIC

NOC—Symptom Control
NIC—Health System Guidance

[ineffective community Therapeutic Regimen Management]

Taxonomy II: Health Promotion—Class 2 Health
  Management (0081)
[Diagnostic Division: Teaching/Learning]
Submitted 1994/Retired from Taxonomy 2009

Definition: Pattern of regulating and integrating into
community processes programs for treatment of illness
and the sequelae of illness that are unsatisfactory for
meeting health-related goals

Related Factors

To be developed
Lack of safety for community members
Economic insecurity
Healthcare not available; unhealthy environment
Education not available for all community members
Lack of means to meet human needs for recognition, fellowship,
  security, and membership

Defining Characteristics

Subjective
Community members or agencies verbalize overburdening of
  resources or inability to meet therapeutic needs of all members

Objective
Deficits in advocates for aggregates
Deficit in community activities for prevention
Illness symptoms above the norm expected for the population;
  unexpected acceleration of illness

Information that appears in brackets has been added by the authors to clarify
and enhance the use of nursing diagnoses.

🌐 Cultural 🧲 Collaborative 🏠 Community/Home Care

Insufficient healthcare resources (e.g., people, programs); unavailable healthcare resources for illness care

Deficits in community for collaboration and development of coalitions to address needs

Desired Outcomes/Evaluation Criteria—Community Will:

- Identify both strengths and limitations affecting community treatment programs for meeting health-related goals.
- Participate in problem-solving of factors interfering with regulating and integrating community programs.
- Report illness symptoms near norm or less than expected for the incidence or prevalence of disease(s).

Actions/Interventions

Nursing Priority No. 1.
To identify causative/precipitating factors:

- Evaluate community healthcare resources for illness or sequelae of illness.
- Note reports from members of the community regarding ineffective or inadequate community functioning.
- Investigate unexpected acceleration of illness in the community.
- Identify strengths and limitations of community resources and community commitment to change.
- Ascertain effect of related factors on community activities.
- Determine knowledge and understanding of treatment regimen.
- Note use of resources available to community for developing and funding programs.

Nursing Priority No. 2.
To assist community to develop strategies to improve community functioning/management:

- Foster cooperative spirit of community without negating individuality of members/groups.
- Involve community in determining and prioritizing healthcare goals **to facilitate planning process.**
- Plan together with community health and social agencies **to problem-solve solutions to identified and anticipated problems and needs.**

Information that appears in brackets has been added by the authors to clarify and enhance the use of nursing diagnoses.

 Diagnostic Studies   Pediatric/Geriatric/Lifespan   Medications **831**

- Identify specific populations at risk or underserved **to actively involve them in process.**
- Create teaching plan, form speakers' bureau **to disseminate information to community members regarding value of treatment and preventive programs.**

Nursing Priority No. 3.

To promote wellness (Teaching/Discharge Considerations):

- Assist community to develop a plan for continuing assessment of community needs and the functioning and effectiveness of plan. **Promotes proactive approach.**
- Encourage community to form partnerships within the community and between the community and the larger society **to aid in long-term planning for anticipated or projected needs and concerns.**

Documentation Focus

Assessment/Reassessment

- Assessment findings, including members' perceptions of community problems, healthcare resources.
- Community use of available resources.

Planning

- Plan of care and who is involved in planning.
- Teaching plan.

Implementation/Evaluation

- Community's response to plan, teaching, and interventions performed.
- Attainment or progress toward desired outcome(s).
- Modifications to plan of care.

Discharge Planning

- Long-term goals and who is responsible for actions to be taken.
- Specific referrals made.

Sample Nursing Outcomes & Interventions Classifications (NOC/NIC) NIC

NOC—Community Competence
NIC—Community Health Development

Information that appears in brackets has been added by the authors to clarify and enhance the use of nursing diagnoses.

Cultural Collaborative Community/Home Care

ineffective family Therapeutic Regimen Management

Taxonomy II: Health Promotion—Class 2 Health
Management (00080)
[Diagnostic Division: Teaching/Learning]
Submitted 1992

Definition: Pattern of regulating and integrating into
family processes a program for treatment of illness and
the sequelae of illness that is unsatisfactory for meeting
specific health goals

Related Factors

Complexity of therapeutic regimen or healthcare system
Decisional conflicts
Economic difficulties
Excessive demands; family conflicts

Defining Characteristics

Subjective
Verbalizes difficulty with therapeutic regimen
Verbalizes desire to manage the illness

Objective
Inappropriate family activities for meeting health goals
Acceleration of illness symptoms of a family member
Failure to take action to reduce risk factors; lack of attention to
illness

Desired Outcomes/Evaluation Criteria—Family Will:

- Identify individual factors affecting regulation/integration of
treatment program.
- Participate in problem solving of factors.
- Verbalize acceptance of need or desire to change actions to
achieve agreed-on outcomes or health goals.
- Demonstrate behaviors and changes in lifestyle necessary to
maintain therapeutic regimen.

Information that appears in brackets has been added by the authors to clarify
and enhance the use of nursing diagnoses.

 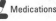

Actions/Interventions

Nursing Priority No. 1.
To identify causative/precipitating factors:

- Ascertain family's perception of efforts to date.
- Evaluate family functioning and activities as related to appropriateness—looking at frequency and effectiveness of family communication, promotion of autonomy, adaptation to meet changing needs, health of home environment and lifestyle, problem-solving abilities, ties to community.
- Note family health goals and agreement of individual members. **Presence of conflict interferes with problem-solving.**
- Determine understanding of and value of the treatment regimen to the family.
- Identify cultural values or religious beliefs affecting view of situation and willingness to make necessary changes.
- Identify availability and use of resources.

Nursing Priority No. 2.
To assist family to develop strategies to improve management of therapeutic regimen:

- Provide information to aid family **in understanding the value of the treatment program.**
- Assist family members to recognize inappropriate family activities. Help the members identify both togetherness and individual needs and behavior **so that effective interactions can be enhanced and perpetuated.**
- Make a plan jointly with family members to deal with complexity of healthcare regimen or system and other related factors. **Enhances commitment to plan, optimizing outcomes.**
- Identify community resources, as needed, using the three strategies of education, problem-solving, and resource linking **to address specific deficits.**

Nursing Priority No. 3.
To promote wellness as related to future health of family members:

- Help family identify criteria to promote ongoing self-evaluation of situation and effectiveness and family progress. **Provides opportunity to be proactive in meeting needs.**
- Make referrals to and/or jointly plan with other health, social, and community resources. **Problems often are multifaceted, requiring involvement of numerous providers and agencies.**

Information that appears in brackets has been added by the authors to clarify and enhance the use of nursing diagnoses.

Cultural Collaborative Community/Home Care

• Provide contact person or case manager for one-to-one assistance, as needed, **to coordinate care, provide support, assist with problem-solving, and so forth.**
- Refer to NDs Caregiver Role Strain; ineffective self Health Management, as indicated.

Documentation Focus

Assessment/Reassessment
- Individual findings, including nature of problem and degree of impairment; family values, health goals, and level of participation and commitment of family members.
- Cultural values, religious beliefs.
- Availability and use of resources.

Planning
- Plan of care and who is involved in planning.
- Teaching plan.

Implementation/Evaluation
- Response to interventions, teaching, and actions performed.
- Attainment or progress toward desired outcome(s).
- Modifications of plan of care.

Discharge Planning
- Long-term needs, plan for meeting, and who is responsible for actions.
- Specific referrals made.

Sample Nursing Outcomes & Interventions Classifications (NOC/NIC) (NIC)

NOC—Family Participation in Professional Care
NIC—Family Involvement Promotion

ineffective **Thermoregulation**

Taxonomy II: Safety/Protection—Class 6 Thermoregulation (00008)
[Diagnostic Division: Safety]
Submitted 1986

Definition: Temperature fluctuation between hypothermia and hyperthermia

---

Information that appears in brackets has been added by the authors to clarify and enhance the use of nursing diagnoses.

Related Factors

Trauma; illness [e.g., cerebral edema, CVA, intracranial surgery, or head injury]

Immaturity; aging [e.g., loss or absence of brown adipose tissue]

Fluctuating environmental temperature

Changes in hypothalamic tissue causing alterations in emission of thermosensitive cells and regulation of heat loss and production

Changes in metabolic rate or activity; changes in level or action of thyroxine and catecholamines

Chemical reactions in contracting muscles

Defining Characteristics

Objective

Fluctuations in body temperature above and below the normal range

Tachycardia

Reduction in body temperature below normal range; cool skin; moderate pallor; mild shivering; piloerection; cyanotic nailbeds; slow capillary refill; hypertension

Warm to touch; flushed skin; increased respiratory rate; seizures

Desired Outcomes/Evaluation Criteria— Client/Caregiver Will:

- Verbalize understanding of individual factors and appropriate interventions.
- Demonstrate techniques and behaviors to correct underlying condition or situation.
- Maintain body temperature within normal limits.

Actions/Interventions

Nursing Priority No. 1.

To identify causative/contributing factors:

- Identify individual factor(s) or underlying condition (e.g., environmental exposure, infectious process, brain injury, effects of drugs or toxins, salt or water depletion, obesity, confined to bed, drug overdose). **Influences choice of interventions.**
- ∞ Note extremes of age (e.g., premature neonate, young child, or aging adult) **as this can directly impact ability to maintain or regulate body temperature.**

Information that appears in brackets has been added by the authors to clarify and enhance the use of nursing diagnoses.

    Cultural   Collaborative   Community/Home Care

- Monitor laboratory studies (e.g., tests indicative of infection, thyroid or other endocrine tests, organ damage, drug screens).

Nursing Priority No. 2.
To assist with measures to correct/treat underlying cause:

- Initiate emergent and/or immediate interventions **to restore or maintain body temperature within normal range,** as indicated in NDs Hypothermia; Hyperthermia; risk for imbalanced Body Temperature.
- Administer fluids, electrolytes, and medications, as appropriate, **to restore or maintain body and organ function.**
- Prepare client for and assist with procedures (e.g., surgical intervention or administering neoplastic agents, antibiotics) **to treat underlying cause of hypothermia or hyperthermia.**

Nursing Priority No. 3.
To promote wellness (Teaching/Discharge Considerations):

- Review causative or related factors and risk factors, if appropriate, with client/SO(s).
- Provide information concerning disease processes, current therapies, and postdischarge precautions, as appropriate to situation.
- Refer to teaching section in NDs Hypothermia; Hyperthermia.

Documentation Focus

Assessment/Reassessment
- Individual findings, including nature of problem, degree of impairment or fluctuations in temperature.

Planning
- Plan of care and who is involved in planning.
- Teaching plan.

Implementation/Evaluation
- Responses to interventions, teaching, and actions performed.
- Attainment or progress toward desired outcome(s).
- Modifications to plan of care.

Discharge Planning
- Long-term needs and who is responsible for actions to be taken.
- Specific referrals made.

Information that appears in brackets has been added by the authors to clarify and enhance the use of nursing diagnoses.

Sample Nursing Outcomes & Interventions Classifications (NOC/NIC) [NIC]

NOC—Thermoregulation
NIC—Temperature Regulation

[disturbed Thought Processes]

Taxonomy II: Perception/Cognition—Class 4 Cognition (00130)
[Diagnostic Division: Neurosensory]
Submitted 1973; Revised 1996/Retired from Taxonomy 2009

Definition: Disruption in cognitive operations and activities

Related Factors

To be developed
[Physiological changes, aging, hypoxia, head injury, malnutrition, infections]
[Biochemical changes, medications, substance abuse]
[Sleep deprivation]
[Psychological conflicts, emotional changes, mental disorders]

Defining Characteristics

Subjective
Ideas of reference, hallucinations, delusions

Objective
Inaccurate interpretation of environment
Inappropriate thinking; egocentricity
Memory deficit; [confabulation]
Hypervigilance; hypovigilance
Cognitive dissonance [decreased ability to grasp ideas, make decisions, problem-solve, use abstract reasoning or conceptualize, calculate; disordered thought sequencing]
Distractibility; [altered attention span]
Inappropriate social behavior

Information that appears in brackets has been added by the authors to clarify and enhance the use of nursing diagnoses.

🌐 Cultural   🐾 Collaborative   🏠 Community/Home Care

Desired Outcomes/Evaluation Criteria—
Client Will:

- Recognize changes in thinking or behavior.
- Verbalize understanding of causative factors when known.
- Identify interventions to deal effectively with situation.
- Demonstrate behaviors and lifestyle changes to prevent or minimize changes in mentation.
- Maintain usual reality orientation.

Actions/Interventions

Nursing Priority No. 1.
To assess causative/contributing factors:

- Identify factors present: for example, acute or chronic brain syndrome (recent stroke, Alzheimer's disease); brain injury, increased intracranial pressure; anoxic event; acute infections, especially in elderly; malnutrition; sleep or sensory deprivation; chronic mental illness, such as schizophrenia.
- Determine alcohol or other drug use (prescription, OTC, or illicit). **Drugs can have direct effects on the brain, or side effects, dose-related effects, and/or cumulative effects that alter thought patterns and sensory perception.**
- Note schedule of drug administration (**may be significant when evaluating cumulative effects or drug interactions).**
- Assess dietary intake and nutritional status.
- Monitor laboratory values for abnormalities, such as metabolic alkalosis, hypokalemia, anemia, elevated ammonia levels, and signs of infection.

Nursing Priority No. 2.
To assess degree of impairment:

- Assist with testing, review results evaluating mental status according to age and developmental capacity, noting extent of impairment in thinking ability, memory (remote and recent), orientation to person, place, time; insight and judgment.
- Assess attention span and distractibility, and ability to make decisions or problem solve. **Determines ability to participate in planning and executing care.**
- Test ability to receive, send, and appropriately interpret communications.
- Note behavior such as untidy personal habits, slowing and/or slurring of speech.

Information that appears in brackets has been added by the authors to clarify and enhance the use of nursing diagnoses.

- Note occurrence of paranoia and delusions, hallucinations.
- Interview SO(s)/caregiver(s) to determine client's usual thinking ability, changes in behavior, length of time problem has existed, and other pertinent information **to provide baseline for comparison over time, and to evaluate effectiveness of interventions.**
- Determine client's anxiety level in relation to situation.
- Assist with in-depth testing of specific cognitive abilities/executive brain functions, as appropriate.

Nursing Priority No. 3.
To prevent further deterioration, maximize level of function:

- Assist with treatment for underlying problems, such as anorexia; brain injury, increased intracranial pressure; sleep disorders; biochemical imbalances. **Cognition or thinking often improves with treatment and correction of medical or psychiatric problems.**
- Establish alternate means for self-expression if unable to communicate verbally. (Refer to ND impaired verbal Communication for related interventions.)
- Monitor and document vital signs periodically, as appropriate.
- Perform periodic neurological and behavioral assessments, as indicated, and compare with baseline. Note changes in level of consciousness and cognition (e.g., increased lethargy, confusion, drowsiness, irritability; changes in ability to communicate and/or appropriateness of thinking and behavior). **Early recognition of changes promotes proactive modifications to plan of care.**
- Reorient to time, place, and person, as needed. **Inability to maintain orientation is a sign of deterioration.**
- Have client write name periodically; keep this record for comparison and report differences.
- Note behavior that may be indicative of potential for violence and take appropriate actions. (Refer to NDs risk for self- or other-directed Violence.)
- Provide safety measures (e.g., side rails, padding, as necessary; close supervision, seizure precautions), as indicated.
- Schedule structured activity and rest periods. **Provides stimulation while reducing fatigue.**
- Monitor medication regimen. Verify that physician is aware of all medications client is taking, noting possible interactions or cumulative effects.

Information that appears in brackets has been added by the authors to clarify and enhance the use of nursing diagnoses.

Cultural Collaborative Community/Home Care

- Encourage family/SO(s) to participate in reorientation and provide ongoing input (e.g., current news and family happenings).
 - Refer to appropriate rehabilitation providers (e.g., cognitive retraining program, speech therapist, psychosocial resources, biofeedback, counselor).

Nursing Priority No. 4.
To create therapeutic milieu and assist client/SO(s) to develop coping strategies—especially when condition is irreversible:

- Provide opportunities for SO(s)/caregivers(s) to ask questions and obtain information.
- Maintain a pleasant, quiet environment and approach client in a slow, calm manner. **Client may respond with anxious or aggressive behaviors if startled or overstimulated.**
- Give simple directions, using short words and simple sentences.
- Listen with regard **to convey interest and worth to individual.**
- Allow ample time for client to respond to questions/comments and make simple decisions.
- Maintain reality-oriented relationship and environment (clocks, calendars, personal items, seasonal decorations).
- Present reality concisely and briefly and do not challenge illogical thinking—**defensive reactions may result.**
- Reduce provocative stimuli, negative criticism, arguments, and confrontations **to avoid triggering fight-or-flight responses.**
- Refrain from forcing activities and communications. **Client may feel threatened and may withdraw or rebel.**
- Respect individuality and personal space.
- Use touch judiciously, respecting personal needs and cultural beliefs, but keeping in mind physical and psychological importance of touch.
- Provide for nutritionally well-balanced diet, incorporating client's preferences as able. Encourage client to eat. Provide pleasant environment and allow sufficient time to eat. **Enhances intake and general well-being.**
- Assist client/SO(s) with grieving process for loss of self or abilities, as in Alzheimer's disease.
- Encourage participation in resocialization activities and groups when available.

Information that appears in brackets has been added by the authors to clarify and enhance the use of nursing diagnoses.

Nursing Priority No. 5.
To promote wellness (Teaching/Discharge Considerations):

- Assist in identifying ongoing treatment needs and rehabilitation program for the individual **to maintain gains and continue progress if able.**
- Emphasize importance of cooperation with therapeutic regimen.
- Promote socialization within individual limitations.
- Identify problems related to aging that are remediable and assist client/SO(s) to seek appropriate assistance and to access resources. **Encourages problem-solving to improve condition rather than accepting the status quo.**
- Help client/SO(s) develop plan of care when problem is progressive or long term. **Advance planning addressing home care, transportation, assistance with care activities, support and respite for caregivers, enhances management of client in home setting.** (Refer to ND Caregiver Role Strain for related interventions.)
- Refer to community resources (e.g., day-care programs, support groups, drug or alcohol rehabilitation, mental health treatment programs).
- Refer to NDs acute Confusion; chronic Confusion; impaired Environmental Interpretation Syndrome; impaired Memory; Self-Care Deficit; Grieving; disturbed Sensory Perception, as appropriate, for additional interventions.

Documentation Focus

Assessment/Reassessment
- Individual findings, including nature of problem, current and previous level of function, effect on independence and lifestyle.
- Results of laboratory tests, diagnostic studies, and mental status or cognitive evaluations.
- SO/family support and participation.
- Availability and use of resources.

Planning
- Plan of care and who is involved in planning.
- Teaching plan.

Implementation/Evaluation
- Response to interventions, teaching, and actions performed.
- Attainment or progress toward desired outcome(s).
- Modifications to plan of care.

Information that appears in brackets has been added by the authors to clarify and enhance the use of nursing diagnoses.

Cultural   Collaborative   Community/Home Care

Discharge Planning

- Long-term needs and who is responsible for actions to be taken.
- Available resources, specific referrals made.

Sample Nursing Outcomes & Interventions Classifications (NOC/NIC) NIC

NOC—Distorted Thought/Self-Control
NIC—Dementia Management

impaired Tissue Integrity

Taxonomy II: Safety/Protection—Class 2 Physical Injury (00044)
[Diagnostic Division: Safety]
Submitted 1986; Revised 1998 (by small group work 1996)

Definition: Damage to mucous membrane, corneal, integumentary, or subcutaneous tissues

Related Factors

Altered circulation
Nutritional factors (e.g., deficit or excess); [metabolic or endocrine dysfunction]
Fluid deficit or excess
Impaired physical mobility
Chemical irritants [including body excretions, secretions, medications]; radiation [including therapeutic radiation]
Temperature extremes
Mechanical (e.g., pressure, shear, friction); [surgery]
Knowledge deficit
Infection

Defining Characteristics

Objective

Damaged tissue (e.g., cornea, mucous membrane, integumentary, subcutaneous)
Destroyed tissue

Information that appears in brackets has been added by the authors to clarify and enhance the use of nursing diagnoses.

 Diagnostic Studies ∞ Pediatric/Geriatric/Lifespan Medications **843**

Desired Outcomes/Evaluation Criteria— Client Will:

- Verbalize understanding of condition and causative factors.
- Identify interventions appropriate for specific condition.
- Demonstrate behaviors and lifestyle changes to promote healing and prevent complications or recurrence.
- Display progressive improvement in wound or lesion healing.

Actions/Interventions

Nursing Priority No. 1.

To identify causative/contributing factors:

- Identify underlying condition or pathology involved in tissue injury (e.g., diabetic neuropathies; peripheral arterial disorders; sensory and perceptual deficits; cognitively impaired, debilitated elderly; emotional or psychological problems; developmental delay; surgery, traumatic injuries; debilitating illness; long-term immobility). **Suggests treatment options, as well as client's desire and ability to protect self, and potential for recurrence of tissue damage.**
- Identify specific behaviors, such as occupational hazards or toxic exposures; sport or leisure activity risks; lifestyle choices (e.g., unsafe sex practices); or use of restraints or prosthetic devices (e.g., limbs, artificial eye, contact lenses, dentures, artificial airway, indwelling catheter).
- Note poor hygiene or health practices (e.g., lack of cleanliness, frequent use of enemas, poor dental care) **that may be impacting tissue health.**
- Determine nutritional status and impact of malnutrition on situation (e.g., pressure points on emaciated and/or elderly client, obesity, lack of activity, slow healing or failure to heal).
- Assess environmental location of home and work or school, as well as recent travel. **Some areas of a country or city may be more susceptible to certain disease conditions orenvironmental pollutants.**
- Note race or ethnic background, familial history for genetic, sociocultural, and religious factors **that may make individual vulnerable to particular condition or impact treatment.**
- Note evidence of deep organ or tissue involvement in client with wound **(e.g., draining fistula through the integumentary and subcutaneous tissue may signal a bone infection).**

Information that appears in brackets has been added by the authors to clarify and enhance the use of nursing diagnoses.

- Assess blood supply and sensation (nerve damage) of affected area. Evaluate pulses and calculate ankle-brachial index **to evaluate actual or potential for impairment of circulation to lower extremities. Result less than 0.9 indicates need for close monitoring and more aggressive intervention (e.g., tighter blood glucose and weight control in diabetic client).**
- Obtain specimens of exudate and lesions for Gram's stain, culture and sensitivity, and so forth, when appropriate.

Nursing Priority No. 2.

To assess degree of impairment:

- Obtain a history of condition (e.g., pressure, venous, or diabetic wound; eye or oral lesions), including whether condition is acute or recurrent; original site/characteristics of wound; duration of problem and changes that have occurred over time.
- Assess skin and tissues, bony prominences, pressure areas and wounds **for comparative baseline:**

  Note color, texture, and turgor.

  Assess areas of least pigmentation for color changes (e.g., sclera, conjunctiva, nailbeds, buccal mucosa, tongue, palms, and soles of feet).

  Note presence, location, and degree of edema (e.g., 4+ pitting).

  Record size (depth, width), color, location, temperature, texture of wounds or lesions.

  Determine degree and depth of injury or damage to integumentary system (involves epidermis, dermis, and/or underlying tissues), extent of tunneling or undermining, if present. *Note:* Full extent of lesions of mucous membranes or subcutaneous tissue may not be discernible.

  Identify stage of ulcers (I–IV) and classify burns using appropriate measuring tool.

  Document with drawings and/or photograph wound, lesion(s), burns, as appropriate.

  Observe for other distinguishing characteristics of surrounding tissue (e.g., exudate; granulation; cyanosis or pallor; tight, shiny skin).

  Describe wound drainage (e.g., amount, color, odor).

- Assist with diagnostic procedures (e.g., x-rays, imaging scans, biopsies, débridement). **May be necessary to determine extent of impairment.**
- Determine psychological effects of condition on client/SO(s). **Can be devastating for client's body or self-image and esteem, especially if condition is severe, disfiguring**

Information that appears in brackets has been added by the authors to clarify and enhance the use of nursing diagnoses.

or chronic, as well as costly and burdensome for SO(s)/
caregiver.

Nursing Priority No. 3.

To assist client to correct/minimize impairment and to promote
healing:

- Modify or eliminate factors contributing to condition, if possible. Assist with treatment of underlying condition(s), as appropriate.
- Inspect lesions or wounds daily, or as appropriate, for changes (e.g., signs of infection, complications, or healing). **Promotes timely intervention and revision of plan of care.**
- Promote optimum nutrition with high-quality protein and sufficient calories, vitamins, and mineral supplements **to facilitate healing.**
- Encourage adequate periods of rest and sleep **to limit metabolic demands, maximize energy available for healing, and meet comfort needs.**
- Limit or avoid use of caffeine, alcohol, and medications affecting REM sleep.
- Provide or assist with oral care (e.g., teaching oral and dental hygiene, avoiding extremes of hot or cold, changing position of ET and nasogastric tubes, lubricating lips) **to prevent damage to mucous membranes.**
- Promote early mobility. Assist with or encourage position changes, active or passive and assistive exercises **to promote circulation and prevent excessive tissue pressure.**
- Provide appropriate protective and healing devices (e.g., eye pads or goggles, heel protectors, padding or cushions, therapeutic beds and mattresses, splints, chronic ulcer dressings, compression wrap).
- Practice aseptic technique for cleansing, dressing, or medicating lesions. **Reduces risk of cross-contamination.**
- Monitor laboratory studies (e.g., CBC, electrolytes, glucose, cultures) **for changes indicative of healing or presence of infection, complications.**
- Protect client from environmental hazards when vision or hearing or cognitive deficits impact safety.
- Advise smoking cessation and refer for assistance or support, if indicated. **Smoking causes vasoconstriction that interferes with healing.**

Nursing Priority No. 4.

To promote wellness (Teaching/Discharge Considerations):

Information that appears in brackets has been added by the authors to clarify
and enhance the use of nursing diagnoses.

- Encourage verbalizations of feelings and expectations regarding condition and potential for recovery of structure and function.
- Help client and family identify effective successful coping mechanisms and implement them **to reduce pain or discomfort and to improve quality of life.**
- Discuss importance of early detection and reporting of changes in condition or any unusual physical discomforts or changes in pain characteristics. **Promotes early intervention and reduces potential for complications.**
- Emphasize need for adequate nutritional and fluid intake **to optimize healing potential.**
- Instruct in dressing changes (technique and frequency) and proper disposal of soiled dressings **to prevent spread of infectious agent.**
- Review medical regimen (e.g., proper use of topical sprays, creams, ointments, soaks, or irrigations).
- Stress importance of follow-up care, as appropriate (e.g., diabetic foot care clinic, wound care specialist or clinic, enterostomal therapist).
- Identify required changes in lifestyle, occupation, or environment **necessitated by limitations imposed by condition or to avoid causative factors.**
- Refer to community or governmental resources, as indicated (e.g., Public Health Department, Occupational Safety and Health Administration [OSHA], National Association for the Prevention of Blindness).
- Refer to NDs dependent on individual situation (e.g., impaired Skin Integrity; impaired Oral Mucous Membrane; risk for perioperative positioning Injury; impaired physical/bed Mobility; disturbed visual Sensory Perception; ineffective peripheral tissue Perfusion; risk for Trauma; risk for Infection).

Documentation Focus

Assessment/Reassessment
- Individual findings, including history of condition, characteristics of wound or lesion, evidence of other organ or tissue involvement.
- Impact on functioning and lifestyle.
- Availability and use of resources.

Planning
- Plan of care and who is involved in planning.
- Teaching plan.

Information that appears in brackets has been added by the authors to clarify and enhance the use of nursing diagnoses.

Implementation/Evaluation
- Responses to interventions, teaching, and actions performed.
- Attainment or progress toward desired outcome(s).
- Modifications to plan of care.

Discharge Planning
- Long-term needs and who is responsible for actions to be taken.
- Specific referrals made.

Sample Nursing Outcomes & Interventions Classifications (NOC/NIC) NIC

NOC—Tissue Integrity: Skin & Mucous Membranes
NIC—Wound Care

---

impaired Transfer Ability

Taxonomy II: Activity/Rest—Class 2 Activity/Exercise (00090)
[Diagnostic Division: Activity/Rest]
Submitted 1998; Revised 2006

Definition: Limitation of independent movement between two nearby surfaces

---

Related Factors

Insufficient muscle strength; deconditioning; neuromuscular impairment; musculoskeletal impairment (e.g., contractures)
Impaired balance
Pain
Obesity
Impaired vision
Lack of knowledge; cognitive impairment
Environment constraints (e.g., bed height, inadequate space, wheelchair type, treatment equipment, restraints)

Defining Characteristics

Subjective or Objective
Inability to transfer: from bed to chair or chair to bed; from chair to car or car to chair; from chair to floor or floor to chair; on or off a toilet or commode; in or out of tub or

---

Information that appears in brackets has been added by the authors to clarify and enhance the use of nursing diagnoses.

shower; from bed to standing or standing to bed; from chair to standing or standing to chair; from standing to floor or floor to standing; between uneven levels

Note: Specify level of independence using a standardized functional scale. [Refer to ND impaired physical Mobility, for suggested functional level classification.]

Desired Outcomes/Evaluation Criteria— Client/Caregiver Will:

- Verbalize understanding of situation and appropriate safety measures.
- Master techniques of transfer successfully.
- Make desired transfer safely.

Actions/Interventions

Nursing Priority No. 1.

To assess causative/contributing factors:

- Determine diagnosis that contributes to transfer problems (e.g., MS, fractures, back injuries, quadriplegia/paraplegia, agedness, dementias, brain injury).
- Note current situations such as surgery, amputation, contractures, traction apparatus, mechanical ventilation, multiple tubings that restrict movement.

Nursing Priority No. 2.

To assess functional ability:

- Evaluate degree of impairment using functional level classification scale of 0 to 4.
- Note emotional or behavioral responses of client/SO(s) to problems of immobility.
- Determine presence and degree of perceptual or cognitive impairment and ability to follow directions.

Nursing Priority No. 3.

To promote optimal level of movement:

- Assist with treatment of underlying condition causing dysfunction.
- Consult with physical therapist, occupational therapist, or rehabilitation team **in identifying balance, gait, and mobility aids/adjunctive devices.**
- Demonstrate and assist with use of side rails, overhead trapeze, transfer boards, transfer or sit-to-stand hoist, specialty

---

Information that appears in brackets has been added by the authors to clarify and enhance the use of nursing diagnoses.

slings, safety grab bars, cane, walker, wheelchair, crutches, as indicated.
* Position devices (e.g., call light, bed-positioning switch) within easy reach on the bed or chair. **Facilitates transfer and allows client to obtain assistance for transfer, as needed.**
* Provide instruction or reinforce information for client and caregivers regarding positioning **to improve or maintain balance when transferring.**
* Monitor body alignment, posture, and balance, and encourage wide base of support when standing to transfer.
* Use full-length mirror, as needed, **to facilitate client's view of own postural alignment.**
* Demonstrate and reinforce safety measures, as indicated, such as transfer board, gait belt, supportive footwear, good lighting, clearing floor of clutter **to avoid possibility of fall and subsequent injury.**

Nursing Priority No. 4.
To promote wellness (Teaching/Discharge Considerations):

* Assist client/caregivers to learn safety measures as individually indicated (e.g., using correct body mechanics for particular transfer, locking wheelchair before transfer, using properly placed and functioning hoists, ascertaining that floor surface is even and clutter-free).
* Refer to appropriate community resources for evaluation and modification of environment (e.g., shower or tub, uneven floor surfaces, steps, use of ramps, standing tables or lifts).

Documentation Focus ─────────────

Assessment/Reassessment
* Individual findings, including level of function and ability to participate in desired transfers.
* Mobility aids or transfer devices used.

Planning
* Plan of care and who is involved in the planning.
* Teaching plan.

Implementation/Evaluation
* Responses to interventions, teaching, and actions performed.
* Attainment or progress toward desired outcome(s).
* Modifications to plan of care.

Information that appears in brackets has been added by the authors to clarify and enhance the use of nursing diagnoses.

Discharge Planning
- Discharge and long-term needs, noting who is responsible for each action to be taken.
- Specific referrals made.
- Sources for and maintenance of assistive devices.

Sample Nursing Outcomes & Interventions Classifications (NOC/NIC) NIC

NOC—Transfer Performance
NIC—Transfer

risk for Trauma

Taxonomy II: Safety/Protection—Class 2 Physical Injury (00038)
[Diagnostic Division: Safety]
Submitted 1980

Definition: Accentuated risk of accidental tissue injury (e.g., wound, burn, fracture)

Risk Factors

Internal
Weakness; balancing difficulties; reduced muscle, hand, or eye coordination
Poor vision
Reduced sensation
Lack of safety education or precautions
Insufficient finances
Cognitive or emotional difficulties
History of previous trauma

External [Includes but Is Not Limited to]
Slippery floors (e.g., wet or highly waxed); unanchored rugs or electric wires
Bathtub without antislip equipment
Use of unsteady ladder or chairs
Obstructed passageways; entering unlighted rooms
Inadequate stair rails; children playing without gates at top of stairs
High beds; inappropriate call-for-aid mechanisms for bedresting client

---

Information that appears in brackets has been added by the authors to clarify and enhance the use of nursing diagnoses.

Unsafe window protection in homes with young children

Pot handles facing toward front of stove; bathing in very hot water (e.g., unsupervised bathing of young children)

Potential igniting gas leaks; delayed lighting of gas appliances

Wearing flowing clothes around open flames; flammable children's clothing or toys

Smoking in bed or near oxygen; grease waste collected on stoves

Children playing with dangerous objects; accessibility of guns

Playing with explosives; experimenting with chemicals; inadequately stored combustibles (e.g., matches, oily rags) or corrosives (e.g., lye); contact with corrosives

Overloaded fuse boxes; faulty electrical plugs; frayed wires; defective appliances; overloaded electrical outlets

Exposure to dangerous machinery; contact with rapidly moving machinery

Struggling with restraints

Contact with intense cold; lack of protection from heat source; overexposure to radiation

Large icicles hanging from the roof

Use of cracked dishware; knives stored uncovered

High-crime neighborhood

Driving a mechanically unsafe vehicle; driving at excessive speeds; driving without necessary visual aids; driving while intoxicated

Children riding in the front seat of car; nonuse or misuse of seat restraints

Unsafe road or walkways; physical proximity to vehicle pathways (e.g., driveways, lanes, railroad tracks)

Misuse [or nonuse] of necessary headgear [e.g., for bicycles, motorcycles, skateboarding, skiing]

> **NOTE:** A risk diagnosis is not evidenced by signs and symptoms, as the problem has not occurred; rather, nursing interventions are directed at prevention.

Desired Outcomes/Evaluation Criteria—Client/Caregiver Will:

- Identify and correct potential risk factors in the environment.
- Demonstrate appropriate lifestyle changes to reduce risk of injury.
- Identify resources to assist in promoting a safe environment.

Information that appears in brackets has been added by the authors to clarify and enhance the use of nursing diagnoses.

 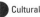 Cultural   Collaborative   Community/Home Care

- Recognize need for and seek assistance to prevent accidents or injuries.

Actions/Interventions

This ND is a compilation of a number of situations that can result in injury. Refer to specific NDs—risk for imbalanced Body Temperature; risk for Contamination; impaired Environmental Interpretation Syndrome; risk for Falls; impaired Home Maintenance; Hyperthermia; Hypothermia; risk for Injury; impaired physical Mobility; risk for impaired Parenting; risk for Poisoning; disturbed Sensory Perception; impaired Skin Integrity; risk for Suffocation; disturbed Thought Processes; impaired Tissue Integrity; risk for self-/other-directed Violence; impaired Walking, as appropriate, for more specific interventions.

Nursing Priority No. 1.

To assess causative/contributing factors:

- Determine factors related to individual situation, as listed in Risk Factors, and extent of risk. **Influences scope and intensity of interventions to manage threat to safety.**
- Note client's age, gender and developmental stage, decision-making ability, and level of cognition and competence. **Affects client's ability to protect self and/or others, and influences choice of interventions and teaching.**
- Ascertain knowledge of safety needs and injury prevention, and motivation to prevent injury in home, community, and work setting.
- Note socioeconomic status and availability and use of resources.
- Assess influence of client's lifestyle and stress on potential for injury.
- Review history of accidents noting circumstances (e.g., time of day, activities coinciding with accident, who was present, type of injury sustained).
- Determine potential for abusive behavior by family members/ SO(s)/peers.
- Review diagnostic studies and laboratory tests for impairments or imbalances **that may result in or exacerbate conditions, such as confusion, tetany, and pathological fractures.**

Information that appears in brackets has been added by the authors to clarify and enhance the use of nursing diagnoses.

Nursing Priority No. 2.

To promote safety measures required by individual situation:

- Implement interventions regarding safety issues when planning for client care and/or discharge from care. **Failure to accurately assess, intervene, and/or refer these issues can place the client at needless risk and create negligence issues for the healthcare practitioner:**

  Orient client to environment.

  Make arrangement for call system for bedridden client in home or hospital setting. Demonstrate use and place device within client's reach.

  Keep bed in low position or place mattress on floor, as appropriate.

  Use and pad side rails, as indicated.

  Provide seizure precautions.

  Lock wheels on bed and movable furniture. Clear travel paths. Provide adequate area lighting.

  Assist with activities and transfers, as needed.

  Provide well-fitting, nonskid footwear.

  Demonstrate and monitor use of assistive devices, such as cane, walker, crutches, wheelchair, safety bars.

  Provide supervision while client is smoking.

  Provide for appropriate disposal of potentially injurious items (e.g., needles, scalpel blades).

   Follow facility protocol and closely monitor use of restraints, when required (e.g., vest, limb, belt, mitten).

Nursing Priority No. 3.

To treat underlying medical/psychiatric condition:

- Assist with treatments for underlying medical, surgical, or psychiatric conditions **to improve cognition and thinking processes, musculoskeletal function, awareness of own safety needs, and general well-being.**
- Provide quiet environment and reduced stimulation, as indicated. **Helps limit confusion or overstimulation for clients at risk for such conditions as seizures, tetany, autonomic hyperreflexia.**
- Refer to counseling or psychotherapy, as needed, especially when individual is "accident-prone" or self-destructive behavior is noted. (Refer to NDs risk for other-/self-directed Violence.)

Information that appears in brackets has been added by the authors to clarify and enhance the use of nursing diagnoses.

Cultural   Collaborative   Community/Home Care

Nursing Priority No. 4.

To promote wellness (Teaching/Discharge Considerations):

- Review client's therapeutic regimen on a continual basis when under direct care (e.g., vital signs, medications, treatment modalities, infusions, nutrition, physical environment) **to prevent healthcare-related complications.**
- Stress importance of obtaining assistance when weak and when problems of balance, coordination, or postural hypotension are present, **to reduce risk of syncope and falls.**
- Encourage use of warm-up and stretching exercises before engaging in athletic activity **to prevent muscle injuries.**
- Recommend use of seat belts; fitted helmets for cyclists, skate-/snowboarders, skiers; approved infant seat; avoidance of hitchhiking; substance abuse programs **to promote transportation and recreation safety.**
- Refer to accident prevention programs (e.g., medication and drug safety, mobility or transfer device training, driving instruction, parenting classes, firearms safety, workplace erogomics).
- Develop fire safety program (e.g., family fire drills; use of smoke detectors; yearly chimney cleaning; purchase of fire-retardant clothing, especially children's nightwear; safe use of in-home oxygen; fireworks safety).
- Problem-solve with client/parent to provide adequate child supervision after school, during working hours, on school holidays; or day program for frail or confused elder.
- Discuss necessary environmental changes (e.g., decals on glass doors to show when they are closed, lowering temperature on hot water heater, adequate lighting of stairways; tamper-proof medication containers, safe chemical and poisons storage) **to prevent or reduce risk of accidents.**
- Identify community resources (e.g., financial) **to assist with necessary corrections or improvements and purchases.**
- Recommend involvement in community self-help programs, such as Neighborhood Watch, Helping Hand.

Documentation Focus

Assessment/Reassessment
- Individual risk factors, past and recent history of injuries, awareness of safety needs.
- Use of safety equipment or procedures.
- Environmental concerns, safety issues.

Information that appears in brackets has been added by the authors to clarify and enhance the use of nursing diagnoses.

Planning
- Plan of care and who is involved in the planning.
- Teaching plan.

Implementation/Evaluation
- Responses to interventions, teaching, and actions performed.
- Attainment or progress toward desired outcome(s).
- Modifications to plan of care.

Discharge Planning
- Long-term needs and who is responsible for actions to be taken.
- Available resources, specific referrals made.

Sample Nursing Outcomes & Interventions Classifications (NOC/NIC) NIC

NOC—Physical Injury Severity
NIC—Environmental Management: Safety

---

risk for vascular Trauma

Taxonomy II: Safety/Protection—Class 2 Physical Injury
[Diagnostic Division: Safety]
Submitted 2008

Definition: At risk for damage to a vein and its surrounding tissues related to the presence of a catheter and/or infused solutions

---

Risk Factors

Insertion site; impaired ability to visualize the insertion site
Catheter type; catheter width
Nature of solution (e.g., concentration, chemical irritant, temperature, pH); infusion rate; length of insertion time

NOTE: A risk diagnosis is not evidenced by signs and symptoms, as the problem has not occurred; rather, nursing interventions are directed at prevention

---

Information that appears in brackets has been added by the authors to clarify and enhance the use of nursing diagnoses.

⊕ Cultural ⊗ Collaborative 🏠 Community/Home Care

Desired Outcomes/Evaluation Criteria— Client Will:

- Identify signs/symptoms to report to healthcare provider.
- Be free of signs/symptoms associated with infusion phlebitis or local infection.
- Develop plan for home therapy and demonstrate appropriate procedures as indicated.

Actions/Interventions

Nursing Priority No. 1.

To assess risk factors:

- Determine presence of medical condition(s) requiring IV therapy (e.g., dehydration, trauma, surgery; long-term antibiotic treatment of severe infections; cancer therapies, pain management when oral drugs not effective or practical).
- Note client's age, body size, and weight. **Very young or elderly client is at risk because of lack of subcutaneous tissue surrounding veins, and veins may be fragile, or ropy, causing difficulties with insertion. Forearm veins may be difficult to see in obese, edematous, or dark-skinned individual.**
- Identify particular issues such as client's emotional state, including fear of needles, mental or developmental status that might interfere with clients ability to cooperate with procedures, IV site choices that interfere with client's mobility, **to prevent or limit potential for vascular damage.**
- Determine type(s) of solutions being used or planned. **Certain infusates are associated with greater risk of vein irritation and pain (e.g., potassium); others are associated with significant risk of tissue injury, especially upon infiltration into surrounding tissues, including certain antibiotics, chemotherapy, or parenteral nutrition.**
- Assess peripheral IV site, when one is already in place, to determine potential for complications. **Reddened, blanched, tight, translucent, or cool skin; swelling; pain; numbness; streak formation; a palpable venous cord or purulent drainage are indicative of problem with IV requiring immediate intervention.**
- Assess central venous access device (CVAD), if present, to determine potential for complications. **Inability to aspirate, slowed or absent solution flow, site pain; engorged veins,**

Information that appears in brackets has been added by the authors to clarify and enhance the use of nursing diagnoses.

or swelling in upper arm, chest wall, neck, or jaw on side
of catheter insertion may indicate vein- or catheter-related
thrombus, requiring immediate intervention.

Nursing Priority No. 2.

To reduce potential complications:

• Determine appropriate site choice:

Inspect and palpate chosen veins to determine size and condition. **Best veins are those that are not scarred, lumpy,
or fragile, to improve ease of cannulation and effectiveness of infusion.**

Identify extremities or sites that have impaired circulation or
injury. **Existing tissue injury, bleeding or edema can inhibit successful IV cannulation, and potentiate risk for
infiltration of infusates.**

Avoid leg veins in adults **due to potential for thrombophlebitis.**

Avoid anticubital veins when using peripheral catheter **because placement there limits client's movement and the
catheter is easily dislodged.**

Avoid inserting needle in vein valve site. **Damage to this
area can cause blood pooling and increase risk of
thrombosis.**

• Use best-practice approach to IV insertion:

Determine best type of access when IV therapy is initiated.
**Peripheral catheter in forearm is recommended for
short-duration, nonirritating solutions of less than 7
days' duration. CVAD is appropriate for infusing many
kinds of solutions over long periods of time, or when
client has suffered multiple peripheral sticks or one extremity is not available (e.g., amputation, dialysis shunt
in one arm).**

Use appropriate needle gauge for chosen vein and solution **to
deliver solution at appropriate rate, to promote hemo-
dilution of fluid(s) at the catheter tip, and to reduce mechanical and chemical irritation to vein wall.**

Clean site and inject 1% lidocaine per agency protocol **to
reduce risk of infection and pain with needle or cannula
insertion.**

Stretch and immobilize skin and tissues **to stabilize vein and
prevent rolling, requiring multiple sticks.**

Insert needle bevel up, during insertion and hold at 3- to 10-
degree angle **to prevent "blowing" the vein by piercing
the back wall.**

Information that appears in brackets has been added by the authors to clarify
and enhance the use of nursing diagnoses.

🌐 Cultural ◎ Collaborative 🏠 Community/Home Care

Release tourniquet immediately when insertion is complete **to prevent intravascular pressure from causing bleeding into surrounding tissues.**

Observe for hematoma development and/or reports of pain and discomfort during insertion, **indicating vein damage with bleeding into tissues.**

Secure needle or cannula with tape or other securing device **to prevent dislodging and to extend catheter dwell time.**

Avoid placing tape entirely around arm to anchor catheter; **can impede venous return and cause pooling of fluid, and infiltration or extravasation into surrounding tissues.**

Utilize transparent dressing over insertion site **to protect from external contaminants and to allow easy observation for potential complications.**

- Adhere to recommended infusions, dilutions, and administration rates for medications or irritating substances such as potassium, **to reduce incidence of tissue irritation and sloughing.**

- Consult with IV/infusion nurse, or other medical provider **to problem-solve issues that arise with IVs and/or for interventions for complications.**

Nursing Priority No. 3.
To promote optimum therapeutic effect:

- Observe IV site on a regular basis and instruct client/caregiver to report any discomfort, bruising, redness, swelling, bleeding or other fluid leaking from site.
- Replace peripheral catheters every 72 to 96 hours (or per agency policy) **to prevent thrombophlebitis and catheter-related infections.**
- Apply pressure to site when IV discontinued for sufficient time **to prevent bleeding, especially in client with coagulopathies or on anticoagulants.**
- Adhere to specific protocols related to infection-control. Refer to ND risk for infection.
- Identify community resources and suppliers as indicated **to support home therapy regimen.**

Documentation Focus

Assessment/Reassessment
- Assessment findings pre- and postinsertion, site choice, use of local anesthetic, type and gauge of needle or cannula inserted, number of sticks required, dressing applied.

Information that appears in brackets has been added by the authors to clarify and enhance the use of nursing diagnoses.

- Type, amount, and rate of solution administered, presence of additives.
- Clients response to procedure.

Planning
- Plan of care, specific interventions, and who is involved in the planning.
- Teaching plan as appropriate.

Implementation/Evaluation
- Attainment or progress toward desired outcome(s).
- Modifications to plan of care.

Discharge Planning
- Long-term needs, identifying who is responsible for actions to be taken.
- Community resources for equipment and supplies for home therapy.
- Specific referrals made.

Sample Nursing Outcomes & Interventions classifications (NOC/NIC) NIC

NOC—Symptom Control
NIC—Intravenous (IV) Insertion

---

impaired Urinary Elimination

Taxonomy II: Elimination and Exchange—Class 1
  Urinary Function (00016)
[Diagnostic Division: Elimination]
Submitted 1973; Revised 2006

Definition: Dysfunction in urine elimination

Related Factors

Multiple causality; sensory motor impairment; anatomical obstruction; UTI; [mechanical trauma; fluid/volume states; psychogenetic factors; surgical diversion]

Defining Characteristics

Subjective
Frequency; urgency
Hesitancy

Information that appears in brackets has been added by the authors to clarify and enhance the use of nursing diagnoses.

Cultural   Collaborative   Community/Home Care

Dysuria
Nocturia [enuresis]

Objective
Incontinence
Retention

Desired Outcomes/Evaluation Criteria— Client Will:

- Verbalize understanding of condition.
- Identify specific causative factors.
- Achieve normal elimination pattern or participate in measures to correct or compensate for defects.
- Demonstrate behaviors and techniques to prevent urinary infection.
- Manage care of urinary catheter, or stoma, and appliance following urinary diversion.

Actions/Interventions

Nursing Priority No. 1.
To assess causative/contributing factors:

- Identify conditions that may be present, such as urinary tract infection, interstitial cystitis or painful bladder syndrome; dehydration; surgery (including urinary diversion); neurological involvement (e.g., MS, stroke, Parkinson's disease, paraplegia/ tetraplegia); mental or emotional dysfunction (e.g., impaired cognition, delirium or confusion, depression, Alzheimer's disease); prostate disorders; recent or multiple pregnancies; pelvic trauma.
- Determine pathology of bladder dysfunction relative to medical diagnosis identified. **For example, in such neurological or demyelinating diseases as MS, problem may be related to inability to store urine, empty the bladder, or both.**
- Assist with physical examination (e.g., cough test for incontinence, palpation for bladder retention or masses, prostate size, observation for urethral stricture).
- Note age and gender of client. **Incontinence and urinary tract infections are more prevalent in women and older adults; painful bladder syndrome (PBS) or interstitial cystitis (IC) is more common in women.**
- Investigate pain, noting location, duration, intensity; presence of bladder spasms; or back or flank pain **to assist in**

Information that appears in brackets has been added by the authors to clarify and enhance the use of nursing diagnoses.

differentiating between bladder and kidney as cause of dysfunction. **Bladder pain located suprapubically, vaginally, in the perineum, low back, or in the medial aspects of the thighs—that is relieved by voiding and often recurs with bladder filling—suggests presence of PBS/IC.**

- Have client complete Pelvic Pain and Urgency/Frequency (PUF) patient symptom survey, as indicated. **Helps in evaluating the presence and severity of PBS/IC symptoms.**
- Note reports of exacerbations and spontaneous remissions of symptoms of urgency and frequency, which may or may not be accompanied by pain, pressure, or spasm. **Clients with PBS/IC void approximately 16 times per day with voided volumes usually less then normal.**
- Determine client's usual daily fluid intake (both amount and beverage choices, use of caffeine). Note condition of skin and mucous membranes, color of urine **to help determine level of hydration.**
- Review medication regimen **for drugs that can alter bladder or kidney function** (e.g., antihypertensive agents [e.g., ACE inhibitors, beta-adrenergic blockers]; anticholinergics [e.g., antihistamines, anti-parkinsonian drugs]; antidepressants or antipsychotics; sedatives, hypnotics, opioids; caffeine and alcohol).
- Send urine specimen (midstream clean-voided or catheterized) for culture and sensitivities in presence of signs of urinary tract infection—cloudy, foul odor; bloody urine.
- Rule out gonorrhea in men when urethritis with a penile discharge is present and there are no bacteria in the urine.
- Obtain specimen for antibody-coated bacteria assay **to diagnose bacterial infection of the kidney or prostate.**
- Assist with potassium sensitivity test (instillation of potassium solution into bladder). **Eighty percent of patients with PBS/IC will react positively.**
- Review laboratory tests for hyperglycemia, hyperparathyroidism, or other metabolic conditions; changes in renal function; culture for presence of infection or sexually transmitted disease (STD), urine cytology for cancer.
- Strain all urine for calculi and describe stones expelled and/ or send to laboratory for analysis.
- Review results of diagnostic studies (e.g., uroflowmetry; cystometogram; postvoid residual; pressure flow and leak point pressure measurement; videourodynamics; electromyography; kidney, ureter, and bladder [KUB] imaging) **to identify presence and type of elimination problem.**

Information that appears in brackets has been added by the authors to clarify and enhance the use of nursing diagnoses.

⊕ Cultural 🔗 Collaborative 🏠 Community/Home Care

Nursing Priority No. 2.

To assess degree of interference/disability:

- Ascertain client's previous pattern of elimination **for comparison with current situation**. Ask about and note reports of problems (e.g., frequency, urgency, painful urination; leaking or incontinence; changes in size and force of urinary stream; problems emptying bladder completely; nocturia or enuresis).
- Ascertain client's/SO's perception of problem and degree of disability (e.g., client is restricting social, employment, or travel activities; having sexual or relationship difficulties; incurring sleep deprivation; experiencing depression).
- Determine cultural factors impacting client's self-image regarding urinary problem (e.g., presence of urostomy and need to empty bag at intervals; painful bladder that interferes with daily activities or employment).
- Have client keep a voiding diary for 3 days to record fluid intake, voiding times, precise urine output, and dietary intake. **Helps determine baseline symptoms, severity of frequency or urgency, and whether diet is a factor (if symptoms worsen).**

Nursing Priority No. 3.

To assist in treating/preventing urinary alteration:

- Refer to specific NDs Urinary Incontinence (specify); Urinary Retention for additional related interventions.
- Encourage fluid intake up to 3000 or more mL/day (within cardiac tolerance), including cranberry juice, **to help maintain renal function, prevent infection and formation of urinary stones, avoid encrustation around catheter, or flush urinary diversion appliance.**
- Discuss possible dietary restrictions (e.g., especially coffee, alcohol, carbonated drinks, citrus, tomatoes, and chocolate) based on individual symptoms.
- Assist with developing toileting routines (e.g., timed voiding, bladder training, prompted voiding, habit retraining), as appropriate. *Note:* Bladder retraining is not recommended for clients with PBS.
- Encourage client to verbalize fears and concerns (e.g., disruption in sexual activity, inability to work). **Open expression allows client to deal with feelings and begin problem solving.**
- Implement and monitor interventions for specific elimination problem (e.g., pelvic floor exercises or other bladder retraining

---

Information that appears in brackets has been added by the authors to clarify and enhance the use of nursing diagnoses.

 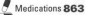

modalities; medication regimen, including antimicrobials [single-dose is frequently being used for UTI], sulfonamides, antispasmodics); and evaluate client's response **to modify treatment, as needed.**

- Discuss possible surgical procedures and medical regimen, as indicated (e.g., client with benign prostatic hypertrophy bladder or prostatic cancer, PBS/IC). **For example, cystoscopy with bladder hydrodistention may be used for PBS/IC, or an electrical stimulator may be implanted to treat chronic urinary urge incontinence, nonobstructive urinary retention, and symptoms of urgency and frequency.**

Nursing Priority No. 4.

To assist in management of long-term urinary alterations:

- Keep bladder deflated by use of an indwelling catheter connected to closed drainage. Investigate alternatives when possible (e.g., intermittent catheterization, surgical interventions, urinary drugs, voiding maneuvers, condom catheter).
- Provide latex-free catheter and care supplies **to reduce risk of latex sensitivity.**
- Check frequently for bladder distention and observe for overflow **to reduce risk of infection and/or autonomic hyperreflexia.**
- Maintain acidic environment of the bladder by the use of agents, such as vitamin C, Mandelamine, when appropriate, **to discourage bacterial growth.**
- Adhere to a regular bladder or diversion appliance emptying schedule **to avoid accidents.**
- Provide for routine diversion appliance care, and assist client to recognize and deal with problems, such as alkaline salt encrustation, ill-fitting appliance, malodorous urine, and infection.

Nursing Priority No. 5.

To promote wellness (Teaching/Discharge Considerations):

- Emphasize importance of keeping area clean and dry **to reduce risk of infection and/or skin breakdown.**
- Instruct female clients with UTI to drink large amounts of fluid, void immediately after intercourse, wipe from front to back, promptly treat vaginal infections, and take showers rather than tub baths **to limit risk or avoid reinfection.**
- Recommend smoking cessation program, as appropriate. **Cigarette smoking can also be a source of bladder irritation.**

Information that appears in brackets has been added by the authors to clarify and enhance the use of nursing diagnoses.

   Cultural Collaborative Community/Home Care

• Encourage SO(s) who participate in routine care to recognize complications (including latex allergy) necessitating medical evaluation or intervention.

• Instruct in proper application and care of appliance for urinary diversion. Encourage liberal fluid intake, avoidance of foods or medications that produce strong odor, use of white vinegar or deodorizer in pouch **to promote odor control.**

• Identify sources for supplies, programs or agencies providing financial assistance **to obtain needed equipment.**

• Recommend avoidance of gas-forming foods in presence of ureterosigmoidostomy **as flatus can cause urinary incontinence.**

• Recommend use of silicone catheter when permanent or long-term catheterization is required.

• Demonstrate proper positioning of catheter drainage tubing and bag **to facilitate drainage and prevent reflux.**

• Refer client/SO(s) to appropriate community resources, such as ostomy specialist, support group, sex therapist, psychiatric clinical nurse specialist, **to deal with changes in body image and function, when indicated.**

Documentation Focus

Assessment/Reassessment
• Individual findings, including previous and current pattern of voiding, nature of problem, effect on desired lifestyle.
• Cultural factors or concerns.

Planning
• Plan of care and who is involved in planning.
• Teaching plan.

Implementation/Evaluation
• Response to interventions, teaching, and actions performed.
• Attainment or progress toward desired outcome(s).
• Modifications to plan of care.

Discharge Planning
• Long-term needs and who is responsible for actions to be taken.
• Available resources and specific referrals made.
• Individual equipment needs and sources.

Information that appears in brackets has been added by the authors to clarify and enhance the use of nursing diagnoses.

Sample Nursing Outcomes & Interventions Classifications (NOC/NIC) NIC

NOC—Urinary Elimination
NIC—Urinary Elimination Management

---

readiness for enhanced Urinary Elimination

Taxonomy II: Elimination and Exchange—Class 1
  Urinary Function (00166)
[Diagnostic Division: Elimination]
Submitted 2002

Definition: A pattern of urinary functions that is sufficient for meeting eliminatory needs and can be strengthened

---

Related Factors

To be developed

Defining Characteristics

Subjective
Expresses willingness to enhance urinary elimination
Positions self for emptying of bladder

Objective
Urine is straw colored, odorless
Amount of output and specific gravity is within normal limits
Fluid intake is adequate for daily needs

Desired Outcomes/Evaluation Criteria— Client Will:

- Verbalize understanding of condition that has potential for altering elimination.
- Achieve improved elimination pattern emptying bladder, voiding in appropriate amounts.
- Alter lifestyle or environment to accommodate individual needs.

Information that appears in brackets has been added by the authors to clarify and enhance the use of nursing diagnoses.

    Cultural   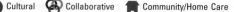 Collaborative   Community/Home Care

Actions/Interventions

Nursing Priority No. 1.

To assess status and adaptive skills being used by client:

- Identify physical conditions (e.g., surgery, childbirth, recent or multiple pregnancies, pelvic trauma, neurogenic bladder from central nervous system disorders or neuropathies [stroke, SCI, diabetes], prostate disease or surgery, mental or emotional dysfunction) **that can impact client's elimination patterns.**
- Determine client's usual pattern of elimination and compare with current situation. Review voiding diary, if indicated. **Provides baseline for future comparison.**
- Observe voiding patterns, time, color, and amount voided, if indicated (e.g., postsurgical or postpartum client) **to document normalization of elimination.**
- Ascertain methods of self-management (e.g., limiting or increasing liquid intake, acting on urge in timely manner, established voiding schedule, regularly spaced cathetrization) **to identify strengths and areas of concern in elimination management**.
- Determine client's usual daily fluid intake. **Both amount and beverage choices are important in managing elimination.**

Nursing Priority No. 2.

To assist client to improve management of urinary elimination:

- Encourage fluid intake, including water and cranberry juice, **to help maintain renal function, prevent infection.**
- Regulate liquid intake at prescheduled times **to promote predictable voiding pattern.** Restrict fluid intake 2 to 3 hours before bedtime **to reduce voiding during the night.**
- Assist with modifying current routines, as appropriate. **Client may benefit from additional information in enhancing success, such as regarding cues or urge to void, adjusting schedule of voiding or catheterization (shorter or longer), relaxation and/or distraction techniques, standing or sitting upright during voiding to ensure that bladder is completely empty, and/or practicing pelvic muscle strengthening exercises.**
- Provide assistance or devices, as indicated (e.g., providing means of summoning assistance; placing bedside commode, urinal, or bedpan within client's reach; using elevated toilet

---

Information that appears in brackets has been added by the authors to clarify and enhance the use of nursing diagnoses.

seats; mobility devices) **when client is frail or mobility impaired.**

- Modify or recommend diet changes, if indicated. **For example, limiting caffeine intake because of its bladder irritant effect; or weight loss to reduce overactive bladder symptoms and incontinence by decreasing pressure on the bladder.**

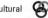• Modify medication regimens, as appropriate (e.g., administer prescribed diuretics in the morning **to lessen nighttime voiding**). Reduce or eliminate use of hypnotics, if possible, **as client may be too sedated to recognize and respond to urge to void.**

• Refer to appropriate resources (e.g., medical supply company, ostomy nurse, rehabilitation team) **for assistance, as desired/ needed to promote self-care.**

Nursing Priority No. 3.
To promote optimum wellness:

• Encourage continuation of successful toileting program and identify possible alterations to meet individual needs (e.g., use of adult briefs for extended outing or travel with limited access to toilet). **Promotes proactive problem solving and supports self-esteem and normalization of social interactions and desired lifestyle activities.**

• Instruct client/SO(s)/caregivers in cues that client needs, such as voiding on routine schedule, showing client location of the bathroom, providing adequate room lighting, signs, color coding of door **to assist client in continued continence, especially when in unfamiliar surroundings.**

• Review with client/SO(s) the signs and symptoms of urinary complications and need for expedient medical follow-up care. **Promotes timely intervention to limit or prevent adverse events.**

Documentation Focus

Assessment/Reassessment
• Indivual findings including adaptive skills being used.

Planning
• Plan of care and who is involved in planning.
• Teaching plan.

Information that appears in brackets has been added by the authors to clarify and enhance the use of nursing diagnoses.

⊕ Cultural ⊛ Collaborative 🏠 Community/Home Care

Implementation/Evaluation
- Responses to treatment plan, interventions, and actions performed.
- Attainment or progress toward desired outcome(s).
- Modifications to plan of care.

Discharge Planning
- Available resources, equipment needs and sources.

Sample Nursing Outcomes & Interventions Classifications (NOC/NIC) `NIC`

NOC—Urinary Elimination
NIC—Urinary Elimination Management

---

functional Urinary Incontinence

Taxonomy II: Elimination—Class 1 Urinary System (00020)
[Diagnostic Division: Elimination]
Submitted 1986; Nursing Diagnosis Extension and Classification (NDEC) Revision 1998

Definition: Inability of usually continent person to reach toilet in time to avoid unintentional loss of urine

---

Related Factors

Altered environmental factors [e.g., poor lighting or inability to locate bathroom]
Neuromuscular limitations
Weakened supporting pelvic structures
Impaired vision or cognition
Psychological factors; [reluctance to call for assistance or use bedpan; fluctuation in mentation]
Increased urine production

Defining Characteristics

Subjective
Senses need to void
Voiding in large amounts

Information that appears in brackets has been added by the authors to clarify and enhance the use of nursing diagnoses.

Objective

Loss of urine before reaching toilet; amount of time required to reach toilet exceeds length of time between sensing urge and uncontrolled voiding

Able to completely empty bladder

May be incontinent only in early morning

Desired Outcomes/Evaluation Criteria—Client/Caregiver Will:

- Verbalize understanding of condition and identify interventions to prevent incontinence.
- Alter environment to accommodate individual needs.
- Report voiding in individually appropriate amounts.
- Urinate at acceptable times and places.

Actions/Interventions

Nursing Priority No. 1.

To assess causative/contributing factors:

- Identify or differentiate client with functional incontinence (e.g., bladder and urethra are functioning normally, but client either cannot get to toilet, or has impaired mental function that interferes with recognizing need to urinate and getting to toilet on time) from other forms of incontinence.
- Evaluate cognition. **Disease process or medications can affect mental status, or orientation to place, recognition of urge to void, and/or its significance.**
- Note presence and type of functional impairments (e.g., poor eyesight, mobility problems, dexterity problems, self-care deficits) **that can hinder ability to get to bathroom.**
- Identify environmental conditions that interfere with timely access to bathroom or successful toileting process. **Unfamiliar surroundings, poor lighting, improperly fitted chair walker, low toilet seat, absence of safety bars, and travel distance to toilet may affect self-care ability.**
- Determine if client is voluntarily postponing urination.

- Review medical history for condition or use of medication or substances known to increase urine output and/or alter bladder tone (e.g., diuretics, alcohol, caffeine).

Nursing Priority No. 2.

To assess degree of interference/disability:

- Determine frequency and timing of continent and incontinent voids. Note time of day or night when incontinence occurs,

---

Information that appears in brackets has been added by the authors to clarify and enhance the use of nursing diagnoses.

Cultural   Collaborative   Community/Home Care

as well as timing issues (e.g., difference between the time it takes to get to bathroom and remove clothing and involuntary loss of urine).
• Ascertain effect on client's lifestyle (including socialization and sexuality) and self-esteem.

Nursing Priority No. 3.
To assist in treating/preventing incontinence:
• Remind client to void when needed and schedule voiding times **to reduce incontinence episodes and promote comfort for client who ambulates slowly because of physical limitations or who has cognitive decline.**
• Administer prescribed diuretics in the morning **to lessen nighttime voidings.**
• Reduce or eliminate use of hypnotics, if possible, **as client may be too sedated to recognize or respond to urge to void.**
• Provide means of summoning assistance (e.g., call light or bell).
• Use night-lights **to mark bathroom location.**
• Provide cues, such as adequate room lighting, signs, color coding of door, **to assist client who is disoriented to find the bathroom.**
• Remove throw rugs, excess furniture in travel path to bathroom.
• Provide bedside commode, urinal, or bedpan, as indicated.
• Adapt clothes for quick removal: Velcro fasteners, full skirts, crotchless panties or no panties, suspenders or elastic waists instead of belts on pants. **Facilitates toileting once urge to void is noted.**
• Schedule voiding for every 3 hours **to minimize bladder pressure.**
• Restrict fluid intake 2 to 3 hours before bedtime **to reduce nighttime voidings.**
• Include physical/occupational therapist in determining ways to alter environment and identifying appropriate assistive devices to meet client's individual needs.

Nursing Priority No. 4.
To promote wellness (Teaching/Discharge Considerations):
• Discuss with client/SO(s) need for prompted and scheduled voidings **to manage continence when client is unable to respond immediately to urge to void.**
• Suggest limiting intake of coffee, tea, and alcohol **because of diuretic effect and impact on voiding pattern.**

Information that appears in brackets has been added by the authors to clarify and enhance the use of nursing diagnoses.

 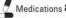

🏠 • Maintain positive regard **to reduce embarrassment associated with incontinence, need for assistance, use of bedpan.**
🏠 • Promote participation in developing long-term plan of care.
• Refer to NDs reflex Urinary Incontinence; stress Urinary Incontinence; total Urinary Incontinence; urge Urinary Incontinence.

Documentation Focus

Assessment/Reassessment
• Current elimination pattern and assessment findings.
• Effect on lifestyle and self-esteem.

Planning
• Plan of care and who is involved in planning.
• Teaching plan.

Implementation/Evaluation
• Response to interventions, teaching, and actions performed.
• Attainment or progress toward desired outcome(s).
• Modifications to plan of care.

Discharge Planning
• Long-term needs and who is responsible for actions to be taken.
• Specific referrals made.

Sample Nursing Outcomes & Interventions Classifications (NOC/NIC) [NIC]

NOC—Urinary Continence
NIC—Prompted Voiding

---

overflow Urinary Incontinence

Taxonomy II: Elimination and Exchange—Class 1 Urinary —Function (00176)
[Diagnostic Division: Elimination]
Submitted 2006

Definition: Involuntary loss of urine associated with overdistention of the bladder

---

Information that appears in brackets has been added by the authors to clarify and enhance the use of nursing diagnoses.

🌐 Cultural ⚛ Collaborative 🏠 Community/Home Care

Related Factors

Bladder outlet obstruction; fecal impaction

Urethral obstruction; severe pelvic prolapse

Detrusor external sphincter dyssynergia; detrusor hypocontractility

Side effects of anticholinergic or decongestant medications; calcium channel blockers

Defining Characteristics

Subjective
Reports involuntary leakage of small volumes of urine

Nocturia

Objective
Bladder distention

High postvoid residual volume

Observed involuntary leakage of small volumes of urine

Desired Outcomes/Evaluation Criteria—Client Will:

- Verbalize understanding of causative factors and appropriate interventions for individual situation.
- Demonstrate techniques or behaviors to alleviate or prevent overflow incontinence.
- Void in sufficient amounts with no palpable bladder distention; experience no post-void residuals greater than 50 mL; have no dribbling or overflow.

Actions/Interventions

Nursing Priority No. 1.
To assess causative/contributing factors:

- Review client's history for: (1) bladder outlet obstruction (e.g., prostatic hypertrophy, urethral stricture, urinary stones or tumors); (2) nonfunctioning detrusor muscle (i.e., sensory or motor paralytic bladder due to underlying neurological disease); or (3) atonic bladder that has lost its muscular tone (i.e., chronic overdistention) **to identify potential for or presence of conditions associated with overflow incontinence.**
- Note client's age and gender. **Urinary incontinence due to overflow bladder is more common in men because of the prevalence of obstructive prostate gland enlargement.**

Information that appears in brackets has been added by the authors to clarify and enhance the use of nursing diagnoses.

- Review medication regimen **for drugs that can cause or exacerbate retention and overflow incontinence (e.g., anticholinergic agents, calcium channel blockers, psychotropics, anesthesia, opiates, sedatives, alpha- and beta-adrenergic blockers, antihistamines, neuroleptics).**

Nursing Priority No. 2.
To determine degree of interference/disability:

- Note client reports of symptoms common to overflow incontinence, such as:

   Feeling no need to urinate, while simultaneously losing urine
   Feeling the urge to urinate, but not being able to
   Feeling as though the bladder is never completely empty
   Passing a dribbling stream of urine, even after spending a long time at the toilet
   Frequently getting up at night to urinate
- Prepare for and assist with urodynamic testing (e.g., uroflowmetry **to assess urine speed and volume;** cystometrogram **to measure bladder pressure and volume;** bladder scan **to measure retention and/or postvoid residual,** leak point pressure).

Nursing Priority No. 3.
To assist in treating/preventing overflow incontinence:

- Collaborate in treatment of underlying conditions (e.g., medications or surgery for prostatic hypertrophy; use of medication, such as terazosin, to relax urinary sphincter; altering dose or discontinuing medications contributing to retention). **If the underlying cause of the overflow problem can be treated or eliminated, client may be able to return to normal voiding pattern.**
- Demonstrate/instruct client/SO(s) in use of gentle massage over bladder (Credé's maneuver). **May facilitate bladder emptying when cause is detrusor weakness.**
- Implement intermittent or continuous catheterization. **Short-term use may be required while acute conditions are treated (e.g., infection, surgery for enlarged prostate); long-term use is required for permanent conditions (e.g., SCI or other neuromuscular conditions resulting in permanent bladder dysfunction).**

Nursing Priority No. 4.
To promote wellness (Teaching/Discharge Considerations):

Information that appears in brackets has been added by the authors to clarify and enhance the use of nursing diagnoses.

 Cultural Collaborative 🏠 Community/Home Care

- Establish regular schedule for bladder emptying whether voiding or using catheter.
- Stress need for adequate fluid intake, including use of acidifying fruit juices or ingestion of vitamin C **to discourage bacterial growth and stone formation.**
- Instruct client/SO(s) in clean intermittent self-catheterization (CISC) techniques.
- Review signs/symptoms of complications requiring prompt medical evaluation/intervention.

Documentation Focus

Assessment/Reassessment
- Current elimination pattern and effect on lifestyle and sleep pattern.

Planning
- Plan of care and who is involved in planning.
- Teaching plan.

Implementation/Evaluation
- Response to interventions, teaching, and actions performed.
- Attainment or progress toward desired outcome(s).
- Modifications to plan of care.

Discharge Planning
- Long-term needs and who is responsible for actions to be taken.
- Specific referrals made.

Sample Nursing Outcomes & Interventions Classifications (NOC/NIC) NIC

NOC—Urinary Continence
NIC—Urinary Retention Care

---

reflex Urinary Incontinence

Taxonomy II: Elimination and Exchange—Class 1
  Urinary Function (00018)
[Diagnostic Division: Elimination]
Submitted 1986; Nursing Diagnosis Extension and
  Classification (NDEC) Revision 1998

Definition: Involuntary loss of urine at somewhat predictable intervals when a specific bladder volume is reached

---

Information that appears in brackets has been added by the authors to clarify and enhance the use of nursing diagnoses.

Related Factors

Tissue damage (e.g., due to radiation cystitis, inflammatory bladder conditions, radical pelvic surgery)

Neurological impairment above level of sacral or pontine micturition center

Defining Characteristics

Subjective

No sensation of bladder fullness, urge to void, or voiding

Sensation of urgency without voluntary inhibition of bladder contraction

Sensations associated with full bladder (e.g., sweating, restlessness, abdominal discomfort)

Objective

Predictable pattern of voiding

Inability to voluntarily inhibit or initiate voiding

Complete emptying with [brain] lesion above pontine micturition center

Incomplete emptying with [spinal cord] lesion above sacral micturition center

Desired Outcomes/Evaluation Criteria— Client Will:

• Verbalize understanding of condition or contributing factors.
• Establish bladder regimen appropriate for individual situation.
• Demonstrate behaviors or techniques to control condition and prevent complications.
• Urinate at acceptable times and places.

Actions/Interventions

Nursing Priority No. 1.

To assess degree of interference/disability:

• Note condition or disease process as listed in Related Factors (e.g., pelvic cancer, radiation, or surgery; CNS disorders, stroke, MS, Parkinson's disease, SCIs, and brain tumors resulting in neurogenic bladder [either hypnotic or spastic]) **affecting bladder storage, emptying, and control.**
• Note whether client experiences any sense of bladder fullness or awareness of incontinence. **Loss of sensation of bladder**

Information that appears in brackets has been added by the authors to clarify and enhance the use of nursing diagnoses.

  Cultural   Collaborative   Community/Home Care

filling can result in overfilling, inadequate emptying (retention), and dribbling. (Refer to NDs acute/chronic Urinary Retention; overflow Urinary Incontinence.)

- Review voiding diary, if available, or record frequency and time of urination. Compare timing of voidings, particularly in relation to liquid intake and medications.
- Measure amount of each voiding **because incontinence often occurs once a specific bladder volume is achieved.**
- Determine actual bladder volume (via bladder scan) in client with incomplete emptying or on scheduled catheterization **when attempting toilet training and to avoid unnecessary catheterizations.**
- Measure or scan postvoid residuals or catheterization volumes. **Determines frequency for emptying bladder and reduces incontinence episodes.**
- Evaluate client's ability to manipulate or use urinary collection device or catheter **to determine long-term need for assistance.**
- Refer to urologist or appropriate specialist for testing of bladder capacity and muscle fibers and sphincter control.

Nursing Priority No. 2.
To assist in managing incontinence:
- Collaborate in treatment of underlying cause or management of reflex incontinence.
- Determine availability and use of resources or assistance.
- Involve client/SO/caregiver in developing plan of care to address specific needs.
- Encourage minimum of 1500 to 2000 mL of fluid intake daily. **Regulating liquid intake at prescheduled times (with and between meals) promotes predictable voiding pattern.**
- Restrict fluids 2 to 3 hours before bedtime **to reduce nighttime voiding.**
- Instruct client, or take to toilet before the expected time of incontinence, **in an attempt to stimulate the reflex for voiding.**
- Instruct in measures, such as pouring warm water over perineum; running water in sink; stimulating or massaging tissues over bladder, lower abdomen, thighs **to stimulate voiding reflexes.**
- Set alarm to awaken during night to maintain schedule, or use external catheter or external collection device, as appropriate.
- Implement continuous catheterization or intermittent self-catheterization using small-lumen straight catheter, if

Information that appears in brackets has been added by the authors to clarify and enhance the use of nursing diagnoses.

 Diagnostic Studies ∞ Pediatric/Geriatric/Lifespan   Medications **877**

condition indicates, **to prevent overdistention with consequent infection and detrusor muscle damage.**

Nursing Priority No. 3.
To promote wellness (Teaching/Discharge Considerations):

- Encourage continuation of regular toileting or bladder program **to limit overdistention and related complications.**
- Suggest use of incontinence pads or pants during day and for social contact, if appropriate, dependent on client's activity level, amount of urine loss, manual dexterity, and cognitive ability.
- Stress importance of perineal care following voiding and frequent changing of incontinence pads, if used.
- Encourage limited intake of coffee, tea, and alcohol **because of diuretic effect, which may affect predictability of voiding pattern.**
- Instruct in proper care of catheter and cleaning techniques **to reduce risk of infection.**
- Review signs/symptoms of urinary complications and need for timely medical follow-up care.

Documentation Focus

Assessment/Reassessment
- Individual findings including degree of disability and effect on lifestyle.
- Availability of resources or support person.

Planning
- Plan of care and who is involved in planning.
- Teaching plan.

Implementation/Evaluation
- Responses to treatment plan, interventions, and actions performed.
- Attainment or progress toward desired outcome(s).
- Modifications to plan of care.

Discharge Planning
- Long-term needs and who is responsible for actions to be taken.
- Available resources, equipment needs and sources.

Information that appears in brackets has been added by the authors to clarify and enhance the use of nursing diagnoses.

⊕ Cultural   ⊛ Collaborative   🏠 Community/Home Care

Sample Nursing Outcomes & Interventions Classifications (NOC/NIC) [NIC]

NOC—Urinary Continence
NIC—Urinary Bladder Training

---

risk for urge **Urinary Incontinence**

Taxonomy II: Elimination and Exchange—Class 1 Urinary Function (00022)
[Diagnostic Division: Elimination]
Submitted 1998 (Nursing Diagnosis Extension and Classification [NDEC])

Definition: At risk for an involuntary loss of urine associated with a sudden, strong sensation or urinary urgency

---

Risk Factors

Effects of medications, caffeine, or alcohol
Detrusor hyperreflexia (e.g., from cystitis, urethritis, tumors, renal calculi, CNS disorders above pontine micturition center)
Impaired bladder contractility; involuntary sphincter relaxation
Ineffective toileting habits
Small bladder capacity

> **NOTE:** A risk diagnosis is not evidenced by signs and symptoms as the problem has not occurred; rather, nursing interventions are directed at prevention.

Desired Outcomes/Evaluation Criteria— Client Will:

- Identify individual risk factors and appropriate interventions.
- Demonstrate behaviors or lifestyle changes to prevent development of problem.

Actions/Interventions

Nursing Priority No. 1.
To assess potential for developing incontinence:

- Identify client with potential for urge incontinence as noted in Risk Factors.
- Note presence of conditions often associated with urgent voiding (e.g., stroke, MS, Parkinson's disease, spinal cord injury,

---

Information that appears in brackets has been added by the authors to clarify and enhance the use of nursing diagnoses.

Alzheimer's disease, obesity, pelvic inflammatory disease, abdominal or pelvic surgeries, urinary tract infections) **affecting bladder capacity; pelvic, bladder, or urethral musculature tone and/or innervation.**

- Determine use or presence of bladder irritants (e.g., significant intake of alcohol or caffeine), **resulting in increased output or concentrated urine.**
- Review client's medication regimen (e.g., diuretics, antipsychotic agents, sedatives) **for use of drugs that increase urine production or that may impair client's recognition of or ability to respond to urge to void.**
- Review history for long-standing habits or medical conditions (e.g., frequent voluntary voiding, impaired mobility, use of sedatives) **that may reduce bladder capacity.**
- Note conditions (e.g., impaired sensory perception or mobility, cognitive impairment or dementia, CNS disorders) **that may affect ability to respond to urge to void.**
- Measure amount of urine voided, especially noting amounts less than 100 mL or greater than 550 mL **to determine bladder capacity and effectiveness of bladder contractions to facilitate emptying.**
- Prepare for, and assist with, appropriate testing (e.g., urinalysis, noninvasive bladder scanning, cystometrogram) **to evaluate voiding pattern, identify potential functional concerns.**

Nursing Priority No. 2.

To prevent occurrence of problem:

- Assist in treatment of underlying conditions that may contribute to urge incontinence.
- Ascertain client's awareness and concerns about developing problem and whether lifestyle might be affected (e.g., daily living activites, socialization, sexual patterns).
- Regulate liquid intake at prescheduled times (with and between meals) **to promote predictable voiding pattern.**
- Establish schedule for voiding (habit training) based on client's usual voiding pattern.
- Provide assistance or devices, as indicated, for clients who are mobility impaired (e.g., providing means of summoning assistance; placing bedside commode, urinal, or bedpan within client's reach).
- Encourage regular pelvic floor strengthening exercises or Kegel exercises.

Information that appears in brackets has been added by the authors to clarify and enhance the use of nursing diagnoses.

  Cultural   Collaborative   Community/Home Care

Nursing Priority No. 3.

To promote wellness (Teaching/Discharge Considerations):

 • Provide information to client/SO(s) about potential for urge incontinence and lifestyle measures to prevent or limit incontinence:

Recommend limiting intake of coffee, tea, and alcohol **because of their irritating effect on the bladder.**

Suggest wearing loose-fitting or especially adapted clothing **to facilitate response to voiding urge.**

 • Emphasize importance of perineal care after each voiding **to reduce risk of ascending infection.**

Documentation Focus

Assessment/Reassessment
• Individual findings, including specific risk factors and pattern of voiding.

Planning
• Plan of care, specific interventions, and who is involved in planning.
• Teaching plan.

Implementation/Evaluation
• Response to interventions, teaching, and actions performed.
• Attainment or progress toward desired outcome(s).
• Modifications to plan of care.

Discharge Planning
• Discharge needs and who is responsible for actions to be taken.
• Specific referrals made.

Sample Nursing Outcomes & Interventions Classifications (NOC/NIC) [NIC]

NOC—Urinary Continence
NIC—Urinary Habit Training

Information that appears in brackets has been added by the authors to clarify and enhance the use of nursing diagnoses.

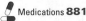

Taxonomy II: Elimination and Exchange—Class 1
 Urinary Function (00017)
[Diagnostic Division: Elimination]
Submitted 1986; Revised 2006

Definition: Sudden leakage of urine with activities that increase intra-abdominal pressure

Related Factors

Degenerative changes in pelvic muscles; weak pelvic muscles
High intra-abdominal pressure [e.g., obesity, gravid uterus]
Intrinsic urethral sphincter deficiency

Defining Characteristics

Subjective

Reported involuntary leakage of small amounts of urine: on exertion [e.g., lifting, impact aerobics]; with sneezing, laughing, or coughing; in the absence of detrusor contraction/an overdistended bladder

Objective

Observed involuntary leakage of small amounts of urine: on exertion [e.g., lifting, impact aerobics]; with sneezing, laughing, or coughing; in the absence of detrusor contraction/an overdistended bladder

Desired Outcomes/Evaluation Criteria—Client Will:

- Verbalize understanding of condition and interventions for bladder conditioning.
- Demonstrate behaviors or techniques to strengthen pelvic floor musculature.
- Remain continent even with increased intra-abdominal pressure.

Actions/Interventions

Nursing Priority No. 1.

To assess causative/contributing factors:

- Identify physiological causes of increased intra-abdominal pressure (e.g., obesity, gravid uterus, repeated heavy lifting);

Information that appears in brackets has been added by the authors to clarify and enhance the use of nursing diagnoses.

🌐 Cultural 🔄 Collaborative 🏠 Community/Home Care

contributing history such as multiple births; bladder or pelvic trauma, fractures; surgery (e.g., radical prostatectomy, bladder or other pelvic surgeries that may damage sphincter muscles); and participation in high-impact athletic or military field activities (particularly women).

- Assess for urine loss (usually small amount) with coughing, sneezing, or sports activities; relaxed pelvic musculature and support, noting inability to start or stop stream while voiding, bulging of perineum when bearing down.
- Review client's medications for those that may cause or exacerbate stress incontinence (e.g., alpha-adrenergic blockers, ACE inhibitors, loop diuretics).

Nursing Priority No. 2.
To assess degree of interference/disability:

- Observe voiding patterns, time and amount voided, and stimulus provoking incontinence. Review voiding diary, if available.
- Prepare for, and assist with, appropriate testing (e.g., urinalysis, noninvasive bladder scanning, cystogram, urodynamics, leak point pressure) **to evaluate functional concerns.**
- Determine effect on lifestyle (including daily activities; participation in sports, exercise or recreation; socialization; sexuality; and self-esteem).
- Ascertain methods of self-management (e.g., regularly timed voiding, limiting liquid intake, using undergarment protection).
- Assess for concomitant urge or functional incontinence, noting whether bladder irritability, reduced bladder capacity, or voluntary overdistention is present. (Refer to appropriate NDs.)

Nursing Priority No. 3.
To assist in treating/preventing incontinence:

- Suggest and implement self-help techniques:

    Practice timed voidings (e.g., every 3 hours during the day) **to keep bladder relatively empty.**

    Void before physical exertion, such as exercise/sports activites, heavy lifting, **to reduce potential for incontinence.**

    Encourage weight loss, as indicated, **to reduce pressure on pelvic organs.**

    Suggest limiting use of coffee, tea, and alcohol **because of diuretic effect.**

Information that appears in brackets has been added by the authors to clarify and enhance the use of nursing diagnoses.

Recommend regular pelvic-floor-strengthening exercises (Kegel exercises).

Suggest starting and stopping stream two or three times during voiding **to isolate muscles involved in voiding process for exercise training.**

Incorporate "bent-knee sit-ups" into exercise program **to increase abdominal muscle tone.**

Restrict intake 2 to 3 hours prior to bedtime **to decrease incontinence during sleep.**

- Assist with medical treatment of underlying urological condition, as indicated (e.g., surgery to reposition bladder or strengthen pelvic musculature; use of vaginal cones; electrical stimulation; biofeedback; medications [e.g., tricylic antidepressants, hormone replacement therapy]).

Nursing Priority No. 4.
To promote wellness (Teaching/Discharge Considerations):

- Discuss participation in incontinence management for activities such as heavy lifting, impact aerobics **that increase intra-abdominal pressure.** Substitute swimming, bicycling, or low-impact exercise.
- Refer to weight-loss program or support group **when obesity is a contributing factor.**
- Suggest use of incontinence pads or pants, as needed. Consider client's activity level, amount of urine loss, physical size, manual dexterity, and cognitive ability **to determine specific product choices best suited to individual situation and needs.**
- Stress importance of perineal care following voiding and frequent changing of incontinence pads **to prevent irritation and infection.** Recommend application of oil-based emollient **to protect skin from irritation.**
- Review use of sympathomimetic drugs, if prescribed, **to improve resting tone of the bladder neck and proximal urethra.**

Documentation Focus

Assessment/Reassessment
- Individual findings including pattern of incontinence and physical factors present.
- Effect on lifestyle and self-esteem.
- Client understanding of condition.

Information that appears in brackets has been added by the authors to clarify and enhance the use of nursing diagnoses.

      Cultural   Collaborative   Community/Home Care

Planning
- Plan of care and who is involved in the planning.
- Teaching plan.

Implementation/Evaluation
- Responses to interventions, teaching, actions performed, and changes that are identified.
- Attainment or progress toward desired outcome(s).
- Modifications to plan of care.

Discharge Planning
- Long-term needs and who is responsible for specific actions.
- Specific referrals made.

Sample Nursing Outcomes & Interventions Classifications (NOC/NIC) NIC

NOC—Urinary Continence
NIC—Pelvic Muscle Exercise

[total Urinary Incontinence]

Taxonomy II: Elimination—Class 1 Urinary System (00021)
[Diagnostic Division: Elimination]
Submitted 1986/Retired from Taxonomy 2009

Definition: Continuous and unpredictable loss of urine

Related Factors

Neuropathy preventing transmission of reflex [signals to the reflex arc] indicating bladder fullness
Neurological dysfunction [e.g., cerebral lesions]
Independent contraction of detrusor reflex
Trauma/disease affecting spinal cord nerves [destruction of sensory or motor neurons below the injury level]
Anatomical (fistula)

Defining Characteristics

Subjective
Constant flow of urine at unpredictable times without uninhibited bladder contractions or spasm, or distention

---

Information that appears in brackets has been added by the authors to clarify and enhance the use of nursing diagnoses.

Nocturia
Lack of bladder or perineal filling [awareness]
Unawareness of incontinence

Objective
Unsuccessful incontinence refractory treatments

Desired Outcomes/Evaluation Criteria— Client/Caregiver Will:

- Verbalize awareness of causative or contributing factors.
- Establish bladder regimen for individual situation.
- Demonstrate behaviors, techniques to manage condition and to prevent complications.
- Manage incontinence so that social functioning is regained or maintained.

Actions/Interventions

Nursing Priority No. 1.
To assess causative/contributing factors:

- Identify client with condition(s) causing actual or potential for total incontinence as listed in Related Factors: High-risk persons include frail elderly; women; those with brain lesions (e.g., stroke, tumors, trauma); SCI (e.g., quadraplegia, paraplegia, herniated disc, pelvic crush injury); chronic neurological diseases (e.g., MS, Parkinson's disease); genitourinary surgery or trauma (e.g., childbirth, radical hysterectomy, perineal resection, prostatectomy); peripheral neuropathy (e.g., diabetes, AIDS, poliomyelitis); and lifestyle issues (e.g., certain medications, fluid intake, mobility limitations).
- Be aware of and note effect of global neurological impairment, neuromuscular trauma from surgery, childbirth, or radiation; or presence of fistula. **Conditions causing injury to nerves supplying the bladder are associated with loss of integrity of lower urinary tract function.**
- Determine if client is aware of incontinence. **Cognitive or developmental issues and/or medical conditions can impair client's awareness and sensory perception of voiding need/process and incontinence.**
- Check for perineal sensation and fecal impaction **to determine whether sensation and reflexes are impaired when neurological condition is present.**

Information that appears in brackets has been added by the authors to clarify and enhance the use of nursing diagnoses.

  Cultural   Collaborative   Community/Home Care

- Determine concomitant chronic retention (e.g., palpate bladder, scan or catheterize for urine volume and residual). **Retention may be associated with outlet obstruction, urge, and overflow incontinence.**
- Assess for continuous involuntary loss of urine at all times and in all positions. **Usually associated with urinary tract fistula or genital malformation.**
- Assist with procedures or tests (e.g., postvoid residual, urine flowmetry, pressure flow study, cystoscopy, cystogram) **to establish diagnosis and identify appropriate interventions.**

Nursing Priority No. 2.
To assess degree of interference/disability:

- Determine client's particular symptoms (e.g., continuous dribbling superimposed upon an otherwise normal voiding pattern, or high-volume urine loss that replaces any detectable pattern of bladder filling, storage, orvoiding). **Influences choice of interventions.**
- Have client/caregiver keep an incontinence chart. Note times of voiding and incontinence. **Determines pattern of urination and whether there is any control.**
- Review history for past interventions regarding alterations in urinary elimination **to ascertain cause for continence failure (e.g., client unable to sustain behavioral management of bladder training program, or medical conditions do not allow for success in voiding efforts).**
- Evaluate client's potential for bladder training or voiding managment program. **Dependent on diagnosed type of incontinence (functional, overflow, reflex, urge).**
- Ascertain effect of condition on lifestyle and self-esteem.

Nursing Priority No. 3.
To assist in preventing/managing incontinence:

- Collaborate in treatment of underlying conditions (e.g., neurological disorders, prostate problems, chronic urinary tract infections, psychiatric disorders) **that contribute to incontinence.**
- Implement bladder training and/or incontinence management, as indicated:

  Provide ready access to bathroom, commode, bedpan, or urinal.

  Encourage adequate fluid intake and regulate time of intake.

  Establish voiding or bladder emptying schedule.

Information that appears in brackets has been added by the authors to clarify and enhance the use of nursing diagnoses.

Use condom catheter or other external device, if tolerated, during the day and absorptive pads during the night, if external device is not tolerated.

Implement intermittent or continuous catheterization appropriate to client's condition (may be of short- or long-term duration).

Refer to NDs functional, stress, urge, reflex, overflow Urinary Incontinence for related interventions.

Administer medications, as indicated.

- Discuss and prepare for surgical intervention depending on underlying cause (e.g., to treat urethral hypermobility, to suspend bladder, repair vaginal walls, remove obstruction, provide artificial sphincter or bladder reservoir).

Nursing Priority No. 4.
To promote wellness (Teaching/Discharge Considerations):

- Assist client/caregiver to identify regular time for bladder program **to establish a predictable elimination program.**
- Suggest use of incontinence pads or adult briefs, as indicated (e.g., during social contacts), **for extra protection and to enhance confidence.**
- Stress importance of pericare after each voiding (using alcohol-free products) and application of oil-based emollient **to protect the skin from irritation.**
- Instruct in proper care of catheter and cleaning technique **to prevent infection.**
- Recommend use of silicone catheter **when long-term or continuous placement is indicated after other measures/bladder training have failed.**
- Encourage self-monitoring of catheter patency and avoidance of reflux of urine. **Reduces risk of infection.**
- Suggest intake of acidifying juices **to discourage bacterial growth and reduce incidence of infection.**

Documentation Focus

Assessment/Reassessment
- Current elimination pattern.
- Assessment findings including effect on lifestyle and self-esteem.

Planning
- Plan of care, specific interventions, and who is involved in planning.
- Teaching plan.

Information that appears in brackets has been added by the authors to clarify and enhance the use of nursing diagnoses.

  Cultural   Collaborative   Community/Home Care

Implementation/Evaluation
- Response to interventions, teaching, and actions performed.
- Attainment or progress toward desired outcome(s).
- Modifications to plan of care.

Discharge Planning
- Discharge plan/long-term needs and who is responsible for actions to be taken.
- Specific referrals made.

Sample Nursing Outcomes & Interventions Classifications (NOC/NIC) (NIC)

NOC—Urinary Continence
NIC—Urinary Incontinence Care

---

urge Urinary Incontinence

Taxonomy II: Elimination and Exchange—Class 1
  Urinary Function (00019)
[Diagnostic Division: Elimination]
Submitted 1986; Revised 2006

Definition: Involuntary passage of urine occurring soon after a strong sense of urgency to void

---

Related Factors

Decreased bladder capacity
Bladder infection; atrophic urethritis or vaginitis
Alcohol or caffeine intake; [increased fluids]
Use of diuretics
Fecal impaction
Detrusor hyperactivity with impaired bladder contractility

Defining Characteristics

Subjective
Reports: urinary urgency; involuntary loss of urine with bladder contractions or spasms; inability to reach toilet in time to avoid urine loss

Objective
Observed inability to reach toilet in time to avoid urine loss

---

Information that appears in brackets has been added by the authors to clarify and enhance the use of nursing diagnoses.

 Diagnostic Studies   Pediatric/Geriatric/Lifespan   Medications **889**

Desired Outcomes/Evaluation Criteria—Client Will:

- Verbalize understanding of condition.
- Demonstrate behaviors or techniques to control or correct situation.
- Report increase in interval between urge and involuntary loss of urine.
- Void every 3 to 4 hours in individually appropriate amounts.

Actions/Interventions

Nursing Priority No. 1.

To assess causative/contributing factors:

- Note presence of conditions often associated with urgent voiding (e.g., stroke, MS, Parkinson's disease, SCI, Alzheimer's disease, obesity, pelvic inflammatory disease, abdominal or pelvic surgeries, recent or lengthy use of indwelling urinary catheter) **affecting bladder capacity; pelvic, bladder, or urethral musculature tone; and/or innervation.**
- Ask client about urgency (more than just normal desire to void). **Urgency (also sometimes called overactive bladder syndrome) is a sudden compelling need to void that is difficult to defer and may be accompanied by leaking or incontinence.**
- Note factors that may affect ability to respond to urge to void in timely manner (e.g., impaired mobility, debilitation, sensory or perceptual impairments).
- Review client's medications and substance use (e.g., diuretics, antipsychotic agents, sedatives, caffeine, alcohol) **for agents that increase urine production or exert a bladder irritant effect.**
- Assess for signs and symptoms of bladder infection (e.g., cloudy, odorous urine; burning pain with voiding; bacteriuria) **associated with acute, painful urgency symptoms.**
- Prepare for and assist with appropriate testing (e.g., pre- or postvoid bladder scanning; pelvic examination for strictures; impaired perineal sensation or musculature; urinalysis; uroflowmetry voiding pressures; cystoscopy; cystometrogram) **to determine anatomical and functional status of bladder and urethra.**
- Assess for concomitant stress or functional incontinence. **Older women often have a mix of stress and urge incontinence, while individuals with dementia or disabling**

Information that appears in brackets has been added by the authors to clarify and enhance the use of nursing diagnoses.

 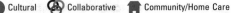 Cultural   Collaborative   Community/Home Care

neurological disorders tend to have urge and functional incontinence. (Refer to NDs stress/functional Urinary Incontinence for additional interventions.)

Nursing Priority No. 2.
To assess degree of interference/disability:

- Record frequency of voiding during a typical 24-hour period.
- Discuss degree of urgency and length of warning time between initial urge and loss of urine.
- Ascertain if client experiences triggers (e.g., sound of running water, putting hands in water, seeing a restroom sign, "key-in-the-lock" syndrome).
- Measure amount of urine voided, especially noting amounts less than 100 mL or greater than 550 mL. **Bladder capacity may be impaired or bladder contractions facilitating emptying may be ineffective.** (Refer to ND [acute/chronic] Urinary Retention.)
- Ascertain effect on lifestyle (including daily activities, socialization, sexuality) and self-esteem.

Nursing Priority No. 3.
To assist in treating/preventing incontinence:

- Collaborate in treating underlying cause and/or managing urge symptoms.
- Administer medications as indicated (e.g., antibiotic for urinary tract infection, or antimuscarinics [e.g., oxybutynin, tolterodine]) **to reduce voiding frequency and urgency by blocking overactive detrusor contractions.**
- Provide assistance or devices, as indicated, for client who is mobility impaired (e.g., provide means of summoning assistance; place bedside commode, urinal, or bedpan within client's reach).
- Offer assistance to cognitively impaired client (e.g., prompt client, or take to bathroom on regularly timed schedule) **to reduce frequency of incontinence episodes and promote comfort.**
- Recommend lifestyle changes:

    Adjust fluid intake to 1500 to 2000 mL/day. Regulate liquid intake at prescheduled times (with and between meals) and limit fluids 2 to 3 hours prior to bedtime **to promote predictable voiding pattern and limit nocturia.**

    Modify diet as indicated (e.g., reduce caffeine, citrus juices, spicy foods, etc.) **to reduce bladder irritation.**

Information that appears in brackets has been added by the authors to clarify and enhance the use of nursing diagnoses.

Manage bowel elimination **to prevent urinary problems associated with constipation or fecal impaction.**

 • Encourage client to participate in behavioral interventions, if able:

Establish voiding schedule (habit and bladder training) based on client's usual voiding pattern and gradually increase time interval.

Recommend consciously delaying voiding by using distraction (e.g., slow deep breaths); self-statements (e.g., "I can wait"); and contracting pelvic muscles when exposed to triggers. **Behavioral techniques for urge suppression.**

Encourage regular pelvic floor strengthening exercises or Kegel exercises as indicated by specific condition.

Instruct client to tighten pelvic floor muscles before arising from bed. **Helps prevent loss of urine as abdominal pressure changes.**

Suggest starting and stopping stream two or more times during voiding **to isolate muscles involved in voiding process for exercise training.**

• Refer to specialists or treament program, as indicated, for additional and specialized interventions (e.g., biofeedback, use of vaginal cones, electronic stimulation therapy, possible surgical interventions).

Nursing Priority No. 4.
To promote wellness (Teaching/Discharge Considerations):

• Encourage comfort measures (e.g., use of incontinence pads or undergarments, wearing loose-fitting or especially adapted clothing) **to prepare for and manage urge incontinence symptoms over the long term, and enhance sense of security and confidence in abilities to be socially active.**

• Emphasize importance of regular perineal care **to prevent skin irritation and incontinence-related dermatitis.**

• Identify signs/symptoms indicating urinary complications and need for timely medical follow-up care.

Documentation Focus

Assessment/Reassessment
• Individual findings, including pattern of incontinence, effect on lifestyle, and self-esteem.

Information that appears in brackets has been added by the authors to clarify and enhance the use of nursing diagnoses.

Planning

- Plan of care, specific interventions, and who is involved in planning.
- Teaching plan.

Implementation/Evaluation

- Response to interventions, teaching, and actions performed.
- Attainment or progress toward desired outcome(s).
- Modifications to plan of care.

Discharge Planning

- Discharge needs and who is responsible for actions to be taken.
- Specific referrals made.

Sample Nursing Outcomes & Interventions Classifications (NOC/NIC) NIC

NOC—Urinary Continence
NIC—Urinary Habit Training

[acute/chronic] Urinary Retention

Taxonomy II: Elimination and Exchange—Class 1 Urinary Function (00023)
[Diagnostic Division: Elimination]
Submitted 1986

Definition: Incomplete emptying of the bladder

Related Factors

High urethral pressure
Inhibition of reflex arc
Strong sphincter; blockage [e.g., benign prostatic hypertrophy—BPH, perineal swelling, trauma]
[Infections; neurological diseases]
[Use of medications with side effect of retention (e.g., atropine, belladonna, psychotropics, antihistamines, opiates)]

Information that appears in brackets has been added by the authors to clarify and enhance the use of nursing diagnoses.

 Diagnostic Studies ∞ Pediatric/Geriatric/Lifespan Medications **893**

Defining Characteristics

Subjective
Sensation of bladder fullness
Dribbling
Dysuria

Objective
Bladder distention
Small or frequent voiding; absence of urine output
Residual urine [150 mL or more]
Overflow incontinence
Reduced stream

Desired Outcomes/Evaluation Criteria— Client Will:

- Verbalize understanding of causative factors and appropriate interventions for individual situation.
- Demonstrate techniques or behaviors to alleviate or prevent retention.
- Void in sufficient amounts with no palpable bladder distention; experience no postvoid residuals greater than 50 mL; have no dribbling or overflow.

Actions/Interventions

Acute

Nursing Priority No. 1.
To assess causative/contributing factors:

- Note presence of pathological conditions (e.g., UTI, neurological disorders or trauma, stone formation, prostate hypertrophy).
- Investigate reports of sudden loss of ability to pass urine or great difficulty passing urine, pain with urination, blood in urine. **May indicate UTI or obstruction.**
- Obtain urine and review results of urinalysis (e.g., presence of red or white blood cells, nitrates, glucose, bacteria) and culture, as indicated, **to determine presence of treatable condition.**
- Review medications, noting those that can cause or exacerbate retention (e.g., psychotropics, anesthesia, opiates, sedatives, alpha- and beta-adrenergic blockers, anticholinergics, antihistamines, neuroleptics).

Information that appears in brackets has been added by the authors to clarify and enhance the use of nursing diagnoses.

 Cultural 🌐 Collaborative 🏠 Community/Home Care

- Examine for fecal impaction, surgical site swelling, postpartal edema, vaginal or rectal packing, enlarged prostate, or other factors (e.g., recent removal of indwelling catheter with urethral swelling or spasm) **that may produce a blockage of the urethra.**
- Determine anxiety level (e.g., **client may be too embarrassed to void in presence of others).**

Nursing Priority No. 2.
To determine degree of interference/disability:

- Ascertain whether client has sensation of bladder fullness, and determine level of discomfort. **Sensation and discomfort can vary, depending on underlying cause of retention.**
- Determine if there has been any significant urine output in the last 6 to 8 hours; presence of frequent/small voidings, and whether dribbling (overflow) is occurring.
- Palpate height of the bladder. Ascertain whether client has sensation of bladder fullness.
- Note recent amount and type of fluid intake.
- Prepare for and assist with urodynamic testing (e.g., cystometrogram **to measure bladder pressure and volume**, bladder scan **to measure retention volume and/or postvoid residual),** or abdominal leak point pressure test.

Nursing Priority No. 3.
To assist in treating/preventing retention:

- Relieve pain by administering appropriate medications and measures **to reduce swelling or treat underlying cause.**
- Assist client to sit upright on bedpan or commode, or stand **to provide functional position of voiding.**
- Provide privacy.
- Use ice techniques, spirits of wintergreen, stroking inner thigh, running water in sink or warm water over perineum **to stimulate reflex arc.**
- Remove blockage if possible (e.g., vaginal packing, bowel impaction). Prepare for more aggressive intervention (e.g., surgery, prostatectomy).
- Catheterize with intermittent or indwelling catheter **to resolve acute retention.**
- Drain bladder with straight catheter per agency protocol. **References are mixed as to need for fractional drainage in increments of 200 mL at a time to prevent possibility of bladder spasm, syncope, or hypotension.**

Information that appears in brackets has been added by the authors to clarify and enhance the use of nursing diagnoses.

- Reduce recurrences by controlling causative or contributing factors when possible (e.g., ice to perineum **to prevent swelling**, use of stool softeners or laxatives, change of medication or dosage).

Nursing Priority No. 4.

To promote wellness (Teaching/Discharge Considerations):

- Encourage client to report problems immediately **so treatment can be instituted promptly.**
- Emphasize need for adequate fluid intake.

Chronic

Nursing Priority No. 1.

To assess causative/contributing factors:

- Review medical history for diagnoses, such as congenital defects, neurological disorders (e.g., MS, polio), prostatic hypertrophy or surgery, birth canal injury or scarring, SCI with lower motor neuron injury **that may suggest detrusor muscle atrophy/dysfunction, or chronic overdistention because of outlet obstruction.**
- Determine presence of weak or absent sensory and/or motor impulses (as with stroke, spinal injury, or diabetes).
- Evaluate customary fluid intake.
- Assess for effects of psychotropics, antihistamines, atropine, belladonna, and so forth.

Nursing Priority No. 2.

To determine degree of interference/disability:

- Measure amount voided and postvoid residuals.
- Determine frequency and timing of voiding, and/or dribbling.
- Note size and force of urinary stream.
- Palpate height of bladder.
- Determine presence of bladder spasms.
- Ascertain effect of condition on functioning and lifestyle.
- Prepare for and assist with urodynamic testing (e.g., uroflowmetry **to assess voiding speed and urine volume,** cystometrogram **to measure bladder pressure and volume,** bladder scan **to measure retention and/or postvoid residual),** or abdominal leak point pressure test.

Nursing Priority No. 3.

To assist in treating/preventing retention:

Information that appears in brackets has been added by the authors to clarify and enhance the use of nursing diagnoses.

      Cultural   Collaborative   Community/Home Care

- Collaborate in treatment of underlying conditions.
- Recommend client void on frequent, timed schedule **to maintain low bladder pressures.**
- Maintain consistent fluid intake **to wash out bacteria or avoid infections, and limit stone formation.**
- Adjust fluid amount and timing, if indicated, **to prevent bladder distention.**
- Demonstrate and instruct client/SO(s) in use of Credé's maneuver **to facilitate emptying of the bladder.**
- Encourage client to use Valsalva's maneuver if appropriate **to increase intra-abdominal pressure.**
- Establish regular voiding or self-catheterization program **to prevent reflux and increased renal pressures.**
- Refer for consideration of advanced or research-based therapies (e.g., implanted sacral, tibial, or pelvic electrical stimulating device) **for long-term management of retention.**

Nursing Priority No. 4.
To promote wellness (Teaching/Discharge Considerations):

- Establish regular schedule for bladder emptying whether voiding or using catheter.
- Stress need for adequate fluid intake, including use of acidifying fruit juices or ingestion of vitamin C, **to discourage bacterial growth and stone formation.**
- Instruct client/SO(s) in clean intermittent self-catheterization (CISC) techniques.
- Review signs/symptoms of complications requiring medical evaluation/intervention.

Documentation Focus

Assessment/Reassessment
- Individual findings, including nature of problem, degree of impairment, and whether client is incontinent.

Planning
- Plan of care and who is involved in planning.
- Teaching plan.

Implementation/Evaluation
- Response to interventions, teaching, and actions performed.
- Attainment or progress toward desired outcome(s).
- Modifications to plan of care.

Information that appears in brackets has been added by the authors to clarify and enhance the use of nursing diagnoses.

Discharge Planning
- Long-term needs and who is responsible for actions to be taken.
- Specific referrals made.

Sample Nursing Outcomes & Interventions Classifications (NOC/NIC) NIC

NOC—Urinary Elimination
NIC—Urinary Retention Care

---

impaired spontaneous Ventilation

Taxonomy II: Activity/Rest—Class 2 Cardiovascular/
   Pulmonary Response (00033)
[Diagnostic Division: Respiration]
Submitted 1992

Definition: Decreased energy reserves results in an
individual's inability to maintain breathing adequate
to support life

Related Factors

Metabolic factors; [hypermetabolic state (e.g., infection), nutritional deficits/depletion of energy stores]
Respiratory muscle fatigue
Airway size or resistance; inadequate secretion management

Defining Characteristics

Subjective
Dyspnea
Apprehension

Objective
Increased metabolic rate
Increased heart rate
Increased restlessness; decreased cooperation
Increased use of accessory muscles
Decreased tidal volume
Decreased PO_2, SaO_2; increased PCO_2

Information that appears in brackets has been added by the authors to clarify
and enhance the use of nursing diagnoses.

🌐 Cultural   🅐 Collaborative   🏠 Community/Home Care

Desired Outcomes/Evaluation Criteria—
Client Will:

- Reestablish and maintain effective respiratory pattern via ventilator with absence of retractions or use of accessory muscles, cyanosis, or other signs of hypoxia; and with ABGs/SaO$_2$ within acceptable range.
- Participate in efforts to wean within individual ability, as appropriate.

Caregiver Will:

- Demonstrate behaviors necessary to maintain respiratory function.

Actions/Interventions

Nursing Priority No. 1.
To determine degree of impairment:

- Identify client with actual or impending respiratory failure (e.g., apnea or slow, shallow breathing; declining mentation or obtunded with need for airway protection).
- Assess spontaneous respiratory pattern, noting rate, depth, rhythm, symmetry of chest movement, use of accessory muscles **to measure work of breathing.**
- Auscultate breath sounds, noting presence or absence and equality of breath sounds, adventitious breath sounds.
- Evaluate ABGs and/or pulse oximetry and capnograpy **to determine presence and degree of arterial hypoxemia (<55%) and hypercapnea (CO$_2$ > 45%), resulting in impaired ventilation requiring ventilatory support.**
- Obtain or review results of pulmonary function studies (e.g., lung volumes, **inspiratory and expiratory pressures, and forced vital capacity), as appropriate, to assess presence and degree of respiratory insufficiency.**
- Investigate etiology of respiratory failure **to determine ventilation needs and most appropriate type of ventilatory support.**
- Review serial chest x-rays and imaging MRI/CT scans results **to diagnose disorder and monitor response to treatment.**
- Note response to respiratory therapy (e.g., bronchodilators, supplemental oxygen, nebulizer or intermittent positive-pressure breathing [IPPB] treatments).

Information that appears in brackets has been added by the authors to clarify and enhance the use of nursing diagnoses.

Nursing Priority No. 2.

To provide/maintain ventilatory support:

- Assist with implementation of ventilatory support, as indicated (e.g., ET or tracheal intubation with mechanical ventilation **to support compromised ventilation**).
- Observe overall breathing pattern, distinguishing between spontaneous respirations and ventilator breaths.
- Count client's respirations for 1 full minute and compare to desired or ventilator set rate.
- Verify that client's respirations are in phase with the ventilator. **Decreases work of breathing; maximizes O₂ delivery.**
- Inflate tracheal or ET tube cuff properly using minimal leak or occlusive technique. Check cuff inflation every 4 to 8 hours and whenever cuff is deflated and reinflated **to prevent risk associated with under- or overinflation.**
- Check tubing for obstruction (e.g., kinking or accumulation of water). Drain tubing as indicated; avoid draining toward client, or back into the reservoir **resulting in contamination and providing medium for growth of bacteria.**
- Check ventilator alarms for proper functioning. Do not turn off alarms, even for suctioning. Remove from ventilator and ventilate manually if source of ventilator alarm cannot be quickly identified and rectified. Verify that alarms can be heard in the nurses' station by care providers.
- Assess ventilator settings routinely and readjust as indicated according to client's primary disease and results of diagnostic testing.
- Verify that oxygen line is in proper outlet/tank; monitor inline oxygen analyzer or perform periodic oxygen analysis.
- Verify tidal volume set to volume needed for individual situation, and proper functioning of spirometer, bellows, or computer readout of delivered volume. Note alterations from desired volume delivery **to determine alteration in lung compliance or leakage through machine/around tube cuff (if used).**
- Monitor airway pressure **for developing complications or equipment problems.**
- Monitor inspiratory and expiratory (I:E) ratio.
- Promote maximal ventilation of alveoli; check sigh rate intervals (usually $1\frac{1}{2}$ to 2 times tidal volume). **Reduces risk of atelectasis, helps mobilize secretions.**
- Note inspired humidity and temperature; maintain hydration **to liquefy secretions, facilitating removal.**

Information that appears in brackets has been added by the authors to clarify and enhance the use of nursing diagnoses.

- Auscultate breath sounds periodically. Investigate frequent crackles or rhonchi that do not clear with coughing or suctioning—**suggestive of developing complications (atelectasis, pneumonia, acute bronchospasm, pulmonary edema).**
- Suction as needed **to clear secretions and maintain airway.**
- Note changes in chest symmetry. **May indicate improper placement of ET tube, development of barotrauma.**
- Keep resuscitation bag at bedside and ventilate manually whenever indicated (e.g., if client is removed from ventilator or when troubleshooting equipment problems).
- Administer sedation as required **to synchronize respirations and reduce work of breathing and energy expenditure, as indicated.**
- Administer and monitor response to medications that promote airway patency and gas exchange.

Nursing Priority No. 3.
To prepare for/assist with weaning process if appropriate:

- Determine physical and psychological readiness to wean, including specific respiratory parameters, absence of infection or cardiac failure, client alert and/or able to sustain spontaneous respiration, nutritional status sufficient to maintain work of breathing.
- Explain weaning activities and techniques, individual plan, and expectations. **Reduces fear of unknown.**
- Elevate head of bed or place in orthopedic chair, if possible, or position **to alleviate dyspnea and to facilitate oxygenation.**
- Assist client in "taking control" of breathing if weaning is attempted or ventilatory support is interrupted during procedure or activity.
- Coach client to take slower, deeper breaths, practice abdominal or pursed-lip breathing, assume position of comfort, and use relaxation techniques **to maximize respiratory function.**
- Assist client to practice effective coughing, secretion management.
- Provide quiet environment, calm approach, undivided attention of nurse. **Promotes relaxation, decreasing energy and oxygen requirements.**
- Involve family/SO(s) as appropriate. Provide diversional activity. **Helps client focus on something other than breathing.**

Information that appears in brackets has been added by the authors to clarify and enhance the use of nursing diagnoses.

- Instruct client in use of energy-saving techniques during care activities **to limit oxygen consumption and fatigue.**
- Acknowledge and provide ongoing encouragement for client's efforts. Communicate hope for successful weaning response (even partial). **Enhances commitment to continue activity, maximizing outcomes.**

Nursing Priority No. 4.

To prepare for discharge on ventilator when indicated:

- Ascertain plan for discharge placement (e.g., return home, short-term in subacute or rehabilitation center, or permanent placement in long-term care facility).
- Determine specific equipment needs. Identify resources for equipment needs and maintenance, and arrange for delivery prior to client discharge.
- Review layout of home, noting size of rooms, doorways, placement of furniture, number and type of electrical outlets, **to identify specific safety needs.**
- Obtain no-smoking signs to be posted in home. Encourage family members to refrain from smoking.
- Have family/SO(s) notify utility companies and fire department about ventilator in home.
- Develop emergency disaster plan to address backup electrical needs and possible evacuation if required.
- Review and provide written or audiovisual materials regarding proper ventilator management, maintenance, and safety **for reference in home setting, enhancing client's/SO's knowledge and level of comfort.**
- Demonstrate airway management techniques and proper equipment cleaning practices.
- Instruct SO(s)/caregivers in other pulmonary physiotherapy measures as indicated (e.g., chest physiotherapy).
- Allow sufficient opportunity for SO(s)/caregivers to practice new skills. Role-play potential crisis situations **to enhance confidence in ability to handle client's needs.**
- Identify signs/symptoms requiring prompt medical evaluation/intervention. **Timely treatment may prevent progression of problem.**
- Provide positive feedback and encouragement for efforts of SO(s)/caregivers. **Promotes continuation of desired behaviors.**
- List names and phone numbers for identified contact persons/resources. **Round-the-clock availability reduces sense of**

Information that appears in brackets has been added by the authors to clarify and enhance the use of nursing diagnoses.

 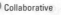 Cultural Collaborative Community/Home Care

isolation and enhances likelihood of obtaining appropriate information or assistance when needed.

Nursing Priority No. 5.

To promote wellness (Teaching/Discharge Considerations):

 • Discuss impact of specific activities on respiratory status and problem solve solutions to maximize weaning effort.

 • Engage client in specialized exercise program **to enhance respiratory muscle strength and general endurance.**

 • Protect client from sources of infection (e.g., monitor health of visitors, roommate(s), caregivers).

 • Recommend involvement in support group; introduce to individuals dealing with similar problems **to provide role models, assistance for problem solving.**

 • Encourage time-out for caregivers **so that they may attend to personal needs, wellness, and growth.**

 • Provide opportunities for client/SO(s) to discuss termination of therapy and other end-of-life decisions.

 • Refer to individual(s) who are ventilator dependent/have managed home ventilation successfully **to encourage hope for the future.**

 • Refer to additional resources (e.g., spiritual advisor, counselor).

Documentation Focus

Assessment/Reassessment
- Baseline findings, subsequent alterations in respiratory function.
- Results of diagnostic testing.
- Individual risk factors and concerns.

Planning
- Plan of care and who is involved in planning.
- Teaching plan.

Implementation/Evaluation
- Client's/SO's responses to interventions, teaching, and actions performed.
- Skill level and assistance needs of SO(s)/family.
- Attainment or progress toward desired outcome(s).
- Modifications to plan of care.

Information that appears in brackets has been added by the authors to clarify and enhance the use of nursing diagnoses.

Discharge Planning

- Discharge plan, including appropriate referrals, action taken, and who is responsible for each action.
- Equipment needs and source.
- Resources for support persons or home care providers.

Sample Nursing Outcomes & Interventions Classifications (NOC/NIC) [NIC]

NOC—Respiratory Status: Ventilation
NIC—Mechanical Ventilation Management: Invasive

---

dysfunctional Ventilatory Weaning Response

Taxonomy II: Activity/Rest—Class 4 Cardiovascular/
   Pulmonary Responses (00034)
[Diagnostic Division: Respiration]
Submitted 1992

Definition: Inability to adjust to lowered levels of mechanical ventilator support that interrupts and prolongs the weaning process

---

Related Factors

Physiological
Ineffective airway clearance
Sleep pattern disturbance
Inadequate nutrition
Uncontrolled pain
Muscle weakness or fatigue; inability to control respiratory
   muscles; immobility

Psychological
Knowledge deficit of the weaning process
Patient's perceived inefficacy about the ability to wean
Decreased motivation, self-esteem
Anxiety; fear; insufficient trust in the nurse
Hopelessness; powerlessness
Unprepared for weaning attempt

Situational
Uncontrolled episodic energy demands
Inappropriate pacing of diminished ventilator support

Information that appears in brackets has been added by the authors to clarify
and enhance the use of nursing diagnoses.

Inadequate social support

Adverse environment (e.g., noisy, active environment; negative events in the room; low nurse:patient ratio; unfamiliar nursing staff)

History of ventilator dependence >4 days

History of multiple unsuccessful weaning attempts

Defining Characteristics

Mild

Subjective

Expressed feelings of increased need for oxygen; breathing discomfort; fatigue; warmth

Queries about possible machine malfunction

Objective

Restlessness

Slight increase of respiratory rate from baseline

Increased concentration on breathing

Moderate

Subjective

Apprehension

Objective

Slight increase from baseline blood pressure (<20 mm Hg, heart rate <20 beats/min)

Baseline increase in respiratory rate (<5 breaths/min); slight respiratory accessory muscle use; decreased air entry on auscultation

Hypervigilance to activities; wide-eyed look

Inability to cooperate or respond to coaching

Diaphoresis

Color changes; pale; slight cyanosis

Severe

Objective

Agitation; decreased level of consciousness

Deterioration in arterial blood gases from current baseline

Increase from baseline blood pressure (≥20 mm Hg), heart rate (≥20 beats/min)

Respiratory rate increases significantly from baseline; full respiratory accessory muscle use; shallow or gasping breaths; paradoxical abdominal breathing

---

Information that appears in brackets has been added by the authors to clarify and enhance the use of nursing diagnoses.

Adventitious breath sounds, audible airway secretions
Asynchronized breathing with the ventilator
Profuse diaphoresis
Cyanosis

Desired Outcomes/Evaluation Criteria—Client Will:

- Actively participate in the weaning process.
- Reestablish independent respiration with ABGs within client's normal range and be free of signs of respiratory failure.
- Demonstrate increased tolerance for activity and participate in self-care within level of ability.

Actions/Interventions

Nursing Priority No. 1.
To identify contributing factors/degree of dysfunction:

- Determine extent and nature of underlying disorders or factors (e.g., preexisting cardiopulmonary diseases, significant trauma, neuromuscular disorders, complications from surgical procedures) **that contribute to client's reliance on mechanical support and can affect future weaning efforts.**
- Note length of time client has been receiving ventilator support. Review previous episodes of extubation and reintubation. **Previous unsuccessful weaning attempts (e.g., due to inability to protect airway or clear secretions; oxygen saturation less than 50% on room air) that can influence future weaning interventions.**
- Assess systemic parameters that may affect readiness for weaning using Burns Weaning Assessment Program (BWAP) or similar checklist (e.g., stability of vital signs, factors that increase metabolic rate [e.g., sepsis, fever]; hydration status; need for/recent use of analgesia or sedation; nutritional state; muscle strength; activity level).
- Ascertain client's alertness and understanding of weaning process, expectations, and concerns. **Client/SO(s) may need specific and repeated instructions during process.**
- Determine psychological readiness, presence and degree of anxiety. Introduce client to individual who has shared similar experiences with successful outcome if desired or indicated **to provide support and encouragement for successful outcome.**

Information that appears in brackets has been added by the authors to clarify and enhance the use of nursing diagnoses.

- Review laboratory studies (e.g., CBC reflecting number and integrity of red blood cells **[affects O$_2$ transport]**, serum albumin and electrolyte levels indicating nutritional status **[to confirm sufficient energy to meet demands of weaning]**).
- Review chest x-ray, pulse oximetry or capnography, and/or ABGs.

Nursing Priority No. 2.

To support weaning process:

- Consult with dietitian, nutritional support team for adjustments in composition of diet **to prevent excessive production of CO$_2$, which could alter respiratory drive.**
- Implement weaning protocols and mode (e.g., spontaneous breathing trials, partial client support [SIMV], or pressure support [PSV] during client's spontaneous breathing); **to determine if client can assume the full work of breathing and to provide support for spontaneous ventilation.**
- Discuss with client/SO(s) individual plan and expectations. Assure client of nurse's presence and assistance during weaning attempts. **May reduce client's anxiety about process and ultimate outcome and enhance willingness to work at spontaneous breathing.**
- Note response to activity/client care during weaning and limit, as indicated. Provide undisturbed rest or sleep periods. Avoid stressful procedures or situations and nonessential activities. **Prevents excessive O$_2$ consumption or demand with increased possibility of weaning failure.**
- Time medications during weaning efforts **to minimize sedative effects.**
- Provide quiet room, calm approach, undivided attention of nurse. **Enhances relaxation, conserving energy.**
- Involve SO(s)/family, as appropriate (e.g., sitting at bedside, providing encouragement, and helping monitor client status).
- Provide diversional activity (e.g., watching TV, reading aloud) **to focus attention away from breathing when not actively working at breathing exercises.**
- Auscultate breath sounds periodically; suction airway, as indicated.
- Acknowledge and provide ongoing encouragement for client's efforts.
- Minimize setbacks, focus client attention on gains and progress to date **to reduce frustration that may further impair progress.**

Information that appears in brackets has been added by the authors to clarify and enhance the use of nursing diagnoses.

- Suspend weaning (take a "holiday") periodically, as individually appropriate (e.g., initially may "rest" 45 or 50 minutes each hour, progressing to a 20-minute rest every 4 hours, then weaning during daytime and resting during night).
- Prepare client/SO(s) for alternative actions when client is unable to resume spontaneous ventilation (e.g., tracheostomy with long-term ventilation support in alternate care setting, palliative care or end-of-life procedures).

Nursing Priority No. 3.
To promote wellness (Teaching/Discharge Considerations):

- Discuss impact of specific activities on respiratory status and problem-solve solutions to maximize weaning effort.
- Engage in rehabilitation program **to enhance respiratory muscle strength and general endurance.**
- Teach client/SO(s) how to protect client from sources of infection (e.g., monitor health of visitors, persons involved in care; avoid crowds during flu season).
- Identify conditions requiring immediate medical intervention **to prevent respiratory failure.**

Documentation Focus

Assessment/Reassessment
- Baseline findings and subsequent alterations.
- Results of diagnostic testing or procedures.
- Individual risk factors.

Planning
- Plan of care, specific interventions, and who is involved in the planning.
- Teaching plan.

Implementation/Evaluation
- Client response to interventions.
- Attainment or progress toward desired outcome(s).
- Modifications to plan of care.

Discharge Planning
- Status at discharge, long-term needs and referrals, indicating who is to be responsible for each action.
- Equipment needs and supplier.

Information that appears in brackets has been added by the authors to clarify and enhance the use of nursing diagnoses.

Sample Nursing Outcomes & Interventions Classifications (NOC/NIC) NIC

NOC—Respiratory Status: Ventilation
NIC—Mechanical Ventilatory Weaning

> **NOTE:** NANDA has separated the diagnosis of Violence into its two elements: "other-directed" and "self-directed." However, the interventions in general address both situations and have been left in one block following the definitions and supporting data of the two diagnoses.

[actual/]risk for other-directed Violence

Taxonomy II: Safety/Protection—Class 3 Violence (00138)
[Diagnostic Division: Safety]
Submitted 1980; Revised 1996

Definition: At risk for behaviors in which an individual demonstrates that he or she can be physically, emotionally, and/or sexually harmful to others

Risk Factors/[Indicators]*

History of:

Violence against others (e.g., hitting, kicking, scratching, biting or spitting, throwing objects at someone; attempted rape, rape, sexual molestation; urinating or defecating on a person)

Threats (e.g., verbal threats against property or person, social threats, cursing, threatening notes or letters, threatening gestures, sexual threats)

Violent antisocial behavior (e.g., stealing, insistent borrowing, insistent demands for privileges, insistent interruption of meetings, refusal to eat or take medication, ignoring instructions)

---

*Although a risk diagnosis does not have defining characteristics (signs and symptoms), the factors identified here can be used to denote an actual diagnosis or as indicators of risk for/escalation of violence.

Information that appears in brackets has been added by the authors to clarify and enhance the use of nursing diagnoses.

✎ Diagnostic Studies   ∞ Pediatric/Geriatric/Lifespan   💊 Medications **909**

Indirect violence (e.g., tearing off clothes, urinating or defecating on floor, stamping feet, temper tantrum, running in corridors, yelling, writing on walls, ripping objects off walls, throwing objects, breaking a window, slamming doors, sexual advances)

Childhood abuse or witnessing family violence

Neurological impairment (e.g., positive EEG, CT, or MRI; neurological findings; head trauma; seizure disorders)

Cognitive impairment (e.g., learning disabilities, attention deficit disorder, decreased intellectual functioning); [organic brain syndrome]

Cruelty to animals; firesetting

Prenatal or perinatal complications

History of substance abuse; pathological intoxication; [toxic reaction to medication]

Psychotic symptomatology (e.g., auditory, visual, command hallucinations; paranoid delusions; loose, rambling, or illogical thought processes); [panic states; rage reactions; catatonic or manic excitement]

Motor vehicle offenses (e.g., frequent traffic violations, use of a motor vehicle to release anger)

Suicidal behavior; impulsivity; availability of weapon(s)

Body language (e.g., rigid posture, clenching of fists and jaw, hyperactivity, pacing, breathlessness, threatening stances)

Hormonal imbalance (e.g., premenstrual syndrome—PMS, postpartal depression or psychosis)

Expressed intent or desire to harm others directly or indirectly

Almost continuous thoughts of violence

[actual/]risk for self-directed Violence

Taxonomy II: Safety/Protection—Class 3 Violence (00140)
[Diagnostic Division: Safety]
Submitted 1994

Definition: At risk for behaviors in which an individual demonstrates that he or she can be physically, emotionally, and/or sexually harmful to self

---

Information that appears in brackets has been added by the authors to clarify and enhance the use of nursing diagnoses.

Cultural   Collaborative   Community/Home Care

Risk Factors/[Indicators]*

Ages 15 to 19 or over 45

Marital status (single, widowed, divorced)

Employment problems (e.g., unemployed, recent job loss or failure); occupation (executive, administrator or owner of business, professional, semiskilled worker)

Conflictual interpersonal relationships

Family background (e.g., chaotic or conflictual, history of suicide)

Sexual orientation (bisexual [active], homosexual [inactive])

Physical health problems (e.g., hypochondriac, chronic or terminal illness)

Mental health problems (e.g., severe depression, [bipolar disorder] psychosis, severe personality disorder, alcoholism or drug abuse)

Emotional problems (e.g., hopelessness, [lifting of depressed mood], despair, increased anxiety, panic, anger, hostility); history of multiple suicide attempts; suicidal ideation; suicidal plan

Lack of personal resources (e.g., poor achievement, poor insight, affect unavailable and poorly controlled)

Lack of social resources (e.g., poor rapport, socially isolated, unresponsive family)

Verbal clues (e.g., talking about death, "better off without me," asking questions about lethal dosages of drugs)

Behavioral clues (e.g., writing forlorn love notes, directing angry messages at an SO who has rejected the person, giving away personal items, taking out a large life insurance policy)

Desired Outcomes/Evaluation Criteria—[Other-Directed or Self-Directed] Client Will:

* Acknowledge realities of the situation.
* Verbalize understanding of why behavior occurs.
* Identify precipitating factors.
* Express realistic self-evaluation and increased sense of self-esteem.

---

*Although a risk diagnosis does not have defining characteristics (signs and symptoms), the factors identified here can be used to denote an actual diagnosis or as indicators of risk for/escalation of violence.

Information that appears in brackets has been added by the authors to clarify and enhance the use of nursing diagnoses.

- Participate in care and meet own needs in an assertive manner.
- Demonstrate self-control as evidenced by relaxed posture, nonviolent behavior.
- Use resources and support systems in an effective manner.

Actions/Interventions

Address both "other-directed" and "self-directed"

Nursing Priority No. 1.
To assess causative/contributing factors:

- Determine underlying dynamics as listed in Risk Factors.
- Ascertain client's perception of self and situation. Note use of defense mechanisms (e.g., denial, projection).
- Observe and listen for early cues of distress or increasing anxiety (e.g., irritability, lack of cooperation, demanding behavior, body posture or expression). **May indicate possibility of loss of control and intervention at this point can prevent a blowup.**
- Identify conditions such as acute or chronic brain syndrome, panic state, hormonal imbalance (e.g., PMS, postpartal psychosis), drug-induced, postanesthesia/postseizure confusion, traumatic brain injury. **These physical conditions may interfere with ability to control own behavior and will need specific interventions to manage.**
- Review laboratory findings (e.g., blood alcohol, blood glucose, ABGs, electrolytes, renal function tests).
- Observe for signs of suicidal/homicidal intent (e.g., perceived morbid or anxious feeling while with the client; warning from the client, "It doesn't matter," "I'd/They'd be better off dead"; mood swings; "accident-prone" or self-destructive behavior; suicidal attempts; possession of alcohol and/or other drug(s) in known substance abuser). (Refer to ND risk for Suicide.)
- Note family history of suicidal or homicidal behavior. **Children who grow up in homes where violence is accepted tend to grow up to use violence as a means of solving problems.**
- Ask directly if the person is thinking of acting on thoughts or feelings **to determine violent intent.**
- Determine availability of homicidal means.
- Assess client coping behaviors already present. *Note:* **Client may believe there are no alternatives other than violence, especially if individual has come from a family background of violence.**

Information that appears in brackets has been added by the authors to clarify and enhance the use of nursing diagnoses.

⊕ Cultural Ⓒ Collaborative ▲ Community/Home Care

- Identify risk factors and assess for indicators of child abuse or neglect: unexplained or frequent injuries, failure to thrive, and so forth.

Nursing Priority No. 2.

To assist client to accept responsibility for impulsive behavior and potential for violence:

- Develop therapeutic nurse-client relationship. Provide consistent caregiver when possible. **Promotes sense of trust, allowing client to discuss feelings openly.**
- Maintain straightforward communication **to avoid reinforcing manipulative behavior.**
- Discuss motivation for change (e.g., failing relationships, job loss, involvement with judicial system). **Crisis situation can provide impetus for change, but requires timely therapeutic intervention to sustain efforts.**
- Help client recognize that client's actions may be in response to own fear **(may be afraid of own behavior or loss of control)**, dependency, and feeling of powerlessness.
- Make time to listen to expressions of feelings. Acknowledge reality of client's feelings and that feelings are OK. (Refer to ND Self-Esteem [specify].)
- Confront client's tendency to minimize situation or behavior. **In domestic violence situations, individual may be remorseful after incident and will apologize and say that it won't happen again.**
- Review factors (feelings and events) involved in precipitating violent behavior.
- Discuss impact of behavior on others and consequences of actions.
- Acknowledge reality of suicide or homicide as an option. Discuss consequences of actions if they were to follow through on intent. Ask how it will help client to resolve problems. **Provides an opportunity for client to look at reality of choices and potential outcomes.**
- Accept client's anger without reacting on emotional basis. Give permission to express angry feelings in acceptable ways and let client know that staff will be available to assist in maintaining control. **Promotes acceptance and sense of safety.**
- Help client identify more appropriate solutions or behaviors (e.g., motor activities, exercise) **to lessen sense of anxiety and associated physical manifestations.**

Information that appears in brackets has been added by the authors to clarify and enhance the use of nursing diagnoses.

- Provide directions for actions client can take, avoiding negatives, such as "do nots."

Nursing Priority No. 3.
To assist client in controlling behavior:

- Contract with client regarding safety of self/others.
- Give client as much control as possible within constraints of individual situation. **Enhances self-esteem, promotes confidence in ability to change behavior.**
- Be truthful when giving information and dealing with client. **Builds trust, enhancing therapeutic relationship; prevents manipulative behavior.**
- Identify current and past successes and strengths. Discuss effectiveness of coping techniques used and possible changes. (Refer to ND ineffective Coping.) **Client is often not aware of positive aspects of life, and once recognized, these can be used as a basis for change.**
- Assist client to distinguish between reality and hallucinations or delusions.
- Approach in positive manner, acting as if the client has control and is responsible for own behavior. Be aware, though, that the client may not have control, especially if under the influence of drugs (including alcohol).
- Maintain distance and do not touch client without permission when situation indicates client does not tolerate such closeness (e.g., posttrauma response).
- Remain calm and state limits on inappropriate behavior (including consequences) in a firm manner.
- Direct client to stay in view of staff/caregiver.
- Administer prescribed medications (e.g., anti-anxiety or antipsychotic), taking care not to oversedate client. **The chemistry of the brain is changed by early violence and has been shown to respond to serotonin, as well as related neurotransmitter systems, which play a role in restraining aggressive impulses.**
- Monitor for possible drug interactions, cumulative effects of drug regimen (e.g., anticonvulsants, antidepressants).
- Give positive reinforcement for client's efforts. **Encourages continuation of desired behaviors.**
- Explore death fantasies when expressed (e.g., "I'll look down and watch them suffer; she'll be sorry") or the idea that death is not final (e.g., "I can come back").

Information that appears in brackets has been added by the authors to clarify and enhance the use of nursing diagnoses.

⊕ Cultural 🅐 Collaborative 🏠 Community/Home Care

Nursing Priority No. 4.

To assist client/SO(s) to correct/deal with existing situation:

* Gear interventions to individual(s) involved, based on age, relationship, and so forth.
* Maintain calm, matter-of-fact, nonjudgmental attitude. **Decreases defensive response.**
* Notify potential victims in the presence of serious homicidal threat in accordance with legal and ethical guidelines. **Various Tarasoff statutes exist in many states requiring mental health professionals to report specific threats to both the individual named and law enforcement.**
* Discuss situation with abused or battered person, providing accurate information about choices and effective actions that can be taken.
* Assist individual to understand that angry, vengeful feelings are appropriate in the situation but need to be expressed and not acted on. (Refer to ND Post-Trauma Syndrome, as psychological responses may be very similar.)
* Identify resources available for assistance (e.g., battered women's shelter, social services).

Nursing Priority No. 5.

To promote safety in event of violent behavior:

* Provide a safe, quiet environment and remove items from the client's environment that could be used to inflict harm to self or others.
* Maintain distance from client who is striking out or hitting and take evasive and controlling actions, as indicated.
* Call for additional staff/security personnel.
* Approach aggressive or attacking client from the front, just out of reach, in a commanding posture with palms down.
* Tell client to *STOP*. **This may be sufficient to help client control own actions.**
* Maintain direct, constant eye contact, when appropriate.
* Speak in a low, commanding voice.
* Provide client with a sense that caregiver is in control of the situation **to provide feeling of safety.**
* Maintain clear route for staff and client and be prepared to move quickly.
* Hold client, using restraints or seclusion, when necessary, until client regains self-control.
* Administer medication, as indicated, **to help client until able to regain self-control.**

Information that appears in brackets has been added by the authors to clarify and enhance the use of nursing diagnoses.

Nursing Priority No. 6.

To promote wellness (Teaching/Discharge Considerations):

- Promote client involvement in planning care within limits of situation, allowing for meeting own needs for enjoyment. **Individuals often believe they are not entitled to pleasure and good things in their lives and need to learn how to meet these needs.**
- Assist client to learn assertive rather than manipulative, nonassertive, or aggressive behavior. **Promotes behaviors that help client to engage in positive social activities with others.**
- Discuss reasons for client's behavior with SO(s). Determine desire and commitment of involved parties to sustain current relationships.
- Develop strategies to help parents learn more effective parenting skills (e.g., parenting classes, appropriate ways of dealing with frustrations). **Developing positive relationships has a powerful effect on helping children learn impulse control.**
- Identify support systems (e.g., family/friends, clergy). **In addition to the client, those around him or her need to learn how to be positive role models and display a broader array of skills for resolving problems.**
- Refer to formal resources, as indicated (e.g., individual or group psychotherapy, substance abuse treatment program, social services, safe house facility, parenting classes).
- Refer to NDs impaired Parenting; family Coping [specify]; Post-Trauma Syndrome.

Documentation Focus

Assessment/Reassessment

- Individual findings, including nature of concern (e.g., suicidal or homicidal), behavioral risk factors and level of impulse control, plan of action and means to carry out plan.
- Client's perception of situation, motivation for change.
- Family history of violence.
- Availability and use of resources.

Planning

- Plan of care and who is involved in the planning.
- Details of contract regarding violence to self/others.
- Teaching plan.

Information that appears in brackets has been added by the authors to clarify and enhance the use of nursing diagnoses.

⊕ Cultural　🅐 Collaborative　🏠 Community/Home Care

Implementation/Evaluation

- Actions taken to promote safety, including notification of parties at risk.
- Response to interventions, teaching, and actions performed.
- Attainment or progress toward desired outcome(s).
- Modifications to plan of care.

Discharge Planning

- Long-term needs and who is responsible for actions to be taken.
- Available resources, specific referrals made.

Sample Nursing Outcomes & Interventions Classifications (NOC/NIC) NIC

other-directed Violence
NOC—Aggression Self-Control
NIC—Anger Control Assistance

self-directed Violence
NOC—Impulse Self-Control
NIC—Behavior Management: Self-Harm

---

impaired Walking

Taxonomy II: Activity/Rest—Class 2 Activity/Exercise (00088)
[Diagnostic Division: Activity/Rest]
Submitted 1998; revised 2006

Definition: Limitation of independent movement within the environment on foot

---

Related Factors

Insufficient muscle strength; neuromuscular impairment; musculoskeletal impairment (e.g., contractures)
Limited endurance; deconditioning
Fear of falling; impaired balance
Impaired vision
Pain
Obesity
Depressed mood; cognitive impairment
Lack of knowledge

Information that appears in brackets has been added by the authors to clarify and enhance the use of nursing diagnoses.

Environmental constraints (e.g., stairs, inclines, uneven surfaces, unsafe obstacles, distances, lack of assistive devices or persons, restraints)

Defining Characteristics

Subjective or Objective

Impaired ability to walk required distances; walk on an incline/decline; walk on uneven surfaces; to navigate curbs, climb stairs

Specify level of independence—refer to ND impaired physical Mobility, for suggested functional level classification

Desired Outcomes/Evaluation Criteria— Client Will:

- Be able to move about within environment as needed or desired within limits of ability or with appropriate adjuncts.
- Verbalize understanding of situation or risk factors and safety measures.

Actions/Interventions

Nursing Priority No. 1.

To assess causative/contributing factors:

- Identify condition or diagnoses that contribute to difficulty walking (e.g., advanced age; acute illness; weakness, chronic illness [e.g., cardiopulmonary disorders, cancer, kidney disease]; recent surgery or trauma; osteo, rheumatoid, or gouty arthritis; leg, hip, or knee trauma or other disorders [e.g., fractures, tendon or ligament injury, amputation]; balance problems [e.g., inner ear infection, brain injury, stroke]; nerve disorders [e.g., MS, Parkinson's disease, cerebral palsy]; spinal abnormalities [disease, trauma, degeneration]; neuropathies [e.g., peripheral, diabetic, alcoholic]; degenerative muscle disorders [e.g., muscular dystrophy, myositis]; vision impairments; foot conditions [e.g., plantar warts, bunions, ingrown toenails, pressure ulcers]; cognitive dysfunction).
- Note client's particular symptoms related to walking (e.g., unable to bear weight, can't walk usual distance, limping, staggering, stiff leg, leg pain, shuffling, asymmetric or unsteady gait).
- Determine ability to follow directions and note emotional/behavioral responses that may be affecting the situation.

Information that appears in brackets has been added by the authors to clarify and enhance the use of nursing diagnoses.

⊕ Cultural ⊛ Collaborative 🏠 Community/Home Care

Nursing Priority No. 2.

To assess functional ability:

- Determine degree of impairment in relation to suggested functional scale (0–4), noting that impairment can be temporary, permanent, or progressive.
- Assist with or review results of mobility testing (e.g., timing of walking over fixed distance, distance walked over set period of time [endurance], limb movement analysis, leg strength and speed of walking, ambulatory activity monitoring) **for differential diagnosis and to guide treatment interventions.**
- Note emotional and behavioral responses of client/SO(s) to problems of mobility.

Nursing Priority No. 3.

To promote safe, optimal level of independence in walking:

- Assist with treatment of underlying condition causing dysfunction, as indicated by individual situation.
- Consult with physical therapist, occupational therapist, or rehabilitation team **for individualized mobility program, and identify and develop appropriate devices (e.g., shoe insert, leg brace to maintain proper foot alignment for walking, quad cane, hemiwalker).**
- Demonstrate use of and help client become comfortable with adjunctive devices (e.g., cane, crutches, walking cast or boot, walker, limb prosthesis, mobility scooter).
- Provide assistance when indicated (e.g., walking on uneven surfaces; client is weak or has to walk a distance; or vision, coordination, or posture are impaired).
- Schedule walking or exercise activities interspersed with adequate rest periods **to reduce fatigue.**
- Provide ample time to perform mobility-related tasks **to reduce risk of falling and manage fatigue or pain.**
- Encourage active and passive exercises. Advance levels of exercise, as able, **to increase stamina and endurance.**
- Provide safety measures, as indicated, including skin and tissue care, environmental management, and fall prevention.

Nursing Priority No. 4.

To promote wellness (Teaching/Discharge Considerations):

- Involve client/SO(s) in care, assisting them to learn ways of managing deficits **to enhance safety for client and SO(s)/ caregivers.**

Information that appears in brackets has been added by the authors to clarify and enhance the use of nursing diagnoses.

- Identify appropriate resources for obtaining and maintaining appliances, equipment, and environmental modifications **to promote mobility.**
- Instruct client/SO(s) in safety measures, as individually indicated (e.g., maintaining safe travel pathway, proper lighting and handrails on stairs) **to reduce risk of falls.**

Documentation Focus

Assessment/Reassessment
- Individual findings, including level of function and ability to participate in specific or desired activities.
- Equipment and assistive device needs.

Planning
- Plan of care and who is involved in the planning.
- Teaching plan.

Implementation/Evaluation
- Responses to interventions, teaching, and actions performed.
- Attainment or progress toward desired outcome(s).
- Modifications to plan of care.

Discharge Planning
- Discharge and long-term needs, noting who is responsible for each action to be taken.
- Specific referrals made.
- Sources for and maintenance of assistive devices.

Sample Nursing Outcomes & Interventions Classifications (NOC/NIC) NIC

NOC—Ambulation
NIC—Exercise Therapy: Ambulation

Wandering [specify sporadic or continuous]

Taxonomy II: Perception/Cognition—Class 2 Orientation (00154)
[Diagnostic Division: Safety]
Submitted 2000

Definition: Meandering, aimless, or repetitive locomotion that exposes the individual to harm; frequently incongruent with boundaries, limits, or obstacles

---

Information that appears in brackets has been added by the authors to clarify and enhance the use of nursing diagnoses.

Related Factors

Cognitive impairment (e.g., memory and recall deficits, disorientation, poor visuoconstructive or visuospatial ability, language defects); sedation

Cortical atrophy

Premorbid behavior (e.g., outgoing, sociable personality; premorbid dementia)

Separation from familiar environment; overstimulating environment

Emotional state (e.g., frustration, anxiety, boredom, depression, agitation)

Physiological state or need (e.g., hunger, thirst, pain, urination, constipation)

Time of day

Defining Characteristics

Objective

Frequent or continuous movement from place to place, often revisiting the same destinations

Persistent locomotion in search of something; scanning or searching behaviors

Haphazard locomotion; fretful locomotion; pacing; long periods of locomotion without an apparent destination

Locomotion into unauthorized or private spaces; trespassing

Locomotion resulting in unintended leaving of a premise

Inability to locate significant landmarks in a familiar setting; getting lost

Locomotion that cannot be easily dissuaded; shadowing a caregiver's locomotion

Hyperactivity

Periods of locomotion interspersed with periods of nonlocomotion (e.g., sitting, standing, sleeping)

Desired Outcomes/Evaluation Criteria— Client Will:

- Be free of injury, or unplanned exits.

Caregiver(s) Will:

- Modify environment, as indicated, to enhance safety.
- Provide for maximal independence of client.

Information that appears in brackets has been added by the authors to clarify and enhance the use of nursing diagnoses.

Actions/Interventions

Nursing Priority No. 1.

To assess degree of impairment/stage of disease process:

- Ascertain history of client's memory loss and cognitive changes.
- Note results of diagnostic testing, confirming diagnosis and type of dementia.
- Evaluate client's mental status during daytime and nighttime, noting when client's confusion is most pronounced and when client sleeps.
- Monitor client's use or need for assistive devices, such as glasses, hearing aids, cane.
- Assess frequency and pattern of wandering behavior (e.g., client may be goal-directed or non–goal-directed, may start wandering in late afternoon or evening [nocturnal]) **to determine individual risks and safety needs.**
- Determine bowel and bladder elimination pattern, timing of incontinence, presence of constipation **for possible correlation to wandering behavior.**
- Identify client's reason for wandering, if possible (e.g., looking for lost item, desire to go home, boredom, need for activity, hunger, thirst, or discomfort).
- Ascertain if client has delusions due to shadows, lights, and noises.

Nursing Priority No. 2.

To assist client/caregiver to deal with situations:

- Provide a structured daily routine. **Decreases wandering behavior and minimizes caregiver stress.**
- Encourage participation in family activities and familiar routines, such as folding laundry, listening to music, shared-walking time outdoors. **Activities and exercises may reduce anxiety and restlessness.**
- Offer drink of water or snack, bring client to bathroom on a regular schedule. **Wandering may at times be expressing a need.**
- Provide safe place for client to wander, away from safety hazards (e.g., hot water, kitchen stove, open stairway) and other, noisy clients. Arrange furniture, remove scatter rugs, electrical cords, and other high-risk items **to accommodate safe wandering.**
- Make sure that doors or gates have alarms or chimes and that alarms are turned on. Provide door and window locks that are

---

Information that appears in brackets has been added by the authors to clarify and enhance the use of nursing diagnoses.

Cultural   Collaborative   Community/Home Care

not within line of sight or easily opened **to prevent unsafe exits.**

🏠• Provide 24-hour supervision and reality orientation. **Client can be awake at any time and fail to recognize day/night routines.**

🏠• Sit with client and visit or reminiscence. Provide TV, radio, music.

• Avoid overstimulation from activities or new partner/roommate during rest periods when client is in a facility.

🏠• Use pressure-sensitive bed or chair alarms **to alert caregivers of movement.**

🏠• Avoid using physical or chemical restraints (sedatives) to control wandering behavior. **May increase agitation, sensory deprivation, and falls; may contribute to wandering behavior.**

• Provide consistent staff as much as possible.

• Provide room near monitoring station; check client location on frequent basis.

Nursing Priority No. 3.
To promote wellness (Teaching/Discharge Considerations):

🏠• Identify problems that are remediable and assist client/SO(s) to seek appropriate assistance and access resources. **Encourages problem solving to improve condition rather than accept the status quo.**

🏠• Notify neighbors about client's condition and request that they contact client's family or local police if they see client outside alone. **Community awareness can prevent/reduce risk of client being lost or hurt.**

🏠• Register client with community or national resources, such as Alzheimer's Association Safe Return Program, **to assist in identification, location, and safe return of individual with wandering behaviors.**

🏠• Help SO(s) develop plan of care when problem is progressive.

Ⓐ• Refer to community resources, such as day-care programs, support groups, respite care.

• Refer to NDs acute Confusion; chronic Confusion; impaired Environmental Interpretation Syndrome; disturbed Sensory Perception (specify); risk for Injury; risk for Falls.

Documentation Focus

Assessment/Reassessment
• Assessment findings, including individual concerns, family involvement, and support factors and availability of resources.

Information that appears in brackets has been added by the authors to clarify and enhance the use of nursing diagnoses.

Planning
- Plan of care and who is involved in planning.
- Teaching plan.

Implementation/Evaluation
- Responses of client/SO(s) to plan interventions and actions performed.
- Attainment or progress toward desired outcome(s).
- Modifications to plan of care.

Discharge Planning
- Long-term needs and who is responsible for actions to be taken.
- Specific referrals made.

Sample Nursing Outcomes & Interventions Classifications (NOC/NIC) NIC

NOC—Safe Wandering
NIC—Elopement Precautions

Information that appears in brackets has been added by the authors to clarify and enhance the use of nursing diagnoses.

Cultural   Collaborative   Community/Home Care

CHAPTER 5

Health Conditions and Client Concerns With Associated Nursing Diagnoses

This chapter presents 440 disorders, health conditions, and life situations reflecting all specialty areas, with associated nursing diagnoses written as client problem/need statements that include the "related to" and "evidenced by" components.

This section will facilitate and help validate the assessment and diagnosis steps of the nursing process. Because the nursing process is perpetual and ongoing, other nursing diagnoses may be appropriate based on changing individual situations. Therefore, the nurse must continually assess, identify, and validate new client needs and evaluate subsequent care. Once the appropriate nursing diagnoses have been selected from this chapter, the reader may refer to Chapter 4, which lists the 206 NANDA diagnoses, and review the diagnostic definition, defining characteristics, and related or risk factors for further validation. This step is necessary to determine if the nursing diagnosis is an accurate match, if more data are required, or if another diagnosis needs to be investigated.

To facilitate access to the health conditions or concerns and nursing diagnoses, the client needs have been listed alphabetically and coded to identify nursing specialty areas.

MS: Medical-Surgical
PED: Pediatric
OB: Obstetric
CH: Community/Home
PSY: Psychiatric/Behavioral
GYN: Gynecological

A separate category for geriatrics has not been made because geriatric concerns and conditions actually are subsumed under the other specialty areas, and elderly persons are susceptible to the majority of these problems.

Abdominal hysterectomy MS
Refer to Hysterectomy

Abdominal perineal resection MS
Also Refer to Surgery, general
disturbed Body Image may be related to presence of surgical wounds,
  possibly evidenced by verbalizations of feelings or perceptions, fear
  of reaction by others, preoccupation with change.
risk for Constipation: risk factors may include decreased physical activity, slowed gastric motility, abdominal muscle weakness, insufficient fluid intake, change in usual foods and/or eating pattern.*
risk for Sexual Dysfunction: risk factors may include altered body structure or function, radical resection, treatment procedures, vulnerability, psychological concern about response of significant other(s)
  [SO(s)], and disruption of sexual response pattern (e.g., erection difficulty).*

Abortion, elective termination OB
risk for decisional Conflict: risk factors may include unclear personal
  values or beliefs, lack of experience or interference with decision
  making, information from divergent sources, deficient support system.*
deficient Knowledge [Learning Need] regarding reproduction, contraception, self-care, Rh factor may be related to lack of exposure or
  recall, or misinterpretation of information, possibly evidenced by
  request for information, statement of misconception, inaccurate follow-through of instructions, development of preventable events or
  complications.
risk for Spiritual Distress/moral Distress: risk factors may include perception of moral or ethical implications of therapeutic procedure,
  time constraints for decision making.*
Anxiety [specify level] may be related to situational or maturational
  crises, unmet needs, unconscious conflict about essential values or
  beliefs, possibly evidenced by increased tension, apprehension, fear
  of unspecific consequences, sympathetic stimulation, focus on self.
acute Pain/impaired Comfort may be related to aftereffects of procedure, drug effect, possibly evidenced by verbal report, distraction
  behaviors, changes in muscle tone, changes in vital signs.
risk for maternal Injury: risk factors may include surgical procedure,
  effects of anesthesia and medications.*

Abortion, spontaneous termination OB
risk for Bleeding: risk factors may include abnormal blood profile (decreased hemoglobin [Hb], altered clotting factors).*
risk for Spiritual Distress: risk factors may include need to adhere to
  personal religious beliefs and practices, blame for loss directed at
  self or God.*
deficient Knowledge [Learning Need] regarding cause of abortion, self-
  care, contraception, future pregnancy may be related to lack of familiarity with new self or healthcare needs, sources for support,

---

*A risk diagnosis is not evidenced by signs and symptoms, as the problem has
not occurred; rather, nursing interventions are directed at prevention.

possibly evidenced by requests for information and statement of concern or misconceptions, development of preventable complications.

Grieving related to perinatal loss, possibly evidenced by crying, expressions of sorrow, or changes in eating habits or sleep patterns.

risk for Sexual Dysfunction: risk factors may include increasing fear of pregnancy and/or repeat loss, impaired relationship with SO(s), self-doubt regarding own femininity.*

Abruptio placentae   OB

risk for Shock: risk factors may include hypotension, hypovolemia.*

Fear related to threat of death (perceived or actual) to fetus and self, possibly evidenced by verbalization of specific concerns, increased tension, sympathetic stimulation.

acute Pain may be related to collection of blood between uterine wall and placenta, uterine contractions, possibly evidenced by verbal reports, abdominal guarding, muscle tension, or alterations in vital signs.

impaired fetal Gas Exchange may be related to altered uteroplacental O_2 transfer, possibly evidenced by alterations in fetal heart rate and movement.

Abscess, brain (acute)   MS

acute Pain may be related to inflammation, edema of tissues, possibly evidenced by reports of headache, restlessness, irritability, and moaning.

risk for Hyperthermia: risk factors may include inflammatory process, hypermetabolic state, and dehydration.*

acute Confusion may be related to physiological changes (e.g., cerebral edema, altered perfusion, fever), possibly evidenced by fluctuation in cognition or level of consciousness, increased agitation, restlessness, hallucinations.

risk for Suffocation/Trauma: risk factors may include development of clonic/tonic muscle activity and changes in consciousness (seizure activity).*

Abscess, skin/tissue   CH/MS

impaired Skin/Tissue Integrity may be related to immunological deficit, infection, possibly evidenced by disruption of skin, destruction of skin layers or tissues, invasion of body structures.

risk for Infection [spread]: risk factors may include broken skin, traumatized tissues, chronic disease, malnutrition, insufficient knowledge.*

Abuse, physical   CH/PSY

Also Refer to Battered child syndrome

risk for Trauma: risk factors may include vulnerable client, recipient of verbal threats, history of physical abuse.*

Powerlessness may be related to abusive relationship, lifestyle of helplessness as evidenced by verbal expressions of having no control, reluctance to express true feelings, apathy, passivity.

---

*A risk diagnosis is not evidenced by signs and symptoms, as the problem has not occurred; rather, nursing interventions are directed at prevention.

---

chronic low Self-Esteem may be related to situational or maturational crisis, overwhelming threat to self, personal vulnerability, inadequate support systems, possibly evidenced by verbalized concern about ability to deal with current situation, chronic worry, anxiety, depression, poor self-esteem, inability to problem-solve, high illness rate, destructive behavior toward self or others.

Sexual Dysfunction may be related to ineffectual or absent role model, vulnerability, physical abuse possibly evidenced by verbalizations, change in sexual behaviors or activities, inability to achieve desired satisfaction.

Abuse, psychological   CH/PSY

ineffective Coping may be related to situational or maturational crisis, overwhelming threat to self, personal vulnerability, inadequate support systems, possibly evidenced by verbalized concern about ability to deal with current situation, chronic worry, anxiety, depression, poor self-esteem, inability to problem-solve, high illness rate, destructive behavior toward self or others.

Powerlessness may be related to abusive relationship, lifestyle of helplessness as evidenced by verbal expressions of having no control, reluctance to express true feelings, apathy, passivity.

Sexual Dysfunction may be related to ineffectual or absent role model, vulnerability, psychological abuse (harmful relationship) possibly evidenced by reported difficulties, inability to achieve desired satisfaction, conflicts involving values, seeking confirmation of desirability.

Achalasia (cardiospasm)   MS

impaired Swallowing may be related to neuromuscular impairment, possibly evidenced by observed difficulty in swallowing or regurgitation.

imbalanced Nutrition: less than body requirements may be related to inability and/or reluctance to ingest adequate nutrients to meet metabolic demands and nutritional needs, possibly evidenced by reported or observed inadequate intake, weight loss, and pale conjunctiva and mucous membranes.

acute Pain may be related to spasm of the lower esophageal sphincter, possibly evidenced by reports of substernal pressure, recurrent heartburn, or gastric fullness (gas pains).

Anxiety [specify level]/Fear may be related to recurrent pain, choking sensation, altered health status, possibly evidenced by verbalizations of distress, apprehension, restlessness, or insomnia.

risk for Aspiration: risk factors may include regurgitation or spillover of esophageal contents.*

deficient Knowledge [Learning Need] regarding condition, prognosis, self-care, and treatment needs may be related to lack of familiarity with pathology and treatment of condition, possibly evidenced by requests for information, statement of concern, or development of preventable complications.

---

*A risk diagnosis is not evidenced by signs and symptoms, as the problem has not occurred; rather, nursing interventions are directed at prevention.

Acidosis, metabolic   MS
Refer to Diabetic ketoacidosis

Acidosis, respiratory   MS
Also Refer to underlying cause or condition

impaired Gas Exchange may be related to ventilation perfusion imbalance (decreased O_2-carrying capacity of blood, altered O_2 supply, alveolar-capillary membrane changes), possibly evidenced by dyspnea with exertion, tachypnea, changes in mentation, irritability, tachycardia, hypoxia, hypercapnia.

Acne   CH/PED
impaired Skin Integrity may be related to secretions, infectious process as evidenced by disruptions of skin surface.

disturbed Body Image may be related to change in visual appearance as evidenced by fear of rejection of others, focus on past appearance, negative feelings about body, change in social involvement.

situational low Self-Esteem may be related to adolescence, negative perception of appearance as evidenced by self-negating verbalizations, expressions of helplessness.

Acquired immune deficiency syndrome   CH
Refer to AIDS

Acromegaly   CH
chronic Pain may be related to soft tissue swelling, joint degeneration, peripheral nerve compression possibly evidenced by verbal reports, altered ability to continue previous activities, changes in sleep pattern, fatigue.

disturbed Body Image may be related to biophysical illness or changes, possibly evidenced by verbalization of feelings, concerns, fear of rejection or of reaction of others, negative comments about body, actual change in structure or appearance, change in social involvement.

risk for Sexual Dysfunction: risk factors may include altered body structure, changes in libido.*

Acute respiratory distress syndrome   MS
Refer to Respiratory distress syndrome, acute

Adams-Stokes syndrome   CH
Refer to Dysrhythmia

ADD   PED/PSY
Refer to Attention deficit disorder

Addiction   CH/PSY
Refer to specific substances; Substance dependence/abuse rehabilitation

Addison's disease   MS
deficient Fluid Volume [hypotonic] may be related to vomiting, diarrhea, increased renal losses, possibly evidenced by delayed capillary refill, poor skin turgor, dry mucous membranes, report of thirst.

---

*A risk diagnosis is not evidenced by signs and symptoms, as the problem has not occurred; rather, nursing interventions are directed at prevention.

---

risk for Electrolyte Imbalance: risk factors may include vomiting, diarrhea, endocrine dysfunction.*

decreased Cardiac Output may be related to hypovolemia and altered electrical conduction (dysrhythmias) and/or diminished cardiac muscle mass, possibly evidenced by alterations in vital signs, changes in mentation, and irregular pulse or pulse deficit.

CH

Fatigue may be related to decreased metabolic energy production, altered body chemistry (fluid, electrolyte, and glucose imbalance), possibly evidenced by unremitting, overwhelming lack of energy, inability to maintain usual routines, decreased performance, impaired ability to concentrate, lethargy, and disinterest in surroundings.

disturbed Body Image may be related to changes in skin pigmentation, mucous membranes, loss of axillary or pubic hair, possibly evidenced by verbalization of negative feelings about body and decreased social involvement.

risk for impaired physical Mobility: risk factors may include neuromuscular impairment (muscle wasting, weakness) and dizziness or syncope.*

imbalanced Nutrition: less than body requirements may be related to glucocorticoid deficiency; abnormal fat, protein, and carbohydrate metabolism; nausea, vomiting, anorexia, possibly evidenced by weight loss, muscle wasting, abdominal cramps, diarrhea, and severe hypoglycemia.

risk for impaired Home Maintenance: risk factors may include effects of disease process, impaired cognitive functioning, and inadequate support systems.*

Adenoidectomy   **PED/MS**
Refer to Tonsillectomy

Adjustment disorder   **PED/PSY**
Refer to Anxiety disorders—PED

Adoption/loss of child custody   **PSY**
risk for complicated Grieving: risk factors may include actual loss of child, expectations for future of child and self, thwarted grieving response to loss.*

risk for Powerlessness: risk factors may include perceived lack of options, no input into decision process, no control over outcome.*

Adrenal crisis, acute   **MS**
Also Refer to Addison's disease; Shock
deficient Fluid Volume [hypotonic] may be related to failure of regulatory mechanism (damage to or suppression of adrenal gland), inability to concentrate urine, possibly evidenced by decreased venous filling and pulse volume and pressure, hypotension, dry mucous membranes, changes in mentation, decreased serum sodium.

---

*A risk diagnosis is not evidenced by signs and symptoms, as the problem has not occurred; rather, nursing interventions are directed at prevention.

acute Pain may be related to effects of disease process, metabolic imbalances, decreased tissue perfusion, possibly evidenced by reports
of severe pain in abdomen, lower back, or legs.

impaired physical Mobility may be related to neuromuscular impairment, decreased muscle strength and control, possibly evidenced by
generalized weakness, inability to perform desired activities or
movements.

risk for Hyperthermia: risk factors may include presence of illness, infectious process, dehydration.*

risk for ineffective Protection: risk factors may include hormone deficiency, drug therapy, nutritional and metabolic deficiencies.*

Adrenalectomy   MS

ineffective tissue Perfusion (specify) may be related to hypovolemia
and vascular pooling (vasodilation), possibly evidenced by diminished pulse, pallor or cyanosis, hypotension, and changes in mentation.

risk for Infection: risk factors may include inadequate primary defenses
(incision, traumatized tissues), suppressed inflammatory response,
invasive procedures.*

deficient Knowledge [Learning Need] regarding condition, prognosis,
self-care and treatment needs may be related to unfamiliarity with
long-term therapy requirements, possibly evidenced by request for
information and statement of concern or misconceptions.

Adrenal insufficiency   CH
Refer to Addison's disease

Affective disorder   PSY
Refer to Bipolar disorder; Depressive disorders, major

Affective disorder, seasonal   PSY
Also Refer to Depressive disorders, major

intermittent ineffective Coping may be related to situational crisis (fall
or winter season), disturbance in pattern of tension release, and inadequate resources available, possibly evidenced by verbalizations
of inability to cope, changes in sleep pattern (too little or too much),
reports of lack of energy, fatigue, lack of resolution of problem,
behavioral changes (irritability, discouragement).

risk for imbalanced Nutrition: more/less than body requirements: risk
factors may include eating in response to internal cues other than
hunger, alteration in usual coping patterns, change in usual activity
level, decreased appetite, lack of energy or interest to prepare food.*

Agoraphobia   PSY
Also Refer to Phobia

Anxiety [panic] may be related to contact with feared situation (public
place, crowds), possibly evidenced by tachycardia, chest pain, dyspnea, gastrointestinal distress, faintness, sense of impending doom.

---

*A risk diagnosis is not evidenced by signs and symptoms, as the problem has
not occurred; rather, nursing interventions are directed at prevention.

Agranulocytosis   MS

risk for infection: risk factors may include suppressed inflammatory response.*

risk for impaired Oral Mucous Membrane: risk factors may include infection.*

risk for imbalanced Nutrition: less than body requirements: risk factors may include inability to ingest food or fluids (lesions of oral cavity).*

AIDS (acquired immunodeficiency syndrome)   MS

Also Refer to HIV positive

risk for Infection [progression to sepsis/onset of new opportunistic infection]: risk factors may include depressed immune system, use of antimicrobial agents, inadequate primary defenses, broken skin, traumatized tissue, malnutrition, environmental exposure, invasive techniques, and chronic disease processes.*

risk for deficient Fluid Volume: risk factors may include excessive losses: copious diarrhea, profuse sweating, vomiting, hypermetabolic state or fever, and restricted intake (nausea, anorexia, lethargy).*

acute/chronic Pain may be related to tissue inflammation or destruction—infections; internal or external cutaneous lesions; rectal excoriation; malignancies; necrosis; peripheral neuropathies, myalgias, and arthralgias, possibly evidenced by verbal reports, self-focusing, or narrowed focus; alteration in muscle tone; paresthesias; paralysis; guarding behaviors; changes in vital signs (acute); restlessness.

risk for ineffective Breathing Pattern/impaired Gas Exchange: risk factors may include muscular impairment—wasting of respiratory musculature, decreased energy, fatigue, decreased lung expansion; retained secretions—tracheobronchial obstruction; infectious or inflammatory process; pain, ventilation perfusion imbalance—*Pneumocystis carinii* pneumonia, other pneumonias, anemia.*

CH

imbalanced Nutrition: less than body requirements may be related to altered ability to ingest, digest, and/or absorb nutrients (nausea, vomiting, hyperactive gag reflex, gastrointestinal disturbances, fatigue); increased metabolic rate and nutritional needs (fever, infection); possibly evidenced by weight loss, decreased subcutaneous fat and muscle mass, lack of interest in food, aversion to eating, altered taste sensation, abdominal cramping, hyperactive bowel sounds, diarrhea, sore and inflamed buccal cavity, abnormal laboratory results—vitamin, mineral, and protein deficiencies; electrolyte imbalances.

Fatigue may be related to decreased metabolic energy production, increased energy requirements (hypermetabolic state), overwhelming psychological or emotional demands, altered body chemistry (side effects of medication, chemotherapy), sleep deprivation possibly evidenced by unremitting or overwhelming lack of energy, inability to maintain usual routines, decreased performance, impaired ability to concentrate, lethargy, listlessness, and disinterest in surroundings.

ineffective Protection may be related to chronic disease affecting immune and neurological systems, inadequate nutrition, drug therapies,

---

*A risk diagnosis is not evidenced by signs and symptoms, as the problem has not occurred; rather, nursing interventions are directed at prevention.

possibly evidenced by deficient immunity, impaired healing, neurosensory alterations, maladaptive stress response, fatigue, anorexia,
disorientation.

PSY

Social Isolation may be related to changes in physical appearance or
mental status, altered state of wellness, perceptions of unacceptable
social or sexual behavior or values, physical isolation, phobic fear
of others (transmission of disease), possibly evidenced by expressed
feelings of aloneness or rejection, absence of supportive SO(s), and
withdrawal from usual activities.

disturbed Thought Processes/chronic Confusion may be related to physiological changes (hypoxemia, central nervous system [CNS] infection by HIV, brain malignancies, and/or disseminated systemic opportunistic infection), altered drug metabolism or excretion,
accumulation of toxic elements (renal failure, severe electrolyte imbalance, hepatic insufficiency), possibly evidenced by clinical evidence of organic impairment, altered attention span, distractibility,
memory deficit, disorientation, cognitive dissonance, delusional
thinking, impaired ability to make decisions or problem-solve, inability to follow complex commands or mental tasks, loss of impulse
control, and altered personality.

AIDS dementia   CH
Also Refer to Dementia, presenile/senile

impaired Environmental Interpretation Syndrome may be related to dementia, depression, possibly evidenced by consistent disorientation,
inability to follow simple directions or instructions, loss of social
functioning from memory decline.

ineffective Protection may be related to chronic disease affecting immune and neurological systems, inadequate nutrition, drug therapies,
possibly evidenced by deficient immunity, impaired healing, neurosensory alterations, maladaptive stress response, fatigue, anorexia,
disorientation.

Alcohol abuse/withdrawal   CH/MS/PSY
Refer to Drug overdose, acute [depressants]; Delirium tremens; Substance dependency/abuse rehabilitation

Alcohol intoxication, acute   MS
Also Refer to Delirium tremens

acute Confusion may be related to substance abuse, hypoxemia, possibly evidenced by hallucinations, exaggerated emotional response,
fluctuation in cognition or level of consciousness, increased agitation.

risk for ineffective Breathing Pattern: direct effect of alcohol toxicity
on respiratory center and/or sedative drugs given to decrease alcohol
withdrawal symptoms, tracheobronchial obstruction, presence of
chronic respiratory problems, inflammatory process, decreased energy, fatigue.*

---

*A risk diagnosis is not evidenced by signs and symptoms, as the problem has
not occurred; rather, nursing interventions are directed at prevention.

---

risk for Aspiration: risk factors may include reduced level of consciousness, depressed cough or gag reflexes, delayed gastric emptying.*

Alcoholism   CH
Refer to Substance dependency/abuse rehabilitation

Aldosteronism, primary   MS
deficient Fluid Volume [isotonic] may be related to increased urinary losses, possibly evidenced by dry mucous membranes, poor skin turgor, dilute urine, excessive thirst, weight loss.

impaired physical Mobility may be related to neuromuscular impairment, weakness, and pain, possibly evidenced by impaired coordination, decreased muscle strength, paralysis, and positive Chvostek's and Trousseau's signs.

risk for decreased Cardiac Output: risk factors may include hypovolemia and altered electrical conduction or dysrhythmias.*

Alkalosis, metabolic   MS
Refer to underlying cause or condition, e.g., Renal dialysis

Alkalosis, respiratory   MS
Also Refer to underlying cause or condition

impaired Gas Exchange may be related to ventilation-perfusion imbalance (decreased O_2 carrying capacity of blood, altered O_2 supply, alveolar-capillary membrane changes), possibly evidenced by dyspnea, tachypnea, changes in mentation, tachycardia, hypoxia, hypocapnia.

Allergies, seasonal   CH
Refer to Hay fever

Alopecia   CH
disturbed Body Image may be related to effects of illness or therapy, or aging process, change in appearance, possibly evidenced by verbalization of feelings, concerns, fear of rejection or reaction of others, focus on past appearance, preoccupation with change, feelings of helplessness.

ALS   CH
Refer to Amyotrophic lateral sclerosis

Alzheimer's disease   CH
Also Refer to Dementia, presenile/senile

risk for Injury/Trauma: risk factors may include inability to recognize or identify danger in environment, disorientation, confusion, impaired judgment, weakness, muscular incoordination, balancing difficulties, altered perception, and seizure activity.*

chronic Confusion related to physiological changes (neuronal degeneration), possibly evidenced by inaccurate interpretation of or response to stimuli, progressive or long-standing cognitive impairment, short-term memory deficit, impaired socialization, altered personality, and clinical evidence of organic impairment.

---

*A risk diagnosis is not evidenced by signs and symptoms, as the problem has not occurred; rather, nursing interventions are directed at prevention.

disturbed Sensory Perception (specify) may be related to altered sensory reception, transmission, and/or integration (neurological disease or deficit), socially restricted environment (homebound, institutionalized), sleep deprivation, possibly evidenced by changes in usual response to stimuli, change in problem-solving abilities, exaggerated emotional responses (anxiety, paranoia, hallucinations), inability to tell position of body parts, diminished or altered sense of taste.

Sleep Deprivation may be related to sensory impairment, changes in activity patterns, psychological stress (neurological impairment), possibly evidenced by wakefulness, disorientation (day/night reversal), increased aimless wandering, inability to identify need or time for sleeping, changes in behavior, lethargy; dark circles under eyes, and frequent yawning.

ineffective Health Maintenance may be related to deterioration affecting ability in all areas, including coordination and communication, cognitive impairment, ineffective individual/family coping, possibly evidenced by reported or observed inability to take responsibility for meeting basic health practices, lack of equipment, financial, or other resources, and impairment of personal support system.

PSY

risk for Stress Overload: risk factors may include inadequate resources, chronic illness, physical demands, threats of violence.*

compromised family Coping/Caregiver Role Strain may be related to disruptive behavior of client, family grief about their helplessness watching loved one deteriorate, prolonged disease or disability progression that exhausts the supportive capacity of SO or family, highly ambivalent family relationships

risk for Relocation Stress Syndrome: risk factors may include little or no preparation for transfer to a new setting, changes in daily routine, sensory impairment, physical deterioration, separation from support systems.*

Amphetamine abuse   **PSY**
Refer to Stimulant abuse

Amputation   **MS**
risk for ineffective peripheral tissue Perfusion: risk factors may include reduced arterial or venous blood flow, tissue edema, hematoma formation, hypovolemia.*

acute Pain may be related to tissue and nerve trauma, psychological impact of loss of body part, possibly evidenced by reports of incisional or phantom pain, observed guarding or protective behavior, narrowed focus or self-focus, and changes in vital signs.

impaired physical Mobility may be related to loss of limb (primarily lower extremity), altered sense of balance, pain or discomfort, possibly evidenced by reluctance to attempt movement; impaired coordination; decreased muscle strength, control, and mass.

---

*A risk diagnosis is not evidenced by signs and symptoms, as the problem has not occurred; rather, nursing interventions are directed at prevention.

---

situational low Self-Esteem may be related to loss of a body part, change in functional abilities, possibly evidenced by verbalization of feelings of powerlessness, grief, preoccupation with loss, negative feelings about body, focus on past strength, function, or appearance; change in usual patterns of responsibility or physical capacity to resume role, fear of rejection or reaction by others, and unwillingness to look at or touch residual limb.

Amyotrophic lateral sclerosis (ALS) MS

impaired physical Mobility may be related to muscle wasting, weakness, possibly evidenced by impaired coordination, limited range of motion, and impaired purposeful movement.

ineffective Breathing Pattern/impaired spontaneous Ventilation may be related to neuromuscular impairment, decreased energy, fatigue, tracheobronchial obstruction, possibly evidenced by shortness of breath, fremitus, respiratory depth changes, and reduced vital capacity.

impaired Swallowing may be related to muscle wasting and fatigue, possibly evidenced by recurrent coughing or choking, and signs of aspiration.

PSY

Powerlessness [specify level] may be related to chronic and debilitating nature of illness, lack of control over outcome, possibly evidenced by expressions of frustration about inability to care for self and depression over physical deterioration.

Grieving may be related to perceived potential loss of self and physiopsychosocial well-being, possibly evidenced by sorrow, choked feelings, expression of distress, changes in eating habits, sleeping patterns, and altered communication patterns or libido.

CH

impaired verbal Communication may be related to physical barrier (neuromuscular impairment), possibly evidenced by impaired articulation, inability to speak in sentences, and use of nonverbal cues (changes in facial expression).

risk for Caregiver Role Strain: risk factors may include illness severity of care receiver, complexity and amount of home-care needs, duration of caregiving required, caregiver is spouse, family/caregiver isolation, lack of respite or recreation for caregiver.*

Anaphylaxis CH

Also Refer to Shock

ineffective Airway Clearance may be related to airway spasm (bronchial), laryngeal edema, possibly evidenced by diminished breath sounds, presence of adventitious sounds, cough ineffective or absent, difficulty vocalizing, wide-eyed.

decreased Cardiac Output may be related to decreased preload, increased capillary permeability (third spacing) and vasodilation,

---

*A risk diagnosis is not evidenced by signs and symptoms, as the problem has not occurred; rather, nursing interventions are directed at prevention.

possibly evidenced by tachycardia, palpitations, changes in blood pressure (BP), anxiety, restlessness.

Anemia   CH

Activity Intolerance may be related to imbalance between O_2 supply (delivery) and demand, possibly evidenced by reports of fatigue and weakness, abnormal heart rate or BP response, decreased exercise or activity level, and exertional discomfort or dyspnea.

imbalanced Nutrition: less than body requirements may be related to failure to ingest or inability to digest food or absorb nutrients necessary for formation of normal red blood cells (RBCs), possibly evidenced by weight loss or weight below normal for age, height, and body build; decreased triceps skinfold measurement, changes in gums or oral mucous membranes, decreased tolerance for activity, weakness, and loss of muscle tone.

deficient Knowledge [Learning Need] regarding condition, prognosis, self-care and treatment needs may be related to inadequate understanding or misinterpretation of dietary and physiological needs, possibly evidenced by inadequate dietary intake, request for information, and development of preventable complications.

Anemia, sickle cell   MS

impaired Gas Exchange may be related to decreased O_2-carrying capacity of blood, reduced RBC life span or premature destruction, abnormal RBC structure, increased blood viscosity, pulmonary congestion—impairment of surface phagocytosis; predisposition to bacterial pneumonia/pulmonary infarcts, possibly evidenced by dyspnea, use of accessory muscles, cyanosis or signs of hypoxia, tachycardia, changes in mentation, and restlessness.

ineffective tissue Perfusion: (specify) may be related to stasis, vaso-occlusive nature of sickling, inflammatory response, atrioventricular (AV) shunts in pulmonary and peripheral circulation, myocardial damage (small infarcts, iron deposits, fibrosis), possibly evidenced by signs and symptoms dependent on system involved, for example: renal—decreased specific gravity and pale urine in face of dehydration; cerebral—paralysis and visual disturbances; peripheral—distal ischemia, tissue infarctions, ulcerations, bone pain; cardiac—angina, palpitations.

                                                                  CH

acute/chronic Pain may be related to intravascular sickling with localized vascular stasis, occlusion, infarction or necrosis and deprivation of O_2 and nutrients, accumulation of noxious metabolites, possibly evidenced by reports of localized, generalized, or migratory joint and/or abdominal or back pain, guarding and distraction behaviors (moaning, crying, restlessness), facial grimacing, narrowed focus, and changes in vital signs.

deficient Knowledge [Learning Need] regarding disease process, genetic factors, prognosis, self-care and treatment needs may be related to lack of exposure or recall, misinterpretation of information, unfamiliarity with resources, possibly evidenced by questions, statement of concern or misconceptions, exacerbation of condition, inadequate follow-through of therapy instructions, and development of preventable complications.

risk for sedentary Lifestyle: risk factors may include lack of interest or motivation, lack of resources, lack of training or knowledge of specific exercise needs, safety concerns or fear of injury.*

PED

delayed Growth and Development may be related to effects and limitations of physical condition, possibly evidenced by altered physical growth and delay or difficulty performing skills typical of age group.

compromised family Coping may be related to chronic nature of disease and disability, family disorganization, presence of other crises or situations impacting significant person/parent, lifestyle restrictions, possibly evidenced by SO expressing preoccupation with own reaction and displaying protective behavior disproportionate to client's ability or need for autonomy.

Aneurysm, abdominal aortic (AAA)   MS
Refer to Aortic aneurysm, abdominal

Aneurysm, cerebral   MS
Refer to Cerebrovascular accident

Angina pectoris   MS
acute Pain may be related to decreased myocardial blood flow, increased cardiac workload/O_2 consumption, possibly evidenced by verbal reports, narrowed focus, distraction behaviors (restlessness, moaning), and autonomic responses (diaphoresis, changes in vital signs).

risk for decreased Cardiac Output: risk factors may include inotropic changes (transient or prolonged myocardial ischemia, effects of medications), alterations in rate, rhythm and electrical conduction, possibly evidenced by changes in hemodynamic readings, dyspnea, restlessness, decreased tolerance for activity, fatigue, diminished peripheral pulses, cool or pale skin, changes in mental status, and continued chest pain.*

Anxiety [specify level] may be related to situational crises, change in health status and/or threat of death, negative self-talk, possibly evidenced by verbalized apprehension, expressed concerns, association of condition with loss of abilities, facial tension, extraneous movements, and focus on self.

CH

Activity Intolerance may be related to imbalance between O_2 supply and demand, possibly evidenced by exertional dyspnea, abnormal pulse or BP response to activity, and electrocardiogram (ECG) changes.

deficient Knowledge [Learning Need] regarding condition, prognosis, self-care and treatment needs may be related to lack of exposure, inaccurate or misinterpretation of information, possibly evidenced by questions, request for information, statement of concern, and inaccurate follow-through of instructions.

---

*A risk diagnosis is not evidenced by signs and symptoms, as the problem has not occurred; rather, nursing interventions are directed at prevention.

risk for sedentary Lifestyle: risk factors may include lack of training or knowledge of specific exercise needs, safety concerns, fear of myocardial injury.*

risk for risk-prone health Behavior: risk factors may include condition requiring long-term therapy, changes in lifestyle, multiple stressors, assault to self-concept, and altered locus of control.*

Anorexia nervosa   MS

imbalanced Nutrition: less than body requirements may be related to psychological restrictions of food intake and/or excessive activity, laxative abuse, possibly evidenced by weight loss, poor skin turgor, decreased muscle tone, denial of hunger, unusual hoarding or handling of food, amenorrhea, electrolyte imbalance, cardiac irregularities, hypotension.

risk for deficient Fluid Volume: risk factors may include inadequate intake of food and liquids, chronic or excessive laxative or diuretic use.*

PSY

disturbed Thought Processes may be related to severe malnutrition, electrolyte imbalance; psychological conflicts, possibly evidenced by impaired ability to make decisions, problem-solve, non-reality-based verbalizations, ideas of reference, altered sleep patterns, altered attention span or distractibility, perceptual disturbances with failure to recognize hunger, fatigue, anxiety, and depression.

disturbed Body Image/chronic low Self-Esteem may be related to morbid fear of obesity, negative perception of body or self, perceived loss of control in some aspect of life, unmet dependency needs, personal vulnerability, dysfunctional family system, possibly evidenced by distorted view of body as fat even in presence of severe emaciation, use of denial, feeling powerless to prevent or make changes, expressions of shame or guilt, overly conforming, dependent on others' opinions.

impaired Parenting may be related to issues of control in family, situational or maturational crises, history of inadequate coping methods possibly evidenced by enmeshed family, dissonance among family members, focus on "identified patient," family developmental tasks not being met, family members acting as enablers, ill-defined family rules, functions, or roles.

Antisocial personality disorder   PSY

risk for other-directed Violence: risk factors may include contempt for authority or rights of others, inability to tolerate frustration, need for immediate gratification, easy agitation, vulnerable self-concept, inability to verbalize feelings, use of maladjusted coping mechanisms including substance use.*

ineffective Coping may be related to very low tolerance for external stress, lack of experience of internal anxiety (e.g., guilt, shame), personal vulnerability, unmet expectations, multiple life changes, possibly evidenced by choice of aggression and manipulation to handle

---

*A risk diagnosis is not evidenced by signs and symptoms, as the problem has not occurred; rather, nursing interventions are directed at prevention.

problems or conflicts, inappropriate use of defense mechanisms (e.g., denial, projection), chronic worry, anxiety, destructive behaviors, high rate of accidents.

chronic low Self-Esteem may be related to lack of positive and/or repeated negative feedback, unmet dependency needs, retarded ego development, dysfunctional family system, possibly evidenced by acting-out behaviors (e.g., substance abuse, sexual promiscuity, feelings of inadequacy, nonparticipation in therapy).

compromised/disabled family Coping may be related to family disorganization or role changes, highly ambivalent family relationships, client providing little support in turn for the primary person(s), history of abuse or neglect in the home, possibly evidenced by expressions of concern or complaints, preoccupation of primary person with own reactions to situation, display of protective behaviors disproportionate to client's abilities, or need for autonomy.

impaired Social Interaction may be related to inadequate personal resources (shallow feelings), immature interests, underdeveloped conscence, unaccepted social values, possibly evidenced by difficulty meeting expectations of others, lack of belief that rules pertain to self, sense of emptiness or inadequacy covered by expressions of self-conceit, arrogance, or contempt; behavior unaccepted by dominant cultural group.

Anxiety disorder, generalized   PSY

Anxiety [specify level]/Powerlessness may be related to real or perceived threat to physical integrity or self-concept (may or may not be able to identify the threat), unconscious conflict about essential values or beliefs and goals of life, unmet needs, negative self-talk, possibly evidenced by sympathetic stimulation, extraneous movements (foot shuffling, hand or arm fidgeting, rocking movements, restlessness), persistent feelings of apprehension and uneasiness, a general anxious feeling that client has difficulty alleviating, poor eye contact, focus on self, impaired functioning, free-floating anxiety, and nonparticipation in decision making.

ineffective Coping may be related to level of anxiety being experienced by the client, personal vulnerability, unmet expectations or unrealistic perceptions, inadequate coping methods and/or support systems, possibly evidenced by verbalization of inability to cope or problem-solve, excessive compulsive behaviors (e.g., smoking, drinking), and emotional or muscle tension, alteration in societal participation, high rate of accidents.

Insomnia may be related to psychological stress, repetitive thoughts, possibly evidenced by reports of difficulty in falling asleep, awakening earlier or later than desired, reports of not feeling rested, dark circles under eyes, and frequent yawning.

risk for compromised family Coping: risk factors may include inadequate or incorrect information or understanding by a primary person, temporary family disorganization and role changes, prolonged disability that exhausts the supportive capacity of SO(s).*

---

*A risk diagnosis is not evidenced by signs and symptoms, as the problem has not occurred; rather, nursing interventions are directed at prevention.

impaired Social Interaction/Social Isolation may be related to low self-concept, inadequate personal resources, misinterpretation of internal or external stimuli, hypervigilance, possibly evidenced by discomfort in social situations, withdrawal from or reported change in pattern of interactions, dysfunctional interactions, expressed feelings of difference from others, sad, dull affect.

Anxiety disorders   PED/PSY

[severe/panic] Anxiety may be related to situational or maturational crisis, internal transmission and contagion, threat to physical integrity or self-concept, unmet needs, dysfunctional family system, independence conflicts possibly evidenced by somatic complaints, nightmares, excessive psychomotor activity, refusal to attend school, persistent worry or fear of catastrophic doom to family or self.

ineffective Coping may be related to situational or maturational crisis, multiple life changes or losses, personal vulnerability, lack of self-confidence possibly evidenced by inability, to problem-solve, persistent or overwhelming fears, inability to meet role expectations, social inhibition, panic attacks.

impaired Social Interaction may be related to excessive self-consciousness, inability to interact with unfamiliar people, altered thought processes possibly evidenced by verbalized or observed discomfort in social situations, inability to receive or communicate a satisfying sense of belonging, caring, or interest; use of unsuccessful social interaction behaviors.

risk for Self-Mutilation/self-directed Violence: risk factors may include panic states, dysfunctional family, history of self-destructive behaviors, emotional disturbance, increasing motor activity.*

compromised/disabled family Coping may be related to situational or developmental crisis (e.g., divorce, addition to the family), unrealistic parental expectations, frequent disruptions in living arrangements, high-risk family situations (neglect or abuse, substance abuse), possibly evidenced by SO reports of frustration with clinging behaviors, emotional lability, harsh or punitive response to tyrannical behaviors, disproportionate protective behaviors.

Anxiolytic abuse   PSY
Refer to Depressant abuse

Aortic aneurysm, abdominal (AAA)   MS

risk for ineffective peripheral tissue Perfusion: risk factors may include interruption of arterial blood flow [embolus formation, spontaneous blockage of aorta].*

risk for Infection: risk factors may include turbulent blood flow through arteriosclerotic lesion.*

acute Pain may be related to vascular enlargement-dissection or rupture, possibly evidenced by verbal coded reports, guarding behavior, facial mask, change in abdominal muscle tone.

---

*A risk diagnosis is not evidenced by signs and symptoms, as the problem has not occurred; rather, nursing interventions are directed at prevention.

Health Conditions and Client Concerns   **941**

Aortic aneurysm repair, abdominal   MS

Also Refer to Surgery, general

Fear related to threat of injury or death, surgical intervention, possibly evidenced by verbal reports, apprehension, decreased self-assurance, increased tension, changes in vital signs.

risk for Bleeding: risk factors may include weakening of vascular wall, failure of vascular repair.*

risk for ineffective renal/peripheral tissue Perfusion: risk factors may include interruption of arterial blood flow, hypovolemia.*

Aortic stenosis   MS

decreased Cardiac Output may be related to structural changes of heart valve, left ventricular outflow obstruction, alteration of afterload (increased left ventricular end-diastolic pressure and systemic vascular resistance [SVR]), alteration in preload or increased atrial pressure and venous congestion, alteration in electrical conduction, possibly evidenced by fatigue, dyspnea, changes in vital signs and hemodynamic parameters, and syncope.

risk for impaired Gas Exchange: risk factors may include alveolar-capillary membrane changes, congestion.*

       CH

risk for acute Pain: risk factors may include episodic ischemia of myocardial tissues and stretching of left atrium.*

Activity Intolerance may be related to imbalance between O_2 supply and demand (decreased or fixed cardiac output), possibly evidenced by exertional dyspnea, reported fatigue or weakness, and abnormal BP or ECG changes or dysrhythmias in response to activity.

Aplastic anemia   CH

Also refer to Anemia

risk for ineffective Protection: risk factors may include abnormal blood profile (leukopenia, thrombocytopenia), drug therapies (antineoplastics, antibiotics, NSAIDs [nonsteroidal anti-inflammatory drugs], anticonvulsants).*

Fatigue may be related to anemia, disease states, malnutrition, possibly evidenced by verbalization of overwhelming lack of energy, inability to maintain usual routines or level of physical activity, tired, decreased libido, lethargy, increase in physical complaints.

Appendicitis   MS

acute Pain may be related to distention of intestinal tissues by inflammation, possibly evidenced by verbal reports, guarding behavior, narrowed focus, and diaphoresis, changes in vital signs.

risk for deficient Fluid Volume: risk factors may include nausea, vomiting, anorexia, and hypermetabolic state.*

risk for Infection: risk factors may include release of pathogenic organisms into peritoneal cavity.*

ARDS   MS

Refer to Respiratory distress syndrome, acute

---

*A risk diagnosis is not evidenced by signs and symptoms, as the problem has not occurred; rather, nursing interventions are directed at prevention.

Arrhythmia, cardiac   MS/CH
Refer to Dysrhythmia, cardiac

Arterial occlusive disease, peripheral   CH
ineffective peripheral tissue Perfusion may be related to decreased arterial blood flow, possibly evidenced by skin discolorations, temperature changes, altered sensation, claudication, delayed healing.
risk for impaired Walking: risk factors may include presence of circulatory problems, pain with activity.*
risk for impaired Skin/Tissue Integrity: risk factors may include altered
  circulation or sensation.*

Arthritis, juvenile rheumatoid   PED/CH
Also Refer to Arthritis, rheumatoid
risk for delayed Development: risk factors may include effects of physical disability and required therapy.*
risk for Social Isolation: risk factors may include delay in accomplishing developmental task, altered state of wellness, and changes in
  physical appearance.*

Arthritis, rheumatoid   CH
acute/chronic Pain may be related to accumulation of fluid, inflammatory process, degeneration of joint, and deformity, possibly evidenced by verbal reports, narrowed focus, guarding or protective
  behaviors, and physical and social withdrawal.
impaired physical Mobility/Walking may be related to musculoskeletal
  deformity, pain or discomfort, decreased muscle strength, possibly
  evidenced by limited range of motion, impaired coordination, reluctance to attempt movement, and decreased muscle strength, control,
  and mass.
Self-Care Deficit [specify] may be related to musculoskeletal impairment, decreased strength and endurance, limited range of motion,
  pain on movement, possibly evidenced by inability to manage activities of daily living (ADLs).
disturbed Body Image/ineffective Role Performance may be related to
  change in body structure or function, impaired mobility or ability to
  perform usual tasks, focus on past strength, function, or appearance,
  possibly evidenced by negative self-talk, feelings of helplessness,
  change in lifestyle or physical abilities, dependence on others for
  assistance, decreased social involvement.

Arthritis, septic   CH
acute Pain may be related to joint inflammation, possibly evidenced by
  verbal or coded reports, guarding behaviors, restlessness, narrowed
  focus.
impaired physical Mobility may be related to joint stiffness, pain or
  discomfort, reluctance to initiate movement, possibly evidenced by
  limited range of motion, slowed movement.
Self-Care Deficit [specify] may be related to musculoskeletal impairment, pain or discomfort, decreased strength, impaired coordination,
  possibly evidenced by inability to perform desired ADLs.

---

*A risk diagnosis is not evidenced by signs and symptoms, as the problem has
not occurred; rather, nursing interventions are directed at prevention.

---

risk for Infection [spread]: risk factors may include presence of infectious process, chronic disease states, invasive procedures.*

Arthroplasty   MS

risk for Infection: risk factors may include breach of primary defenses (surgical incision), stasis of body fluids at operative site, and altered inflammatory response.*

risk for Bleeding: risk factors may include surgical procedure, trauma to vascular area.*

impaired physical Mobility may be related to decreased strength, pain, musculoskeletal changes, possibly evidenced by impaired coordination and reluctance to attempt movement.

acute Pain may be related to tissue trauma, local edema, possibly evidenced by verbal reports, narrowed focus, guarded movement, and diaphoresis, changes in vital signs.

Arthroscopy, knee   MS

deficient Knowledge [Learning Need] regarding procedure, outcomes, and self-care needs may be related to unfamiliarity with information or resources, misinterpretations, possibly evidenced by questions and requests for information, misconceptions.

risk for impaired Walking: risk factors may include joint stiffness, discomfort, prescribed movement restrictions, use of assistive devices (crutches) for ambulation.*

Asthma   MS

Also Refer to Emphysema

ineffective Airway Clearance may be related to increased production and retained pulmonary secretions, bronchospasm, decreased energy, fatigue, possibly evidenced by wheezing, difficulty breathing, changes in depth and rate of respirations, use of accessory muscles, and persistent ineffective cough with or without sputum production.

impaired Gas Exchange may be related to altered delivery of inspired O_2 and air trapping, possibly evidenced by dyspnea, restlessness, reduced tolerance for activity, cyanosis, and changes in arterial blood gases (ABGs) and vital signs.

Anxiety [specify level] may be related to perceived threat of death, possibly evidenced by apprehension, fearful expression, and extraneous movements.

                                                            CH

Activity Intolerance may be related to imbalance between O_2 supply and demand, possibly evidenced by fatigue and exertional dyspnea.

risk for Contamination: risk factors may include presence of atmospheric pollutants, environmental contaminants in the home (e.g., smoking or secondhand tobacco smoke).

Athlete's foot   CH

impaired Skin Integrity may be related to fungal invasion, humidity, secretions, possibly evidenced by disruption of skin surface, reports of painful itching.

---

*A risk diagnosis is not evidenced by signs and symptoms, as the problem has not occurred; rather, nursing interventions are directed at prevention.

risk for Infection [spread]: risk factors may include multiple breaks in skin, exposure to moist and warm environment.*

Atrial fibrillation   CH
Also refer to Dysrhythmias

Activity Intolerance may be related to imbalance between oxygen supply and demand possibly evidenced by dyspnea, dizziness, presyncope or syncopal episodes.

risk for ineffective cerebral tissue Perfusion: risk factors may include interruption of arterial flow (microemboli).*

Atrial flutter   CH
Refer to Dysrhythmias

Atrial tachycardia   CH
Refer to Dysrhythmias

Attention deficit disorder (ADD)   PED/PSY
ineffective Coping may be related to situational or maturational crisis, retarded ego development, low self-concept, possibly evidenced by easy distraction by extraneous stimuli, shifting between uncompleted activities.

chronic low Self-Esteem may be related to retarded ego development, lack of positive or repeated negative feedback, negative role models, possibly evidenced by lack of eye contact, derogatory self-comments, hesitance to try new tasks, inadequate level of confidence.

deficient Knowledge [Learning Need] regarding condition, prognosis, therapy may be related to misinformation or misinterpretations, unfamiliarity with resources, possibly evidenced by verbalization of problems or misconceptions, poor school performance, unrealistic expectations of medication regimen.

Autistic disorder   PED/PSY
impaired Social Interaction may be related to abnormal response to sensory input or inadequate sensory stimulation, organic brain dysfunction, delayed development of secure attachment or trust, lack of intuitive skills to comprehend and accurately respond to social cues, disturbance in self-concept, possibly evidenced by lack of responsiveness to others, lack of eye contact or facial responsiveness, treating persons as objects, lack of awareness of feelings in others, indifference or aversion to comfort, affection, or physical contact, failure to develop cooperative social play and peer friendships in childhood.

impaired verbal Communication may be related to inability to trust others, withdrawal into self, organic brain dysfunction, abnormal interpretation or response to and/or inadequate sensory stimulation, possibly evidenced by lack of interactive communication mode, no use of gestures or spoken language, absent or abnormal nonverbal communication, lack of eye contact or facial expression, peculiar patterns of speech (form, content, or speech production), and impaired ability to initiate or sustain conversation despite adequate speech.

---

*A risk diagnosis is not evidenced by signs and symptoms, as the problem has not occurred; rather, nursing interventions are directed at prevention.

Health Conditions and Client Concerns   **945**

risk for Self-Mutilation: risk factors may include organic brain dysfunction, inability to trust others, disturbance in self-concept, inadequate sensory stimulation or abnormal response to sensory input (sensory overload), history of physical, emotional, or sexual abuse, and response to demands of therapy, realization of severity of condition.*

disturbed personal Identity may be related to organic brain dysfunction, lack of development of trust, maternal deprivation, fixation at presymbiotic phase of development, possibly evidenced by lack of awareness of the feelings or existence of others, increased anxiety resulting from physical contact with others, absent or impaired imitation of others, repeating what others say, persistent preoccupation with parts of objects, obsessive attachment to objects, marked distress over changes in environment, autoerotic or ritualistic behaviors, self-touching, rocking, swaying.

compromised/disabled family Coping may be related to family members unable to express feelings, excessive guilt, anger, or blaming among family members regarding child's condition, ambivalent or dissonant family relationships, prolonged coping with problem exhausting supportive ability of family members, possibly evidenced by denial of existence or severity of disturbed behaviors, preoccupation with personal emotional reaction to situation, rationalization that problem will be outgrown, attempts to intervene with child are achieving increasingly ineffective results, family withdraws from or becomes overly protective of child.

Barbiturate abuse   CH/PSY
Refer to Depressant abuse

Battered child syndrome   PED/CH
Also refer to Abuse

risk for Trauma: risk factors may include dependent position in relationship(s), vulnerability (e.g., congenital problems, chronic illness), history of previous abuse or neglect, lack of or nonuse of support systems by caregiver(s).*

interrupted Family Processes/impaired Parenting may be related to poor role model, unrealistic expectations, presence of stressors, and lack of support, possibly evidenced by verbalization of negative feelings, inappropriate caretaking behaviors, and evidence of physical or psychological trauma to child.

PSY

chronic low Self-Esteem may be related to deprivation and negative feedback of family members, personal vulnerability, feelings of abandonment, possibly evidenced by lack of eye contact, withdrawal from social contacts, discounting own needs, nonassertive or passive, indecisive or overly conforming behaviors.

Post-Trauma Syndrome may be related to sustained or recurrent physical or emotional abuse; possibly evidenced by acting-out behavior,

---

*A risk diagnosis is not evidenced by signs and symptoms, as the problem has not occurred; rather, nursing interventions are directed at prevention.

development of phobias, poor impulse control, and emotional numbness.

ineffective Coping may be related to situational or maturational crisis, overwhelming threat to self, personal vulnerability, inadequate support systems, possibly evidenced by verbalized concern about ability to deal with current situation, chronic worry, anxiety, depression, poor self-esteem, inability to problem-solve, high illness rate, destructive behavior toward self or others.

Benign prostatic hyperplasia   CH/MS

[acute/chronic] Urinary Retention/overflow Urinary Incontinence may be related to mechanical obstruction (enlarged prostate), decompensation of detrusor musculature, inability of bladder to contract adequately, possibly evidenced by frequency, hesitancy, inability to empty bladder completely, incontinence or dribbling, nocturia, bladder distention, residual urine.

acute Pain may be related to mucosal irritation, bladder distention, colic, urinary infection, and radiation therapy, possibly evidenced by verbal reports (bladder or rectal spasm), narrowed focus, altered muscle tone, grimacing, distraction behaviors, restlessness, and changes in vital signs.

risk for deficient Fluid Volume/Electrolyte Imbalance: risk factors may include postobstructive diuresis, renal or endocrine dysfunction.*

Fear/Anxiety [specify level] may be related to change in health status (possibility of surgical procedure, malignancy); embarrassment or loss of dignity associated with genital exposure before, during, and after treatment, and concern about sexual ability, possibly evidenced by increased tension, apprehension, worry, expressed concerns regarding perceived changes, and fear of unspecific consequences.

Bipolar disorder   PSY

risk for other-directed Violence: risk factors may include irritability, impulsive behavior, delusional thinking, angry response when ideas are refuted or wishes denied, manic excitement, with possible indicators of threatening body language or verbalizations, increased motor activity, overt and aggressive acts, hostility.*

imbalanced Nutrition: less than body requirements may be related to inadequate intake in relation to metabolic expenditures, possibly evidenced by body weight 20% or more below ideal weight, observed inadequate intake, inattention to mealtimes, and distraction from task of eating, laboratory evidence of nutritional deficits or imbalances.

risk for Poisoning [lithium toxicity]: risk factors may include narrow therapeutic range of drug, client's ability (or lack of) to follow through with medication regimen and monitoring, and denial of need for information or therapy.*

Insomnia may be related to psychological stress, lack of recognition of fatigue or need to sleep, hyperactivity, possibly evidenced by denial of need to sleep, interrupted nighttime sleep, one or more nights without sleep, changes in behavior and performance, increasing irritability, restlessness, and dark circles under eyes.

---

*A risk diagnosis is not evidenced by signs and symptoms, as the problem has not occurred; rather, nursing interventions are directed at prevention.

disturbed Sensory Perception (specify)/Stress Overload may be related to decrease in sensory threshold, endogenous chemical alteration, psychological stress, sleep deprivation, possibly evidenced by increased distractibility and agitation, anxiety, disorientation, poor concentration, auditory or visual hallucination, bizarre thinking, and motor incoordination.

interrupted Family Processes may be related to situational crises (illness, economics, change in roles), euphoric mood and grandiose ideas or actions of client, manipulative behavior and limit testing, client's refusal to accept responsibility for own actions, possibly evidenced by statements of difficulty coping with situation, lack of adaptation to change, or not dealing constructively with illness, ineffective family decision-making process, failure to send and receive clear messages, and inappropriate boundary maintenance.

Bone cancer   MS/CH

Also refer to Myeloma, multiple; Amputation

acute Pain may be related to bone destruction, pressure on nerves, possibly evidenced by verbal or coded report, protective behavior, changes in vital signs.

risk for Trauma: risk factors may include increased bone fragility, general weakness, balancing difficulties.*

Borderline personality disorder   PSY

risk for self-/other-directed Violence/Self-Mutilation: risk factors may include use of projection as a major defense mechanism, pervasive problems with negative transference, feelings of guilt or need to "punish" self, distorted sense of self, inability to cope with increased psychological or physiological tension in a healthy manner.*

Anxiety [severe to panic] may be related to unconscious conflicts (experience of extreme stress), perceived threat to self-concept, unmet needs, possibly evidenced by easy frustration and feelings of hurt, abuse of alcohol or other drugs, transient psychotic symptoms, and performance of self-mutilating acts.

chronic low Self-Esteem/disturbed personal Identity may be related to lack of positive feedback, unmet dependency needs, retarded ego development or fixation at an earlier level of development, possibly evidenced by difficulty identifying self or defining self-boundaries, feelings of depersonalization, extreme mood changes, lack of tolerance of rejection or of being alone, unhappiness with self, striking out at others, performance of ritualistic self-damaging acts, and belief that punishing self is necessary.

Social Isolation may be related to immature interests, unaccepted social behavior, inadequate personal resources, and inability to engage in satisfying personal relationships, possibly evidenced by alternating clinging and distancing behaviors, difficulty meeting expectations of others, experiencing feelings of difference from others, expressing interests inappropriate to developmental age, and exhibiting behavior unaccepted by dominant cultural group.

---

*A risk diagnosis is not evidenced by signs and symptoms, as the problem has not occurred; rather, nursing interventions are directed at prevention.

Botulism (food-borne)   MS

deficient Fluid Volume [isotonic] may be related to active losses—vomiting, diarrhea, decreased intake—nausea, dysphagia, possibly evidenced by reports of thirst, dry skin and mucous membranes, decreased BP and urine output, change in mental state, increased hematocrit (Hct).

impaired physical Mobility may be related to neuromuscular impairment, possibly evidenced by limited ability to perform gross or fine motor skills.

Anxiety [specify level]/Fear may be related to threat of death, interpersonal transmission, possibly evidenced by expressed concerns, apprehension, awareness of physiological symptoms, focus on self.

risk for impaired spontaneous Ventilation: risk factors may include neuromuscular impairment, presence of infectious process.*

CH

Contamination may be related to lack of proper precautions in food storage or preparation as evidenced by gastrointestinal and neurological effects of exposure to biological agent.*

Brain tumor   MS

acute Pain may be related to pressure on brain tissues, possibly evidenced by reports of headache, facial mask of pain, narrowed focus, and changes in vital signs.

disturbed Thought Processes may be related to altered circulation to and/or destruction of brain tissue, possibly evidenced by memory loss, personality changes, impaired ability to make decisions or conceptualize, and inaccurate interpretation of environment.

disturbed Sensory Perception (specify) may be related to compression or displacement of brain tissue, disruption of neuronal conduction, possibly evidenced by changes in visual acuity, alterations in sense of balance, gait disturbance, and paresthesia.

risk for deficient Fluid Volume: risk factors may include recurrent vomiting from irritation of vagal center in medulla and decreased intake.*

Self-Care Deficit [specify] may be related to sensory or neuromuscular impairment interfering with ability to perform tasks, possibly evidenced by unkempt and disheveled appearance, body odor, and verbalization or observation of inability to perform ADLs.

Breast cancer   MS/CH

Also refer to Cancer

Anxiety [specify level] may be related to change in health status, threat of death, stress, interpersonal transmission, possibly evidenced by expressed concerns, apprehension, uncertainty, focus on self, diminished productivity.

deficient Knowledge [Learning Need] regarding diagnosis, prognosis, and treatment options may be related to lack of exposure or unfamiliarity with information resources, information misinterpretation, cognitive limitation, anxiety, possibly evidenced by verbalizations, statements of misconceptions, inappropriate behaviors.

---

*A risk diagnosis is not evidenced by signs and symptoms, as the problem has not occurred; rather, nursing interventions are directed at prevention.

---

risk for disturbed Body Image: risk factors may include significance of body part with regard to sexual perceptions.*

risk for Sexual Dysfunction: risk factors may include health-related changes, medical treatments, concern about relationship with SO.*

Bronchitis   CH

ineffective Airway Clearance may be related to excessive, thickened mucus secretions, possibly evidenced by presence of rhonchi, tachypnea, and ineffective cough.

Activity Intolerance [specify level] may be related to imbalance between O_2 supply and demand, general weakness, exhaustion—interruption in usual sleep pattern due to cough, discomfort, dyspnea, possibly evidenced by reports of fatigue, dyspnea, and abnormal vital sign response to activity.

acute Pain may be related to inflammation of lung parenchyma, persistent cough, cellular reactions to circulating toxins, aching associated with fever, possibly evidenced by reports of pleuritic chest pain, guarding affected area, distraction behaviors, and restlessness.

Bronchopneumonia   MS/CH

Also refer to Bronchitis

ineffective Airway Clearance may be related to tracheal bronchial inflammation, edema formation, increased sputum production, pleuritic pain, decreased energy, fatigue, possibly evidenced by changes in rate and depth of respirations, abnormal breath sounds, use of accessory muscles, dyspnea, cyanosis, effective or ineffective cough—with or without sputum production.

impaired Gas Exchange may be related to alveolar-capillary membrane changes—inflammatory effects, ventilation-perfusion mismatch—collection of secretions affecting O_2 exchange across alveolar membrane, and hypoventilation, altered release of oxygen at cellular level—fever, shifting oxyhemogloblin curve, possibly evidenced by restlessness, changes in mentation, dyspnea, tachycardia, pallor, cyanosis, and ABGs or oximetry evidence of hypoxia.

risk for Infection [spread]: risk factors may include decreased ciliary action, stasis of secretions, presence of existing infection, immunosuppression, chronic disease, malnutrition.*

Bulimia nervosa   PSY/MS

Also refer to Anorexia nervosa

impaired Dentition may be related to dietary habits, poor oral hygiene, chronic vomiting, possibly evidenced by erosion of tooth enamel, multiple caries, abraded teeth.

impaired Oral Mucous Membrane may be related to malnutrition or vitamin deficiency, poor oral hygiene, chronic vomiting, possibly evidenced by sore, inflamed buccal mucosa, swollen salivary glands, ulcerations of mucosa, reports of constant sore mouth or throat.

risk for deficient Fluid Volume/Bleeding: risk factors may include consistent self-induced vomiting, chronic or excessive laxative or diuretic use, esophageal erosion or tear (Mallory-Weiss syndrome).*

---

*A risk diagnosis is not evidenced by signs and symptoms, as the problem has not occurred; rather, nursing interventions are directed at prevention.

---

deficient Knowledge [Learning Need] regarding condition, prognosis, complication, treatment may be related to lack of exposure or recall, unfamiliarity with information about condition, learned maladaptive coping skills, possibly evidenced by verbalization of misconception of relationship of current situation and bingeing and purging behaviors, distortion of body image, verbalized need for information, desire to change behaviors.

Burns (dependent on type, degree, and
severity of the injury)   MS/CH

risk for deficient Fluid Volume/Bleeding: risk factors may include loss of fluids through wounds, capillary damage and evaporation, hypermetabolic state, insufficient intake, hemorrhagic losses.*

risk for ineffective Airway Clearance: risk factors may include tracheobronchial obstruction—mucosal edema and loss of ciliary action with smoke inhalation; circumferential full-thickness burns of the neck, thorax, and chest, with compression of the airway or limited chest excursion, trauma—direct upper airway injury by flame, steam, chemicals, or gases; fluid shifts, pulmonary edema, decreased lung compliance.*

risk for Infection: risk factors may include loss of protective dermal barrier, traumatized tissue, necrosis, decreased Hb, suppressed inflammatory response, environmental exposure, invasive procedures.*

acute/chronic Pain may be related to destruction of skin, tissues, and nerves; edema formation, and manipulation of injured tissues, possibly evidenced by verbal reports, narrowed focus, distraction and guarding behaviors, facial mask of pain, and changes in vital signs.

risk for imbalanced Nutrition: less than body requirements: risk factors may include hypermetabolic state as much as 50% to 60% higher than normal proportional to the severity of injury, protein catabolism, anorexia, restricted oral intake.*

Post-Trauma Syndrome may be related to life-threatening event, possibly evidenced by reexperiencing the event, repetitive dreams or nightmares, psychic or emotional numbness, and sleep disturbance.

ineffective Protection may be related to extremes of age, inadequate nutrition, anemia, impaired immune system, possibly evidenced by impaired healing, deficient immunity, fatigue, anorexia.

                                                                  PED

deficient Diversional Activity may be related to long-term hospitalization, frequent lengthy treatments, and physical limitations, possibly evidenced by expressions of boredom, restlessness, withdrawal, and requests for something to do.

risk for delayed Development: risk factors may include effects of physical disability, separation from SO(s), and environmental deficiencies.*

---

*A risk diagnosis is not evidenced by signs and symptoms, as the problem has not occurred; rather, nursing interventions are directed at prevention.

Bursitis

acute/chronic Pain may be related to inflammation of affected joint, possibly evidenced by verbal reports, guarding behavior, and narrowed focus.

impaired physical Mobility may be related to inflammation and swelling of joint, and pain, possibly evidenced by diminished range of motion, reluctance to attempt movement, and imposed restriction of movement by medical treatment.

Calculi, urinary

acute Pain may be related to increased frequency or force of ureteral contractions, tissue trauma, edema formation, cellular ischemia, possibly evidenced by reports of sudden, severe, colicky pain, guarding and distraction behaviors, self-focus, and changes in vital signs.

impaired Urinary Elimination may be related to stimulation of the bladder by calculi, renal or ureteral irritation, mechanical obstruction of urinary flow, inflammation, possibly evidenced by urgency and frequency, oliguria, hematuria.

risk for deficient Fluid Volume: risk factors may include stimulation of renal-intestinal reflexes—nausea, vomiting, and diarrhea, changes in urinary output, postobstructive diuresis.*

risk for Infection: risk factors may include stasis of urine.*

deficient Knowledge [Learning Need] regarding condition, prognosis, self-care, and treatment needs may be related to lack of exposure or recall and information misinterpretation, possibly evidenced by requests for information, statements of concern, and recurrence or development of preventable complications.

Cancer

Also refer to Chemotherapy

Fear/death Anxiety may be related to situational crises, threat to or change in health or socioeconomic status, role functioning, interaction patterns, threat of death, separation from family, interpersonal transmission of feelings, possibly evidenced by expressed concerns, feelings of inadequacy or helplessness, insomnia, increased tension, restlessness, focus on self, sympathetic stimulation.

Grieving may be related to potential loss of physiological well-being (body part or function), change in lifestyle, perceived potential death, possibly evidenced by anger, sadness, withdrawal, choked feelings, changes in eating or sleep patterns, activity level, libido, and communication patterns.

acute/chronic Pain may be related to the disease process (compression of nerve tissue, infiltration of nerves or their vascular supply, obstruction of a nerve pathway, inflammation), or side effects of therapeutic agents, possibly evidenced by verbal reports, self-focusing or narrowed focus, alteration in muscle tone, facial mask of pain, distraction or guarding behaviors, autonomic responses, and restlessness.

Fatigue may be related to decreased metabolic energy production, increased energy requirements (hypermetabolic state), overwhelming

---

*A risk diagnosis is not evidenced by signs and symptoms, as the problem has not occurred; rather, nursing interventions are directed at prevention.

psychological or emotional demands, and altered body chemistry—side effects of medications, chemotherapy, radiation therapy, biotherapy, possibly evidenced by unremitting or overwhelming lack of energy, inability to maintain usual routines, decreased performance, impaired ability to concentrate, lethargy, listlessness, and disinterest in surroundings.

impaired Home Maintenance may be related to debilitation, lack of resources, and/or inadequate support systems, possibly evidenced by verbalization of problem, request for assistance, and lack of necessary equipment or aids.

PSY/PED

risk for interrupted Family Processes: risk factors may include situational or transitional crises—long-term illness, change in roles or economic status; developmental—anticipated loss of a family member.*

readiness for enhanced family Coping may be related to individual's needs being sufficiently gratified and adaptive tasks effectively addressed, enabling goals of self-actualization to surface, possibly evidenced by verbalizations of impact of crisis on own values, priorities, goals, or relationships.

Candidiasis   CH

Also refer to Thrush

impaired Skin/Tissue Integrity may be related to infectious lesions, possibly evidenced by disruption of skin surfaces and mucous membranes.

acute Pain/impaired Comfort may be related to exposure of irritated skin and mucous membranes to excretions (urine, feces), possibly evidenced by verbal or coded reports, restlessness, guarding behaviors.

risk for Sexual Dysfunction: risk factors include presence of infectious process and vaginal discomfort.*

Cannabis abuse   CH

Refer to Stimulant abuse

Cardiac catheterization   MS

Anxiety [specify level] may be related to threat to or change in health status, stress, family heredity possibly evidenced by expressed concerns, apprehension, uncertainty, focus on self.

risk for decreased Cardiac Output: risk factors may include altered heart rate and rhythm (vasovagal response, ventricular dysrhythmias), decreased myocardial contractility (ischemia).*

risk for ineffective tissue Perfusion (specify): risk factors may include mechanical reduction of arterial blood flow, local hematoma formation, thrombosis, emboli, allergic dye response.*

Cardiac surgery   MS/PED

risk for decreased Cardiac Output: risk factors may include altered myocardial contractility secondary to temporary factors—ventricular

---

*A risk diagnosis is not evidenced by signs and symptoms, as the problem has not occurred; rather, nursing interventions are directed at prevention.

wall surgery, recent myocardial infarction, response to certain medications or drug interactions; altered preload—hypovolemia, and afterload—systemic vascular resistance; altered heart rate or rhythm—dysrhythmias.*

risk for Bleeding/deficient Fluid Volume [isotonic]: risk factors may include intraoperative bleeding with inadequate blood replacement; bleeding related to insufficient heparin reversal, fibrinolysis, or platelet destruction; or volume depletion effects of intraoperative or postoperative diuretic therapy. *

risk for impaired Gas Exchange: risk factors may include alveolar-capillary membrane changes (atelectasis), intestinal edema, inadequate function or premature discontinuation of chest tubes, and diminished O_2-carrying capacity of the blood.*

acute Pain/impaired Comfort may be related to tissue inflammation or trauma, edema formation, intraoperative nerve trauma, and myocardial ischemia, possibly evidenced by reports of incisional discomfort, pain in chest and donor site; paresthesia or pain in hand, arm, shoulder; anxiety, restlessness, irritability; distraction behaviors; and changes in heart rate and BP.

impaired Skin/Tissue Integrity related to mechanical trauma (surgical incisions, puncture wounds) and edema evidenced by disruption of skin surface and tissues.

Cardiogenic shock   MS
Refer to Shock, cardiogenic

Cardiomyopathy   CH/MS
decreased Cardiac Output may be related to altered contractility, possibly evidenced by dyspnea, fatigue, chest pain, dizziness, syncope.

Activity Intolerance may be related to imbalance between O_2 supply and demand, possibly evidenced by weakness, fatigue, dyspnea, abnormal heart rate and BP response to activity, ECG changes.

ineffective Role Performance may be related to changes in physical health, stress, demands of job/life, possibly evidenced by change in usual patterns of responsibility, role strain, change in capacity to resume role.

Carotid endarterectomy   MS
Also refer to Surgery, general

risk for ineffective cerebral tissue Perfusion: risk factors may include interruption of arterial flow (wound hematoma, emboli), pressure changes with edema formation (hyperperfusion syndrome).*

Carpal tunnel syndrome   CH/MS
acute/chronic Pain may be related to pressure on median nerve, possibly evidenced by verbal reports, reluctance to use affected extremity, guarding behaviors, expressed fear of reinjury, altered ability to continue previous activities.

impaired physical Mobility may be related to neuromuscular impairment and pain, possibly evidenced by decreased hand strength, weakness, limited range of motion, and reluctance to attempt movement.

---

*A risk diagnosis is not evidenced by signs and symptoms, as the problem has not occurred; rather, nursing interventions are directed at prevention.

risk for Peripheral Neurovascular Dysfunction: risk factors may include mechanical compression (e.g., brace, repetitive tasks or motions), immobilization.*

deficient Knowledge [Learning Need] regarding condition, prognosis, treatment, and safety needs may be related to lack of exposure or recall, information misinterpretation, possibly evidenced by questions, statements of concern, request for information, inaccurate follow-through of instructions, development of preventable complications.

Casts   CH/MS

Also refer to Fractures

risk for Peripheral Neurovascular Dysfunction: risk factors may include presence of fracture(s), mechanical compression (cast), tissue trauma, immobilization, vascular obstruction.*

risk for impaired Skin Integrity: risk factors may include pressure of cast, moisture or debris under cast, objects inserted under cast to relieve itching, and altered sensation or circulation.*

Self-Care Deficit [specify] may be related to impaired ability to perform self-care tasks, possibly evidenced by statements of need for assistance and observed difficulty in performing ADLs.

Cataract   CH

disturbed visual Sensory Perception may be related to altered sensory reception or status of sense organs, and therapeutically restricted environment (surgical procedure, patching), possibly evidenced by diminished acuity, visual distortions, and change in usual response to stimuli.

risk for Trauma: risk factors may include poor vision, reduced hand-eye coordination.*

Anxiety [specify level]/Fear may be related to alteration in visual acuity, threat of permanent loss of vision/independence, possibly evidenced by expressed concerns, apprehension, and feelings of uncertainty.

deficient Knowledge [Learning Need] regarding ways of coping with altered abilities, therapy choices, lifestyle changes may be related to lack of exposure or recall, misinterpretation, or cognitive limitations, possibly evidenced by requests for information, statement of concern, inaccurate follow-through of instructions, development of preventable complications.

Cat scratch disease   CH

acute Pain may be related to effects of circulating toxins (fever, headache, and lymphadenitis), possibly evidenced by verbal reports, guarding behavior, and changes in vital signs.

Hyperthermia may be related to inflammatory process, possibly evidenced by increased body temperature, flushed warm skin, tachypnea, and tachycardia.

---

*A risk diagnosis is not evidenced by signs and symptoms, as the problem has not occurred; rather, nursing interventions are directed at prevention.

Cellulitis CH/MS

risk for Infection [abscess, bacteremia]: risk factors may inlcude broken skin, chronic disease, presence of pathogens, insufficient knowledge to avoid exposure to pathogens.*

acute Pain/impaired Comfort may be related to inflammatory process, circulating toxins possibly evidenced by reports of localized pain or headache, guarding behaviors, restlessness, changes in vital signs.

impaired Tissue Integrity may be related to trauma, inflammation and/ or invasion of tissues by infectious bacterial agent, or altered circulation; possibly evidenced by redness, warmth, edema, tenderness or pain under the surface of skin, or deep in tissues.

Cerebrovascular accident (CVA) MS

ineffective cerebral tissue Perfusion may be related to interruption of blood flow (occlusive disorder, hemorrhage, cerebral vasospasm or edema), possibly evidenced by altered level of consciousness, changes in vital signs, changes in motor or sensory responses, restlessness, memory loss, as well as sensory, language, intellectual, and emotional deficits.

impaired physical Mobility may be related to neuromuscular involvement (weakness, paresthesia, flaccid or hypotonic paralysis, spastic paralysis), perceptual or cognitive impairment, possibly evidenced by inability to purposefully move involved body parts, limited range of motion, impaired coordination, and/or decreased muscle strength or control.

impaired verbal [and/or written] Communication may be related to impaired cerebral circulation, neuromuscular impairment, loss of facial/ oral muscle tone and control, generalized weakness, fatigue, possibly evidenced by impaired articulation, does not or cannot speak (dysarthria), inability to modulate speech, find and/or name words, identify objects and/or inability to comprehend written or spoken language, inability to produce written communication.

Self-Care Deficit [specify] may be related to neuromuscular impairment, decreased strength or endurance, loss of muscle control or coordination, perceptual or cognitive impairment, pain, discomfort, and depression, possibly evidenced by stated or observed inability to perform ADLs, requests for assistance, disheveled appearance, and incontinence.

risk for impaired Swallowing: risk factors may include muscle paralysis and perceptual impairment.*

risk for unilateral Neglect: risk factors may include sensory loss of part of visual field with perceptual loss of corresponding body segment.*

CH

impaired Home Maintenance may be related to condition of individual family member, insufficient finances, family organization or planning; unfamiliarity with resources, and inadequate support systems, possibly evidenced by members expressing difficulty in managing home in a comfortable manner, requesting assistance with home

---

*A risk diagnosis is not evidenced by signs and symptoms, as the problem has not occurred; rather, nursing interventions are directed at prevention.

maintenance, disorderly surroundings, and overtaxed family members.

situational low Self-Esteem/disturbed Body Image/ineffective Role Performance may be related to biophysical, psychosocial, and cognitive or perceptual changes, possibly evidenced by actual change in structure and/or function, change in usual patterns of responsibility/physical capacity to resume role, and verbal or nonverbal response to actual or perceived change.

risk for complicated Grieving: risk factors may include preloss psychological symptoms, predisposition for anxiety and feelings of inadequacy, frequency of major life events.*

Cervix, dysfunctional **OB**

Refer to Dilation of cervix, premature

Cesarean birth **OB**

Also refer to Cesarean birth, unplanned; Cesarean birth, postpartal

deficient Knowledge [Learning Need] regarding surgical procedure and expectation, postoperative routines and therapy, and self-care needs may be related to lack of information/misinterpretation, possibly evidenced by statements of concern, questions, and misconceptions.

risk for deficient Fluid Volume/Bleeding: risk factors may include restrictions of oral intake, blood loss; pregnancy-related complications.*

risk for impaired Attachment: risk factors may include separation, existing health conditions of mother or infant, lack of privacy.*

Cesarean birth, postpartal **OB**

Also refer to Postpartal period

risk for impaired Attachment: risk factors may include developmental transition or gain of a family member, situational crisis (e.g., surgical intervention, physical complications interfering with initial acquaintance and interaction, negative self-appraisal).*

acute Pain/impaired Comfort may be related to surgical trauma, effects of anesthesia, hormonal effects, bladder or abdominal distention, possibly evidenced by verbal reports (e.g., incisional pain, cramping, afterpains, spinal headache), guarding or distraction behaviors, irritability, facial mask of pain.

risk for situational low Self-Esteem: risk factors may include perceived "failure" at life event, maturational transition, perceived loss of control in unplanned delivery.*

risk for Injury: risk factors may include biochemical or regulatory functions (e.g., orthostatic hypotension, development of pregnancy-induced hypertension or eclampsia), effects of anesthesia, thromboembolism, abnormal blood profile (anemia or excessive blood loss, rubella sensitivity, Rh incompatibility), tissue trauma.*

risk for Infection: risk factors may include tissue trauma, broken skin, decreased Hb, invasive procedures and/or increased environmental exposure, prolonged rupture of amniotic membranes, malnutrition.*

---

*A risk diagnosis is not evidenced by signs and symptoms, as the problem has not occurred; rather, nursing interventions are directed at prevention.

Self-Care Deficit (specify) may be related to effects of anesthesia, decreased strength and endurance, physical discomfort, possibly evidenced by verbalization of inability to perform desired ADL(s).

Cesarean birth, unplanned OB
Also refer to Cesarean birth, postpartal

deficient Knowledge [Learning Need] regarding underlying procedure, pathophysiology, and self-care needs may be related to incomplete or inadequate information, possibly evidenced by request for information, verbalization of concerns or misconceptions, and inappropriate or exaggerated behavior.

Anxiety [specify level] may be related to actual or perceived threat to mother/fetus, emotional threat to self-esteem, unmet needs or expectations, interpersonal transmission, possibly evidenced by increased tension, apprehension, feelings of inadequacy, sympathetic stimulation, and narrowed focus, restlessness.

Powerlessness may be related to interpersonal interaction, perception of illness-related regimen, lifestyle of helplessness, possibly evidenced by verbalization of lack of control, lack of participation in care or decision making, passivity.

risk for impaired fetal Gas Exchange: risk factors may include altered blood flow to placenta and/or through umbilical cord.*

risk for acute Pain: risk factors may include increased or prolonged contractions, psychological reaction.*

risk for Infection: risk factors may include invasive procedures, rupture of amniotic membranes, break in skin, decreased Hb, exposure to pathogens.*

Chemotherapy MS/CH
Also refer to Cancer

risk for deficient Fluid Volume: risk factors may include gastrointestinal losses (vomiting, diarrhea); interference with adequate intake (stomatitis, anorexia), losses through abnormal routes (indwelling tubes, wounds, fistulas), hypermetabolic state.*

imbalanced Nutrition: less than body requirements may be related to inability to ingest adequate nutrients—nausea, stomatitis, gastric irritation, taste distortions, and fatigue; hypermetabolic state, poorly controlled pain, possibly evidenced by weight loss (wasting), aversion to eating, reported altered taste sensation, sore and inflamed buccal cavity, diarrhea and/or constipation.

impaired Oral Mucous Membrane may be related to side effects of therapeutic agents or radiation, dehydration, and malnutrition, possibly evidenced by ulcerations, leukoplakia, decreased salivation, and reports of pain.

disturbed Body Image may be related to anatomical or structural changes, loss of hair and weight, possibly evidenced by negative feelings about body, preoccupation with change, feelings of helplessness or hopelessness, and change in social environment.

ineffective Protection may be related to inadequate nutrition, drug or radiation therapy, abnormal blood profile, disease state (cancer),

---

*A risk diagnosis is not evidenced by signs and symptoms, as the problem has not occurred; rather, nursing interventions are directed at prevention.

possibly evidenced by impaired healing, deficient immunity, anorexia, fatigue.

readiness for enhanced Hope may be related to expectations of therapeutic interventions, results of diagnostic procedures as evidenced by expressed desire to enhance belief in possibilities and sense of meaning to life.

Cholecystectomy   MS

acute Pain may be related to interruption in skin and tissue layers with mechanical closure (sutures or staples) and invasive procedures (including T-tube, nasogastric [NG] tube), possibly evidenced by verbal reports, guarding or distraction behaviors, and changes in vital signs.

ineffective Breathing Pattern may be related to pain, muscular impairment, decreased energy, fatigue, possibly evidenced by fremitus, tachypnea, and decreased respiratory depth and vital capacity, holding breath, reluctance to cough.

risk for deficient Fluid Volume/Bleeding: risk factors may include losses from vomiting or NG aspiration, medically restricted intake, altered coagulation.*

Cholelithiasis   CH

acute Pain may be related to obstruction or ductal spasm, inflammatory process, tissue ischemia, necrosis, possibly evidenced by verbal reports, guarding or distraction behaviors, self- or narrowed focus, and changes in vital signs.

risk for imbalanced Nutrition: less than body requirements: risk factors may include self-imposed or prescribed dietary restrictions, nausea and vomiting, dyspepsia, pain; loss of nutrients; impaired fat digestion—obstruction of bile flow.*

deficient Knowledge [Learning Need] regarding pathophysiology, therapy choices, and self-care needs may be related to lack of information or recall, misinterpretation, possibly evidenced by verbalization of concerns, questions, and recurrence of condition.

Chronic obstructive lung disease   CH/MS

ineffective Airway Clearance may be related to bronchospasm, increased production of tenacious secretions, retained secretions, and decreased energy, fatigue, possibly evidenced by presence of wheezes, crackles, tachypnea, dyspnea, changes in depth of respirations, use of accessory muscles, persistent cough, and chest x-ray findings.

impaired Gas Exchange may be related to altered O_2 delivery (obstruction of airways by secretions or bronchospasm, air trapping) and alveoli destruction, possibly evidenced by dyspnea, restlessness, confusion, abnormal ABG values—hypoxia, hypercapnia, changes in vital signs, and reduced tolerance for activity.

Activity Intolerance may be related to imbalance between O_2 supply and demand, and generalized weakness, possibly evidenced by verbal reports of fatigue, exertional dyspnea, and abnormal vital sign response.

---

*A risk diagnosis is not evidenced by signs and symptoms, as the problem has not occurred; rather, nursing interventions are directed at prevention.

---

imbalanced Nutrition: less than body requirements may be related to inability to ingest adequate nutrients (dyspnea, fatigue, medication side effects, sputum production, anorexia), possibly evidenced by weight loss, reported altered taste sensation, decreased muscle mass or subcutaneous fat, poor muscle tone, and aversion to eating/lack of interest in food.

risk for Infection: risk factors may include decreased ciliary action, stasis of secretions, and debilitated state or malnutrition.*

Circumcision   PED

deficient Knowledge [Learning Need] regarding surgical procedure, prognosis, and treatment may be related to lack of exposure, misinterpretation, unfamiliarity with information resources, possibly evidenced by request for information, verbalization of concern/misconceptions, inaccurate follow-through of instructions.

acute Pain may be related to trauma to/edema of tender tissues, possibly evidenced by crying, changes in sleep pattern, refusal to eat.

impaired urinary Elimination may be related to tissue injury or inflammation or development of urethral fistula, possibly evidenced by edema, difficulty voiding.

risk for Bleeding: risk factors may include decreased clotting factors immediately after birth, previously undiagnosed problems with bleeding or clotting.*

risk for Infection: risk factors may include immature immune system, invasive procedure, tissue trauma, environmental exposure.*

Cirrhosis   MS/CH

Also refer to Substance dependence/abuse rehabilitation; Hepatitis, acute viral

risk for impaired Liver Function: risk factors may include viral infection, alcohol abuse.*

imbalanced Nutrition: less than body requirements may be related to inability to ingest or absorb nutrients (anorexia, nausea, indigestion, early satiety), abnormal bowel function, impaired storage of vitamins, possibly evidenced by aversion to eating, observed lack of intake, poor muscle tone, muscle wasting, weight loss, and imbalances in nutritional studies.

excess Fluid Volume may be related to compromised regulatory mechanism (e.g., syndrome of inappropriate antidiuretic hormone [SIADH], decreased plasma proteins, malnutrition) and excess sodium and/or fluid intake, possibly evidenced by generalized or abdominal edema, weight gain, dyspnea, BP changes, positive hepatojugular reflex, change in mentation, altered electrolytes, changes in urine specific gravity, and pleural effusion.

risk for impaired Skin Integrity: risk factors may include altered circulation and metabolic state, poor skin turgor, skeletal prominence, presence of edema or ascites, and accumulation of bile salts in skin.*

risk for Bleeding: risk factors may include abnormal blood profile, altered clotting factors—decreased production of prothrombin, fibrinogen, and factors VIII, IX, and X; impaired vitamin K absorption;

---

*A risk diagnosis is not evidenced by signs and symptoms, as the problem has not occurred; rather, nursing interventions are directed at prevention.

release of thromboplastin, portal hypertension, development of esophageal varices.*

risk for acute Confusion: risk factors may include alcohol abuse, increased serum ammonia level, and inability of liver to detoxify certain enzymes or drugs.*

Self-Esteem (specify)/disturbed Body Image may be related to biophysical changes, altered physical appearance, uncertainty of prognosis, changes in role function, personal vulnerability, self-destructive behavior (alcohol-induced disease), possibly evidenced by verbalization of changes in lifestyle, fear of rejection/reaction of others, negative feelings about body or abilities, and feelings of helplessness, hopelessness, powerlessness.

risk for ineffective Protection: risk factors may include abnormal blood profile (altered clotting factors), portal hypertension, development of esophageal varices.*

Cocaine hydrochloride poisoning, acute　　　MS
Also refer to Stimulant abuse; Substance dependence/abuse rehabilitation

ineffective Breathing Pattern may be related to pharmacological effects on respiratory center of the brain, possibly evidenced by tachypnea, altered depth of respiration, shortness of breath, and abnormal ABGs.

risk for decreased Cardiac Output: risk factors may include drug effect on myocardium (degree dependent on drug purity and quality used), alterations in electrical rate, rhythm, or conduction, preexisting myocardiopathy.*

CH

risk for impaired Liver Function: risk factors may include cocaine abuse.*

imbalanced Nutrition: less than body requirements may be related to anorexia, insufficient or inappropriate use of financial resources, possibly evidenced by reported inadequate intake, weight loss or less than normal weight gain, lack of interest in food, poor muscle tone, signs or laboratory evidence of vitamin deficiencies.

risk for Infection: risk factors may include injection techniques, impurities of drugs, localized trauma/nasal septum damage, malnutrition, altered immune state.*

PSY

ineffective Coping may be related to personal vulnerability, negative role modeling, inadequate support systems, ineffective or inadequate coping skills with substitution of drug, possibly evidenced by use of harmful substance despite evidence of undesirable consequences.

disturbed Sensory Perception (specify) may be related to exogenous chemical, altered sensory reception, transmission, or integration (hallucination), altered status of sense organs, possibly evidenced by responding to internal stimuli from hallucinatory experiences, bizarre thinking, anxiety, panic, changes in sensory acuity (sense of smell or taste).

---

*A risk diagnosis is not evidenced by signs and symptoms, as the problem has not occurred; rather, nursing interventions are directed at prevention.

Coccidioidomycosis (San Joaquin/ Valley Fever)

CH

acute Pain may be related to inflammation, possibly evidenced by verbal reports, distraction behaviors, and narrowed focus.

Fatigue may be related to decreased energy production, states of discomfort, possibly evidenced by reports of overwhelming lack of energy, inability to maintain usual routine, emotional lability or irritability, impaired ability to concentrate, and decreased endurance or libido.

deficient Knowledge [Learning Need] regarding nature and course of disease, therapy and self-care needs may be related to lack of information, possibly evidenced by statements of concern and questions.

Colitis, ulcerative

MS

Diarrhea may be related to inflammation or malabsorption of the bowel, presence of toxins, segmental narrowing of the lumen, possibly evidenced by increased bowel sounds and peristalsis, frequent watery stools (acute phase), changes in stool color, abdominal pain, urgency, cramping.

acute/chronic Pain may be related to inflammation of the intestines, hyperperistalsis, prolonged diarrhea, and anal/rectal irritation, fissures, fistulas, possibly evidenced by verbal reports, guarding or distraction behaviors—restlessness, self-focusing.

risk for deficient Fluid Volume: risk factors may include excessive losses through normal routes—severe frequent diarrhea, vomiting; capillary plasma loss; hypermetabolic state—inflammation, fever; restricted intake—nausea, anorexia.*

CH

imbalanced Nutrition: less than body requirements may be related to altered intake or absorption of nutrients—medically restricted intake, fear that eating may cause diarrhea; and hypermetabolic state, possibly evidenced by weight loss, decreased subcutaneous fat and muscle mass, poor muscle tone, hyperactive bowel sounds, steatorrhea, pale conjunctiva and mucous membranes, and aversion to eating.

ineffective Coping may be related to chronic nature and indefinite outcome of disease, multiple stressors repeated over time, situational crisis, personal vulnerability, severe pain, inadequate sleep, lack of or ineffective support systems, possibly evidenced by verbalization of inability to cope, discouragement, anxiety, preoccupation with physical self, chronic worry, emotional tension, depression, and recurrent exacerbation of symptoms.

risk for Powerlessness: risk factors may include unresolved dependency conflicts, feelings of insecurity or resentment, repression of anger and aggressive feelings, lacking a sense of control in stressful situations, sacrificing own wishes for others, and retreat from aggression or frustration.*

---

*A risk diagnosis is not evidenced by signs and symptoms, as the problem has not occurred; rather, nursing interventions are directed at prevention.

Colostomy   MS

risk for impaired Skin Integrity: risk factors may include absence of sphincter at stoma, character and flow of effluent and flatus from stoma, reaction to product or removal of adhesive, and improperly fitting or care of appliance.*

risk for Diarrhea/Constipation: risk factors may include interruption or alteration of normal bowel function/placement of ostomy, changes in dietary or fluid intake, and effects of medication.*

C

CH

deficient Knowledge [Learning Need] regarding changes in physiological function, and self-care and treatment needs may be related to lack of exposure or recall, information misinterpretation, possibly evidenced by questions, statement of concern, and inaccurate follow-through of instruction or performance of ostomy care, development of preventable complications.

disturbed Body Image may be related to biophysical changes (presence of stoma, loss of control of bowel elimination) and psychosocial factors (altered body structure, disease process—cancer, colitis, and associated treatment regimen, possibly evidenced by verbalization of change in perception of self, negative feelings about body, fear of rejection/reaction of others, not touching or looking at stoma, and refusal to participate in care.

impaired Social Interaction may be related to fear of embarrassing situation secondary to altered bowel control with loss of contents, odor, possibly evidenced by reduced participation and verbalized or observed discomfort in social situations.

risk for Sexual Dysfunction: risk factors may include altered body structure and function, radical resection and treatment procedures, vulnerability, psychological concern about response of SO(s), and disruption of sexual response pattern—erection difficulty.*

Coma   MS

risk for Suffocation: risk factors may include cognitive impairment/loss of protective reflexes and purposeful movement.*

risk for deficient Fluid Volume/imbalanced Nutrition: less than body requirements: risk factors may include inability to ingest food or fluids, increased needs—hypermetabolic state.*

[total] Self-Care Deficit may be related to cognitive impairment and absence of purposeful activity, evidenced by inability to perform ADLs.

risk for ineffective cerebral tissue Perfusion: risk factors may include reduced or interrupted arterial or venous blood flow (direct injury, edema formation, space-occupying lesions), metabolic alterations, effects of drug or alcohol overdose, hypoxia, anoxia.*

risk for Infection: risk factors may include may include stasis of body fluids (oral, pulmonary, urinary), invasive procedures, and nutritional deficits.*

Coma, diabetic   MS

Refer to Diabetic ketoacidosis; Coma

---

*A risk diagnosis is not evidenced by signs and symptoms, as the problem has not occurred; rather, nursing interventions are directed at prevention.

Complex regional pain syndrome   MS

acute/chronic Pain may be related to continued nerve stimulation, possibly evidenced by verbal reports, distraction or guarding behaviors, narrowed focus, changes in sleep patterns, and altered ability to continue previous activities.

ineffective peripheral tissue Perfusion may be related to reduction of arterial blood flow (arteriole vasoconstriction), possibly evidenced by reports of pain, decreased skin temperature and pallor, diminished arterial pulsations, and tissue swelling.

disturbed tactile Sensory Perception may be related to altered sensory reception (neurological deficit, pain), possibly evidenced by change in usual response to stimuli, abnormal sensitivity of touch, physiological anxiety, and irritability.

risk for ineffective Role Performance: risk factors may include situational crisis, chronic disability, debilitating pain.*

risk for compromised family Coping: risk factors may include temporary family disorganization and role changes and prolonged disability that exhausts the supportive capacity of SO(s).*

Concussion, brain   CH

acute Pain may be related to trauma to or edema of cerebral tissue, possibly evidenced by reports of headache, guarding or distraction behaviors, and narrowed focus.

risk for deficient Fluid Volume: risk factors may include vomiting, decreased intake, and hypermetabolic state (fever).*

risk for disturbed Thought Processes: risk factors may include trauma to or edema of cerebral tissue.*

deficient Knowledge [Learning Need] regarding condition, treatment/safety needs, and potential complications may be related to lack of recall, misinterpretation, cognitive limitation, possibly evidenced by questions or statement of concerns, development of preventable complications.

Conduct disorder (childhood, adolescence)   PSY/PED

risk for self-/other-directed Violence: risk factors may include retarded ego development, antisocial character, poor impulse control, dysfunctional family system, loss of significant relationships, history of suicidal or acting-out behaviors.*

defensive Coping may be related to inadequate coping strategies, maturational crisis, multiple life changes or losses, lack of control of impulsive actions, and personal vulnerability, possibly evidenced by inappropriate use of defense mechanisms, inability to meet role expectations, poor self-esteem, failure to assume responsibility for own actions, hypersensitivity to slight or criticism, and excessive smoking, drinking, or drug use.

disturbed Thought Processes may be related to physiological changes, lack of appropriate psychological conflict, biochemical changes, as evidenced by tendency to interpret the intentions or actions of others as blaming and hostile, deficits in problem-solving skills, with physical aggression the solution most often chosen.

---

*A risk diagnosis is not evidenced by signs and symptoms, as the problem has not occurred; rather, nursing interventions are directed at prevention.

chronic low Self-Esteem may be related to life choices perpetuating failure, personal vulnerability, possibly evidenced by self-negating verbalizations, anger, rejection of positive feedback, frequent lack of success in life events.

compromised/disabled family Coping may be related to excessive guilt, anger, or blaming among family members regarding child's behavior; parental inconsistencies; disagreements regarding discipline, limit setting, and approaches; and exhaustion of parental resources (prolonged coping with disruptive child), possibly evidenced by unrealistic parental expectations, rejection or overprotection of child; and exaggerated expressions of anger, disappointment, or despair regarding child's behavior or ability to improve or change.

impaired Social Interaction may be related to retarded ego development, developmental state (adolescence), lack of social skills, low self-concept, dysfunctional family system, and neurological impairment, possibly evidenced by dysfunctional interaction with others (difficulty waiting turn in games or group situations, not seeming to listen to what is being said), difficulty playing quietly and maintaining attention to task or play activity, often shifting from one activity to another and interrupting or intruding on others.

Congestive heart failure MS
Refer to Heart failure, chronic

Conn's syndrome MS/CH
Refer to Aldosteronism, primary

Constipation CH
Constipation may be related to weak abdominal musculature, gastrointestinal obstructive lesions, pain on defecation, diagnostic procedures, pregnancy, possibly evidenced by change in character and frequency of stools, feeling of abdominal or rectal fullness or pressure, changes in bowel sounds, abdominal distention.

impaired Comfort may be related to abdominal fullness or pressure, straining to defecate, and trauma to delicate tissues, possibly evidenced by verbal reports, reluctance to defecate, and distraction behaviors.

deficient Knowledge [Learning Need] regarding dietary needs, bowel function, and medication effect may be related to lack of information, misconceptions, possibly evidenced by development of problem and verbalization of concerns or questions.

Coronary artery bypass surgery MS
risk for decreased Cardiac Output: risk factors may include decreased myocardial contractility, diminished circulating volume (preload), alterations in electrical conduction, and increased SVR (afterload).*

acute Pain may be related to direct chest tissue and bone trauma, invasive tubes and lines, donor site incision, tissue inflammation and edema formation, intraoperative nerve trauma, possibly evidenced

---

*A risk diagnosis is not evidenced by signs and symptoms, as the problem has not occurred; rather, nursing interventions are directed at prevention.

by verbal reports, changes in vital signs, and distraction behaviors (restlessness), irritability.

disturbed Sensory Perception (specify) may be related to restricted environment (postoperative or acute), sleep deprivation, effects of medications, continuous environmental sounds and activities, and psychological stress of procedure, possibly evidenced by disorientation, alterations in behavior, exaggerated emotional responses, and visual or auditory distortions.

CH

ineffective Role Performance may be related to situational crises (dependent role), recuperative process, uncertainty about future, possibly evidenced by delay or alteration in physical capacity to resume role, change in usual role or responsibility, change in self or others' perception of role.

Crohn's disease   MS/CH

Also refer to Colitis, ulcerative

imbalanced Nutrition: less than body requirements may be related to intestinal pain after eating, decreased transit time through bowel, fear that eating may cause diarrhea possibly evidenced by weight loss, decreased subcutaneous fat and muscle mass, poor muscle tone, aversion to eating, and observed lack of intake.

Diarrhea may be related to inflammation, irritation—particular dietary intake, malabsorption of the bowel, presence of toxins, segmental narrowing of the lumen, possibly evidenced by hyperactive bowel sounds, increased peristalsis, cramping, and frequent loose liquid stools.

deficient Knowledge [Learning Need] regarding condition, nutritional needs, and prevention of recurrence may be related to misinterpretation of information, lack of recall, unfamiliarity with resources, possibly evidenced by statements of concern, questions, inaccurate follow-through of instructions, and development of preventable complications or exacerbation of condition.

Croup   PED/CH

ineffective Airway Clearance may be related to presence of thick, tenacious mucus and swelling or spasms of the epiglottis, possibly evidenced by harsh, brassy cough; tachypnea, use of accessory breathing muscles, and presence of wheezes.

deficient Fluid Volume [isotonic] may be related to decreased ability or aversion to swallowing, presence of fever, and increased respiratory losses, possibly evidenced by dry mucous membranes, poor skin turgor, and scanty, concentrated urine.

Croup, membranous   PED/CH

Also refer to Croup

risk for Suffocation: risk factors may include inflammation of larynx with formation of false membrane.*

---

*A risk diagnosis is not evidenced by signs and symptoms, as the problem has not occurred; rather, nursing interventions are directed at prevention.

Anxiety [specify level]/Fear may be related to change in environment, perceived threat to self (difficulty breathing), and transmission of anxiety of adults, possibly evidenced by restlessness, facial tension, glancing about, and sympathetic stimulation.

C-Section   OB

Refer to Cesarean birth; Cesarean birth, unplanned

Cushing's syndrome   CH/MS
risk for excess Fluid Volume: risk factors may include compromised regulatory mechanism (fluid and sodium retention).*

risk for Infection: risk factors may include immunosuppressed inflammatory response, skin and capillary fragility, and negative nitrogen balance.*

imbalanced Nutrition: less than body requirements may be related to inability to utilize nutrients (disturbance of carbohydrate metabolism), possibly evidenced by decreased muscle mass and increased resistance to insulin.

Self-Care Deficit [specify] may be related to muscle wasting, generalized weakness, fatigue, and demineralization of bones, possibly evidenced by statements of or observed inability to complete or perform ADLs.

disturbed Body Image may be related to change in structure or appearance (effects of disease process, drug therapy), possibly evidenced by negative feelings about body, feelings of helplessness, and changes in social involvement.

Sexual Dysfunction may be related to loss of libido, impotence, and cessation of menses, possibly evidenced by verbalization of concerns and/or dissatisfaction with and alteration in relationship with SO.

risk for Trauma [fractures]: risk factors may include increased protein breakdown, negative protein balance, demineralization of bones.*

CVA   MS/CH

Refer to Cerebrovascular accident

Cystic fibrosis   CH/PED
ineffective Airway Clearance may be related to excessive production of thick mucus and decreased ciliary action, possibly evidenced by abnormal breath sounds, ineffective cough, cyanosis, and altered respiratory rate and depth.

risk for Infection: risk factors may include stasis of respiratory secretions and development of atelectasis.*

imbalanced Nutrition: less than body requirements may be related to impaired digestive process and absorption of nutrients, possibly evidenced by failure to gain weight, muscle wasting, and retarded physical growth.

deficient Knowledge [Learning Need] regarding pathophysiology of condition, medical management, and available community resources may be related to insufficient information, misconceptions, possibly evidenced by statements of concern and questions, inaccurate follow-through of instructions, development of preventable complications.

---

*A risk diagnosis is not evidenced by signs and symptoms, as the problem has not occurred; rather, nursing interventions are directed at prevention.

compromised family Coping may be related to chronic nature of disease and disability, inadequate or incorrect information or understanding by a primary person, possibly evidenced by significant person attempting assistive or supportive behaviors with less than satisfactory results, protective behavior disproportionate to client's abilities, or need for autonomy.

Cystitis CH

acute Pain may be related to inflammation and bladder spasms, possibly evidenced by verbal reports, distraction behaviors, and narrowed focus.

impaired Urinary Elimination may be related to inflammation or irritation of bladder, possibly evidenced by frequency, nocturia, and dysuria.

deficient Knowledge [Learning Need] regarding condition, treatment, and prevention of recurrence may be related to inadequate information, misconceptions, possibly evidenced by statements of concern and questions, recurrent infections.

Cytomegalic inclusion disease CH

Refer to Cytomegalovirus infection

Cytomegalovirus (CMV) infection CH

risk for disturbed visual Sensory Perception: risk factors may include inflammation of the retina.*

risk for fetal Infection: risk factors may include transplacental exposure, contact with blood or body fluids.*

Deep Vein Thrombosis (DVT) CH/MS

Refer to Thrombophlebitis

Degenerative joint disease CH

Refer to Arthritis, rheumatoid

Dehiscence (abdominal) MS

impaired Skin Integrity may be related to altered circulation, altered nutritional state (obesity, malnutrition), and physical stress on incision, possibly evidenced by poor or delayed wound healing and disruption of skin surface or wound closure.

risk for Infection: risk factors may include inadequate primary defenses (separation of incision, traumatized intestines, environmental exposure).*

risk for impaired Tissue Integrity: risk factors may include exposure of abdominal contents to external environment.*

Fear/[severe] Anxiety may be related to crises, perceived threat of death, possibly evidenced by fearfulness, restless behaviors, and sympathetic stimulation.

deficient Knowledge [Learning Need] regarding condition, prognosis, and treatment needs may be related to lack of information or recall, misinterpretation of information, possibly evidenced by development of preventable complication, requests for information, and statement of concern.

---

*A risk diagnosis is not evidenced by signs and symptoms, as the problem has not occurred; rather, nursing interventions are directed at prevention.

Dehydration PED/CH

deficient Fluid Volume [specify] may be related to etiology as defined by specific situation, possibly evidenced by dry mucous membranes, poor skin turgor, decreased pulse volume and pressure, and thirst.

risk for impaired Oral Mucous Membrane: risk factors may include dehydration and decreased salivation.*

deficient Knowledge [Learning Need] regarding fluid needs may be related to lack of information, misinterpretation, possibly evidenced by questions, statement of concern, and inadequate follow-through of instructions, development of preventable complications.

Delirium tremens (acute alcohol withdrawal) MS/PSY

[severe to panic] Anxiety/Fear may be related to cessation of alcohol intake, physiological withdrawal, threat to self-concept, perceived threat of death, possibly evidenced by increased tension, apprehension, feelings of inadequacy, shame, self-disgust, or remorse; fear of unspecified consequences, identifies object of fear.

disturbed Sensory Perception (specify) may be related to exogenous factors—alcohol consumption and sudden cessation; endogenous—electrolyte imbalance, elevated ammonia and blood urea nitrogen (BUN); sleep deprivation, and psychological stress, possibly evidenced by disorientation, restlessness, irritability, exaggerated emotional responses, bizarre thinking, and visual or auditory distortions or hallucinations.

risk for decreased Cardiac Output: risk factors may include direct effect of alcohol on heart muscle, altered SVR, presence of dysrhythmias.*

risk for Trauma: risk factors may include alterations in balance, reduced muscle coordination, cognitive impairment, and involuntary clonic/tonic muscle activity.*

imbalanced Nutrition: less than body requirements may be related to poor dietary intake, effects of alcohol on organs involved in digestion, interference with absorption or metabolism of nutrients and amino acids, possibly evidenced by reports of inadequate food intake, altered taste sensation, lack of interest in food, debilitated state, decreased subcutaneous fat and muscle mass, signs or laboratory findings of mineral and electrolyte deficiency.

Delivery, precipitous/out of hospital OB

Also refer to Labor, precipitous; Labor stages I–II

risk for deficient Fluid Volume: risk factors may include presence of nausea, vomiting, lack of intake, excessive vascular loss.*

risk for Infection: risk factors may include broken or traumatized tissue, increased environmental exposure, rupture of amniotic membranes.*

risk for fetal Injury: risk factors may include rapid descent and pressure changes, compromised circulation, environmental exposure.*

Delusional disorder PSY

risk for self-/other-directed Violence: risk factors may include perceived threats of danger, increased feelings of anxiety, acting out in an irrational manner.*

---

*A risk diagnosis is not evidenced by signs and symptoms, as the problem has not occurred; rather, nursing interventions are directed at prevention.

[severe] Anxiety may be related to inability to trust, possibly evidenced by rigid delusional system, frightened of other people and own hostility.

Powerlessness may be related to lifestyle of helplessness, feelings of inadequacy, interpersonal interaction, possibly evidenced by verbal expressions of no control or influence over situation(s), use of paranoid delusions, aggressive behavior to compensate for lack of control.

disturbed Thought Processes may be related to psychological conflicts, increasing anxiety or fear, possibly evidenced by interference with ability to think clearly or logically, fragmentation and autistic thinking, delusions, beliefs and behaviors of suspicion or violence.

impaired Social Interaction may be related to mistrust of others, delusional thinking, lack of knowledge or skills to enhance mutuality, possibly evidenced by discomfort in social situations, difficulty in establishing relationships with others, expression of feelings of rejection, no sense of belonging.

Dementia, presenile/senile   CH/PSY
Also refer to Alzheimer's disease

impaired Memory may be related to neurological disturbances, possibly evidenced by observed experiences of forgetting, inability to determine if a behavior was performed, inability to perform previously learned skills, inability to recall factual information or recent or past events.

Fear may be related to decreases in functional abilities, public disclosure of disabilities, further mental or physical deterioration, possibly evidenced by social isolation, apprehension, irritability, defensiveness, suspiciousness, aggressive behavior.

Self-Care Deficit [specify] may be related to cognitive decline, physical limitations, frustration over loss of independence, depression, possibly evidenced by impaired ability to perform ADLs.

risk for Trauma: risk factors may include changes in muscle coordination or balance, impaired judgment, seizure activity.*

risk for sedentary Lifestyle: risk factors may include lack of interest or motivation, lack of resources, lack of training or knowledge of specific exercise needs, safety concerns or fear of injury.*

risk for Caregiver Role Strain: risk factors may include illness severity of care receiver, duration of caregiving required, complexity or amount of caregiving tasks, care receiver exhibiting deviant or bizarre behavior; family/caregiver isolation, lack of respite or recreation, spouse is caregiver.*

Grieving may be related to awareness of something "being wrong," predisposition for anxiety and feelings of inadequacy, family perception of potential loss of loved one, possibly evidenced by expressions of distress, anger at potential loss, choked feelings, crying, alteration in activity level, communication patterns, eating habits, and sleep patterns.

---

*A risk diagnosis is not evidenced by signs and symptoms, as the problem has not occurred; rather, nursing interventions are directed at prevention.

Depressant abuse   **CH/PSY**

Also refer to Drug overdose, acute (depressants)

<u>ineffective Denial</u> may be related to weak, underdeveloped ego, unmet self-needs, possibly evidenced by inability to admit impact of condition on life, minimizes symptoms or problem, refuses healthcare attention.

<u>ineffective Coping</u> may be related to weak ego, possibly evidenced by abuse of chemical agents, lack of goal-directed behavior, inadequate problem-solving, destructive behavior toward self.

<u>imbalanced Nutrition: less than body requirements</u> may be related to use of substance in place of nutritional food, possibly evidenced by loss of weight, pale conjunctiva and mucous membranes, electrolyte imbalances, anemias.

<u>risk for Injury:</u> risk factors may include changes in sleep, decreased concentration, loss of inhibitions.*

**Depressive disorders, major
depression, dysthymia**   **PSY**

<u>risk for self-directed Violence:</u> risk factors may include depressed mood and feeling of worthlessness and hopelessness.*

[moderate to severe] <u>Anxiety/disturbed Thought Processes</u> may be related to psychological conflicts, unconscious conflict about essential values or goals of life, unmet needs, threat to self-concept, sleep deprivation, interpersonal transmission or contagion, possibly evidenced by reports of nervousness or fearfulness, feelings of inadequacy; agitation, angry or tearful outbursts, rambling and discoordinated speech, restlessness, hand rubbing or wringing, tremulousness, poor memory or concentration, decreased ability to grasp ideas, impaired ability to make decisions, numerous or repetitious physical complaints without organic cause, ideas of reference, hallucinations, delusions.

<u>Insomnia</u> may be related to biochemical alterations (decreased serotonin), unresolved fears and anxieties, and inactivity, possibly evidenced by difficulty in falling or remaining asleep, early morning awakening or awakening later than desired, reports of not feeling rested, physical signs (e.g., dark circles under eyes, excessive yawning).

<u>Social Isolation/impaired Social Interaction</u> may be related to alterations in mental status or thought processes (depressed mood), inadequate personal resources, decreased energy, inertia, difficulty engaging in satisfying personal relationships, feelings of worthlessness, low self-concept, inadequacy or absence of significant purpose in life, and knowledge or skill deficit about social interactions, possibly evidenced by decreased involvement with others, expressed feelings of difference from others, remaining in home/room/bed, refusing invitations or suggestions for social involvement, and dysfunctional interaction with peers, family, and/or others.

<u>interrupted Family Processes</u> may be related to situational crises of illness of family member with change in roles or responsibilities,

---

*A risk diagnosis is not evidenced by signs and symptoms, as the problem has not occurred; rather, nursing interventions are directed at prevention.

developmental crises (e.g., loss of family member or relationship), possibly evidenced by statements of difficulty coping with situation, family system not meeting needs of its members, difficulty accepting or receiving help appropriately, ineffective family decision-making process, and failure to send and to receive clear messages.

risk for impaired Religiosity: risk factors may include ineffective support or coping, lack of social interaction, depression.*

risk for Injury [effects of electroconvulsive therapy (ECT)]: risk factors may include effects of therapy on the cardiovascular, respiratory, musculoskeletal, and nervous systems; and pharmacological effects of anesthesia.*

Depression, postpartum   OB/PSY
Also refer to Depressive disorders

risk for impaired Attachment: risk factors may include anxiety associated with the parent role, inability to meet personal needs, perceived guilt regarding relationship with infant.*

risk for other-directed Violence: risk factors may include hopelessness, increased anxiety, mood swings, despondency, severe depression or psychosis. *

Dermatitis, seborrheic   CH

impaired Skin Integrity may be related to chronic inflammatory condition of the skin, possibly evidenced by disruption of skin surface with dry or moist scales, yellowish crusts, erythema, and fissures.

Diabetes mellitus   CH/PED

deficient Knowledge [Learning Need] regarding disease process, treatment, and individual care needs may be related to unfamiliarity with information, lack of recall, misinterpretation, possibly evidenced by requests for information, statements of concern, misconceptions, inadequate follow-through of instructions, or development of preventable complications.

risk for unstable blood Glucose Level: risk factors may include lack of adherence to diabetes management, medication management, inadequate blood glucose monitoring, physical activity level, health status, stress, rapid growth periods.*

risk for risk-prone health Behavior: risk factors may include all-encompassing change in lifestyle, self-concept requiring lifelong adherence to therapeutic regimen and internal altered locus of control.*

risk for Infection: risk factors may include decreased leukocyte function, circulatory changes, and delayed healing.*

risk for disturbed Sensory Perception (specify): risk factors may include endogenous chemical alteration (glucose, insulin, and/or electrolyte imbalance).*

compromised family Coping may be related to inadequate or incorrect information or understanding by primary person(s), other situational or developmental crises or situations the significant person(s) may be facing, lifelong condition requiring behavioral changes impacting family, possibly evidenced by family expressions of confusion about

---

*A risk diagnosis is not evidenced by signs and symptoms, as the problem has not occurred; rather, nursing interventions are directed at prevention.

what to do, verbalizations that they are having difficulty coping with situation, family does not meet physical or emotional needs of its members; SO(s) preoccupied with personal reaction (e.g., guilt, fear), display protective behavior disproportionate (too little or too much) to client's abilities or need for autonomy.

Diabetic ketoacidosis   CH/MS

<u>deficient Fluid Volume [specify]</u> may be related to hyperosmolar urinary losses, gastric losses and inadequate intake, possibly evidenced by increased urinary output, dilute urine; reports of weakness, thirst, sudden weight loss, hypotension, tachycardia, delayed capillary refill, dry mucous membranes, poor skin turgor.

<u>unstable blood Glucose Level</u> may be related to medication management, lack of diabetes management, inadequate blood glucose moitoring, presence of infection, possibly evidenced by elevated serum glucose level, presence of ketones in urine, nausea, weight loss, blurred vision, irritability.

<u>Fatigue</u> may be related to decreased metabolic energy production, altered body chemistry (insufficient insulin), increased energy demands (hypermetabolic state—infection), possibly evidenced by overwhelming lack of energy, inability to maintain usual routines, decreased performance, impaired ability to concentrate, listlessness.

<u>risk for Infection:</u> risk factors may include high glucose levels, decreased leukocyte function, stasis of body fluids, invasive procedures, alterations in circulation.*

Dialysis, general   CH

Also refer to Dialysis, peritoneal; Hemodialysis

<u>imbalanced Nutrition: less than body requirements</u> may be related to inadequate ingestion of nutrients—dietary restrictions, anorexia, nausea, vomiting, stomatitis, sensation of feeling full with continuous ambulatory peritoneal dialysis (CAPD); loss of peptides and amino acids (building blocks for proteins) during dialysis, possibly evidenced by reported inadequate intake, aversion to eating, altered taste sensation, poor muscle tone, weakness, sore and inflamed buccal cavity, pale conjunctiva and mucous membranes.

<u>Grieving</u> may be related to actual or perceived loss, chronic and/or fatal illness, and thwarted grieving response to a loss, possibly evidenced by verbal expression of distress or unresolved issues, denial of loss, altered eating habits, sleep and dream patterns, activity levels, libido, crying, labile affect; feelings of sorrow, guilt, and anger.

<u>disturbed Body Image/situational low Self-Esteem</u> may be related to situational crisis and chronic illness with changes in usual roles and body image, possibly evidenced by verbalization of changes in lifestyle, focus on past function, negative feelings about body, feelings of helplessness and powerlessness, extension of body boundary to incorporate environmental objects (e.g., dialysis setup), change in social involvement, overdependence on others for care, not taking responsibility for self-care, lack of follow-through, and self-destructive behavior.

---

*A risk diagnosis is not evidenced by signs and symptoms, as the problem has not occurred; rather, nursing interventions are directed at prevention.

Self-Care Deficit [specify] may be related to perceptual or cognitive impairment (accumulated toxins), intolerance to activity, decreased strength and endurance, pain, discomfort, possibly evidenced by reported inability to perform ADLs, disheveled or unkempt appearance, strong body odor.

Powerlessness may be related to illness-related regimen and healthcare environment, possibly evidenced by verbal expression of having no control, depression over physical deterioration, nonparticipation in care, anger, and passivity.

compromised/disabled family Coping may be related to inadequate or incorrect information or understanding by a primary person, temporary family disorganization and role changes, client providing little support in turn for the primary person, and prolonged disease and disability progression that exhausts the supportive capacity of significant persons, possibly evidenced by expressions of concern or reports about response of SO(s)/family to client's health problem, preoccupation of SO(s) with own personal reactions, display of intolerance or rejection, and protective behavior disproportionate (too little or too much) to client's abilities or need for autonomy.

Dialysis, peritoneal   MS/CH
Also refer to Dialysis, general

risk for excess Fluid Volume: risk factors may include inadequate osmotic gradient of dialysate, fluid retention—malpositioned, kinked, or clotted catheter; bowel distention, peritonitis, scarring of peritoneum; excessive PO or IV intake.*

risk for Trauma: risk factors may include improper placement during insertion or manipulation of catheter.*

acute Pain/impaired Comfort may be related to catheter irritation, improper catheter placement, presence of edema, abdominal distention, inflammation or infection, rapid infusion or infusion of cold or acidic dialysate, possibly evidenced by verbal reports, guarding or distraction behaviors, and self-focus.

risk for Infection [peritoneal]: risk factors may include contamination of catheter or infusion system, skin contaminants, sterile peritonitis (response to composition of dialysate).*

risk for ineffective Breathing Pattern: risk factors may include increased abdominal pressure restricting diaphragmatic excursion, rapid infusion of dialysate, pain or discomfort, inflammatory process—atelectasis/pneumonia.*

Diaper rash   PED
Refer to Candidiasis

Diarrhea   PED/CH
deficient Knowledge [Learning Need] regarding causative and contributing factors, and therapeutic needs may be related to lack of information, misconceptions, possibly evidenced by statements of concern, questions, and development of preventable complications.

---

*A risk diagnosis is not evidenced by signs and symptoms, as the problem has not occurred; rather, nursing interventions are directed at prevention.

risk for deficient Fluid Volume: risk factors may include excessive losses through gastrointestinal tract, altered intake.*

acute Pain may be related to abdominal cramping and irritation or excoriation of skin, possibly evidenced by verbal reports, facial grimacing, and changes in vital signs.

impaired Skin Integrity may be related to effects of excretions on delicate tissues, possibly evidenced by reports of discomfort and disruption of skin surface or destruction of skin layers.

Digitalis toxicity   MS/CH

decreased Cardiac Output may be related to altered myocardial contractility or electrical conduction, properties of digitalis (long half-life and narrow therapeutic range), concurrent medications, age and general health status, and electrolyte and acid-base balance, possibly evidenced by changes in rate, rhythm, or conduction (development or worsening of dysrhythmias); changes in mentation, worsening of heart failure, elevated serum drug levels.

risk for imbalanced Fluid Volume: risk factors may include excessive losses from vomiting or diarrhea, decreased intake, nausea, decreased plasma proteins, malnutrition, continued use of diuretics; excess sodium and fluid retention.*

deficient Knowledge [Learning Need] regarding condition/therapy and self-care needs may be related to information misinterpretation and lack of recall, possibly evidenced by inaccurate follow-through of instructions and development of preventable complications.

risk for disturbed Thought Processes: risk factors may include physiological effects of toxicity, reduced cerebral perfusion.*

Dilation and curettage (D and C)   OB/GYN
Also refer to Abortion, elective or spontaneous termination

deficient Knowledge [Learning Need] regarding surgical procedure, possible postprocedural complications, and therapeutic needs may be related to lack of exposure or unfamiliarity with information, possibly evidenced by requests for information and statements of concern, misconceptions.

Dilation of cervix, premature   OB
Also refer to Labor, preterm

Anxiety [specify level] may be related to situational crisis, threat of death or fetal loss, possibly evidenced by increased tension, apprehension, feelings of inadequacy, sympathic stimulation, and repetitive questioning.

risk for disrupted Maternal/Fetal Dyad: risk factors may include surgical intervention, use of tocolytic drugs.*

risk for fetal Injury: risk factors may include premature delivery, surgical procedure.*

Grieving may be related to perceived potential fetal loss, possibly evidenced by expression of distress, guilt, anger, choked feelings.

---

*A risk diagnosis is not evidenced by signs and symptoms, as the problem has not occurred; rather, nursing interventions are directed at prevention.

Dislocation/subluxation of joint   CH

acute Pain may be related to lack of continuity of bone/joint, muscle spasms, edema, possibly evidenced by verbal or coded reports, guarded or protective behaviors, narrowed focus, changes in vital signs.

risk for Injury: risk factors may include nerve impingement, improper fitting of splint device.*

impaired physical Mobility may be related to immobilization device, activity restrictions, pain, edema, decreased muscle strength, possibly evidenced by limited range of motion, limited ability to perform motor skills, gait changes.

Disseminated intravascular coagulation (DIC)   MS

risk for deficient Fluid Volume: risk factors may include failure of regulatory mechanism (coagulation process) and active loss—hemorrhage.*

ineffective tissue Perfusion (specify) may be related to alteration of arterial or venous flow (microemboli throughout circulatory system, and hypovolemia), possibly evidenced by changes in respiratory rate and depth, changes in mentation, decreased urinary output, and development of acral cyanosis or focal gangrene.

Anxiety [specify level]/Fear may be related to sudden change in health status/threat of death, interpersonal transmission or contagion, possibly evidenced by sympathetic stimulation, restlessness, focus on self, and apprehension.

risk for impaired Gas Exchange: risk factors may include reduced O_2-carrying capacity, development of acidosis, fibrin deposition in microcirculation, and ischemic damage of lung parenchyma.*

acute Pain may be related to bleeding into joints/muscles, with hematoma formation, and ischemic tissues with areas of acral cyanosis or focal gangrene, possibly evidenced by verbal reports, narrowed focus, alteration in muscle tone, guarding or distraction behaviors, restlessness, changes in vital signs.

Dissociative disorders   PSY

[severe/panic] Anxiety/Fear may be related to a maladaptation or ineffective coping continuing from early life, unconscious conflict(s), threat to self-concept, unmet needs, or phobic stimulus, possibly evidenced by maladaptive response to stress (e.g., dissociating self or fragmentation of the personality), increased tension, feelings of inadequacy, and focus on self, projection of personal perceptions onto the environment.

risk for self-/other-directed Violence: risk factors may include dissociative state/conflicting personalities, depressed mood, panic states, and suicidal or homicidal behaviors.*

disturbed personal Identity may be related to psychological conflicts (dissociative state), childhood trauma or abuse, threat to physical integrity or self-concept, and underdeveloped ego, possibly evidenced by alteration in perception or experience of the self, loss of one's own sense of reality or the external world, poorly differentiated

---

*A risk diagnosis is not evidenced by signs and symptoms, as the problem has not occurred; rather, nursing interventions are directed at prevention.

ego boundaries, confusion about sense of self, confusion regarding purpose or direction in life, memory loss, presence of more than one personality within the individual.

compromised family Coping may be related to multiple stressors repeated over time, prolonged progression of disorder that exhausts the supportive capacity of significant person(s), family disorganization and role changes, high-risk family situation, possibly evidenced by family/SO(s) describing inadequate understanding or knowledge that interferes with assistive or supportive behaviors, relationship and marital conflict.

Diverticulitis   CH

acute Pain may be related to inflammation of intestinal mucosa, abdominal cramping, and presence of fever or chills, possibly evidenced by verbal reports, guarding or distraction behaviors, changes in vital signs, and narrowed focus.

Diarrhea/Constipation may be related to altered structure or function and presence of inflammation, possibly evidenced by signs and symptoms dependent on specific problem (e.g., increase or decrease in frequency of stools and change in consistency).

deficient Knowledge [Learning Need] regarding disease process, potential complications, therapeutic and self-care needs may be related to lack of information/misconceptions, possibly evidenced by statements of concern, request for information, and development of preventable complications.

risk for Powerlessness: risk factors may include chronic nature of disease process and recurrent episodes despite cooperation with medical regimen.*

Down syndrome   PED/CH

Also refer to Mental retardation

delayed Growth and Development may be related to effects of physical or mental disability, possibly evidenced by altered physical growth, delay or inability in performing skills and self-care or self-control activities appropriate for age.

risk for Trauma: risk factors may include cognitive difficulties and poor muscle tone or coordination, weakness.*

imbalanced Nutrition: less than body requirements may be related to poor muscle tone and protruding tongue, possibly evidenced by weak and ineffective sucking or swallowing and observed lack of adequate intake with weight loss or failure to gain.

interrupted Family Processes may be related to situational or maturational crises requiring incorporation of new skills into family dynamics, possibly evidenced by confusion about what to do, verbalized difficulty coping with situation, unexamined family myths.

risk for complicated Grieving: risk factors may include loss of "the perfect child," chronic condition requiring long-term care, and unresolved feelings.*

risk for impaired Attachment: risk factors may include ill infant/child who is unable to effectively initiate parental contact due to altered behavioral organization, inability of parents to meet personal needs.*

---

*A risk diagnosis is not evidenced by signs and symptoms, as the problem has not occurred; rather, nursing interventions are directed at prevention.

risk for Social Isolation: risk factors may include withdrawal from usual social interactions and activities, assumption of total child care, and becoming overindulgent or overprotective.*

Drug overdose, acute (depressants)　　　MS/PSY
Also refer to Substance dependence/abuse rehabilitation

ineffective Breathing Pattern/impaired Gas Exchange may be related to neuromuscular impairment or CNS depression, decreased lung expansion, possibly evidenced by changes in respirations, cyanosis, and abnormal ABGs.

risk for Trauma/Suffocation/Poisoning: risk factors may include CNS depression or agitation, hypersensitivity to the drug(s), psychological stress.*

risk for self-/other-directed Violence: risk factors may include suicidal behaviors, toxic reactions to drug(s).*

risk for Infection: risk factors may include drug injection techniques, impurities in injected drugs, localized trauma; malnutrition, altered immune state.*

Drug withdrawal　　　CH/MS
disturbed Thought Processes may be related to substance abuse and cessation, sleep deprivation, malnutrition possibly evidenced by inaccurate interpretation of environment, inappropriate or non-reality-based thinking, paranoia.

risk for Injury: risk factors may include CNS agitation (depressants).*

risk for Suicide: risk factors may include alcohol or other substance abuse, legal or disciplinary problems, depressed mood (stimulants).*

acute Pain/impaired Comfort may be related to biochemical changes associated with cessation of drug use possibly evidenced by reports of muscle aches, fever, diaphoresis, rhinorrhea, lacrimation, malaise.

Self-Care Deficit (specify) may be related to perceptual or cognitive impairment, therapeutic management (restraints) possibly evidenced by inability to meet own physical needs.

Insomnia may be related to cessation of substance use, fatigue possibly evidenced by reports of insomnia/hypersomnia, decreased ability to function, increased irritability.

Fatigue may be related to altered body chemistry (drug withdrawal), sleep deprivation, malnutrition, poor physical condition possibly evidenced by verbal reports of overwhelming lack of energy, inability to maintain usual level of physical activity, inability to restore energy after sleep, compromised concentration.

Duchenne's muscular dystrophy　　　PED/CH
Refer to Muscular dystrophy [Duchenne's]

DVT　　　CH/MS
Refer to Thrombophlebitis

Dysmenorrhea　　　GYN
acute Pain may be related to exaggerated uterine contractibility, possibly evidenced by verbal reports, guarding or distraction behaviors, narrowed focus, and changes in vital signs.

---

*A risk diagnosis is not evidenced by signs and symptoms, as the problem has not occurred; rather, nursing interventions are directed at prevention.

risk for Activity Intolerance: risk factors may include severity of pain and presence of secondary symptoms (nausea, vomiting, syncope, chills), depression.*

ineffective Coping may be related to chronic, recurrent nature of problem, anticipatory anxiety, and inadequate coping methods, possibly evidenced by muscular tension, headaches, general irritability, chronic depression, and verbalization of inability to cope, report of poor self-concept.

Dysrhythmia, cardiac   MS

risk for decreased Cardiac Output: risk factors may include altered electrical conduction and reduced myocardial contractility.*

deficient Knowledge [Learning Need] regarding medical condition and therapy needs may be related to lack of information or recall, misinterpretation, and unfamiliarity with information resources, possibly evidenced by questions, statement of misconception, failure to improve on previous regimen, and development of preventable complications.

risk for Poisoning, [digitalis toxicity]: risk factors may include limited range of therapeutic effectiveness, lack of education or proper precautions, reduced vision, cognitive limitations.*

Eating disorders   CH/PSY

Refer to Anorexia nervosa; Bulimia nervosa; Obesity

Eclampsia   OB

Also refer to Pregnancy-induced hypertension

Anxiety [specify]/Fear may be related to situational crisis, threat of change in health status or death (self/fetus), separation from support system, interpersonal contagion possibly evidenced by expressed concerns, apprehension, increased tension, decreased self-assurance, difficulty concentrating.

risk for maternal Injury: risk factors may include tissue edema, hypoxia, tonic-clonic convulsions, abnormal blood profile and/or clotting factors.*

impaired physical Mobility may be related to prescribed bedrest, discomfort, anxiety possibly evidenced by difficulty turning, postural instability.

risk for Self-Care Deficit (specify): risk factors may include weakness, discomfort, physical restrictions.*

Ectopic pregnancy (tubal)   OB

Also refer to Abortion, spontaneous termination

acute Pain may be related to distention or rupture of fallopian tube, possibly evidenced by verbal reports, guarding or distraction behaviors, facial mask of pain, and diaphoresis, changes in vital signs.

risk for Bleeding/deficient Fluid Volume [isotonic]: risk factors may include pregnancy-related complications, hemorrhagic losses and decreased or restricted intake.*

Anxiety [specify level]/Fear may be related to threat of death and possible loss of ability to conceive, possibly evidenced by increased

---

*A risk diagnosis is not evidenced by signs and symptoms, as the problem has not occurred; rather, nursing interventions are directed at prevention.

tension, apprehension, sympathetic stimulation, restlessness, and focus on self.

Eczema (dermatitis) CH
acute Pain/impaired Comfort may be related to cutaneous inflammation and irritation, possibly evidenced by verbal reports, irritability, and scratching.

risk for Infection: risk factors may include broken skin and tissue trauma.*

Social Isolation may be related to alterations in physical appearance, possibly evidenced by expressed feelings of rejection and decreased interaction with peers.

Edema, pulmonary MS
excess Fluid Volume may be related to decreased cardiac functioning, excessive fluid/sodium intake, possibly evidenced by dyspnea, presence of crackles (rales), pulmonary congestion on x-ray, restlessness, anxiety, and increased central venous pressure (CVP) and pulmonary pressures.

impaired Gas Exchange may be related to altered blood flow and decreased alveolar/capillary exchange (fluid collection or shifts into interstitial space or alveoli), possibly evidenced by hypoxia, restlessness, and confusion.

Anxiety [specify level]/Fear may be related to perceived threat of death (inability to breathe), possibly evidenced by responses ranging from apprehension to panic state, restlessness, and focus on self.

Emphysema CH/MS
impaired Gas Exchange may be related to alveolar-capillary membrane changes and destruction, possibly evidenced by dyspnea, restlessness, changes in mentation, abnormal ABG values.

ineffective Airway Clearance may be related to increased production or retained tenacious secretions, decreased energy level, and muscle wasting, possibly evidenced by abnormal breath sounds (rhonchi), ineffective cough, changes in rate and depth of respirations, and dyspnea.

Activity Intolerance may be related to imbalance between O_2 supply and demand, possibly evidenced by reports of fatigue, weakness, exertional dyspnea, and abnormal vital sign response to activity.

imbalanced Nutrition: less than body requirements may be related to inability to ingest food (shortness of breath, anorexia, generalized weakness, medication side effects), possibly evidenced by lack of interest in food, reported altered taste, loss of muscle mass and tone, fatigue, and weight loss.

risk for Infection: risk factors may include inadequate primary defenses (stasis of body fluids, decreased ciliary action), chronic disease process, and malnutrition.*

Powerlessness may be related to illness-related regimen and healthcare environment, possibly evidenced by verbal expression of having no

---

*A risk diagnosis is not evidenced by signs and symptoms, as the problem has not occurred; rather, nursing interventions are directed at prevention.

control, depression over physical deterioration, nonparticipation in therapeutic regimen, anger, and passivity.

Encephalitis MS

risk for ineffective cerebral tissue Perfusion: risk factors may include cerebral edema altering or interrupting cerebral arterial or venous blood flow, hypovolemia, exchange problems at cellular level (acidosis).*

Hyperthermia may be related to increased metabolic rate, illness, and dehydration, possibly evidenced by increased body temperature, flushed, warm skin; and increased pulse and respiratory rates.

acute Pain may be related to inflammation or irritation of the brain and cerebral edema, possibly evidenced by verbal reports of headache, photophobia, distraction behaviors, restlessness, and changes in vital signs.

risk for Trauma/Suffocation: risk factors may include restlessness, clonic/tonic activity, altered sensorium, cognitive impairment, generalized weakness, ataxia, vertigo.*

Endocarditis MS

risk for decreased Cardiac Output: risk factors may include inflammation of lining of heart and structural change in valve leaflets.*

Anxiety [specify level] may be related to change in health status and threat of death, possibly evidenced by apprehension, expressed concerns, and focus on self.

acute Pain may be related to generalized inflammatory process and effects of embolic phenomena, possibly evidenced by verbal reports, narrowed focus, distraction behaviors, and changes in vital signs.

risk for Activity Intolerance: risk factors may include imbalance between O$_2$ supply and demand, debilitating condition.*

risk for ineffective tissue Perfusion (specify): risk factors may include embolic interruption of arterial flow (embolization of thrombi or valvular vegetations).*

Endometriosis GYN

acute/chronic Pain may be related to pressure of concealed bleeding, formation of adhesions, possibly evidenced by verbal reports (pain between or with menstruation), guarding or distraction behaviors, and narrowed focus.

Sexual Dysfunction may be related to pain secondary to presence of adhesions, possibly evidenced by verbalization of problem, and altered relationship with partner.

deficient Knowledge [Learning Need] regarding pathophysiology of condition and therapy needs may be related to lack of information/misinterpretations, possibly evidenced by statements of concern and misconceptions.

Enteral feeding MS/CH

imbalanced Nutrition: less than body requirements may be related to conditions that interfere with nutrient intake or increase nutrient need

---

*A risk diagnosis is not evidenced by signs and symptoms, as the problem has not occurred; rather, nursing interventions are directed at prevention.

or metabolic demand—cancer and associated treatments, anorexia, surgical procedures, dysphagia, or decreased level of consciousness, possibly evidenced by body weight 10% or more under ideal, decreased subcutaneous fat or muscle mass, poor muscle tone, changes in gastric motility and stool characteristics.

risk for Infection: risk factors may include invasive procedure with surgical placement of feeding tube, malnutrition, chronic disease, improper preparation, handling or contamination of the feeding solution.*

risk for Aspiration: risk factors may include presence of feeding tube, bolus tube feedings, increased intragastric pressure, delayed gastric emptying, medication administration.*

risk for imbalanced Fluid Volume: risk factors may include active loss or failure of regulatory mechanisms specific to underlying disease process or trauma, inability to obtain or ingest fluids.*

Fatigue may be related to decreased metabolic energy production, increased energy requirements—hypermetabolic state, healing process; altered body chemistry—medications, chemotherapy, possibly evidenced by overwhelming lack of energy, inability to maintain usual routines/accomplish routine tasks, lethargy, impaired ability to concentrate.

Enteritis   MS/CH
Refer to Colitis, ulcerative; Crohn's disease

Epididymitis   MS
acute Pain may be related to inflammation, edema formation, and tension on the spermatic cord, possibly evidenced by verbal reports, guarding or distraction behaviors (restlessness), and changes in vital signs.

risk for Infection, [spread]: risk factors may include presence of inflammation, infectious process, insufficient knowledge to avoid spread of infection.*

deficient Knowledge [Learning Need] regarding pathophysiology, outcome, and self-care needs may be related to lack of information, misinterpretations, possibly evidenced by statements of concern, misconceptions, and questions.

Epilepsy   CH
Refer to Seizure disorder

Erectile dysfunction   CH
Sexual Dysfunction may be related to altered body function possibly evidenced by reports of disruption of sexual response pattern, inability to achieve desired satisfaction.

situational low Self-Esteem may be related to functional impairment; rejection of other(s).

Failure to thrive, infant/child   PED
imbalanced Nutrition: less than body requirements may be related to inability to ingest, digest, or absorb nutrients (defects in organ

---

*A risk diagnosis is not evidenced by signs and symptoms, as the problem has not occurred; rather, nursing interventions are directed at prevention.

function or metabolism, genetic factors), physical deprivation, psychosocial factors, possibly evidenced by lack of appropriate weight gain or weight loss, poor muscle tone, pale conjunctiva, and laboratory tests reflecting nutritional deficiency.

delayed Growth and Development may be related to inadequate caretaking (physical or emotional neglect or abuse), indifference, inconsistent responsiveness, multiple caretakers, environmental and stimulation deficiencies, possibly evidenced by altered physical growth, flat affect, listlessness, decreased response, delay or difficulty in performing skills or self-control activities appropriate for age group.

risk for impaired Parenting: risk factors may include lack of knowledge, inadequate bonding, unrealistic expectations for self or infant, and lack of appropriate response of child to relationship.*

deficient Knowledge [Learning Need] regarding pathophysiology of condition, nutritional needs, growth and development expectations, and parenting skills may be related to lack of information, misinformation or misinterpretation, possibly evidenced by verbalization of concerns, questions, and misconceptions, or development of preventable complications.

Fatigue syndrome, chronic   CH

Fatigue may be related to disease state, inadequate sleep, possibly evidenced by verbalization of unremitting and overwhelming lack of energy, inability to maintain usual routines, listless, compromised concentration.

chronic Pain may be related to chronic physical disability, possibly evidenced by verbal reports of headache, sore throat, arthralgias, abdominal pain, muscle aches, altered ability to continue previous activities, changes in sleep pattern.

Self-Care Deficit [specify] may be related to tiredness, pain/discomfort, possibly evidenced by reports of inability to perform desired ADLs.

risk for ineffective Role Performance: risk factors may include health alterations, stress.*

Fetal alcohol syndrome   PED

risk for Injury [CNS damage]: risk factors may include external chemical factors (alcohol intake by mother), placental insufficiency, fetal drug withdrawal in utero or postpartum, and prematurity.*

disorganized Infant Behavior may be related to prematurity, environmental overstimulation, lack of containment or boundaries, possibly evidenced by change from baseline physiological measures, tremors, startles, twitches, hyperextension of arms and legs, deficient self-regulatory behaviors, deficient response to visual or auditory stimuli.

risk for impaired Parenting: risk factors may include mental and/or physical illness, inability of mother to assume the overwhelming task of unselfish giving and nurturing, presence of stressors (financial or legal problems), lack of available or ineffective role model, interruption of bonding process, lack of appropriate response of child to relationship.*

---

*A risk diagnosis is not evidenced by signs and symptoms, as the problem has not occurred; rather, nursing interventions are directed at prevention.

ineffective [maternal] Coping may be related to personal vulnerability, low self-esteem, inadequate coping skills, and multiple stressors (repeated over period of time), possibly evidenced by inability to meet basic needs, fulfill role expectations, or problem-solve, and excessive use of drug(s).

dysfunctional Family Processes may be related to lack of or insufficient support from others, mother's drug problem and treatment status, together with poor coping skills, lack of family stability, overinvolvement of parents with children and multigenerational addictive behaviors, possibly evidenced by abandonment, rejection, neglectful relationships with family members, and decisions and actions by family that are detrimental.

F

Fetal demise OB

Grieving may be related to death of fetus/infant (wanted or unwanted), possibly evidenced by verbal expressions of distress, anger, loss, crying, alteration in eating habits or sleep pattern.

situational low Self-Esteem may be related to perceived "failure" at a life event, possibly evidenced by negative self-appraisal in response to life event in a person with a previous positive self-evaluation, verbalization of negative feelings about the self (helplessness, uselessness), difficulty making decisions.

risk for Spiritual Distress: risk factors may include loss of loved one, low self-esteem, poor relationships, challenged belief and value system (birth is supposed to be the beginning of life, not of death) and intense suffering.*

Fibromyalgia syndrome, primary CH

acute/chronic Pain may be related to idiopathic diffuse condition possibly evidenced by reports of achy pain in fibrous tissues (muscles, tendons, ligaments), muscle stiffness or spasm, disturbed sleep, guarding behaviors, fear of reinjury or exacerbation, restlessness, irritability, self-focusing, reduced interaction with others.

Fatigue may be related to disease state, stress, anxiety, depression, sleep deprivation possibly evidenced by verbalization of overwhelming lack of energy, inability to maintain usual routines or desired level of physical activity, tired, feelings of guilt for not keeping up with responsibilities, increase in physical complaints, listless.

risk for Hopelessness: risk factors may include chronic debilitating physical condition, prolonged activity restriction (possibly self-induced) creating isolation, lack of specific therapeutic cure, prolonged stress.*

Fractures MS/CH

Also refer to Casts; Traction

risk for Trauma [additional injury]: risk factors may include loss of skeletal integrity, movement of skeletal fragments, use of traction apparatus, and so on.*

---

*A risk diagnosis is not evidenced by signs and symptoms, as the problem has not occurred; rather, nursing interventions are directed at prevention.

acute Pain may be related to muscle spasms, movement of bone fragments, soft tissue trauma, edema, traction or immobility device, stress, and anxiety, possibly evidenced by verbal reports, distraction behaviors, self-focusing or narrowed focus, facial mask of pain, guarding or protective behavior, alteration in muscle tone, and changes in vital signs.

risk for Peripheral Neurovascular Dysfunction: risk factors may include reduction or interruption of blood flow (direct vascular injury, tissue trauma, excessive edema, thrombus formation, hypovolemia).*

impaired physical Mobility may be related to musculoskeletal impairment, pain, discomfort, restrictive therapies—extremity immobilization, bedrest; and psychological immobility, possibly evidenced by inability to purposefully move within the physical environment, imposed restrictions, reluctance to attempt movement, limited range of motion, and decreased muscle strength or control.

risk for impaired Gas Exchange: risk factors may include altered blood flow, blood or fat emboli, alveolar-capillary membrane changes (interstitial pulmonary edema, congestion).*

deficient Knowledge [Learning Need] regarding healing process, therapy requirements, potential complications, and self-care needs may be related to lack of exposure or recall, misinterpretation of information, possibly evidenced by statements of concern, questions, and misconceptions.

Frostbite MS/CH

impaired Tissue Integrity may be related to altered circulation and thermal injury, possibly evidenced by damaged or destroyed tissue.

acute Pain may be related to diminished circulation with tissue ischemia or necrosis, and edema formation, possibly evidenced by verbal reports, guarding or distraction behaviors, narrowed focus, and changes in vital signs.

risk for Infection: risk factors may include traumatized tissue or tissue destruction, altered circulation, and compromised immune response in affected area.*

Gallstones CH
Refer to Cholelithiasis

Gangrene, dry MS

ineffective peripheral tissue Perfusion may be related to interruption in arterial flow, possibly evidenced by cool skin temperature, change in color (black), atrophy of affected part, and presence of pain.

acute Pain may be related to tissue hypoxia and necrotic process, possibly evidenced by verbal reports, guarding or distraction behaviors, narrowed focus, and changes in vital signs.

Gas, lung irritant MS/CH

ineffective Airway Clearance may be related to irritation and inflammation of airway, possibly evidenced by marked cough, abnormal breath sounds (wheezes), dyspnea, and tachypnea.

---

*A risk diagnosis is not evidenced by signs and symptoms, as the problem has not occurred; rather, nursing interventions are directed at prevention.

Health Conditions and Client Concerns **985**

risk for impaired Gas Exchange: risk factors may include irritation and inflammation of alveolar membrane (dependent on type of agent and length of exposure).*

Anxiety [specify level] may be related to change in health status and threat of death, possibly evidenced by verbalizations, increased tension, apprehension, and sympathetic stimulation.

Gastritis, acute   MS

acute Pain may be related to irritation or inflammation of gastric mucosa, possibly evidenced by verbal reports, guarding or distraction behaviors, and changes in vital signs.

risk for deficient Fluid Volume [isotonic]/Bleeding: risk factors may include excessive losses through vomiting and diarrhea, reluctance to ingest or restrictions of oral intake; gastrointestinal disorder, continued bleeding.*

Gastritis, chronic   CH

risk for imbalanced Nutrition: less than body requirements: risk factors may include inability to ingest adequate nutrients (prolonged nausea, vomiting, anorexia, epigastric pain).*

deficient Knowledge [Learning Need] regarding pathophysiology, psychological factors, therapy needs, and potential complications may be related to lack of information or recall, unfamiliarity with information resources, information misinterpretation, possibly evidenced by verbalization of concerns, questions, and continuation of problem or development of preventable complications.

Gastroenteritis   MS

Diarrhea may be related to toxins, contaminants, travel, infectious process, parasites possibly evidenced by at least three loose, liquid stools/day, hyperactive bowel sounds, abdominal pain.

risk for deficient Fluid Volume: risk factors may include excessive losses (diarrhea, vomiting), hypermetabolic state (infection), decreased intake (nausea, anorexia), extremes of age or weight.*

risk for Infection [transmission]: risk factors may include insufficient knowledge to prevent contamination (inappropriate hand hygiene and food handling).*

Gastroesophageal reflux disease (GERD)   CH

acute/chronic Pain may be related to acidic irritation of mucosa, muscle spasm, recurrent vomiting possibly evidenced by reports of heartburn, distraction behaviors.

impaired Swallowing may be related to GERD, esophageal defects, achalasia possibly evidenced by reports of heartburn or epigastric pain, "something stuck" when swallowing, food refusal or volume limiting, nighttime coughing or awakening.

risk for imbalanced Nutrition: less than body requirements: risk factors may include limiting intake, recurrent vomiting.*

risk for Insomnia: risk factors may include nighttime heartburn, regurgitation of stomach contents.*

---

*A risk diagnosis is not evidenced by signs and symptoms, as the problem has not occurred; rather, nursing interventions are directed at prevention.

risk for Aspiration: risk factors may include incompetent lower esophageal sphincter, regurgitation of gastric acid.*

Gender identity disorder   PSY
(For individuals experiencing persistent and marked distress regarding
uncertainty about issues relating to personal identity, e.g., sexual
orientation and behavior.)

Anxiety [specify level] may be related to unconscious or conscious
conflicts about essential values and beliefs (ego-dystonic gender
identification), threat to self-concept, unmet needs, possibly evidenced by increased tension, helplessness, hopelessness, feelings of
inadequacy, uncertainty, insomnia and focus on self, and impaired
daily functioning.

ineffective Role Performance/disturbed personal Identity may be related
to crisis in development in which person has difficulty knowing or
accepting to which sex he or she belongs or is attracted, sense of
discomfort and inappropriateness about anatomical sex characteristics, possibly evidenced by confusion about sense of self, purpose or
direction in life, sexual identification or preference, verbalization of
desire to be or insistence that person is the opposite sex, change in
self-perception of role, and conflict in roles.

ineffective Sexuality Pattern may be related to ineffective or absent role
models and conflict with sexual orientation and/or preferences, lack
of or impaired relationship with an SO, possibly evidenced by verbalizations of discomfort with sexual orientation or role, and lack of
information about human sexuality.

risk for compromised/disabled family Coping: risk factors may include
inadequate or incorrect information or understanding, SO unable to
perceive or to act effectively in regard to client's needs, temporary
family disorganization and role changes, and client providing little
support in turn for primary person.*

readiness for enhanced family Coping may be related to individual's
basic needs being sufficiently gratified and adaptive tasks effectively
addressed to enable goals of self-actualization to surface, possibly
evidenced by family member's attempts to describe growth or impact
of crisis on own values, priorities, goals, or relationships, family
member is moving in direction of health-promoting and enriching
lifestyle that supports client's search for self and choosing experiences that optimize wellness.

Genetic disorder   CH/OB
Anxiety may be related to presence of specific risk factors (e.g., exposure to teratogens), situational crisis, threat to self-concept, conscious or unconscious conflict about essential values and life goals,
possibly evidenced by increased tension, apprehension, uncertainty,
feelings of inadequacy, expressed concerns.

deficient Knowledge [Learning Need] regarding purpose and process
of genetic counseling may be related to lack of awareness of rami-
fications of diagnosis, process necessary for analyzing available options, and information misinterpretation, possibly evidenced by

G

*A risk diagnosis is not evidenced by signs and symptoms, as the problem has
not occurred; rather, nursing interventions are directed at prevention.

verbalization of concerns, statement of misconceptions, request for information.

risk for interrupted Family Processes: risk factors may include situational crisis, individual/family vulnerability, difficulty reaching agreement regarding options.*

Spiritual Distress may be related to intense inner conflict about the outcome, normal grieving for the loss of the "perfect" child, anger that is often directed at God or greater power, religious beliefs and moral convictions, possibly evidenced by verbalization of inner conflict about beliefs, questioning of the moral and ethical implications of therapeutic choices, viewing situation as punishment, anger, hostility, and crying.

risk for complicated Grieving: risk factors may include preloss psychological symptoms, predisposition for anxiety and feelings of inadequacy, frequency of major life events.*

G

Gigantism CH
Refer to Acromegaly

Glaucoma CH
disturbed visual Sensory Perception may be related to altered sensory reception–increased intraocular pressure, atrophy of optic nerve head, possibly evidenced by progressive loss of visual field.

Anxiety [specify level] may be related to change in health status, presence of pain, possibility or reality of loss of vision, unmet needs, and negative self-talk, possibly evidenced by apprehension, uncertainty, and expressed concern regarding changes in life event.

Glomerulonephritis PED
excess Fluid Volume may be related to failure of regulatory mechanism (inflammation of glomerular membrane inhibiting filtration), possibly evidenced by weight gain, edema or anasarca, intake greater than output, and blood pressure changes.

acute Pain may be related to effects of circulating toxins and edema or distention of renal capsule, possibly evidenced by verbal reports, guarding or distraction behaviors, and changes in vital signs.

imbalanced Nutrition: less than body requirements may be related to anorexia and dietary restrictions, possibly evidenced by aversion to eating, reported altered taste, weight loss, and decreased intake.

deficient Diversional Activity may be related to treatment modality or restrictions, fatigue, and malaise, possibly evidenced by statements of boredom, restlessness, and irritability.

risk for disproportionate Growth: risk factors may include infection, malnutrition, chronic illness.*

Goiter CH
disturbed Body Image may be related to visible swelling in neck, possibly evidenced by verbalization of feelings, fear of reaction of others, actual change in structure, change in social involvement.

Anxiety may be related to change in health status and progressive growth of mass, perceived threat of death.

---

*A risk diagnosis is not evidenced by signs and symptoms, as the problem has not occurred; rather, nursing interventions are directed at prevention.

risk for imbalanced Nutrition: less than body requirements: risk factors may include decreased ability to ingest or difficulty swallowing.*

risk for ineffective Airway Clearance: risk factors may include tracheal compression or obstruction.*

Gonorrhea   CH
Also refer to Sexually transmitted disease (STD)

risk for Infection [dissemination, bacteremia]: risk factors may include presence of infectious process in highly vascular area and lack of recognition of disease process.*

acute Pain may be related to irritation or inflammation of mucosa and effects of circulating toxins, possibly evidenced by verbal reports of genital or pharyngeal irritation, perineal or pelvic pain, guarding or distraction behaviors.

deficient Knowledge [Learning Need] regarding disease cause, transmission, therapy, and self-care needs may be related to lack of information, misinterpretation, denial of exposure, possibly evidenced by statements of concern, questions, misconceptions, and inaccurate follow-through of instructions, development of preventable complications.

Gout   CH
acute Pain may be related to inflammation of joint(s), possibly evidenced by verbal reports, guarding or distraction behaviors, and changes in vital signs.

impaired physical Mobility may be related to joint pain and inflammation, possibly evidenced by reluctance to attempt movement, limited range of motion, and therapeutic restriction of movement.

deficient Knowledge [Learning Need] regarding cause, treatment, and prevention of condition may be related to lack of information or misinterpretation, possibly evidenced by statements of concern, questions, misconceptions, and inaccurate follow-through of instructions.

Guillain-Barré syndrome (acute polyneuritis)   MS
risk for ineffective Breathing Pattern/Airway Clearance: risk factors may include weakness or paralysis of respiratory muscles, impaired gag or swallow reflexes, decreased energy, fatigue.*

disturbed Sensory Perceptual (specify) may be related to altered sensory reception, transmission, or integration (altered status of sense organs, sleep deprivation), therapeutically restricted environment, endogenous chemical alterations (electrolyte imbalance, hypoxia), and psychological stress, possibly evidenced by reported or observed change in usual response to stimuli, altered communication patterns, and measured change in sensory acuity and motor coordination.

impaired physical Mobility may be related to neuromuscular impairment, pain or discomfort, possibly evidenced by impaired coordination, partial or complete paralysis, decreased muscle strength and control.

---

*A risk diagnosis is not evidenced by signs and symptoms, as the problem has not occurred; rather, nursing interventions are directed at prevention.

Anxiety [specify level]/Fear may be related to situational crisis, change in health status or threat of death, possibly evidenced by increased tension, restlessness, helplessness, apprehension, uncertainty, fearfulness, focus on self, and sympathetic stimulation.

risk for Disuse Syndrome: risk factors include paralysis and pain.*

Hallucinogen abuse   **CH/PSY**

Also refer to Substance dependence/abuse rehabilitation

disturbed Thought Processes may be related to physiological changes associated with drug use, impaired judgment, memory loss, possibly evidenced by inaccurate interpretation of environment, bizarre thinking, disorientation, inability to make decisions, unpredictable behavior, distractibility, non–reality based thinking.

Anxiety/Fear may be related to situational crisis, threat to or change in health status, perceived threat of death, inexperience or unfamiliarity with effects of drug possibly evidenced by assumptions of "losing my mind or control," apprehension, preoccupation with feelings of impending doom, sympathetic stimulation.

Self-Care Deficit (specify) may be related to perceptual or cognitive impairment, therapeutic management (restraints) possibly evidenced by inability to meet own physical needs.

Hay fever   **CH**

impaired Comfort may be related to irritation or inflammation of upper airway mucous membranes and conjunctiva, possibly evidenced by verbal reports, irritability, and restlessness.

deficient Knowledge [Learning Need] regarding underlying cause, appropriate therapy, and required lifestyle changes may be related to lack of information, possibly evidenced by statements of concern, questions, and misconceptions.

Heart failure, chronic   **MS**

decreased Cardiac Output may be related to altered myocardial contractility, inotropic changes; alterations in rate, rhythm, and electrical conduction; and structural changes (valvular defects, ventricular aneurysm), possibly evidenced by tachycardia, dysrhythmias, changes in blood pressure, extra heart sounds, decreased urine output, diminished peripheral pulses, cool, ashen skin; orthopnea, crackles; dependent or generalized edema and chest pain.

excess Fluid Volume may be related to reduced glomerular filtration rate, increased antidiuretic hormone production, and sodium and water retention, possibly evidenced by orthopnea and abnormal breath sounds, S_3 heart sound, jugular vein distention, positive hepatojugular reflex, weight gain, hypertension, oliguria, generalized edema.

risk for impaired Gas Exchange: risk factors may include alveolar-capillary membrane changes (fluid collection or shifts into interstitial space or alveoli).*

                                                            CH

Activity Intolerance may be related to imbalance between O_2 supply and demand, generalized weakness, and prolonged bedrest, sedentary

---

*A risk diagnosis is not evidenced by signs and symptoms, as the problem has not occurred; rather, nursing interventions are directed at prevention.

lifestyle, possibly evidenced by reported or observed weakness, fatigue, changes in vital signs, presence of dysrhythmias, dyspnea, pallor, and diaphoresis.

risk for impaired Skin Integrity: risk factors may include prolonged chair or bedrest, edema, vascular pooling, decreased tissue perfusion.*

deficient Knowledge [Learning Need] regarding cardiac function/ disease process, therapy and self-care needs may be related to lack of information or misinterpretation, possibly evidenced by questions, statements of concern, misconceptions; development of preventable complications or exacerbations of condition.

Heatstroke   MS
Hyperthermia may be related to prolonged exposure to hot environment, vigorous activity with failure of regulating mechanism of the body, possibly evidenced by high body temperature (>105°F [40.6°C]), flushed, hot skin; tachycardia, and seizure activity.

decreased Cardiac Output may be related to functional stress of hypermetabolic state, altered circulating volume and venous return, and direct myocardial damage secondary to hyperthermia, possibly evidenced by decreased peripheral pulses, dysrhythmias, tachycardia, and changes in mentation.

Hemodialysis   MS/CH
Also refer to Dialysis, general

risk for Injury [loss of vascular access]: risk factors may include clotting or thrombosis, infection, disconnection and hemorrhage.*

risk for deficient Fluid Volume/Bleeding: risk factors may include excessive fluid losses or shifts via ultrafiltration, fluid restrictions, altered coagulation, disconnection of shunt.*

risk for excess Fluid Volume: risk factors may include rapid or excessive fluid intake—IV, blood, plasma expanders, saline given to support BP during procedure.*

ineffective Protection may be related to chronic disease state, drug therapy, abnormal blood profile, inadequate nutrition, possibly evidenced by altered clotting, impaired healing, deficient immunity, fatigue, anorexia.

Hemophilia   PED
risk for deficient Fluid Volume [isotonic]: risk factors may include impaired coagulation/hemorrhagic losses.*

risk for acute/chronic Pain: risk factors may include nerve compression from hematomas, nerve damage, or hemorrhage into joint space.*

risk for impaired physical Mobility: risk factors may include joint hemorrhage, swelling, degenerative changes, and muscle atrophy.*

ineffective Protection may be related to abnormal blood profile, possibly evidenced by altered clotting.

compromised family Coping may be related to prolonged nature of condition that exhausts the supportive capacity of significant

---

*A risk diagnosis is not evidenced by signs and symptoms, as the problem has not occurred; rather, nursing interventions are directed at prevention.

person(s), possibly evidenced by protective behaviors disproportionate to client's abilities or need for autonomy.

Hemorrhoidectomy   MS/CH

acute Pain may be related to edema or swelling, and tissue trauma, possibly evidenced by verbal reports, guarding or distraction behaviors, focus on self, and changes in vital signs.

risk for Urinary Retention: risk factors may include perineal trauma, edema or swelling, and pain.*

deficient Knowledge [Learning Need] regarding therapeutic treatment and potential complications may be related to lack of information or misconceptions, possibly evidenced by statements of concern and questions.

Hemorrhoids   CH/OB

acute Pain may be related to inflammation and edema of prolapsed varices, possibly evidenced by verbal reports, and guarding or distraction behaviors.

Constipation may be related to pain on defecation and reluctance to defecate, possibly evidenced by frequency less than usual pattern, and hard, formed stools.

Hemothorax   MS

Also refer to Pneumothorax

risk for Trauma/Suffocation: risk factors may include concurrent disease or injury process, dependence on external device (chest drainage system), and lack of safety education or precautions.*

Anxiety [specify level] may be related to change in health status and threat of death, possibly evidenced by increased tension, restlessness, expressed concern, sympathetic stimulation, and focus on self.

Hepatitis, acute viral   MS/CH

impaired Liver Function related to viral infection as evidenced by jaundice, hepatic enlargement, abdominal pain, marked elevations in serum liver function tests.

Fatigue may be related to decreased metabolic energy production, discomfort, altered body chemistry—changes in liver function, effect on target organs, possibly evidenced by reports of lack of energy, inability to maintain usual routines, decreased performance, and increased physical complaints.

imbalanced Nutrition: less than body requirements may be related to inability to ingest adequate nutrients—nausea, vomiting, anorexia, hypermetabolic state, altered absorption and metabolism, possibly evidenced by aversion to eating or lack of interest in food, altered taste sensation, observed lack of intake, and weight loss.

acute Pain/impaired Comfort may be related to inflammation and swelling of the liver, arthralgias, urticarial eruptions, and pruritus, possibly evidenced by verbal reports, guarding or distraction behaviors, focus on self, and changes in vital signs.

---

*A risk diagnosis is not evidenced by signs and symptoms, as the problem has not occurred; rather, nursing interventions are directed at prevention.

risk for Infection: risk factors may include inadequate secondary defenses and immunosuppression, malnutrition, insufficient knowledge to avoid exposure to pathogens.*

risk for impaired Tissue Integrity: risk factors may include bile salt accumulation in the tissues.*

risk for impaired Home Management: risk factors may include debilitating effects of disease process and inadequate support systems (family, financial, role model).*

deficient Knowledge [Learning Need] regarding disease process and transmission, treatment needs, and future expectations may be related to lack of information or recall, misinterpretation, unfamiliarity with resources, possibly evidenced by questions, statement of concerns, misconceptions, inaccurate follow-through of instructions, or development of preventable complications.

Hernia, hiatal   CH

chronic Pain may be related to regurgitation of acidic gastric contents, possibly evidenced by verbal reports, facial grimacing, and focus on self.

deficient Knowledge [Learning Need] regarding pathophysiology, prevention of complications and self-care needs may be related to lack of information, misconceptions, possibly evidenced by statements of concern, questions, and recurrence of condition.

Herniated nucleus pulposus (ruptured
intervertebral disk)   CH/MS

acute/chronic Pain may be related to nerve compression or irritation and muscle spasms, possibly evidenced by verbal reports, guarding or distraction behaviors, preoccupation with pain, self-focus or narrowed focus, changes in vital signs when pain is acute, altered muscle tone or function, changes in eating or sleeping patterns and libido, physical or social withdrawal.

impaired physical Mobility may be related to pain (muscle spasms), discomfort, therapeutic restrictions—bedrest, traction, or braces; muscular impairment, and depressive mood state, possibly evidenced by reports of pain on movement, reluctance to attempt or difficulty with purposeful movement, decreased muscle strength, impaired coordination, and limited range of motion.

deficient Diversional Activity may be related to length of recuperation period and therapy restrictions, physical limitations, pain, and depression, possibly evidenced by statements of boredom, disinterest, "nothing to do," restlessness, irritability, withdrawal.

Heroin withdrawal   CH/MS

acute Pain/impaired Comfort may be related to cessation of drug, muscle tremors/twitching, possibly evidenced by reports of muscle aches, hot or cold flashes, diaphoresis, lacrimation, rhinorrhea, drug cravings.

severe Anxiety may be related to CNS hyperactivity possibly evidenced by apprehension, pervasive anxious feelings, jittery, restlessness, weakness, insomnia, anorexia.

---

*A risk diagnosis is not evidenced by signs and symptoms, as the problem has not occurred; rather, nursing interventions are directed at prevention.

risk for ineffective self Health Management: risk factors may include protracted withdrawal, economic difficulties, family or social support deficits, perceived barriers or benefits.*

Herpes, herpes simplex   CH
acute Pain may be related to presence of localized inflammation and open lesions, possibly evidenced by verbal reports, distraction behaviors, and restlessness.

risk for [secondary] Infection: risk factors may include broken or traumatized tissue, altered immune response, and untreated infection or treatment failure.*

risk for Sexual Dysfunction: risk factors may include lack of knowledge, values conflict, and/or fear of transmitting the disease.*

Herpes zoster (shingles)   CH
acute Pain may be related to inflammation and local lesions along sensory nerve(s), possibly evidenced by verbal reports, guarding or distraction behaviors, narrowed focus, restlessness, and changes in vital signs.

deficient Knowledge [Learning Need] regarding pathophysiology, therapeutic needs, and potential complications may be related to lack of information, misinterpretation, possibly evidenced by statements of concern, questions, and misconceptions.

High-altitude pulmonary edema (HAPE)   MS
Also refer to Mountain sickness, acute

impaired Gas Exchange may be related to ventilation perfusion imbalance, alveolar-capillary membrane changes, altered O_2 supply, possibly evidenced by dyspnea, confusion, cyanosis, tachycardia, abnormal ABGs.

excess Fluid Volume may be related to compromised regulatory mechanism, possibly evidenced by shortness of breath, anxiety, edema, abnormal breath sounds, pulmonary congestion.

High-altitude sickness   MS
Refer to Mountain sickness, acute; High-altitude pulmonary edema

HIV infection   CH
Also refer to AIDS

risk-prone health Behavior may be related to life-threatening, stigmatizing condition or disease, assault to self-esteem, altered locus of control, inadequate support systems, possibly evidenced by verbalization of nonacceptance or denial of diagnosis, failure to take action that prevents health problems.

deficient Knowledge [Learning Need] regarding disease, prognosis, and treatment needs may be related to lack of exposure or recall, information misinterpretation, unfamiliarity with information resources, or cognitive limitation, possibly evidenced by statement of misconception, request for information, inappropriate or exaggerated behaviors (hostile, agitated, hysterical, apathetic), inaccurate

*A risk diagnosis is not evidenced by signs and symptoms, as the problem has not occurred; rather, nursing interventions are directed at prevention.

follow-through of instructions, or development of preventable complications.

risk for ineffective self Health Management: risk factors may include complexity of healthcare system and access to care, economic difficulties; complexity of therapeutic regimen—confusing or difficult dosing schedule, duration of regimen; mistrust of regimen and/or healthcare personnel—client and provider interactions; health beliefs or cultural influences, perceived seriousness, susceptibility, or benefits of therapy; decisional conflicts, powerlessness.*

risk for complicated Grieving: risk factors may include preloss psychological symptoms, predisposition for anxiety and feelings of inadequacy, frequency of major life events.*

Hodgkin's disease   CH/MS
Also refer to Cancer; Chemotherapy

Anxiety [specify level]/Fear may be related to threat of self-concept and threat of death, possibly evidenced by apprehension, insomnia, focus on self, and increased tension.

deficient Knowledge [Learning Need] regarding diagnosis, pathophysiology, treatment, and prognosis may be related to lack of information/misinterpretation, possibly evidenced by statements of concern, questions, and misconceptions.

acute Pain/impaired Comfort may be related to manifestations of inflammatory response (fever, chills, night sweats) and pruritus, possibly evidenced by verbal reports, distraction behaviors, and focus on self.

risk for ineffective Breathing Pattern/Airway Clearance: risk factors may include tracheobronchial obstruction (enlarged mediastinal nodes and/or airway edema).*

Hospice/End-of-life care   CH
acute/chronic Pain may be related to biological, physical, psychological agent; chronic physical disability, possibly evidenced by verbal or coded report, preoccupation with pain, changes in appetite/eating, sleep pattern, altered ability to continue desired activities, guarded or protective behaviors, restlessness, irritability, narrowed focus—altered time perception, impaired thought processes.

Activity Intolerance/Fatigue may be related to generalized weakness, bedrest or immobility, pain, progressive disease state or debilitating condition, depressive state, imbalance between O_2 supply and demand, possibly evidenced by inability to maintain usual routine, verbalized lack of desire or interest in activity, decreased performance, lethargy.

Grieving/death Anxiety may be related to anticipated loss of physiological well-being, change in body function, perceived threat of death or dying process, possibly evidenced by changes in communication pattern, denial of potential loss; choked feelings, anger, fear of loss of physical or mental abilities; negative death images or unpleasant thoughts about any event related to death or dying; anticipated pain related to dying; powerlessness over issues related to dying, worrying about impact of one's own death on SO(s), being the cause of other's

---

*A risk diagnosis is not evidenced by signs and symptoms, as the problem has not occurred; rather, nursing interventions are directed at prevention.

grief and suffering, concerns of overworking the caregiver as terminal illness incapacitates.

compromised/disabled family Coping/Caregiver Role Strain may be related to prolonged disease/disability progression, temporary family disorganization and role changes, unrealistic expectations, inadequate or incorrect information or understanding by primary person, possibly evidenced by client expressing despair about family reactions or lack of involvement, history of poor relationship between caregiver and care receiver; altered caregiver health status; SO attempting assistive or supportive behaviors with less than satisfactory results, apprehension about future regarding caregiver's ability to provide care; SO describing preoccupation about personal reactions; displaying intolerance, abandonment, rejection; family behaviors that are detrimental to well-being.

risk for Spiritual Distress: risk factors may include physical or psychological stress, energy-consuming anxiety; situational losses; blocks to self-love, low self-esteem, inability to forgive.*

risk for moral Distress: risk factors may include conflict among decision makers, cultural conflicts, end-of-life decisions, loss of autonomy, physical distance of decision makers.*

Hydrocephalus   PED/MS

ineffective cerebral tissue Perfusion may be related to decreased arterial or venous blood flow (compression of brain tissue), possibly evidenced by changes in mentation, restlessness, irritability, reports of headache, pupillary changes, and changes in vital signs.

disturbed visual Sensory Perception may be related to pressure on sensory or motor nerves, possibly evidenced by reports of double vision, development of strabismus, nystagmus, pupillary changes, and optic atrophy.

risk for impaired physical Mobility: risk factors may include neuromuscular impairment, decreased muscle strength, and impaired coordination.*

risk for decreased Intracranial Adaptive Capacity: risk factors may include brain injury, changes in perfusion pressure or intracranial pressure.*

CH

risk for Infection: risk factors may include invasive procedure, presence of shunt.*

deficient Knowledge [Learning Need] regarding condition, prognosis, and long-term therapy needs and medical follow-up may be related to lack of information, misperceptions, possibly evidenced by questions, statement of concern, request for information, and inaccurate follow-through of instruction, or development of preventable complications.

Hyperactivity disorder   PED/PSY

defensive Coping may be related to mild neurological deficits, dysfunctional family system, abuse or neglect, possibly evidenced by denial of obvious problems, projection of blame or responsibility, grandiosity, difficulty in reality testing perceptions.

---

*A risk diagnosis is not evidenced by signs and symptoms, as the problem has not occurred; rather, nursing interventions are directed at prevention.

impaired Social Interaction may be related to retarded ego development, negative role models, neurological impairment, possibly evidenced by discomfort in social situations; interrupts or intrudes on others, difficulty waiting turn in games or group activities, difficulty maintaining attention to task.

disabled family Coping may be related to excessive guilt, anger, or blaming among family members, parental inconsistencies, disagreements regarding discipline, limit-setting, approaches; exhaustion of parental expectations, possibly evidenced by unrealistic parental expectations, rejection or overprotection of child, exaggerated expression of feelings, despair regarding child's behavior.

Hyperbilirubinemia   PED

neonatal Jaundice may be related to, difficulty transitioning to extrauterine life, feeding pattern not well established, abnormal weight loss, possibly evidenced by abnormal blood profile—elevated BUN, yellow-orange skin/sclera.

risk for Injury [effects of treatment]: risk factors may include physical properties of phototherapy and effects on body regulatory mechanisms, invasive procedure (exchange transfusion), abnormal blood profile, chemical imbalances.*

deficient Knowledge [Learning Need] regarding condition prognosis, treatment and safety needs may be related to lack of exposure or recall and information misinterpretation, possibly evidenced by questions, statement of concern, and inaccurate follow-through of instructions, or development of preventable complications.

Hyperemesis gravidarum   OB

deficient Fluid Volume [isotonic] may be related to excessive gastric losses and reduced intake, possibly evidenced by dry mucous membranes, decreased, concentrated urine; decreased pulse volume and pressure, thirst, and hemoconcentration.

risk for Electrolyte Imbalance: risk factors may include vomiting, dehydration.*

imbalanced Nutrition: less than body requirements may be related to inability to ingest, digest, or absorb nutrients (prolonged vomiting), possibly evidenced by reported inadequate food intake, lack of interest in food or aversion to eating, and weight loss.

risk for ineffective Coping: risk factors may include situational or maturational crisis (pregnancy, change in health status, projected role changes, concern about outcome).*

Hypertension   CH

deficient Knowledge [Learning Need] regarding condition, therapeutic regimen, and potential complications may be related to lack of information or recall, misinterpretation, cognitive limitations, and/or denial of diagnosis, possibly evidenced by statements of concern, questions, and misconceptions, inaccurate follow-through of instructions, and lack of BP control.

---

*A risk diagnosis is not evidenced by signs and symptoms, as the problem has not occurred; rather, nursing interventions are directed at prevention.

risk-prone health Behavior may be related to condition requiring change in lifestyle, altered locus of control, and absence of feelings, denial of illness, possibly evidenced by verbalization of nonacceptance of health status change and lack of movement toward independence.

risk for Activity Intolerance: risk factors may include generalized weakness, imbalance between oxygen supply and demand.*

risk for Sexual Dysfunction: risk factors may include side effects of medication.*

MS

risk for decreased Cardiac Output: risk factors may include increased afterload (vasoconstriction), fluid shifts, hypovolemia, myocardial ischemia, ventricular hypertrophy or rigidity.*

acute Pain may be related to increased cerebrovascular pressure, possibly evidenced by verbal reports (throbbing pain located in suboccipital region, present on awakening and disappearing spontaneously after being up and about), reluctance to move head, avoidance of bright lights and noise, increased muscle tension.

Hypertension, pulmonary   CH/MS
Refer to Pulmonary hypertension

Hyperthyroidism   CH
Also refer to Thyrotoxicosis

Fatigue may be related to hypermetabolic imbalance with increased energy requirements, irritability of CNS, and altered body chemistry, possibly evidenced by verbalization of overwhelming lack of energy to maintain usual routine, decreased performance, emotional lability or irritability, and impaired ability to concentrate.

Anxiety [specify level] may be related to increased stimulation of the CNS (hypermetabolic state, pseudocatecholamine effect of thyroid hormones), possibly evidenced by increased feelings of apprehension, overexcitement or distress, irritability or emotional lability, shakiness, restless movements, tremors.

risk for imbalanced Nutrition: less than body requirements: risk factors may include inability to ingest adequate nutrients for hypermetabolic rate and constant activity level, impaired absorption of nutrients—vomiting, diarrhea), hyperglycemia, relative insulin insufficiency.*

risk for impaired Tissue Integrity: risk factors may include periorbital edema, altered protective mechanisms of eye—reduced ability to blink; eye dryness.*

Hypoglycemia   CH
disturbed Thought Processes may be related to inadequate glucose for cellular brain function and effects of endogenous hormone activity, possibly evidenced by irritability, changes in mentation, memory loss, altered attention span, and emotional lability.

risk for unstable blood Glucose Level: risk factors may include dietary intake, lack of adherence to diabetes management, inadequate blood glucose monitoring, medication management.*

---

*A risk diagnosis is not evidenced by signs and symptoms, as the problem has not occurred; rather, nursing interventions are directed at prevention.

deficient Knowledge [Learning Need] regarding pathophysiology of condition, therapy, and self-care needs may be related to lack of information or recall, misinterpretations, possibly evidenced by development of hypoglycemia and statements of questions, misconceptions.

Hypoparathyroidism (acute)   MS

risk for Injury: risk factors may include neuromuscular excitability or tetany and formation of renal stones.*

acute Pain may be related to recurrent muscle spasms and alteration in reflexes, possibly evidenced by verbal reports, distraction behaviors, and narrowed focus.

risk for ineffective Airway Clearance: risk factors may include spasm of the laryngeal muscles.*

Anxiety [specify level] may be related to threat to, or change in, health status, physiological responses.

Hypothermia (systemic)   CH
Also refer to Frostbite

Hypothermia may be related to exposure to cold environment, inadequate clothing, age extremes (very young or elderly), damage to hypothalamus, consumption of alcohol or medications causing vasodilation, possibly evidenced by reduction in body temperature below normal range, shivering, cool skin, pallor.

deficient Knowledge [Learning Need] regarding risk factors, treatment needs, and prognosis may be related to lack of information or recall, misinterpretation, possibly evidenced by statement of concerns, misconceptions, occurrence of problem, and development of complications.

Hypothyroidism   CH
Also refer to Myxedema

impaired physical Mobility may be related to weakness, fatigue, muscle aches, altered reflexes, and mucin deposits in joints and interstitial spaces, possibly evidenced by decreased muscle strength or control, and impaired coordination.

Fatigue may be related to decreased metabolic energy production, possibly evidenced by verbalization of unremitting or overwhelming lack of energy, inability to maintain usual routines, impaired ability to concentrate, decreased libido, irritability, listlessness, decreased performance, increase in physical complaints.

disturbed Sensory Perception (specify) may be related to mucin deposits and nerve compression, possibly evidenced by paresthesias of hands and feet or decreased hearing.

Constipation may be related to decreased physical activity, slowed peristalsis, possibly evidenced by frequency less than usual pattern, decreased bowel sounds, hard dry stools, and development of fecal impaction.

---

*A risk diagnosis is not evidenced by signs and symptoms, as the problem has not occurred; rather, nursing interventions are directed at prevention.

Hysterectomy GYN/MS

Also refer to Surgery, general

acute Pain may be related to tissue trauma and abdominal incision, edema or hematoma formation, possibly evidenced by verbal reports, guarding or distraction behaviors, and changes in vital signs.

risk for impaired Urinary Elimination/[acute] Urinary Retention: risk factors may include mechanical trauma, surgical manipulation, presence of localized edema or hematoma, or nerve trauma with temporary bladder atony.*

risk for Sexual Dysfunction: risk factors may include concerns regarding altered body function or structure, perceived changes in femininity, changes in hormone levels, loss of libido, and changes in sexual response pattern.*

risk for complicated Grieving: risk factors may include preloss psychological symptoms, predisposition for anxiety and feelings of inadequacy, frequency of major life events. *

Ileocolitis MS/CH

Refer to Crohn's disease

Ileostomy MS/CH

Refer to Colostomy

Ileus MS

acute Pain may be related to distention or edema, and ischemia of intestinal tissue, possibly evidenced by verbal reports, guarding or distraction behaviors, narrowed focus, and changes in vital signs.

Diarrhea/Constipation may be related to presence of obstruction or changes in peristalsis, possibly evidenced by changes in frequency and consistency or absence of stool, alterations in bowel sounds, presence of pain, and cramping.

risk for deficient Fluid Volume: risk factors may include increased intestinal losses (vomiting and diarrhea), and decreased intake.*

Impetigo PED/CH

impaired Skin Integrity may be related to presence of infectious process and pruritus, possibly evidenced by open or crusted lesions.

acute Pain may be related to inflammation and pruritus, possibly evidenced by verbal reports, distraction behaviors, and self-focusing.

risk for [secondary] Infection: risk factors may include broken skin, traumatized tissue, altered immune response, and virulence and contagious nature of causative organism.*

risk for Infection [transmission]: risk factors may include virulent nature of causative organism, insufficient knowledge to prevent infection of others.*

Infection, prenatal OB

Also refer to AIDS

risk for maternal/fetal Infection: risk factors may include inadequate primary defenses (e.g., broken skin, stasis of body fluids), inadequate

---

*A risk diagnosis is not evidenced by signs and symptoms, as the problem has not occurred; rather, nursing interventions are directed at prevention.

secondary defenses (e.g., decreased Hb, immunosuppression), inadequate acquired immunity, environmental exposure, malnutrition, rupture of amniotic membranes.*

deficient Knowledge regarding treatment/prevention, prognosis of condition may be related to lack of exposure to information and/or unfamiliarity with resources, misinterpretation possibly evidenced by verbalization of problem, inaccurate follow-through of instructions, development of preventable complications or continuation of infectious process.

impaired Comfort may be related to body response to infective agent, properties of infection (e.g., skin or tissue irritation, development of lesions), possibly evidenced by verbal reports, restlessness, withdrawal from social contacts.

Inflammatory bowel disease   CH
Refer to Colitis, ulcerative; Crohn's disease

Infertility   CH
situational low Self-Esteem may be related to functional impairment (inability to conceive), unrealistic self-expectations, sense of failure possibly evidenced by self-negating verbalizations, expressions of helplessness, perceived inability to deal with situation.

chronic Sorrow may be related to perceived physical disability (inability to conceive) possibly evidenced by expressions of anger, disappointment, emptiness, self-blame, helplessness, sadness, feelings interfering with client's ability to achieve maximum well-being.

risk for Spiritual Distress: risk factors may include energy-consuming anxiety, low self-esteem, deteriorating relationship with SO, viewing situation as deserved or punishment for past behaviors.*

Influenza   CH
acute Pain/impaired Comfort may be related to inflammation and effects of circulating toxins, possibly evidenced by verbal reports, distraction behaviors, and narrowed focus.

risk for deficient Fluid Volume: risk factors may include excessive gastric losses, hypermetabolic state, and altered intake.*

Hyperthermia may be related to effects of circulating toxins and dehydration, possibly evidenced by increased body temperature, warm, flushed skin; and tachycardia.

risk for ineffective Breathing: risk factors may include response to infectious process, decreased energy, fatigue.*

Insulin shock   MS/CH
Refer to Hypoglycemia

Intestinal obstruction   MS
Refer to Ileus

Irritable bowel syndrome   CH
acute Pain may be related to abnormally strong intestinal contractions, increased sensitivity of intestine to distention, hypersensitivity to

---

*A risk diagnosis is not evidenced by signs and symptoms, as the problem has not occurred; rather, nursing interventions are directed at prevention.

hormones gastrin and cholecystokinin, skin or tissue irritation, perirectal excoriation, possibly evidenced by verbal reports, guarding behavior, expressive behavior (restlessness, moaning, irritability).

Constipation may be related to motor abnormalities of longitudinal muscles and changes in frequency and amplitude of contractions, dietary restrictions, stress, possibly evidenced by change in bowel pattern, decreased frequency, sensation of incomplete evacuation, abdominal pain, distention.

Diarrhea may be related to motor abnormalities of longitudinal muscles and changes in frequency and amplitude of contractions, possibly evidenced by precipitous passing of liquid stool on rising or immediately after eating, rectal urgency, incontinence, bloating.

Kawasaki disease   PED

Hyperthermia may be related to increased metabolic rate and dehydration, possibly evidenced by increased body temperature greater than normal range, flushed skin, increased respiratory rate, and tachycardia.

acute Pain may be related to inflammation and edema or swelling of tissues, possibly evidenced by verbal reports, restlessness, guarding behaviors, and narrowed focus.

impaired Skin Integrity may be related to inflammatory process, altered circulation, and edema formation, possibly evidenced by disruption of skin surface, including macular rash and desquamation.

impaired Oral Mucous Membrane may be related to inflammatory process, dehydration, and mouth breathing, possibly evidenced by pain, hyperemia, and fissures of lips.

risk for decreased Cardiac Output: risk factors may include structural changes, inflammation of coronary arteries and alterations in rate, rhythm, or conduction.*

Kidney stone(s)   CH

Refer to Calculi, urinary

Labor, induced/augmented   OB

deficient Knowledge [Learning Need] regarding procedure, treatment needs, and possible outcomes may be related to lack of exposure/recall, information misinterpretation, and unfamiliarity with information resources, possibly evidenced by questions, statements of concern/misconception, and exaggerated behaviors.

risk for maternal Injury: risk factors may include adverse effects or response to therapeutic interventions.*

risk for impaired fetal Gas Exchange: risk factors may include altered placental perfusion or cord prolapse.*

acute Pain may be related to altered characteristics of chemically stimulated contractions, psychological concerns, possibly evidenced by verbal reports, increased muscle tone, distraction or guarding behaviors, and narrowed focus.

---

*A risk diagnosis is not evidenced by signs and symptoms, as the problem has not occurred; rather, nursing interventions are directed at prevention.

Labor, precipitous   **OB**

Anxiety [specify level] may be related to situational crisis, threat to self or fetus, interpersonal transmission, possibly evidenced by increased tension; scared, fearful, restless, jittery; sympathetic stimulation.

risk for impaired Skin/Tissue Integrity: risk factors may include rapid progress of labor, lack of necessary equipment.*

acute Pain may be related to occurrence of rapid, strong muscle contractions; psychological issues, possibly evidenced by verbalizations of inability to use learned pain-management techniques, sympathetic stimulation, distraction behaviors (e.g., moaning, restlessness).

Labor, preterm   **OB/CH**

Activity Intolerance may be related to muscle or cellular hypersensitivity, possibly evidenced by continued uterine contractions or irritability.

risk for Poisoning: risk factors may include dose-related toxic or side effects of tocolytics.*

risk for fetal Injury: risk factors may include delivery of premature or immature infant.*

Anxiety [specify level] may be related to situational crisis, perceived or actual threats to self or fetus, and inadequate time to prepare for labor, possibly evidenced by increased tension, restlessness, expressions of concern, and changes in vital signs.

deficient Knowledge [Learning Need] regarding preterm labor treatment needs and prognosis may be related to lack of information and misinterpretation, possibly evidenced by questions, statements of concern, misconceptions, inaccurate follow-through of instruction, and development of preventable complications.

Labor, stage I (active phase)   **OB**

acute Pain/impaired Comfort may be related to contraction-related hypoxia, dilation of tissues, and pressure on adjacent structures combined with stimulation of both parasympathetic and sympathetic nerve endings, possibly evidenced by verbal reports, guarding or distraction behaviors (restlessness), muscle tension, and narrowed focus.

impaired Urinary Elimination may be related to altered intake, dehydration, fluid shifts, hormonal changes, hemorrhage, severe intrapartal hypertension, mechanical compression of bladder, and effects of regional anesthesia, possibly evidenced by changes in amount or frequency of voiding, urinary retention, slowed progression of labor, and reduced sensation.

risk for ineffective [individual/couple] Coping : risk factors may include situational crises, personal vulnerability, use of ineffective coping mechanisms, inadequate support systems, and pain.*

Labor, stage II (expulsion)   **OB**

acute Pain may be related to strong uterine contractions, tissue stretching/ dilation and compression of nerves by presenting part of the fetus, and bladder distention, possibly evidenced by verbalizations, facial

---

*A risk diagnosis is not evidenced by signs and symptoms, as the problem has not occurred; rather, nursing interventions are directed at prevention.

grimacing, guarding or distraction behaviors (restlessness), narrowed focus, and diaphoresis.

Cardiac Output [fluctuation] may be related to changes in SVR, fluctuations in venous return (repeated or prolonged Valsalva's maneuvers, effects of anesthesia or medications, dorsal recumbent position occluding the inferior vena cava and partially obstructing the aorta), possibly evidenced by decreased venous return, changes in vital signs (BP, pulse), urinary output, fetal bradycardia.

risk for impaired fetal Gas Exchange: risk factors may include mechanical compression of head or cord, maternal position or prolonged labor affecting placental perfusion, and effects of maternal anesthesia, hyperventilation.*

risk for impaired Skin/Tissue Integrity: risk factors may include untoward stretching or lacerations of delicate tissues (precipitous labor, hypertonic contractile pattern, adolescence, large fetus) and application of forceps.*

risk for Fatigue: risk factors may include pregnancy, stress, anxiety, sleep deprivation, increased physical exertion, anemia, environmental humidity or temperature, lights.*

Laminectomy, lumbar   MS
Also refer to Surgery, general

ineffective tissue Perfusion (specify) may be related to diminished or interrupted blood flow—edema of operative site, hematoma formation; hypovolemia, possibly evidenced by paresthesia, numbness, decreased range of motion or muscle strength.

risk for [spinal] Trauma: risk factors may include temporary weakness of spinal column, balancing difficulties, changes in muscle tone or coordination.*

acute Pain may be related to traumatized tissues—surgical manipulation, harvesting bone graft, localized inflammation, and edema, possibly evidenced by altered muscle tone, verbal reports, and distraction or guarding behaviors, changes in vital signs, diaphoresis, pallor.

impaired physical Mobility may be related to imposed therapeutic restrictions, neuromuscular impairment, and pain, possibly evidenced by limited range of motion, decreased muscle strength or control, impaired coordination, and reluctance to attempt movement.

risk for [acute] Urinary Retention: risk factors may include pain and swelling in operative area and reduced mobility/restrictions of position.*

Laryngectomy   MS
Also refer to Cancer; Chemotherapy

ineffective Airway Clearance may be related to partial or total removal of the glottis, temporary or permanent change to neck breathing, edema formation, and copious and thick secretions, possibly evidenced by dyspnea or difficulty breathing, changes in rate and depth of respiration, use of accessory respiratory muscles, weak or ineffective cough, abnormal breath sounds, and cyanosis.

---

*A risk diagnosis is not evidenced by signs and symptoms, as the problem has not occurred; rather, nursing interventions are directed at prevention.

impaired Skin/Tissue Integrity may be related to surgical removal of tissues and grafting, effects of radiation or chemotherapeutic agents, altered circulation or reduced blood supply, compromised nutritional status, edema formation, and pooling or continuous drainage of secretions, possibly evidenced by disruption of skin and tissue surface and destruction of skin and tissue layers.

impaired Oral Mucous Membrane may be related to dehydration or absence of oral intake, decreased saliva production, poor or inadequate oral hygiene, pathological condition (oral cancer), mechanical trauma (oral surgery), difficulty swallowing and pooling or drooling of secretions, and nutritional deficits, possibly evidenced by xerostomia (dry mouth), oral discomfort, thick, mucoid saliva; decreased saliva production, dry and crusted or coated tongue, inflamed lips, absent teeth and gums, poor dental health and halitosis.

CH

impaired verbal Communication may be related to anatomical deficit (removal of vocal cords), physical barrier (tracheostomy tube), and required voice rest, possibly evidenced by inability to speak, change in vocal characteristics, and impaired articulation.

risk for Aspiration: risk factors may include impaired swallowing, facial and neck surgery, presence of tracheostomy, tube feedings.*

Laryngitis **CH/PED**
Refer to Croup

Latex allergy **CH**
latex Allergy Response may be related to no immune mechanism response, possibly evidenced by contact dermatitis—erythema, blisters; delayed hypersensitivity—eczema, irritation; hypersensitivity—generalized edema, wheezing, bronchospasm, hypotension, cardiac arrest.

Anxiety [specify level]/Fear may be related to threat of death, possibly evidenced by expressed concerns, hypervigilance, restlessness, focus on self.

risk for risk-prone health Behavior: risk factors may include health status requiring change in occupation.*

Lead poisoning, acute **PED/CH**
Also refer to Lead poisoning, chronic

Contamination may be related to flaking or peeling paint (young children), improperly lead-glazed ceramic pottery, unprotected contact with lead (e.g., battery manufacture or recycling, bronzing, soldering or welding), imported herbal products or medicinals, possibly evidenced by abdominal cramping, headache, irritability, decreased attentiveness, constipation, tremors.

risk for Trauma: risk factors may include loss of coordination, altered level of consciousness, clonic or tonic muscle activity, neurological damage.*

risk for deficient Fluid Volume: risk factors may include excessive vomiting, diarrhea, or decreased intake.*

---

*A risk diagnosis is not evidenced by signs and symptoms, as the problem has not occurred; rather, nursing interventions are directed at prevention.

---

deficient Knowledge [Learning Need] regarding sources of lead and prevention of poisoning may be related to lack of information/ misinterpretation, possibly evidenced by statements of concern, questions, and misconceptions.

Lead poisoning, chronic   CH
Also refer to Lead poisoning, acute

Contamination may be related to flaking or peeling paint (young children), improperly lead-glazed ceramic pottery, unprotected contact with lead (e.g., battery manufacture or recycling, bronzing, soldering or welding), imported herbal products or medicinals, possibly evidenced by chronic abdominal pain, headache, personality changes, cognitive deficits, seizures, neuropathy.

imbalanced Nutrition: less than body requirements may be related to decreased intake (chemically induced changes in the gastrointestinal tract), possibly evidenced by anorexia, abdominal discomfort, reported metallic taste, and weight loss.

disturbed Thought Processes may be related to deposition of lead in CNS and brain tissue, possibly evidenced by personality changes, learning disabilities, and impaired ability to conceptualize and reason.

chronic Pain may be related to deposition of lead in soft tissues and bone, possibly evidenced by verbal reports, distraction behaviors, and focus on self.

Leukemia, acute   MS
Also refer to Chemotherapy

risk for Infection: risk factors may include inadequate secondary defenses (alterations in mature white blood cells [WBCs], increased number of immature lymphocytes, immunosuppression, and bone marrow suppression), invasive procedures, and malnutrition.*

Anxiety [specify level]/Fear may be related to change in health status, threat of death, and situational crisis, possibly evidenced by sympathetic stimulation, apprehension, feelings of helplessness, focus on self, and insomnia.

Activity Intolerance [specify level] may be related to reduced energy stores, increased metabolic rate, imbalance between O_2 supply and demand—anemia, hypoxia; therapeutic restrictions–isolation, bedrest; effect of drug therapy, possibly evidenced by generalized weakness, reports of fatigue and exertional dyspnea, abnormal heart rate or BP response.

acute Pain may be related to physical agents (infiltration of tissues/ organs/CNS, expanding bone marrow) and chemical agents (antileukemic treatments), psychological manifestations—anxiety, fear possibly evidenced by verbal reports (abdominal discomfort, arthralgia, bone pain, headache), distraction behaviors, narrowed focus, and changes in vital signs.

risk for deficient Fluid Volume/Bleeding: risk factors may include excessive losses (vomiting, diarrhea, coagulopathy), decreased intake

---

*A risk diagnosis is not evidenced by signs and symptoms, as the problem has not occurred; rather, nursing interventions are directed at prevention.

(nausea, anorexia), increased fluid need (hypermetabolic state/fever), predisposition for kidney stone formation, tumor lysis syndrome.*

Leukemia, chronic   MS
risk for Infection: risk factors may include inadequate secondary defenses (alterations in mature WBCs, increased number of immature lymphocytes, immunosuppression, and bone marrow suppression), invasive procedures, and malnutrition.*

ineffective Protection may be related to abnormal blood profiles, drug therapy—cytotoxic agents, steroids; radiation treatments possibly evidenced by deficient immunity, impaired healing, altered clotting, weakness.

Fatigue may be related to disease state, anemia possibly evidenced by verbalizations, inability to maintain usual routines, listlessness.

imbalanced Nutrition: less than body requirements may be related to inability to ingest nutrients possibly evidenced by lack of interest in food, anorexia, weight loss, abdominal fullness, pain.

Long-term care   CH
Also refer to condition requiring or contributing to need for facility placement

Anxiety [specify level]/Fear may be related to change in health status, role functioning, interaction patterns, socioeconomic status, environment; unmet needs, recent life changes, and loss of friends/SO(s), possibly evidenced by apprehension, restlessness, insomnia, repetitive questioning, pacing, purposeless activity, expressed concern regarding changes in life events, and focus on self.

Grieving may be related to perceived, actual or potential loss of physiopsychosocial well-being, personal possessions, and SO(s), as well as cultural beliefs about aging and debilitation, possibly evidenced by denial of feelings, depression, sorrow, guilt, alterations in activity level, sleep patterns, eating habits, and libido.

risk for Poisoning [drug toxicity]: risk factors may include effects of aging (reduced metabolism, impaired circulation, precarious physiological balance, presence of multiple diseases and organ involvement), and use of multiple prescribed and over-the-counter (OTC) drugs.*

impaired Memory/disturbed Thought Processes may be related to physiological changes of aging (loss of cells and brain atrophy, decreased blood supply), altered sensory input, pain, effects of medications, and psychological conflicts (disrupted life pattern), possibly evidenced by slower reaction times, memory loss, altered attention span, disorientation, inability to follow, altered sleep patterns, and personality changes.

Insomnia may be related to internal factors (illness, psychological stress, inactivity) and external factors (environmental changes, facility routines), possibly evidenced by reports of difficulty in falling asleep/not feeling rested, interrupted sleep, awakening earlier than desired, change in behavior or performance, increasing irritability, and listlessness.

L

---

*A risk diagnosis is not evidenced by signs and symptoms, as the problem has not occurred; rather, nursing interventions are directed at prevention.

risk for Sexual Dysfunction: risk factors may include biopsychosocial alteration of sexuality, interference in psychological/physical well-being, self-image, and lack of privacy/SO(s).*

risk for Relocation Stress Syndrome: risk factors may include temporary or permanent move that may be voluntary or involuntary, lack of predeparture counseling, multiple losses, feeling of powerlessness, lack of or inappropriate use of support system, changes in psychosocial or physical health status.*

risk for impaired Religiosity: risk factors may include life transition, ineffective support or coping, lack of social interaction, depression.*

Lupus erythematosus, systemic (SLE)   CH

Fatigue may be related to inadequate energy production or increased energy requirements (chronic inflammation), overwhelming psychological or emotional demands, states of discomfort, and altered body chemistry (including effects of drug therapy), possibly evidenced by reports of unremitting and overwhelming lack of energy, inability to maintain usual routines, decreased performance, lethargy, and decreased libido.

acute Pain may be related to widespread inflammatory process affecting connective tissues, blood vessels, serosal surfaces and mucous membranes, possibly evidenced by verbal reports, guarding or distraction behaviors, self-focusing, and changes in vital signs.

impaired Skin/Tissue Integrity may be related to chronic inflammation, edema formation, and altered circulation, possibly evidenced by presence of skin rash or lesions, ulcerations of mucous membranes, and photosensitivity.

disturbed Body Image may be related to presence of chronic condition with rash, lesions, ulcers, purpura, mottled erythema of hands, alopecia, loss of strength, and altered body function, possibly evidenced by hiding body parts, negative feelings about body, feelings of helplessness, and change in social involvement.

Lyme disease   CH/MS

acute/chronic Pain may be related to systemic effects of toxins, presence of rash, urticaria, and joint swelling or inflammation, possibly evidenced by verbal reports, guarding behaviors, autonomic responses, and narrowed focus.

Fatigue may be related to increased energy requirements, altered body chemistry, and states of discomfort evidenced by reports of overwhelming lack of energy, inability to maintain usual routines, decreased performance, lethargy, and malaise.

risk for decreased Cardiac Output: risk factors may include alteration in cardiac rate, rhythm, or conduction.*

Macular degeneration   CH

disturbed visual Sensory Perception may be related to altered sensory reception, possibly evidenced by reported or measured change in sensory acuity, change in usual response to stimuli.

---

*A risk diagnosis is not evidenced by signs and symptoms, as the problem has not occurred; rather, nursing interventions are directed at prevention.

Anxiety [specify level]/Fear may be related to situational crisis, threat to or change in health status and role function, possibly evidenced by expressed concerns, apprehension, feelings of inadequacy, diminished productivity, impaired attention.

risk for impaired Home Maintenance: risk factors may include impaired cognitive functioning, inadequate support systems.*

risk for impaired Social Interaction: risk factors may include limited physical mobility, environmental barriers.*

Mallory-Weiss syndrome   MS
Also refer to Achalasia

risk for deficient Fluid Volume [isotonic]: risk factors may include excessive vascular losses, presence of vomiting, and reduced intake.*

deficient Knowledge [Learning Need] regarding causes, treatment, and prevention of condition may be related to lack of information or misinterpretation, possibly evidenced by statements of concern, questions, and recurrence of problem.

Mastectomy   MS
impaired Skin/Tissue Integrity may be related to surgical removal of skin and tissue, altered circulation, presence of edema, drainage, changes in skin elasticity and sensation, and tissue destruction (radiation), possibly evidenced by disruption of skin surface and destruction of skin layers and subcutaneous tissues.

impaired physical Mobility may be related to neuromuscular impairment, pain, and edema formation, possibly evidenced by reluctance to attempt movement, limited range of motion, and decreased muscle mass and strength.

bathing/dressing Self-Care Deficit may be related to temporary decreased range of motion of one or both arms, possibly evidenced by statements of inability to perform or complete self-care tasks.

disturbed Body Image/situational low Self-Esteem may be related to loss of body part denoting femininity, fear of rejection or reaction of others, behaviors inconsistent with self-value system possibly evidenced by not looking at or touching area, self-negating verbalizations, preoccupation with loss, and change in social involvement or relationship.

risk for complicated Grieving: risk factors may include preloss psychological symptoms, predisposition for anxiety and feelings of inadequacy, frequency of major life events.*

Mastitis   OB/GYN
acute Pain may be related to erythema and edema of breast tissues, possibly evidenced by verbal reports, guarding or distraction behaviors, self-focusing, changes in vital signs.

risk for Infection [spread/abscess formation]: risk factors may include traumatized tissues, stasis of fluids, and insufficient knowledge to prevent complications.*

deficient Knowledge [Learning Need] regarding pathophysiology, treatment, and prevention may be related to lack of information or

M

---

*A risk diagnosis is not evidenced by signs and symptoms, as the problem has not occurred; rather, nursing interventions are directed at prevention.

misinterpretation, possibly evidenced by statements of concern, questions, and misconceptions.

risk for ineffective Breastfeeding: risk factors may include inability to feed on affected side or interruption in breastfeeding.*

Mastoidectomy   PED/MS

risk for Infection [spread]: risk factors may include preexisting infection, surgical trauma, and stasis of body fluids in close proximity to brain.*

acute Pain may be related to inflammation, tissue trauma, and edema formation, possibly evidenced by verbal reports, distraction behaviors, restlessness, self-focusing, and changes in vital signs.

disturbed auditory Sensory Perception may be related to presence of surgical packing, edema, and surgical disturbance of middle ear structures, possibly evidenced by reported/tested hearing loss in affected ear.

Measles   CH/PED

acute Pain may be related to inflammation of mucous membranes, conjunctiva, and presence of extensive skin rash with pruritus, possibly evidenced by verbal reports, distraction behaviors, self-focusing, and changes in vital signs.

Hyperthermia may be related to presence of viral toxins and inflammatory response, possibly evidenced by increased body temperature, flushed, warm skin; and tachycardia.

risk for [secondary] Infection: risk factors may include altered immune response and traumatized dermal tissues.*

deficient Knowledge [Learning Need] regarding condition, transmission, and possible complications may be related to lack of information, misinterpretation, possibly evidenced by statements of concern, questions, misconceptions, and development of preventable complications.

Melanoma, malignant   MS/CH

Refer to Cancer; Chemotherapy

Meningitis, acute meningococcal   MS

risk for Infection [spread]: risk factors may include hematogenous dissemination of pathogen, stasis of body fluids, suppressed inflammatory response (medication-induced), and exposure of others to pathogens.*

risk for ineffective cerebral tissue Perfusion: risk factors may include cerebral edema altering or interrupting cerebral arterial or venous blood flow, hypovolemia, exchange problems at cellular level (acidosis).*

Hyperthermia may be related to infectious process (increased metabolic rate) and dehydration, possibly evidenced by increased body temperature, warm, flushed skin; and tachycardia.

acute Pain may be related to inflammation or irritation of the meninges with spasm of extensor muscles (neck, shoulders, and back), possibly

---

*A risk diagnosis is not evidenced by signs and symptoms, as the problem has not occurred; rather, nursing interventions are directed at prevention.

evidenced by verbal reports, guarding or distraction behaviors, narrowed focus, photophobia, and changes in vital signs.

risk for Trauma/Suffocation: risk factors may include alterations in level of consciousness, possible development of clonic-tonic muscle activity (seizures), and generalized weakness, prostration, ataxia, vertigo.*

Meniscectomy   MS/CH

impaired Walking may be related to pain, joint instability, and imposed medical restrictions of movement, possibly evidenced by impaired ability to move about environment as needed or desired.

deficient Knowledge [Learning Need] regarding postoperative expectations, prevention of complications, and self-care needs may be related to lack of information, possibly evidenced by statements of concern, questions, and misconceptions.

Menopause   GYN

ineffective Thermoregulation may be related to fluctuation of hormonal levels, possibly evidenced by skin flushed/warm to touch, diaphoresis, night sweats, cold hands or feet.

Fatigue may be related to change in body chemistry, lack of sleep, depression, possibly evidenced by reports of lack of energy, tired, inability to maintain usual routines, decreased performance.

risk for Sexual Dysfunction: risk factors may include perceived altered body function, changes in physical response, myths or inaccurate information, impaired relationship with SO.*

risk for stress Urinary Incontinence: risk factors may include degenerative changes in pelvic muscles and structural support.*

readiness for enhanced self Health Management may be related to maturational change, possibly evidenced by expressed desire for management of life cycle changes, increased control of health practice.

Mental retardation   CH

Also refer to Down syndrome

impaired verbal Communication may be related to developmental delay, impairment of cognitive and motor abilities, possibly evidenced by impaired articulation, difficulty with phonation, and inability to modulate speech or find appropriate words (dependent on degree of retardation).

risk for Self-Care Deficit [specify]: risk factors may include impaired cognitive ability and motor skills.*

risk for imbalanced Nutrition: more than body requirements: risk factors may include decreased metabolic rate coupled with impaired cognitive development, dysfunctional eating patterns, and sedentary activity level.*

risk for sedentary Lifestyle: risk factors may include lack of interest or motivation, lack of resources, lack of training or knowledge of specific exercise needs, safety concerns, fear of injury. *

impaired Social Interaction may be related to impaired thought processes, communication barriers, and knowledge or skill deficit about

---

*A risk diagnosis is not evidenced by signs and symptoms, as the problem has not occurred; rather, nursing interventions are directed at prevention.

ways to enhance mutuality, possibly evidenced by dysfunctional interactions with peers, family, and/or SO(s), and verbalized or observed discomfort in social situation.

compromised family Coping may be related to chronic nature of condition and degree of disability that exhausts supportive capacity of SO(s), other situational or developmental crises or situations SO(s) may be facing, unrealistic expectations of SO(s), possibly evidenced by preoccupation of SO with personal reaction, SO(s) withdraw(s) or enter(s) into limited interaction with individual, protective behavior disproportionate (too much or too little) to client's abilities or need for autonomy.

impaired Home Maintenance may be related to impaired cognitive functioning, insufficient finances/family organization or planning, lack of knowledge, and inadequate support systems, possibly evidenced by requests for assistance, expression of difficulty in maintaining home, disorderly surroundings, and overtaxed family members.

risk for Sexual Dysfunction: risk factors may include biopsychosocial alteration of sexuality, ineffectual or absent role models, misinformation or lack of knowledge, lack of SO(s), and lack of appropriate behavior control.*

Metabolic syndrome   CH/MS

risk for unstable blood Glucose Level: risk factors may include dietary intake, weight gain, physical activity level.*

sedentary Lifestyle may be related to deficient knowledge of health benefits of physical exercise, lack of interest/motivation or resources; possibly evidenced by verbalized preference for activities low in physical activity, choice of a daily routine lacking physical exercise.

compromised family Coping may be related to chronic nature of condition and degree of disability that exhausts supportive capacity of SO(s), other situational or developmental crises or situations SO(s) may be facing, unrealistic expectations of SO(s), possibly evidenced by preoccupation of SO with personal reaction, SO(s) withdraw(s) or enter(s) into limited interaction with individual, protective behavior disproportionate (too much or too little) to client's abilities or need for autonomy.

impaired Home Maintenance may be related to impaired cognitive functioning, insufficient finances and family organization or planning, lack of knowledge, and inadequate support systems, possibly evidenced by requests for assistance, expression of difficulty in maintaining home, disorderly surroundings, and overtaxed family members.

risk for ineffective tissue Perfusion (specify): risk factors may include arterial plaque formation (elevated triglycerides, low levels of HDL), prothrombotic state, proinflammatory state.*

Miscarriage   OB
Refer to Abortion, spontaneous termination

---

*A risk diagnosis is not evidenced by signs and symptoms, as the problem has not occurred; rather, nursing interventions are directed at prevention.

Mitral stenosis   MS/CH

Activity Intolerance may be related to imbalance between O_2 supply
   and demand, possibly evidenced by reports of fatigue, weakness,
   exertional dyspnea, and tachycardia.

impaired Gas Exchange may be related to altered blood flow, possibly
   evidenced by restlessness, hypoxia, and cyanosis (orthopnea/parox-
   ysmal nocturnal dyspnea).

decreased Cardiac Output may be related to impeded blood flow as
   evidenced by jugular vein distention, peripheral or dependent edema,
   orthopnea, paroxysmal nocturnal dyspnea.

deficient Knowledge [Learning Need] regarding pathophysiology, therapeutic needs, and potential complications may be related to lack of
   information or recall, misinterpretation, possibly evidenced by statements of concern, questions, inaccurate follow-through of instructions, and development of preventable complications.

Mononucleosis, infectious   CH

Fatigue may be related to decreased energy production, states of discomfort, and increased energy requirements (inflammatory process),
   possibly evidenced by reports of overwhelming lack of energy, inability to maintain usual routines, lethargy, and malaise.

acute Pain/impaired Comfort may be related to inflammation of lym-
   phoid and organ tissues, irritation of oropharyngeal mucous membranes, and effects of circulating toxins, possibly evidenced by verbal reports, distraction behaviors, and self-focusing.

Hyperthermia may be related to inflammatory process, possibly evidenced by increased body temperature, warm, flushed skin; and
   tachycardia.

deficient Knowledge [Learning Need] regarding disease transmission,
   self-care needs, medical therapy, and potential complications may
   be related to lack of information, misinterpretation, possibly evidenced by statements of concern, misconceptions, and inaccurate
   follow-through of instructions.

Mood disorders   PSY
Refer to Depressive disorders

Mountain sickness, acute (AMS)   CH/MS

acute Pain may be related to reduced O_2 tension, possibly evidenced by
   reports of headache.

Fatigue may be related to stress, increased physical exertion, sleep deprivation, possibly evidenced by overwhelming lack of energy, inability to restore energy even after sleep, compromised concentration, decreased performance.

risk for deficient Fluid Volume: risk factors may include increased water loss (e.g., overbreathing dry air), exertion, altered fluid intake
   (nausea).*

Multiple personality   PSY
Refer to Dissociative disorders

---

*A risk diagnosis is not evidenced by signs and symptoms, as the problem has
not occurred; rather, nursing interventions are directed at prevention.

Multiple sclerosis CH

Fatigue may be related to decreased energy production or increased energy requirements to perform activities, psychological or emotional demands, pain or discomfort, medication side effects, possibly evidenced by verbalization of overwhelming lack of energy, inability to maintain usual routine, decreased performance, impaired ability to concentrate, increase in physical complaints.

disturbed visual, kinesthetic, tactile Sensory Perception may be related to delayed or interrupted neuronal transmission, possibly evidenced by impaired vision, diplopia, disturbance of vibratory or position sense, paresthesias, numbness, and blunting of sensation.

impaired physical Mobility may be related to neuromuscular impairment; discomfort or pain; sensoriperceptual impairments; decreased muscle strength, control and/or mass; deconditioning, as evidenced by limited ability to perform motor skills; limited range of motion; gait changes, postural instability.

Powerlessness/Hopelessness may be related to illness-related regimen, unpredictability of disease, and lifestyle of helplessness, possibly evidenced by verbal expressions of having no control or influence over the situation, depression over physical deterioration that occurs despite client compliance with regimen, nonparticipation in care or decision making when opportunities are provided, passivity, decreased verbalization and affect, isolating behaviors.

impaired Home Maintenance may be related to effects of debilitating disease, impaired cognitive and/or emotional functioning, insufficient finances, and inadequate support systems, possibly evidenced by reported difficulty, observed disorderly surroundings, and poor hygienic conditions.

compromised/disabled family Coping may be related to situational crises/temporary family disorganization and role changes, client providing little support in turn for SO(s), prolonged disease or disability progression that exhausts the supportive capacity of SO(s), feelings of guilt, anxiety, hostility, despair, and highly ambivalent family relationships, possibly evidenced by client expressing or confirming concern or report about SO's response to client's illness, SO(s) preoccupied with own personal reactions, intolerance, abandonment, neglectful care of the client, and distortion of reality regarding client's illness.

Mumps PED/CH

acute Pain may be related to presence of inflammation, circulating toxins, and enlargement of salivary glands, possibly evidenced by verbal reports, guarding or distraction behaviors, self-focusing, and changes in vital signs.

Hyperthermia may be related to inflammatory process (increased metabolic rate) and dehydration, possibly evidenced by increased body temperature, warm, flushed skin; and tachycardia.

risk for deficient Fluid Volume: risk factors may include hypermetabolic state and painful swallowing, with decreased intake.*

---

*A risk diagnosis is not evidenced by signs and symptoms, as the problem has not occurred; rather, nursing interventions are directed at prevention.

Muscular dystrophy (Duchenne's)   **PED/CH**

impaired physical Mobility may be related to musculoskeletal impairment or weakness, possibly evidenced by decreased muscle strength, control, and mass, limited range of motion, and impaired coordination.

delayed Growth and Development may be related to effects of physical disability, possibly evidenced by altered physical growth and altered ability to perform self-care or self-control activities appropriate to age.

risk for imbalanced Nutrition: more than body requirements: risk factors may include sedentary lifestyle and dysfunctional eating patterns.*

compromised family Coping may be related to situational crisis, emotional conflicts around issues about hereditary nature of condition and prolonged disease or disability that exhausts supportive capacity of family members, possibly evidenced by preoccupation with personal reactions regarding disability and displaying protective behavior disproportionate (too little or too much) to client's abilities or need for autonomy.

Myasthenia gravis   **MS**

ineffective Breathing Pattern/Airway Clearance may be related to neuromuscular weakness and decreased energy, fatigue, possibly evidenced by dyspnea, changes in rate and depth of respiration, ineffective cough, and adventitious breath sounds.

impaired verbal Communication may be related to neuromuscular weakness, fatigue, and physical barrier (intubation), possibly evidenced by facial weakness, impaired articulation, hoarseness, and inability to speak.

impaired Swallowing may be related to neuromuscular impairment of laryngeal or pharyngeal muscles, and muscular fatigue, possibly evidenced by reported or observed difficulty swallowing, coughing, choking, and evidence of aspiration.

Anxiety [specify level]/Fear may be related to situational crisis, threat to self-concept, change in health or socioeconomic status or role function; separation from support systems, lack of knowledge, and inability to communicate, possibly evidenced by expressed concerns, increased tension, restlessness, apprehension, sympathetic stimulation, crying, focus on self, uncooperative behavior, withdrawal, anger, and noncommunication.

CH

deficient Knowledge [Learning Need] regarding drug therapy, potential for crisis (myasthenic or cholinergic), and self-care management may be related to inadequate information, misinterpretation, possibly evidenced by statements of concern, questions, and misconceptions; development of preventable complications.

impaired physical Mobility may be related to neuromuscular impairment, possibly evidenced by reports of progressive fatigability with repetitive or prolonged muscle use, impaired coordination, and decreased muscle strength/control.

---

*A risk diagnosis is not evidenced by signs and symptoms, as the problem has not occurred; rather, nursing interventions are directed at prevention.

disturbed visual Sensory Perception may be related to neuromuscular impairment, possibly evidenced by visual distortions (diplopia) and motor incoordination.

Myeloma, multiple   MS/CH
Also refer to Cancer

acute/chronic Pain may be related to destruction of tissues or bone, side effects of therapy, possibly evidenced by verbal or coded reports, guarding or protective behaviors, changes in appetite or weight, sleep; reduced interaction with others.

impaired physical Mobility may be related to loss of integrity of bone structure, pain, deconditioning, depressed mood, possibly evidenced by verbalizations, limited range of motion, slowed movement, gait changes.

risk for ineffective Protection: risk factors may include presence of cancer, drug therapies, radiation treatments, inadequate nutrition.*

Myocardial infarction   MS
Also refer to Myocarditis

acute Pain may be related to ischemia of myocardial tissue, possibly evidenced by verbal reports, guarding or distraction behaviors (restlessness), facial mask of pain, self-focusing, and diaphoresis, changes in vital signs.

Anxiety [specify level]/Fear may be related to threat of death, threat of change of health status, role functioning and lifestyle; interpersonal transmission or contagion, possibly evidenced by increased tension, fearful attitude, apprehension, expressed concerns or uncertainty, restlessness, sympathetic stimulation, and somatic complaints.

risk for decreased Cardiac Output: risk factors may include changes in rate and electrical conduction, reduced preload/increased SVR and altered muscle contractility/depressant effects of some medications, infarcted or dyskinetic muscle, structural defects.*

                                                        CH
risk for sedentary Lifestyle: risk factors may include lack of resources, lack of training or knowledge of specific exercise needs, safety concerns, fear of injury.*

Myocarditis   MS
Also refer to Myocardial infarction

Activity Intolerance may be related to imbalance in O_2 supply and demand (myocardial inflammation or damage), cardiac depressant effects of certain drugs, and enforced bedrest, possibly evidenced by reports of fatigue, exertional dyspnea, tachycardia and palpitations in response to activity, ECG changes—dysrhythmias, and generalized weakness.

risk for decreased Cardiac Output: risk factors may include degeneration of cardiac muscle.*

deficient Knowledge [Learning Need] regarding pathophysiology of condition, outcomes, treatment, and self-care needs and lifestyle

---

*A risk diagnosis is not evidenced by signs and symptoms, as the problem has not occurred; rather, nursing interventions are directed at prevention.

changes may be related to lack of information, misinterpretation, possibly evidenced by statements of concern, misconceptions, inaccurate follow-through of instructions, and development of preventable complications.

Myringotomy   **PED/MS**
Refer to Mastoidectomy

Myxedema   **CH**
Also refer to Hypothyroidism
disturbed Body Image may be related to change in structure or function (loss of hair, thickening of skin, masklike facial expression, enlarged tongue, menstrual and reproductive disturbances), possibly evidenced by negative feelings about body, feelings of helplessness, and change in social involvement.
imbalanced Nutrition: more than body requirements may be related to decreased metabolic rate and activity level, possibly evidenced by weight gain greater than ideal for height and frame.
risk for decreased Cardiac Output: risk factors may include altered electrical conduction and myocardial contractility.*

Neglect/Abuse   **CH/PSY**
Refer to Abuse; Battered child syndrome

Neonatal, normal newborn   **PED**
risk for impaired Gas Exchange: risk factors may include prenatal or intrapartal stressors, excess production of mucus, or cold stress.*
risk for Hypothermia: risk factors may include large body surface in relation to mass, limited amounts of insulating subcutaneous fat, nonrenewable sources of brown fat and few white fat stores, thin epidermis with close proximity of blood vessels to the skin, inability to shiver, and movement from a warm uterine environment to a much cooler environment.*
risk for impaired Attachment: risk factors may include developmental transition (gain of a family member), anxiety associated with the parent role, lack of privacy (healthcare interventions, intrusive family/visitors).*
risk for imbalanced Nutrition: less than body requirements: risk factors may include rapid metabolic rate, high caloric requirement, increased insensible water losses through pulmonary and cutaneous routes, fatigue, and a potential for inadequate or depleted glucose stores.*
risk for Infection: risk factors may include inadequate secondary defenses (inadequate acquired immunity, e.g., deficiency of neutrophils and specific immunoglobulins), and inadequate primary defenses (e.g., environmental exposure, broken skin, traumatized tissues, decreased ciliary action).*

Neonatal, premature newborn   **PED**
impaired Gas Exchange may be related to alveolar-capillary membrane changes (inadequate surfactant levels), altered blood flow (immaturity

---

*A risk diagnosis is not evidenced by signs and symptoms, as the problem has not occurred; rather, nursing interventions are directed at prevention.

of pulmonary arteriole musculature), altered O_2 supply (immaturity of CNS and neuromuscular system, tracheobronchial obstruction), altered O_2-carrying capacity of blood (anemia), and cold stress, possibly evidenced by respiratory difficulties, inadequate oxygenation of tissues, and acidemia.

ineffective Breathing Pattern may be related to immaturity of the respiratory center, poor positioning, drug-related depression and metabolic imbalances, decreased energy, fatigue, possibly evidenced by dyspnea, tachypnea, periods of apnea, nasal flaring and use of accessory muscles, cyanosis, abnormal ABGs, and tachycardia.

risk for ineffective Thermoregulation: risk factors may include immature CNS development (temperature regulation center), decreased ratio of body mass to surface area, decreased subcutaneous fat, limited brown fat stores, inability to shiver or sweat, poor metabolic reserves, muted response to hypothermia, and frequent medical or nursing manipulations and interventions.*

risk for deficit Fluid Volume: risk factors may include extremes of age and weight, excessive fluid losses (thin skin, lack of insulating fat, increased environmental temperature, immature kidney, and failure to concentrate urine).*

risk for disorganized Infant Behavior: risk factors may include prematurity (immaturity of CNS system, hypoxia), lack of containment or boundaries, pain, overstimulation, separation from parents.*

Nephrectomy   MS

acute Pain may be related to surgical tissue trauma with mechanical closure (suture), possibly evidenced by verbal reports, guarding or distraction behaviors, self-focusing, and changes in vital signs.

risk for deficient Fluid Volume: risk factors may include excessive vascular losses and restricted intake.*

ineffective Breathing Pattern may be related to incisional pain with decreased lung expansion, possibly evidenced by tachypnea, fremitus, changes in respiratory depth and chest expansion, and changes in ABGs.

Constipation may be related to reduced dietary intake, decreased mobility, gastrointestinal obstruction (paralytic ileus), and incisional pain with defecation, possibly evidenced by decreased bowel sounds, reduced frequency/amount of stool, and hard, formed stool.

Nephrolithiasis   MS/CH
Refer to Calculi, urinary

Nephrotic syndrome   MS/CH

excess Fluid Volume may be related to compromised regulatory mechanism with changes in hydrostatic or oncotic vascular pressure and increased activation of the renin-angiotensin-aldosterone system, possibly evidenced by edema, anasarca, effusions, ascites, weight gain, intake greater than output, and BP changes.

imbalanced Nutrition: less than body requirements may be related to excessive protein losses and inability to ingest adequate nutrients

---

*A risk diagnosis is not evidenced by signs and symptoms, as the problem has not occurred; rather, nursing interventions are directed at prevention.

(anorexia), possibly evidenced by weight loss and muscle wasting (may be difficult to assess due to edema), lack of interest in food, and observed inadequate intake.

risk for Infection: risk factors may include chronic disease and steroidal suppression of inflammatory responses.*

risk for impaired Skin Integrity: risk factors may include presence of edema and activity restrictions.*

Neuralgia, trigeminal   CH

acute Pain may be related to neuromuscular impairment with sudden violent muscle spasm, possibly evidenced by verbal reports, guarding or distraction behaviors, self-focusing, and changes in vital signs.

deficient Knowledge [Learning Need] regarding control of recurrent episodes, medical therapies, and self-care needs may be related to lack of information or recall and misinterpretation, possibly evidenced by statements of concern, questions, and exacerbation of condition.

Neuritis   CH

acute/chronic Pain may be related to nerve damage usually associated with a degenerative process, possibly evidenced by verbal reports, guarding or distraction behaviors, self-focusing, and changes in vital signs.

deficient Knowledge [Learning Need] regarding underlying causative factors, treatment, and prevention may be related to lack of information, misinterpretation, possibly evidenced by statements of concern, questions, and misconceptions.

Nonketotic hyperglycemic-
hyperosmolar coma   MS

deficient Fluid Volume may be related to excessive renal losses, inadequate oral intake, extremes of age, presence of infection possibly evidenced by sudden weight loss, dry skin and mucous membranes, poor skin turgor, hypotension, increased pulse, fever, change in mental status (confusion to coma).

imbalanced Nutrition: less than body requirements may be related to decreased preload (hypovolemia), altered heart rhythm (hyper or hypokalemia) possibly evidenced by decreased hemodynamic pressures (e.g., CVP), ECG changes, dysrhythmias.

decreased Cardiac Output may be related to inadequate utilization of nutrients (insulin deficiency), decreased oral intake, hypermetabolic state, possibly evidenced by recent weight loss, imbalance between glucose and insulin levels.

risk for Trauma: risk factors may include weakness, cognitive limitations or altered consciousness, loss of large- or small-muscle coordination (risk for seizure activity).*

Obesity   CH

imbalanced Nutrition: more than body requirements may be related to food intake that exceeds body needs, psychosocial factors, socioeconomic

---

*A risk diagnosis is not evidenced by signs and symptoms, as the problem has not occurred; rather, nursing interventions are directed at prevention.

status, possibly evidenced by weight of 20% or more over optimum body weight, excess body fat by skinfold or other measurements, reported or observed dysfunctional eating patterns, intake more than body requirements.

sedentary Lifestyle may be related to lack of interest or motivation, lack of resources, lack of training or knowledge of specific exercise needs, safety concerns, fear of injury, possibly evidenced by demonstration of physical deconditioning, choice of a daily routine lacking physical exercise.

Activity Intolerance may be related to imbalance between O_2 supply and demand, and sedentary lifestyle, possibly evidenced by fatigue or weakness, exertional discomfort, and abnormal heart rate or BP response.

risk for Sleep Deprivation: risk factors may include inadequate daytime activity, discomfort, sleep apnea.*

PSY

disturbed Body Image/chronic low Self-Esteem may be related to view of self in contrast to societal values; family or subcultural encouragement of overeating; control, sex, and love issues; perceived failure at ability to control weight, possibly evidenced by negative feelings about body; fear of rejection or reaction of others; feeling of hopelessness, powerlessness; and lack of follow-through with treatment plan.

impaired Social Interaction may be related to self-concept disturbance, absence of or ineffective supportive SO(s), limited mobility, possibly evidenced by reluctance to participate in social gatherings, verbalized or observed discomfort in social situations, dysfunctional interactions with others, feelings of rejection.

Obsessive-compulsive disorder   PSY

[severe] Anxiety may be related to earlier life conflicts possibly evidenced by repetitive actions, recurring thoughts, decreased social and role functioning.

risk for impaired Skin/Tissue Integrity: risk factors may include repetitive behaviors related to cleansing (e.g., hand washing, brushing teeth, showering).*

risk for ineffective Role Performance: risk factors may include psychological stress, health-illness problems.*

Opioid abuse   CH/PSY
Refer to Depressant abuse

Organic brain syndrome   CH
Refer to Alzheimer's disease

Osteoarthritis (degenerative joint disease)   CH
Refer to Arthritis, rheumatoid
(Although this is a degenerative process versus the inflammatory process of rheumatoid arthritis, nursing concerns are the same.)

---

*A risk diagnosis is not evidenced by signs and symptoms, as the problem has not occurred; rather, nursing interventions are directed at prevention.

Osteomyelitis   MS/CH

acute Pain may be related to inflammation and tissue necrosis, possibly evidenced by verbal reports, guarding or distraction behaviors, self-focus, and changes in vital signs.

Hyperthermia may be related to increased metabolic rate and infectious process, possibly evidenced by increased body temperature and warm, flushed skin.

ineffective [bone] tissue Perfusion may be related to inflammatory reaction with thrombosis of vessels, destruction of tissue, edema, and abscess formation, possibly evidenced by bone necrosis, continuation of infectious process, and delayed healing.

risk for impaired Walking: risk factors may include inflammation and tissue necrosis, pain, joint instability.*

deficient Knowledge [Learning Need] regarding pathophysiology of condition, long-term therapy needs, activity restriction, and prevention of complications may be related to lack of information, misinterpretation, possibly evidenced by statements of concern, questions, and misconceptions, and inaccurate follow-through of instructions.

Osteoporosis   CH

risk for Trauma: risk factors may include loss of bone density and integrity increasing risk of fracture with minimal or no stress.*

acute/chronic Pain may be related to vertebral compression on spinal nerve, muscles, and ligaments; spontaneous fractures, possibly evidenced by verbal reports, guarding or distraction behaviors, self-focus, and changes in sleep pattern.

impaired physical Mobility may be related to pain and musculoskeletal impairment, possibly evidenced by limited range of motion, reluctance to attempt movement, expressed fear of reinjury, and imposed restrictions or limitations.

Palsy, cerebral (spastic hemiplegia)   PED/CH

impaired physical Mobility may be related to muscular weakness or hypertonicity, increased deep tendon reflexes, tendency to contractures, and underdevelopment of affected limbs, possibly evidenced by decreased muscle strength, control, mass; limited range of motion; and impaired coordination.

compromised family Coping may be related to permanent nature of condition, situational crisis, emotional conflicts, temporary family disorganization, and incomplete information or understanding of client's needs, possibly evidenced by verbalized anxiety or guilt regarding client's disability, inadequate understanding and knowledge base, and displaying protective behaviors disproportionate (too little or too much) to client's abilities or need for autonomy.

delayed Growth and Development may be related to effects of physical disability, possibly evidenced by altered physical growth, delay or difficulty in performing skills (motor, social, expressive), and altered ability to perform self-care or self-control activities appropriate to age.

---

*A risk diagnosis is not evidenced by signs and symptoms, as the problem has not occurred; rather, nursing interventions are directed at prevention.

Health Conditions and Client Concerns   **1021**

Pancreatitis

acute Pain may be related to obstruction of pancreatic or biliary ducts,
chemical contamination of peritoneal surfaces by pancreatic exudate,
autodigestion of pancreas, extension of inflammation to the retro-
peritoneal nerve plexus, possibly evidenced by verbal reports, guarding or distraction behaviors, self-focusing, grimacing, changes in vital signs, and alteration in muscle tone.

risk for deficient Fluid Volume/Bleeding: risk factors may include
excessive gastric losses (vomiting, nasogastric suctioning), increase in size of vascular bed (vasodilation, effects of kinins), third-
space fluid transudation, ascites formation, alteration of clotting
process.*

risk for unstable blood Glucose Level: risk factors may include decreased insulin production, increased glucagon release, physical
health status, stress.*

imbalanced Nutrition: less than body requirements may be related to
vomiting, decreased oral intake, prescribed dietary restrictions, altered ability to digest nutrients (loss of digestive enzymes), possibly
evidenced by reported inadequate food intake, aversion to eating,
reported altered taste sensation, weight loss, and reduced muscle
mass.

risk for Infection: risk factors may include inadequate primary defenses
(stasis of body fluids, altered peristalsis, change in pH secretions),
immunosuppression, nutritional deficiencies, tissue destruction, and
chronic disease.*

Paranoid personality disorder

risk for self-/other-directed Violence: risk factors may include perceived threats of danger, paranoid delusions, and increased feelings
of anxiety.*

[severe] Anxiety may be related to inability to trust (has not mastered
task of trust versus mistrust), possibly evidenced by rigid delusional
system (serves to provide relief from stress that justifies the delu-
sion), frightened of other people and own hostility.

Powerlessness may be related to feelings of inadequacy, lifestyle of
helplessness, maladaptive interpersonal interactions (e.g., misuse of
power, force, abusive relationships), sense of severely impaired self-
concept, and belief that individual has no control over situation(s),
possibly evidenced by paranoid delusions, use of aggressive behavior
to compensate, and expressions of recognition of damage paranoia
has caused self and others.

disturbed Thought Processes may be related to psychological conflicts, increased anxiety and fear, possibly evidenced by difficulties
in the process and character of thought, interference with the ability
to think clearly and logically, delusions, fragmentation, and autistic
thinking.

compromised family Coping may be related to temporary or sustained
family disorganization or role changes, prolonged progression of
condition that exhausts the supportive capacity of SO(s), possibly

---

*A risk diagnosis is not evidenced by signs and symptoms, as the problem has
not occurred; rather, nursing interventions are directed at prevention.

evidenced by family system not meeting physical, emotional, or spiritual needs of its members; inability to express or to accept wide range of feelings, inappropriate boundary maintenance, SO(s) describe(s) preoccupation with personal reactions.

Paraplegia   MS/CH
Also refer to Quadriplegia

impaired Transfer Ability may be related to loss of muscle function and control, injury to upper extremity joints (overuse).

disturbed kinesthetic/tactile Sensory Perception: may be related to neurological deficit with loss of sensory reception and transmission, psychological stress, possibly evidenced by reported or measured change in sensory acuity, change in usual response to stimuli, anxiety, disorientation, bizarre thinking; exaggerated emotional responses.

reflex Urinary Incontinence/impaired Urinary Elimination may be related to disruption of bladder innervation, bladder atony, fecal impaction possibly evidenced by bladder distention, retention, incontinence or overflow, urinary tract infections (UTIs), kidney stone formation, renal dysfunction.

situational low Self-Esteem may be related to situational crisis, loss of body functions, change in physical abilities, perceived loss of self/identity, possibly evidenced by negative feelings about body or self, feelings of helplessness, powerlessness, delay in taking responsibility for self-care or participation in therapy, and change in social involvement.

Sexual Dysfunction may be related to loss of sensation, altered function, and vulnerability, possibly evidenced by seeking of confirmation of desirability, verbalization of concern, alteration in relationship with SO, and change in interest in self or others.

Parathyroidectomy   MS
acute Pain may be related to presence of surgical incision and effects of calcium imbalance (bone pain, tetany), possibly evidenced by verbal reports, guarding or distraction behaviors, self-focus, and changes in vital signs.

risk for excess Fluid Volume: risk factors may include preoperative renal involvement, stress-induced release of antidiuretic hormone, and changing calcium and electrolyte levels.*

risk for ineffective Airway Clearance: risk factors may include edema formation and laryngeal nerve damage.*

deficient Knowledge [Learning Need] regarding postoperative care, complications, and long-term needs may be related to lack of information or recall, misinterpretation, possibly evidenced by statements of concern, questions, and misconceptions.

Parenteral feeding   MS/CH
imbalanced Nutrition: less than body requirements may be related to conditions that interfere with nutrient intake or increase nutrient need or metabolic demand—cancer and associated treatments, anorexia,

---

*A risk diagnosis is not evidenced by signs and symptoms, as the problem has not occurred; rather, nursing interventions are directed at prevention.

---

surgical procedures, dysphagia, or decreased level of consciousness, possibly evidenced by body weight 10% or more under ideal, decreased subcutaneous fat or muscle mass, poor muscle tone.

risk for Infection: risk factors may include insertion of venous catheter, malnutrition, chronic disease, improper preparation or handling of feeding solution.*

risk for Injury [multifactor]: risk factors may include catheter-related complications (air emboli, septic thrombophlebitis).*

risk for imbalanced Fluid Volume: risk factors may include active loss or failure of regulatory mechanisms specific to underlying disease process or trauma, complications of therapy—high glucose solutions/hyperglycemia—hyperosmolar nonketotic coma and severe dehydration; inability to obtain or ingest fluids.*

Fatigue may be related to decreased metabolic energy production, increased energy requirements—hypermetabolic state, healing process; altered body chemistry—medications, chemotherapy; possibly evidenced by overwhelming lack of energy, inability to maintain usual routines/accomplish routine tasks, lethargy, impaired ability to concentrate.

Parkinson's disease CH

impaired Walking may be related to neuromuscular impairment (muscle weakness, tremors, bradykinesia) and musculoskeletal impairment (joint rigidity), possibly evidenced by inability to move about the environment as desired, increased occurrence of falls.

impaired Swallowing may be related to neuromuscular impairment, muscle weakness, possibly evidenced by reported or observed difficulty in swallowing, drooling, evidence of aspiration (choking, coughing).

impaired verbal Communication may be related to muscle weakness and incoordination, possibly evidenced by impaired articulation, difficulty with phonation, and changes in rhythm and intonation.

risk for Stress Overload: risk factors may include inadequate resources, chronic illness, physical demands.*

Caregiver Role Strain may be related to illness, severity of care receiver, psychological or cognitive problems in care receiver, caregiver is spouse, duration of caregiving required, lack of respite or recreation for caregiver, possibly evidenced by feeling stressed, depressed, worried; lack of resources or support, family conflict.

Pelvic inflammatory disease OB/GYN/CH

risk for Infection [spread]: risk factors may include presence of infectious process in highly vascular pelvic structures, delay in seeking treatment.*

acute Pain may be related to inflammation, edema, and congestion of reproductive and pelvic tissues, possibly evidenced by verbal reports, guarding or distraction behaviors, self-focus, and changes in vital signs.

Hyperthermia may be related to inflammatory process and hypermetabolic state, possibly evidenced by increased body temperature; warm, flushed skin; and tachycardia.

*A risk diagnosis is not evidenced by signs and symptoms, as the problem has not occurred; rather, nursing interventions are directed at prevention.

risk for situational low Self-Esteem: risk factors may include perceived stigma of physical condition (infection of reproductive system).*

deficient Knowledge [Learning Need] regarding cause, complications of condition, therapy needs, and transmission of disease to others may be related to lack of information, misinterpretation, possibly evidenced by statements of concern, questions, misconceptions, and development of preventable complications.

Periarteritis nodosa   MS/CH
Refer to Polyarteritis [nodosa]

Pericarditis   MS
acute Pain may be related to tissue inflammation and presence of effusion, possibly evidenced by verbal reports of pain affected by movement or position, guarding or distraction behaviors, self-focus, and changes in vital signs.

Activity Intolerance may be related to imbalance between O_2 supply and demand (restriction of cardiac filling and ventricular contraction, reduced cardiac output), possibly evidenced by reports of weakness, fatigue, exertional dyspnea, abnormal heart rate or BP response, and signs of heart failure.

risk for decreased Cardiac Output: risk factors may include accumulation of fluid (effusion) restricted cardiac filling and contractility.*

Anxiety [specify level] may be related to change in health status and perceived threat of death, possibly evidenced by increased tension, apprehension, restlessness, and expressed concerns.

Perinatal loss/death of child   OB/CH
Grieving may be related to death of fetus or infant, possibly evidenced by verbal expressions of distress, anger, loss, guilt; crying, change in eating habits or sleep.

situational low Self-Esteem may be related to perceived failure at a life event, inability to meet personal expectations, possibly evidenced by negative self-appraisal in response to situation or personal actions, expressions of helplessness, hopelessness, evaluation of self as unable to deal with situation.

risk for ineffective Role Performance: risk factors may include stress, family conflict, inadequate support system.*

risk for interrupted Family Processes: risk factors may include situational crisis, developmental transition [loss of child], family roles shift.*

risk for Spiritual Distress: risk factors may include blame for loss directed at self or God, intense suffering, alienation from SO or support systems.*

Peripheral arterial occlusive disease   CH
Refer to Arterial occlusive disease

Peripheral vascular disease (atherosclerosis)   CH
ineffective peripheral tissue Perfusion may be related to reduction or interruption of arterial or venous blood flow, possibly evidenced by

P

*A risk diagnosis is not evidenced by signs and symptoms, as the problem has not occurred; rather, nursing interventions are directed at prevention.

changes in skin temperature and color, lack of hair growth, BP and pulse changes in extremity, presence of bruits, and reports of claudication.

Activity Intolerance may be related to imbalance between O_2 supply and demand, possibly evidenced by reports of muscle fatigue, weakness and exertional discomfort (claudication).

risk for impaired Skin/Tissue Integrity: risk factors may include altered circulation with decreased sensation and impaired healing.*

Peritonitis   MS

risk for Infection [spread/septicemia]: risk factors may include inadequate primary defenses (broken skin, traumatized tissue, altered peristalsis), inadequate secondary defenses (immunosuppression), and invasive procedures.*

deficient Fluid Volume [mixed] may be related to fluid shifts from extracellular, intravascular, and interstitial compartments into intestines and/or peritoneal space, excessive gastric losses (vomiting, diarrhea, NG suction), fever, hypermetabolic state, and restricted intake, possibly evidenced by dry mucous membranes; poor skin turgor; delayed capillary refill; weak peripheral pulses; diminished urinary output; dark, concentrated urine; hypotension; and tachycardia.

acute Pain may be related to chemical irritation of parietal peritoneum, trauma to tissues, abdominal distention—accumulation of fluid in abdominal or peritoneal cavity, possibly evidenced by verbal reports, muscle guarding, rebound tenderness, distraction behaviors, facial mask of pain, self-focus, changes in vital signs.

risk for imbalanced Nutrition: less than body requirements: risk factors may include nausea, vomiting, intestinal dysfunction, metabolic abnormalities, increased metabolic needs.*

Pheochromocytoma   MS

Anxiety [specify level] may be related to excessive physiological (hormonal) stimulation of the sympathetic nervous system, situational crises, threat to or change in health status, possibly evidenced by apprehension, shakiness, restlessness, focus on self, fearfulness, diaphoresis, and sense of impending doom.

deficient Fluid Volume [mixed] may be related to excessive gastric losses (vomiting, diarrhea), hypermetabolic state, diaphoresis, and hyperosmolar diuresis, possibly evidenced by hemoconcentration, dry mucous membranes, poor skin turgor, thirst, and weight loss.

decreased Cardiac Output/ineffective tissue Perfusion (specify) may be related to altered preload—decreased blood volume, altered SVR, and increased sympathetic activity (excessive secretion of catecholamines), possibly evidenced by cool, clammy skin; change in BP (hypertension, postural hypotension), visual disturbances, severe headache, and angina.

deficient Knowledge [Learning Need] regarding pathophysiology of condition, outcome, preoperative and postoperative care needs may be related to lack of information or recall, possibly evidenced by statements of concern, questions, and misconceptions.

---

*A risk diagnosis is not evidenced by signs and symptoms, as the problem has not occurred; rather, nursing interventions are directed at prevention.

Phlebitis CH
Refer to Thrombophlebitis

Phobia PSY
Also refer to Anxiety disorder, generalized

Fear may be related to learned irrational response to natural or innate origins (phobic stimulus), unfounded morbid dread of a seemingly harmless object or situation, possibly evidenced by sympathetic stimulation and reactions ranging from apprehension to panic, withdrawal from or total avoidance of situations that place individual in contact with feared object.

impaired Social Interaction may be related to intense fear of encountering feared object, activity or situation; and anticipated loss of control, possibly evidenced by reported change of style or pattern of interaction, discomfort in social situations, and avoidance of phobic stimulus.

Placenta previa OB
risk for deficient Fluid Volume: risk factors may include excessive vascular losses (vessel damage and inadequate vasoconstriction).*

impaired fetal Gas Exchange: may be related to altered blood flow, altered O_2-carrying capacity of blood (maternal anemia), and decreased surface area of gas exchange at site of placental attachment, possibly evidenced by changes in fetal heart rate or activity and release of meconium.

Fear may be related to threat of death (perceived or actual) to self or fetus, possibly evidenced by verbalization of specific concerns, increased tension, sympathetic stimulation.

risk for deficient Diversional Activity: risk factors may include imposed activity restrictions, bedrest.*

Pleurisy CH
acute Pain may be related to inflammation or irritation of the parietal pleura, possibly evidenced by verbal reports, guarding or distraction behaviors, self-focus, and changes in vital signs.

ineffective Breathing Pattern may be related to pain on inspiration, possibly evidenced by decreased respiratory depth, tachypnea, and dyspnea.

risk for Infection [pneumonia]: risk factors may include stasis of pulmonary secretions, decreased lung expansion, and ineffective cough.*

Pneumonia CH/MS
Refer to Bronchitis; Bronchopneumonia

Pneumothorax MS
Also refer to Hemothorax

ineffective Breathing Pattern may be related to decreased lung expansion (fluid and air accumulation), musculoskeletal impairment, pain, inflammatory process, possibly evidenced by dyspnea, tachypnea,

---

*A risk diagnosis is not evidenced by signs and symptoms, as the problem has not occurred; rather, nursing interventions are directed at prevention.

altered chest excursion, respiratory depth changes, use of accessory muscles and nasal flaring, cough, cyanosis, and abnormal ABGs.

risk for decreased Cardiac Output: risk factors may include compression or displacement of cardiac structures.*

acute Pain may be related to irritation of nerve endings within pleural space by foreign object (chest tube), possibly evidenced by verbal reports, guarding or distraction behaviors, self-focus, and changes in vital signs.

Polyarteritis (nodosa)   MS/CH

ineffective tissue Perfusion (specify) may be related to reduction or interruption of blood flow, possibly evidenced by organ tissue infarctions, changes in organ function, and development of organic psychosis.

Hyperthermia may be related to widespread inflammatory process, possibly evidenced by increased body temperature and warm, flushed skin.

acute Pain may be related to inflammation, tissue ischemia, and necrosis of affected area, possibly evidenced by verbal reports, guarding or distraction behaviors, self-focus, and changes in vital signs.

Grieving may be related to perceived loss of self, possibly evidenced by expressions of sorrow and anger, altered sleep and/or eating patterns, changes in activity level, and libido.

Polycythemia vera   CH

Activity Intolerance may be related to imbalance between O_2 supply and demand, possibly evidenced by reports of fatigue, weakness.

ineffective tissue Perfusion (specify) may be related to reduction or interruption of arterial or venous blood flow (insufficiency, thrombosis, or hemorrhage), possibly evidenced by pain in affected area, impaired mental ability, visual disturbances, and color changes of skin or mucous membranes.

Polyradiculitis   MS
Refer to Guillain-Barré syndrome

Postoperative recovery period   MS

ineffective Breathing Pattern may be related to neuromuscular and perceptual or cognitive impairment, decreased lung expansion and energy, and tracheobronchial obstruction, possibly evidenced by changes in respiratory rate and depth, reduced vital capacity, apnea, cyanosis, and noisy respirations.

risk for imbalanced Body Temperature: risk factors may include exposure to cool environment, effect of medications/anesthetic agents, extremes of age or weight, and dehydration.*

disturbed Sensory Perception (specify)/disturbed Thought Processes may be related to chemical alteration (use of pharmaceutical agents, hypoxia), therapeutically restricted environment, excessive sensory stimuli and physiological stress, possibly evidenced by changes in usual response to stimuli, motor incoordination; impaired ability to

---

*A risk diagnosis is not evidenced by signs and symptoms, as the problem has not occurred; rather, nursing interventions are directed at prevention.

concentrate, reason, and make decisions; and disorientation to person, place, and time.

risk for deficient Fluid Volume: risk factors may include restriction of oral intake, loss of fluid through abnormal routes (indwelling tubes, drains) and normal routes (vomiting, loss of vascular integrity, changes in clotting ability), extremes of age and weight.*

acute Pain may be related to disruption of skin, tissue, and muscle integrity; musculoskeletal/bone trauma; and presence of tubes and drains, possibly evidenced by verbal reports, alteration in muscle tone, facial mask of pain, distraction or guarding behaviors, narrowed focus, and changes in vital signs.

impaired Skin/Tissue Integrity may be related to mechanical interruption of skin and tissues, altered circulation, effects of medication, accumulation of drainage, and altered metabolic state, possibly evidenced by disruption of skin surface, skin layers, and tissues.

risk for Infection: risk factors may include broken skin, traumatized tissues, stasis of body fluids, presence of pathogens or contaminants, environmental exposure, and invasive procedures.*

Postpartal period   OB/CH

readiness for enhanced Family Processes may be related to developmental transition and gain of a family member possibly evidenced by expressing willingness to enhance family dynamics.

risk for deficient Fluid Volume/Bleeding: risk factors may include excessive blood loss during delivery, reduced intake, inadequate replacement, nausea, vomiting, increased urine output, and insensible losses.*

acute Pain/impaired Comfort may be related to tissue trauma and edema, muscle contractions, bladder fullness, and physical or psychological exhaustion, possibly evidenced by reports of cramping (afterpains), self-focusing, alteration in muscle tone, distraction behaviors, and changes in vital signs.

impaired Urinary Elimination may be related to hormonal effects (fluid shifts, continued elevation in renal plasma flow), mechanical trauma, tissue edema, and effects of medication and anesthesia, possibly evidenced by frequency, dysuria, urgency, incontinence, or retention.

Constipation may be related to decreased muscle tone associated with diastasis recti, prenatal effects of progesterone, dehydration, excess analgesia or anesthesia, pain (hemorrhoids, episiotomy, or perineal tenderness), prelabor diarrhea and lack of intake, possibly evidenced by frequency less than usual pattern, hard-formed stool, straining at stool, decreased bowel sounds, and abdominal distention.

Insomnia may be related to pain or discomfort, intense exhilaration and excitement, anxiety, exhausting process of labor and delivery, and needs/demands of family members, possibly evidenced by verbal reports of difficulty in falling or staying asleep, dissatisfaction with sleep, lack of energy, nonrestorative sleep.

risk for impaired Attachment/Parenting: risk factors may include lack of support between or from SO(s), ineffective or no role model,

---

*A risk diagnosis is not evidenced by signs and symptoms, as the problem has not occurred; rather, nursing interventions are directed at prevention.

anxiety associated with the parental role, unrealistic expectations, presence of stressors (e.g., financial, housing, employment).*

Posttraumatic stress disorder   PSY

Post-Trauma Syndrome related to having experienced a traumatic life event, possibly evidenced by reexperiencing the event, somatic reactions, psychic or emotional numbness, altered lifestyle, impaired sleep, self-destructive behaviors, difficulty with interpersonal relationships, development of phobia, poor impulse control/irritability, and explosiveness.

risk for other-directed Violence: risk factors may include startle reaction, an intrusive memory causing a sudden acting out of a feeling as if the event were occurring, use of alcohol or other drugs to ward off painful effects and produce psychic numbing, breaking through the rage that has been walled off, response to intense anxiety or panic state, and loss of control.*

ineffective Coping may be related to personal vulnerability, inadequate support systems, unrealistic perceptions, unmet expectations, overwhelming threat to self, and multiple stressors repeated over a period of time, possibly evidenced by verbalization of inability to cope or difficulty asking for help, muscular tension, headaches, chronic worry, and emotional tension.

complicated Grieving may be related to actual or perceived object loss (loss of self as seen before the traumatic incident occurred, as well as other losses incurred in/after the incident), loss of physiopsychosocial well-being, thwarted grieving response to a loss, and lack of resolution of previous grieving responses, possibly evidenced by verbal expression of distress at loss, anger, sadness, labile affect; alterations in eating habits, sleep/dream patterns, libido; reliving of past experiences, expression of guilt, and alterations in concentration.

interrupted Family Processes may be related to situational crisis, failure to master developmental transitions, possibly evidenced by expressions of confusion about what to do and that family is having difficulty coping; family system not meeting physical, emotional, or spiritual needs of its members; not adapting to change or dealing with traumatic experience constructively; and ineffective family decision-making process.

Pregnancy (prenatal period) 1st trimester   OB/CH

risk for imbalanced Nutrition: less than body requirements: risk factors may include changes in appetite, insufficient intake (nausea, vomiting, inadequate financial resources and nutritional knowledge), meeting increased metabolic demands (increased thyroid activity associated with the growth of fetal and maternal tissues).*

impaired Comfort may be related to hormonal influences, physical changes, possibly evidenced by verbal reports (nausea, breast changes, leg cramps, hemorrhoids, nasal stuffiness), alteration in muscle tone, inability to relax.

risk for disturbed Maternal/Fetal Dyad: risk factors may include environmental and hereditary factors and problems of maternal well-

---

*A risk diagnosis is not evidenced by signs and symptoms, as the problem has not occurred; rather, nursing interventions are directed at prevention.

being that directly affect the developing fetus (e.g., malnutrition, substance use).*

[maximally compensated] Cardiac Output may be related to increased fluid volume and maximal cardiac effort, hormonal effects of progesterone and relaxin (places the client at risk for hypertension and/ or circulatory failure), and changes in peripheral resistance (afterload), possibly evidenced by variations in BP and pulse, syncopal episodes, presence of pathological edema.

readiness for enhanced family Coping may be related to situational or maturational crisis with anticipated changes in family structure and roles, needs sufficiently met and adaptive tasks effectively addressed to enable goals of self-actualization to surface, as evidenced by movement toward health-promoting and enriching lifestyle, choosing experiences that optimize pregnancy experience and wellness.

risk for Constipation: risk factors may include changes in dietary and fluid intake, smooth muscle relaxation, decreased peristalsis, and effects of medications (e.g., iron).*

Fatigue/Insomnia may be related to increased carbohydrate metabolism, altered body chemistry, increased energy requirements to perform ADLs, discomfort, anxiety, inactivity, possibly evidenced by reports of overwhelming lack of energy, inability to maintain usual routines, difficulty falling asleep, dissatisfaction with sleep, decreased quality of life.

risk for ineffective Role Performance: risk factors may include maturational crisis, developmental level, history of maladaptive coping, absence of support systems.*

deficient Knowledge [Learning Need] regarding normal physiological/ psychological changes and self-care needs may be related to lack of information or recall, and misinterpretation of normal physiological and psychological changes and their impact on the client/family, possibly evidenced by questions, statements of concern, misconceptions, and inaccurate follow-through of instructions, development of preventable complications.

Pregnancy (prenatal period) 2nd trimester   OB/CH
Also Refer to Pregnancy 1st trimester

risk for disturbed Body Image: risk factors may include perception of biophysical changes, response of others.*

ineffective Breathing Pattern may be related to impingement of the diaphragm by enlarging uterus, possibly evidenced by reports of shortness of breath, dyspnea, and changes in respiratory depth.

risk for [decompensated] Cardiac Output: risk factors may include increased circulatory demand, changes in preload (decreased venous return) and afterload (increased peripheral vascular resistance), and ventricular hypertrophy.*

risk for excess Fluid Volume: risk factors may include changes in regulatory mechanisms, sodium and water retention.

Sexual Dysfunction may be related to conflict regarding changes in sexual desire and expectations, fear of physical injury to woman or

---

*A risk diagnosis is not evidenced by signs and symptoms, as the problem has not occurred; rather, nursing interventions are directed at prevention.

fetus, possibly evidenced by reported difficulties, limitations, or changes in sexual behaviors or activities.

Pregnancy (prenatal period) 3rd trimester   OB/CH

Also Refer to Pregnancy 1st and 2nd trimester

deficient Knowledge [Learning Need] regarding preparation for labor and delivery, infant care may be related to lack of exposure or experience, misinterpretations of information, possibly evidenced by request for information, statement of concerns, misconceptions.

impaired Urinary Elimination may be related to uterine enlargement, increased abdominal pressure, fluctuation of renal blood flow, and glomerular filtration rate (GFR), possibly evidenced by urinary frequency, urgency, dependent edema.

risk for ineffective Coping/compromised family Coping: risk factors may include situational or maturational crisis, personal vulnerability, unrealistic perceptions, absent or insufficient support systems.*

risk for disturbed Maternal/Fetal Dyad: risk factors may include presence of hypertension, infection, substance use or abuse, altered immune system, abnormal blood profile, tissue hypoxia, premature rupture of membranes.*

Pregnancy, adolescent   OB/CH

Also refer to Pregnancy, prenatal period

interrupted Family Processes may be related to situational or developmental transition (economic, change in roles, gain of a family member), possibly evidenced by family expressing confusion about what to do, unable to meet physical, emotional, or spiritual needs of the members; family inability to adapt to change or to deal with traumatic experience constructively, does not demonstrate respect for individuality and autonomy of its members, ineffective family decision-making process, and inappropriate boundary maintenance.

Social Isolation may be related to alterations in physical appearance, perceived unacceptable social behavior, restricted social sphere, stage of adolescence, and interference with accomplishing developmental tasks, possibly evidenced by expressions of feelings of aloneness, rejection, or difference from others; uncommunicative, withdrawn, no eye contact, seeking to be alone, unacceptable behavior, and absence of supportive SO(s).

situational/chronic low Self-Esteem may be related to situational or maturational crisis, biophysical changes, and fear of failure at life events, absence of support systems, possibly evidenced by self-negating verbalizations, expressions of shame, guilt, fear of rejection or reaction of other, hypersensitivity to criticism, and lack of follow-through or nonparticipation in prenatal care.

deficient Knowledge [Learning Need] regarding pregnancy, developmental or individual needs, future expectations may be related to lack of exposure, information misinterpretation, unfamiliarity with information resources, lack of interest in learning, possibly evidenced by questions, statement of concern, misconception, sense of

---

*A risk diagnosis is not evidenced by signs and symptoms, as the problem has not occurred; rather, nursing interventions are directed at prevention.

vulnerability, denial of reality, inaccurate follow-through of instruction, and development of preventable complications.

risk for impaired Parenting: may be related to chronological age and developmental stage; unmet social, emotional, or maturational needs of parenting figures; unrealistic expectation of self/infant/partner; ineffective role model or social support; lack of role identity; and presence of stressors (e.g., financial, social).*

Pregnancy, high-risk   OB/CH
Also refer to Pregnancy 1st, 2nd, 3rd trimester

Anxiety [specify level] may be related to situational crisis, threat of maternal or fetal death (perceived or actual), interpersonal transmission and contagion, possibly evidenced by increased tension, apprehension, feelings of inadequacy, somatic complaints, difficulty sleeping.

deficient Knowledge [Learning Need] regarding high-risk situation/preterm labor may be related to lack of exposure to or misinterpretation of information, unfamiliarity with individual risks and own role in risk prevention and management, possibly evidenced by request for information, statement of concerns, misconceptions, inaccurate follow-through of instructions.

risk of maternal Injury: risk factors may include preexisting medical conditions, complications of pregnancy.*

risk for Activity Intolerance: risk factors may include presence of circulatory or respiratory problems, uterine irritability.*

risk for ineffective self Health Management: risk factors may include client value system, health beliefs and cultural influences, issues of control, presence of anxiety, complexity of therapeutic regimen, economic difficulties, perceived susceptibility.*

Pregnancy-induced hypertension
(preeclampsia)   OB/CH
Also refer to Eclampsia

deficient Fluid Volume [isotonic] may be related to a plasma protein loss, decreasing plasma colloid osmotic pressure allowing fluid shifts out of vascular compartment, possibly evidenced by edema formation, sudden weight gain, hemoconcentration, nausea, vomiting, epigastric pain, headaches, visual changes, decreased urine output.

decreased Cardiac Output may be related to hypovolemia/decreased venous return, increased SVR, possibly evidenced by variations in BP and hemodynamic readings, edema, shortness of breath, change in mental status.

risk for disturbed Maternal/Fetal Dyad: risk factors may include vasospasm of spiral arteries and relative hypovolemia.*

deficient Knowledge [Learning Need] regarding pathophysiology of condition, therapy, self-care and nutritional needs, and potential complications may be related to lack of information or recall, misinterpretation, possibly evidenced by statements of concern, questions, misconceptions, inaccurate follow-through of instructions, or development of preventable complications.

---

*A risk diagnosis is not evidenced by signs and symptoms, as the problem has not occurred; rather, nursing interventions are directed at prevention.

Premenstrual tension syndrome (PMS)   GYN/CH/PSY

chronic/acute Pain may be related to cyclic changes in female hormones affecting other systems (e.g., vascular congestion or spasms), vitamin deficiency, fluid retention, possibly evidenced by increased tension, apprehension, jitteriness, verbal reports, distraction behaviors, somatic complaints, self-focusing, physical and social withdrawal.

excess Fluid Volume may be related to abnormal alterations of hormonal levels, possibly evidenced by edema formation, weight gain, and periodic changes in emotional status, irritability.

Anxiety [specify level] may be related to cyclic changes in female hormones affecting other systems, possibly evidenced by feelings of inability to cope or loss of control, depersonalization, increased tension, apprehension, jitteriness, somatic complaints, and impaired functioning.

deficient Knowledge [Learning Need] regarding pathophysiology of condition and self-care/treatment needs may be related to lack of information, misinterpretation, possibly evidenced by statements of concern, questions, misconceptions, and continuation of condition, exacerbating symptoms.

Pressure ulcer or sore   CH

Also refer to Ulcer, decubitus

ineffective peripheral tissue Perfusion may be related to reduced or interrupted blood flow, possibly evidenced by presence of inflamed, necrotic lesion.

deficient Knowledge [Learning Need] regarding cause/prevention of condition and potential complications may be related to lack of information, misinterpretation, possibly evidenced by statements of concern, questions, misconceptions, and inaccurate follow-through of instructions.

Preterm labor   OB/CH

Refer to Labor, preterm

Prostatectomy   MS

impaired Urinary Elimination may be related to mechanical obstruction (blood clots, edema, trauma, surgical procedure, pressure or irritation of catheter and balloon) and loss of bladder tone, possibly evidenced by dysuria, frequency, dribbling, incontinence, retention, bladder fullness, suprapubic discomfort.

risk for Bleeding/deficient Fluid Volume: risk factors may include trauma to highly vascular area with excessive vascular losses, restricted intake, postobstructive diuresis.*

acute Pain may be related to irritation of bladder mucosa and tissue trauma or edema, possibly evidenced by verbal reports (bladder spasms), distraction behaviors, self-focus, and changes in vital signs.

disturbed Body Image may be related to perceived threat of altered body or sexual function, possibly evidenced by preoccupation with change or loss, negative feelings about body, and statements of concern regarding functioning.

---

*A risk diagnosis is not evidenced by signs and symptoms, as the problem has not occurred; rather, nursing interventions are directed at prevention.

risk for Sexual Dysfunction: risk factors may include situational crisis
(incontinence, leakage of urine after catheter removal, involvement
of genital area) and threat to self-concept or change in health status.*

Pruritus

impaired Comfort/acute Pain may be related to cutaneous hyperesthesia
and inflammation, possibly evidenced by verbal reports, distraction
behaviors, and self-focus.
risk for impaired Skin Integrity: risk factors may include mechanical
trauma (scratching) and development of vesicles or bullae that may
rupture.*

Psoriasis

impaired Skin Integrity may be related to increased epidermal cell pro-
liferation and absence of normal protective skin layers, possibly evidenced by scaling papules and plaques.
disturbed Body Image may be related to cosmetically unsightly skin
lesions, possibly evidenced by hiding affected body part, negative
feelings about body, feelings of helplessness, and change in social
involvement.

Pulmonary edema

impaired Gas Exchange may be related to alveolar-capillary membrane
changes (fluid collection or shifts into interstitial space or alveoli)
possibly evidenced by dyspnea, restlessness, irritability, abnormal
rate/depth of respirations, lethargy, confusion.
[moderate to severe] Anxiety may be related to change in health status,
threat of death, interpersonal transmission possibly evidenced by expressed concerns, distressed, apprehension, extraneous movement.
risk for impaired spontaneous Ventilation: risk factors may include respiratory muscle fatigue, problems with secretion management.*

Pulmonary edema, high-altitude
Refer to High-altitude pulmonary edema

Pulmonary embolus

ineffective Breathing Pattern may be related to tracheobronchial obstruction (inflammation, copious secretions, or active bleeding), decreased
lung expansion, inflammatory process, possibly evidenced by changes
in depth and/or rate of respiration, dyspnea, use of accessory muscles,
altered chest excursion, abnormal breath sounds (crackles, wheezes),
and cough (with or without sputum production).
impaired Gas Exchange may be related to altered blood flow to alveoli
or to major portions of the lung, alveolar-capillary membrane changes
(atelectasis, airway or alveolar collapse, pulmonary edema or effusion,
excessive secretions or active bleeding), possibly evidenced by pro-
found dyspnea, restlessness, apprehension, somnolence, cyanosis, and
changes in ABGs or pulse oximetry (hypoxemia and hypercapnia).
ineffective [pulmonary] tissue Perfusion may be related to interruption
of blood flow (arterial or venous), exchange problems at alveolar

---

*A risk diagnosis is not evidenced by signs and symptoms, as the problem has
not occurred; rather, nursing interventions are directed at prevention.

level or at tissue level (acidotic shifting of the oxyhemoglobin curve), possibly evidenced by radiology or laboratory findings of ventilation/perfusion mismatch, dyspnea, and central cyanosis.

Fear/Anxiety [specify level] may be related to severe dyspnea and inability to breathe normally, perceived threat of death, threat to or change in health status, physiological response to hypoxemia and acidosis, and concern regarding unknown outcome of situation, possibly evidenced by restlessness, irritability, withdrawal or attack behavior, sympathetic stimulation (cardiovascular excitation, pupil dilation, sweating, vomiting, diarrhea), crying, voice quivering, and impending sense of doom.

Pulmonary hypertension CH/MS

impaired Gas Exchange may be related to changes in alveolar membrane, increased pulmonary vascular resistance, possibly evidenced by dyspnea, irritability, decreased mental acuity, somnolence, abnormal ABGs.

decreased Cardiac Output may be related to increased pulmonary vascular resistance, decreased blood return to left side of heart, possibly evidenced by increased heart rate, dyspnea, fatigue.

Activity Intolerance may be related to imbalance between O_2 supply and demand, possibly evidenced by reports of weakness, fatigue, abnormal vital signs with activity.

Anxiety may be related to change in health status, stress, threat to self-concept, possibly evidenced by expressed concerns, uncertainty, awareness of physiological symptoms, diminished productivity or ability to problem-solve.

Purpura, idiopathic thrombocytopenic CH

ineffective Protection may be related to abnormal blood profile, drug therapy (corticosteroids or immunosuppressive agents), possibly evidenced by altered clotting, fatigue, deficient immunity.

Activity Intolerance may be related to decreased O_2-carrying capacity/imbalance between O_2 supply and demand, possibly evidenced by reports of fatigue, weakness.

deficient Knowledge [Learning Need] regarding therapy choices, outcomes, and self-care needs may be related to lack of information/misinterpretation, possibly evidenced by statements of concern, questions, and misconceptions.

Pyelonephritis MS

acute Pain may be related to acute inflammation of renal tissues, possibly evidenced by verbal reports, guarding/distraction behaviors, self-focus, and changes in vital signs.

Hyperthermia may be related to inflammatory process and increased metabolic rate, possibly evidenced by increase in body temperature; warm, flushed skin; tachycardia; and chills.

impaired Urinary Elimination may be related to inflammation or irritation of bladder mucosa, possibly evidenced by dysuria, urgency, and frequency.

deficient Knowledge [Learning Need] regarding therapy needs and prevention may be related to lack of information, misinterpretation, possibly evidenced by statements of concern, questions, misconceptions, and recurrence of condition.

P

Quadriplegia

Also refer to Paraplegia

ineffective Breathing Pattern may be related to neuromuscular impairment of innervation of diaphragm—lesions at or above C5, complete or mixed loss of intercostal muscle function, reflex abdominal spasms, gastric distention, possibly evidenced by decreased respiratory depth, dyspnea, cyanosis, and abnormal ABGs.

risk for Trauma [additional spinal injury]: risk factors may include temporary weakness or instability of spinal column.*

Grieving may be related to perceived loss of self, anticipated alterations in lifestyle and expectations, and limitation of future options or choices, possibly evidenced by expressions of distress, anger, sorrow, choked feelings, and changes in eating habits, sleep, communication patterns.

[total] Self-Care Deficit related to neuromuscular impairment, evidenced by inability to perform self-care tasks.

Bowel Incontinence/Constipation may be related to disruption of nerve innervation, perceptual impairment, changes in dietary and fluid intake, change in activity level, side effects of medication possibly evidenced by inability to evacuate bowel voluntarily; increased abdominal pressure or distention; dry, hard-formed stool; change in bowel sounds.

impaired bed/wheelchair Mobility may be related to loss of muscle function and control possibly evidenced by inability to reposition self, impaired ability to operate wheelchair.

risk for Autonomic Dysreflexia: risk factors may include altered nerve function (spinal cord injury at T6 or above), bladder, bowel, or skin stimulation (tactile, pain, thermal).*

impaired Home Maintenance may be related to permanent effects of injury, inadequate or absent support systems and finances, and lack of familiarity with resources, possibly evidenced by expressions of difficulties, requests for information and assistance, outstanding debts or financial crisis, and lack of necessary aids and equipment.

Rape

deficient Knowledge [Learning Need] regarding required medical and legal procedures, prophylactic treatment for individual concerns (STDs, pregnancy), community resources and supports may be related to lack of information, possibly evidenced by statements of concern, questions, misconceptions, and exacerbation of symptoms.

Rape-Trauma Syndrome (acute phase) related to actual or attempted sexual penetration without consent, possibly evidenced by wide range of emotional reactions, including anxiety, fear, anger, embarrassment, and multisystem physical complaints.

risk for impaired Tissue Integrity: risk factors may include forceful sexual penetration and trauma to fragile tissues.*

ineffective Coping may be related to personal vulnerability, unmet expectations, unrealistic perceptions, inadequate support systems or

R

---

*A risk diagnosis is not evidenced by signs and symptoms, as the problem has not occurred; rather, nursing interventions are directed at prevention.

coping methods, multiple stressors repeated over time, overwhelming threat to self, possibly evidenced by verbalizations of inability to cope or difficulty asking for help, muscular tension, headaches, emotional tension, chronic worry.

Sexual Dysfunction may be related to biopsychosocial alteration of sexuality (stress of post-trauma response), vulnerability, loss of sexual desire, impaired relationship with SO, possibly evidenced by alteration in achieving sexual satisfaction, change in interest in self or others, preoccupation with self.

Raynaud's phenomenon   CH

acute/chronic Pain may be related to vasospasm or altered perfusion of affected tissues, ischemia or destruction of tissues, possibly evidenced by verbal reports, guarding of affected parts, self-focusing, and restlessness.

ineffective peripheral tissue Perfusion may be related to periodic reduction of arterial blood flow to affected areas, possibly evidenced by pallor, cyanosis, coolness, numbness, paresthesia, slow healing of lesions.

deficient Knowledge [Learning Need] regarding pathophysiology of condition, potential for complications, therapy and self-care needs may be related to lack of information, misinterpretation, possibly evidenced by statements of concern, questions, and misconceptions; development of preventable complications.

Reflex sympathetic dystrophy (RSD)   CH
Refer to Complex regional pain syndrome

Regional enteritis   CH
Refer to Crohn's disease

Renal failure, acute   MS
excess Fluid Volume may be related to compromised regulatory mechanisms–decreased kidney function, possibly evidenced by weight gain, edema or anasarca, intake greater than output, venous congestion, changes in BP and CVP, and altered electrolyte levels, decreased Hb and Hct; pulmonary congestion on x-ray.

risk for imbalanced Nutrition: less than body requirements: risk factors may include inability to ingest or digest adequate nutrients–anorexia, nausea, vomiting, ulcerations of oral mucosa, and increased metabolic needs; protein catabolism, therapeutic dietary restrictions.*

risk for Infection: risk factors may include depression of immunological defenses, invasive procedures and devices, and changes in dietary intake, malnutrition.*

risk for acute Confusion: risk factors may include accumulation of toxic waste products and altered cerebral perfusion.*

Renal failure, chronic   CH/MS
Also refer to Dialysis, general
risk for decreased Cardiac Output: risk factors may include fluid imbalances affecting circulating volume, myocardial workload,

R

---

*A risk diagnosis is not evidenced by signs and symptoms, as the problem has not occurred; rather, nursing interventions are directed at prevention.

systemic vascular resistance; alterations in rate, rhythm, cardiac conduction—electrolyte imbalances, hypoxia; accumulation of toxins—urea; soft-tissue calcification—deposits of calcium phosphate.*

risk for Bleeding: risk factors may include abnormal blood profile—suppressed erythropoietin production or secretion, decreased RBC production and survival, altered clotting factors; increased capillary fragility.*

disturbed Thought Processes may be related to accumulation of toxins—urea, ammonia; metabolic acidosis, hypoxia, electrolyte imbalances, calcifications in brain possibly evidenced by disorientation, memory deficit, altered attention span, decreased ability to grasp ideas, impaired ability to make decisions or problem-solve, changes in sensorium, irritability, psychosis.

risk for impaired Skin Integrity: risk factors may include altered metabolic state and circulation (anemia with tissue ischemia), altered sensation (peripheral neuropathy), decreased skin turgor, reduced activity or immobility, accumulation of toxins in the skin.*

risk for impaired Oral Mucous Membrane: risk factors may include decreased or lack of salivation, fluid restrictions, chemical irritation, conversion of urea in saliva to ammonia.*

Renal transplantation   MS

risk for excess Fluid Volume: risk factors may include compromised regulatory mechanism (implantation of new kidney requiring adjustment period for optimal functioning).*

disturbed Body Image may be related to failure and subsequent replacement of body part and medication-induced changes in appearance, possibly evidenced by preoccupation with loss or change, negative feelings about body, and focus on past strength or function.

Fear may be related to potential for transplant rejection or failure and threat of death, possibly evidenced by increased tension, apprehension, concentration on source, and verbalizations of concern.

risk for Infection: risk factors may include broken skin, traumatized tissue, stasis of body fluids, immunosuppression, invasive procedures, nutritional deficits, and chronic disease.*

CH

risk for ineffective Coping/compromised family Coping: risk factors may include situational crises, family disorganization and role changes, prolonged disease exhausting supportive capacity of SO(s)/family, therapeutic restrictions, long-term therapy needs.*

Respiratory distress syndrome, acute   MS

ineffective Airway Clearance may be related to loss of ciliary action, increased amount and viscosity of secretions, and increased airway resistance, possibly evidenced by presence of dyspnea, changes in depth and rate of respiration, use of accessory muscles for breathing, wheezes and crackles, cough with or without sputum production.

impaired Gas Exchange may be related to changes in pulmonary capillary permeability with edema formation, alveolar hypoventilation

---

*A risk diagnosis is not evidenced by signs and symptoms, as the problem has not occurred; rather, nursing interventions are directed at prevention.

---

and collapse, with intrapulmonary shunting, possibly evidenced by tachypnea, use of accessory muscles, cyanosis, hypoxia per ABGs or oximetry, anxiety, and changes in mentation.

risk for deficient Fluid Volume: risk factors may include active loss from diuretic use and restricted intake.*

risk for decreased Cardiac Output: risk factors may include alteration in preload (hypovolemia, vascular pooling, diuretic therapy, and increased intrathoracic pressure, use of ventilator and positive end-expiratory pressure [PEEP]).*

Anxiety [specify level]/Fear may be related to physiological factors (effects of hypoxemia), situational crisis, change in health status and threat of death possibly evidenced by increased tension, apprehension, restlessness, focus on self, and sympathetic stimulation.

risk for [barotrauma] Injury: risk factors may include increased airway pressure associated with mechanical ventilation (PEEP).*

Respiratory distress syndrome
(premature infant)   PED

Also refer to Neonatal, premature newborn

impaired Gas Exchange may be related to alveolar-capillary membrane changes (inadequate surfactant levels), altered O$_2$ supply (tracheobronchial obstruction, atelectasis), altered blood flow (immaturity of pulmonary arteriole musculature), altered O$_2$-carrying capacity of blood (anemia), and cold stress, possibly evidenced by tachypnea, use of accessory muscles—retractions, expiratory grunting, pallor, or cyanosis, abnormal ABGs, and tachycardia.

impaired spontaneous Ventilation may be related to respiratory muscle fatigue and metabolic factors, possibly evidenced by dyspnea, increased metabolic rate, restlessness, use of accessory muscles, and abnormal ABGs.

risk for Infection: risk factors may include inadequate primary defenses (decreased ciliary action, stasis of body fluids, traumatized tissues), inadequate secondary defenses (deficiency of neutrophils and specific immunoglobulins), invasive procedures, and malnutrition (absence of nutrient stores, increased metabolic demands).*

risk for ineffective gastrointestinal Perfusion: risk factors may include persistent fetal circulation and exchange problems.*

risk for impaired Attachment: risk factors may include premature or ill infant who is unable to effectively initiate parental contact (altered behavioral organization), separation, physical barriers, anxiety associated with the parental role and demands of infant.*

Retinal detachment   CH

disturbed visual Sensory Perception related to decreased sensory reception, possibly evidenced by visual distortions, decreased visual field, and changes in visual acuity.

deficient Knowledge [Learning Need] regarding therapy, prognosis, and self-care needs may be related to lack of information or misconceptions, possibly evidenced by statements of concern and questions.

---

*A risk diagnosis is not evidenced by signs and symptoms, as the problem has not occurred; rather, nursing interventions are directed at prevention.

risk for impaired Home Maintenance: risk factors may include visual
limitations activity restrictions.*

Reye's syndrome   PED

deficient Fluid Volume [isotonic] may be related to failure of regulatory
mechanism (diabetes insipidus), excessive gastric losses (pernicious
vomiting), and altered intake, possibly evidenced by increased/dilute
urine output, sudden weight loss, decreased venous filling, dry mucous membranes, decreased skin turgor, hypotension, and tachycardia.

ineffective cerebral tissue Perfusion may be related to diminished arterial or venous blood flow and hypovolemia, possibly evidenced by
memory loss, altered consciousness, and restlessness or agitation.

risk for Trauma: risk factors may include generalized weakness, reduced coordination, and cognitive deficits.*

ineffective Breathing Pattern may be related to decreased energy and
fatigue, cognitive impairment, tracheobronchial obstruction, and inflammatory process (aspiration pneumonia), possibly evidenced by
tachypnea, abnormal ABGs, cough, and use of accessory muscles.

Rheumatic fever   PED

acute Pain may be related to migratory inflammation of joints, possibly
evidenced by verbal reports, guarding or distraction behaviors, self-
focus, and changes in vital signs.

Hyperthermia may be related to inflammatory process, hypermetabolic
state, possibly evidenced by increased body temperature; warm,
flushed skin; and tachycardia.

Activity Intolerance may be related to generalized weakness, joint pain,
medical restrictions, and bedrest, possibly evidenced by reports of
fatigue, exertional discomfort, and abnormal heart rate in response
to activity.

risk for decreased Cardiac Output: risk factors may include cardiac
inflammation or enlargement and altered contractility.*

Rickets (osteomalacia)   PED

delayed Growth and Development may be related to dietary deficiencies
or indiscretions, malabsorption syndrome, and lack of exposure to
sunlight, possibly evidenced by altered physical growth and delay or
difficulty in performing motor skills typical for age.

deficient Knowledge [Learning Need] regarding cause, pathophysiology, therapy needs, and prevention may be related to lack of information, possibly evidenced by statements of concern, questions, misconceptions, and inaccurate follow-through of instructions.

Ringworm, tinea   CH

Also refer to Athlete's Foot

impaired Skin Integrity may be related to fungal infection of the dermis,
possibly evidenced by disruption of skin surfaces—presence of lesions.

deficient Knowledge [Learning Need] regarding infectious nature, therapy, and self-care needs may be related to lack of information,

*A risk diagnosis is not evidenced by signs and symptoms, as the problem has
not occurred; rather, nursing interventions are directed at prevention.

misinformation, possibly evidenced by statements of concern, questions, and recurrence or spread.

Rubella PED/CH

acute Pain/impaired Comfort may be related to inflammatory effects of viral infection and presence of desquamating rash, possibly evidenced by verbal reports, distraction behaviors, restlessness.

deficient Knowledge [Learning Need] regarding contagious nature, possible complications, and self-care needs may be related to lack of information, misinterpretations, possibly evidenced by statements of concern, questions, and inaccurate follow-through of instructions.

Scabies CH

impaired Skin Integrity may be related to presence of invasive parasite and development of pruritus, possibly evidenced by disruption of skin surface and inflammation.

deficient Knowledge [Learning Need] regarding communicable nature, possible complications, therapy, and self-care needs may be related to lack of information, misinterpretation, possibly evidenced by questions and statements of concern about spread to others.

Scarlet fever PED

Hyperthermia may be related to effects of circulating toxins, possibly evidenced by increased body temperature; warm, flushed skin; and tachycardia.

acute Pain/impaired Comfort may be related to inflammation of mucous membranes and effects of circulating toxins (malaise, fever), possibly evidenced by verbal reports, distraction behaviors, guarding (decreased swallowing), and self-focus.

risk for deficient Fluid Volume: risk factors may include hypermetabolic state (hyperthermia) and reduced intake.*

Schizophrenia (schizophrenic disorders) PSY/CH

disturbed Thought Processes may be related to disintegration of thinking processes, impaired judgment, presence of psychological conflicts, disintegrated ego boundaries, sleep disturbance, ambivalence and concomitant dependence, possibly evidenced by impaired ability to reason or problem-solve, inappropriate affect, presence of delusional system, command hallucinations, obsessions, ideas of reference, cognitive dissonance.

Social Isolation may be related to alterations in mental status, mistrust of others, delusional thinking, unacceptable social behaviors, inadequate personal resources, and inability to engage in satisfying personal relationships, possibly evidenced by difficulty in establishing relationships with others, dull affect, uncommunicative or withdrawn behavior, seeking to be alone, inadequate or absent significant purpose in life, and expression of feelings of rejection.

ineffective Health Maintenance/impaired Home Maintenance may be related to impaired cognitive or emotional functioning, altered ability to make deliberate and thoughtful judgments, altered communication,

S

---

*A risk diagnosis is not evidenced by signs and symptoms, as the problem has not occurred; rather, nursing interventions are directed at prevention.

and lack or inappropriate use of material resources, possibly evidenced by inability to take responsibility for meeting basic health practices in any or all functional areas and demonstrated lack of adaptive behaviors to internal or external environmental changes, disorderly surroundings, accumulation of dirt and unwashed clothes, repeated hygienic disorders.

risk for self-/other-directed Violence: risk factors may include disturbances of thinking or feeling (depression, paranoia, suicidal ideation), lack of development of trust and appropriate interpersonal relationships, catatonic or manic excitement, toxic reactions to drugs (alcohol).*

ineffective Coping may be related to personal vulnerability, inadequate support system(s), unrealistic perceptions, inadequate coping methods, and disintegration of thought processes, possibly evidenced by impaired judgment, cognition, and perception; diminished problem-solving or decision-making capacities; poor self-concept; chronic anxiety; depression; inability to perform role expectations; and alteration in social participation.

interrupted Family Processes/disabled family Coping may be related to ambivalent family system or relationships, change of roles, and difficulty of family member in coping effectively with client's maladaptive behaviors, possibly evidenced by deterioration in family functioning, ineffective family decision-making process, difficulty relating to each other, client's expressions of despair at family's lack of reaction or involvement, neglectful relationships with client, extreme distortion regarding client's health problem including denial about its existence or severity, or prolonged overconcern.

Self-Care Deficit [specify] may be related to perceptual and cognitive impairment, immobility (withdrawal, isolation, and decreased psychomotor activity), and side effects of psychotropic medications, possibly evidenced by inability or difficulty in areas of feeding self, keeping body clean, dressing appropriately, toileting self, and/or changes in bowel or bladder elimination.

Sciatica   CH

acute/chronic Pain may be related to peripheral nerve root compression, possibly evidenced by verbal reports, guarding or distraction behaviors, and self-focus.

impaired physical Mobility may be related to neurological pain and muscular involvement, possibly evidenced by reluctance to attempt movement and decreased muscle strength and mass.

Scleroderma   CH

Also refer to Lupus erythematosus, systemic—SLE

impaired physical Mobility may be related to musculoskeletal impairment and associated pain, possibly evidenced by decreased strength, decreased range of motion, and reluctance to attempt movement.

ineffective tissue Perfusion (specify) may be related to reduced arterial blood flow (arteriolar vasoconstriction), possibly evidenced by

---

*A risk diagnosis is not evidenced by signs and symptoms, as the problem has not occurred; rather, nursing interventions are directed at prevention.

changes in skin temperature and color, ulcer formation, and changes in organ function (cardiopulmonary, gastrointestinal, renal).

imbalanced Nutrition: less than body requirements may be related to inability to ingest, digest, or absorb adequate nutrients (sclerosis of the tissues rendering mouth immobile, decreased peristalsis of esophagus or small intestine, atrophy of smooth muscle of colon), possibly evidenced by weight loss, decreased intake, and reported or observed difficulty swallowing.

risk-prone health Behavior may be related to disability requiring change in lifestyle, inadequate support systems, assault to self-concept, and altered locus of control, possibly evidenced by verbalization of non-acceptance of health status change and lack of movement toward independence or future-oriented thinking.

disturbed Body Image may be related to skin changes with induration, atrophy, and fibrosis, loss of hair, and skin and muscle contractures, possibly evidenced by verbalization of negative feelings about body, focus on past strength or function or appearance, fear of rejection or reaction by others, hiding body part, and change in social involvement.

Scoliosis   PED

disturbed Body Image may be related to altered body structure, use of therapeutic device(s), and activity restrictions, possibly evidenced by negative feelings about body, change in social involvement, and preoccupation with situation or refusal to acknowledge problem.

deficient Knowledge [Learning Need] regarding pathophysiology of condition, therapy needs, and possible outcomes may be related to lack of information, misinterpretation, possibly evidenced by statements of concern, questions, misconceptions, and inaccurate follow-through of instructions.

risk-prone health Behavior may be related to lack of comprehension of long-term consequences of behavior, possibly evidenced by minimization of health status change, failure to take action, and evidence of failure to improve.

Seizure disorder   CH

deficient Knowledge [Learning Need] regarding condition and medication control may be related to lack of information, misinterpretations, scarce financial resources, possibly evidenced by questions, statements of concern, misconceptions, incorrect use of anticonvulsant medication, recurrent episodes or uncontrolled seizures.

chronic low Self-Esteem/disturbed personal Identity may be related to stigma associated with condition, perception of being out of control or helpless, possibly evidenced by verbalization about changed lifestyle, fear of rejection, negative feelings about "brain" or self, change in usual pattern of responsibility, denial of problem resulting in lack of follow-through or nonparticipation in therapy.

impaired Social Interaction may be related to unpredictable nature of condition and self-concept disturbance, possibly evidenced by decreased self-assurance, verbalization of concern, discomfort in social situations, inability to receive or communicate a satisfying sense of belonging or caring, and withdrawal from social contacts and activities.

risk for Trauma/Suffocation: risk factors may include weakness, balancing difficulties, cognitive limitations, altered consciousness, loss of large or small-muscle coordination (during seizure).*

Sepsis   MS

Also refer to Sepsis, puerperal

risk for deficient Fluid Volume: risk factors may include marked increase in vascular compartment, massive vasodilation, capillary permeability, vascular shifts to interstitial space, and reduced intake.*

risk for decreased Cardiac Output: risk factors may include decreased preload—venous return and circulating volume; altered afterload—increased systemic vascular resistance; negative inotropic effects of hypoxia, complement activation, and lysosomal hydrolase.*

risk for impaired Gas Exchange: risk factors may include effects of endotoxins on the respiratory center in the medulla—hyperventilation and respiratory alkalosis; hypoventilation; changes in vascular resistance, alveolar-capillary membrane changes—increased capillary permeability leading to pulmonary congestion; interference with oxygen delivery and utilization in the tissues—endotoxin-induced damage to the cells and capillaries.*

risk for Shock: risk factors may include infection/sepsis, hypovolemia—fluid shifts/third spacing; hypotension, hypoxemia.*

Sepsis, puerperal   OB

Also refer to Sepsis

risk for Infection [spread/septic shock]: risk factors may include presence of infection, broken skin, and/or traumatized tissues, rupture of amniotic membranes, high vascularity of involved area, stasis of body fluids, invasive procedures, and/or increased environmental exposure, chronic disease (e.g., diabetes, anemia, malnutrition), altered immune response, and untoward effect of medications (e.g., opportunistic or secondary infection).*

Hyperthermia may be related to inflammatory process, hypermetabolic state, dehydration, effect of circulating endotoxins on the hypothalamus, possibly evidenced by increase in body temperature; warm, flushed skin; increased respiratory rate; and tachycardia.

risk for impaired Attachment: risk factors may include interruption in bonding process, physical illness, perceived threat to own survival.*

risk for ineffective peripheral tissue Perfusion: risk factors may include interruption or reduction of blood flow (presence of infectious thrombi).*

S

Serum sickness   CH

acute Pain may be related to inflammation of the joints and skin eruptions, possibly evidenced by verbal reports, guarding or distraction behaviors, and self-focus.

deficient Knowledge [Learning Need] regarding nature of condition, treatment needs, potential complications, and prevention of recurrence may be related to lack of information, misinterpretation,

---

*A risk diagnosis is not evidenced by signs and symptoms, as the problem has not occurred; rather, nursing interventions are directed at prevention.

possibly evidenced by statements of concern, questions, misconceptions, and inaccurate follow-through of instructions.

Sexually transmitted disease (STD)　　　　GYN/CH
risk for Infection [transmission]: risk factors may include contagious nature of infecting agent and insufficient knowledge to avoid exposure to or transmission of pathogens.*

impaired Skin/Tissue Integrity may be related to invasion of or irritation by pathogenic organism(s), possibly evidenced by disruptions of skin or tissues and inflammation of mucous membranes.

deficient Knowledge [Learning Need] regarding condition, prognosis/complications, therapy needs, and transmission may be related to lack of information, misinterpretation, lack of interest in learning, possibly evidenced by statements of concern, questions, misconceptions; inaccurate follow-through of instructions; and development of preventable complications.

Shock　　　　MS
Also refer to Shock, cardiogenic; Shock, hypovolemic/hemorrhagic

ineffective tissue Perfusion (specify) may be related to changes in circulating volume and/or vascular tone, possibly evidenced by changes in skin color and temperature and pulse pressure, reduced blood pressure, changes in mentation, and decreased urinary output.

Anxiety [specify level] may be related to change in health status and threat of death, possibly evidenced by increased tension, apprehension, sympathetic stimulation, restlessness, and expressions of concern.

Shock, cardiogenic　　　　MS
Also refer to Shock

decreased Cardiac Output may be related to structural damage, decreased myocardial contractility, and presence of dysrhythmias, possibly evidenced by ECG changes, variations in hemodynamic readings, jugular vein distention, cold or clammy skin, diminished peripheral pulses, and decreased urinary output.

risk for impaired Gas Exchange: risk factors may include ventilation perfusion imbalance, alveolar-capillary membrane changes.*

Shock, hypovolemic/hemorrhagic　　　　MS
Also refer to Shock

deficient Fluid Volume [isotonic] may be related to excessive vascular loss, inadequate intake or replacement, possibly evidenced by hypotension, tachycardia, decreased pulse volume and pressure, change in mentation, and decreased, concentrated urine.

Shock, septic　　　　MS
Refer to Sepsis

Sick sinus syndrome　　　　MS
Also refer to Dysrhythmia, cardiac

decreased Cardiac Output may be related to alterations in rate, rhythm, and electrical conduction, possibly evidenced by ECG evidence of

---

*A risk diagnosis is not evidenced by signs and symptoms, as the problem has not occurred; rather, nursing interventions are directed at prevention.

dysrhythmias, reports of palpitations or weakness, changes in mentation or consciousness, and syncope.

risk for Trauma: risk factors may include changes in cerebral perfusion with altered consciousness, loss of balance.*

SLE   CH
Refer to Lupus erythematosus, systemic

Smallpox   MS
risk of Infection [spread]: risk factors may include contagious nature of organism, inadequate acquired immunity, presence of chronic disease, immunosuppression.*

deficient Fluid Volume may be related to hypermetabolic state, decreased intake (pharyngeal lesions, nausea), increased losses (vomiting), fluid shifts from vascular bed, possibly evidenced by reports of thirst, decreased BP, venous filling and urinary output; dry mucous membranes, decreased skin turgor, change in mental state, elevated Hct.

impaired Tissue Integrity may be related to immunological deficit, possibly evidenced by disruption of skin surface, cornea, mucous membranes.

Anxiety [specify level]/Fear may be related to threat of death, interpersonal transmission and contagion, separation from support system, possibly evidenced by expressed concerns, apprehension, restlessness, focus on self.

        CH

interrupted Family Processes may be related to temporary family disorganization, situational crisis, change in health status of family member, possibly evidenced by changes in satisfaction with family, stress-reduction behaviors, mutual support; expression of isolation from community resources.

ineffective community Coping may be related to human-made disaster (bioterrorism), inadequate resources for problem solving, possibly evidenced by deficits of community participation, high illness rate, excessive community conflicts, expressed vulnerability or powerlessness.

Snow blindness   CH
disturbed visual Sensory Perception may be related to altered status of sense organ (irritation of the conjunctiva, hyperemia), possibly evidenced by intolerance to light (photophobia) and decreased or loss of visual acuity.

acute Pain may be related to irritation and vascular congestion of the conjunctiva, possibly evidenced by verbal reports, guarding or distraction behaviors, and self-focus.

Anxiety [specify level] may be related to situational crisis and threat to or change in health status, possibly evidenced by increased tension, apprehension, uncertainty, worry, restlessness, and focus on self.

***

*A risk diagnosis is not evidenced by signs and symptoms, as the problem has not occurred; rather, nursing interventions are directed at prevention.

Somatoform disorders   PSY

ineffective Coping may be related to severe level of anxiety that is repressed, personal vulnerability, unmet dependency needs, fixation in earlier level of development, retarded ego development, and inadequate coping skills, possibly evidenced by verbalized inability to cope or problem-solve, high illness rate, multiple somatic complaints of several years' duration, decreased functioning in social and occupational settings, narcissistic tendencies with total focus on self and physical symptoms, demanding behaviors, history of "doctor shopping," and refusal to attend therapeutic activities.

chronic Pain may be related to severe level of repressed anxiety, low self-concept, unmet dependency needs, history of self or loved one having experienced a serious illness, possibly evidenced by verbal reports of severe or prolonged pain, guarded movement or protective behaviors, facial mask of pain, fear of reinjury, altered ability to continue previous activities, social withdrawal, demands for therapy or medication.

disturbed Sensory Perception (specify) may be related to psychological stress (narrowed perceptual fields, expression of stress as physical problems), poor quality of sleep, presence of chronic pain, possibly evidenced by reported change in voluntary motor or sensory function (paralysis, anosmia, aphonia, deafness, blindness, loss of touch or pain sensation), *la belle indifférence* (lack of concern over functional loss).

impaired Social Interaction may be related to inability to engage in satisfying personal relationships, preoccupation with self and physical symptoms, altered state of wellness, chronic pain, and rejection by others, possibly evidenced by preoccupation with own thoughts, sad or dull affect, absence of supportive SO(s), uncommunicative or withdrawn behavior, lack of eye contact, and seeking to be alone.

Spinal cord injury (SCI)   MS/CH
Refer to Paraplegia; Quadriplegia

Sprain of ankle or foot   CH

acute Pain may be related to trauma to and swelling in joint, possibly evidenced by verbal reports, guarding or distraction behaviors, self-focusing, and changes in vital signs.

impaired Walking may be related to musculoskeletal injury, pain, and therapeutic restrictions, possibly evidenced by reluctance to attempt movement, inability to move about environment easily.

Stapedectomy   MS

risk for Trauma: risk factors may include increased middle-ear pressure with displacement of prosthesis and balancing difficulties, dizziness.*

risk for Infection: risk factors may include surgically traumatized tissue, invasive procedures, and environmental exposure to upper respiratory infections.*

---

*A risk diagnosis is not evidenced by signs and symptoms, as the problem has not occurred; rather, nursing interventions are directed at prevention.

acute Pain may be related to surgical trauma, edema formation, and presence of packing, possibly evidenced by verbal reports, guarding or distraction behaviors, and self-focus.

STD **CH**
Refer to Sexually transmitted disease

Stimulant abuse **CH**
Also refer to Cocaine hydrochloride poisoning, acute; Substance dependence/abuse rehabilitation

imbalanced Nutrition: less than body requirements may be related to anorexia, insufficient or inappropriate use of financial resources, possibly evidenced by reported inadequate intake, weight loss or less than normal weight gain; lack of interest in food, poor muscle tone, signs or laboratory evidence of vitamin deficiencies.

risk for Infection: risk factors may include injection techniques, impurities of drugs; localized trauma or nasal septum damage, malnutrition, altered immune state.*

Insomnia may be related to CNS sensory alterations, psychological stress possibly evidenced by constant alertness, racing thoughts preventing rest, denial of need to sleep, reported inability to stay awake, initial insomnia then hypersomnia.

PSY
Fear/Anxiety [specify] may be related to paranoid delusions associated with stimulant use possibly evidenced by feelings or beliefs that others are conspiring against or are about to attack or kill client.

ineffective Coping may be related to personal vulnerability, negative role modeling, inadequate support systems; ineffective or inadequate coping skills with substitution of drug, possibly evidenced by use of harmful substance despite evidence of undesirable consequences.

disturbed Sensory Perception (specify) may be related to exogenous chemical, altered sensory reception, transmission, or integration (hallucination), altered status of sense organs, possibly evidenced by responding to internal stimuli from hallucinatory experiences, bizarre thinking, anxiety or panic changes in sensory acuity (sense of smell/ taste).

Substance dependence/abuse rehabilitation **PSY/CH**
(following acute detoxification)

ineffective Denial may be related to threat of unpleasant reality, lack of emotional support from others, overwhelming stress, possibly evidenced by lack of acceptance that drug use is causing the present situation, delay in seeking or refusal of healthcare attention to the detriment of health, use of manipulation to avoid responsibility for self, projection of blame or responsibility for problems.

ineffective Coping may be related to personal vulnerability, negative role modeling, inadequate support systems, previous ineffective or inadequate coping skills with substitution of drug(s), possibly evidenced by impaired adaptive behavior and problem-solving skills,

---

*A risk diagnosis is not evidenced by signs and symptoms, as the problem has not occurred; rather, nursing interventions are directed at prevention.

decreased ability to handle stress of illness or hospitalization, financial affairs in disarray, employment or school difficulties—losing time on job or not maintaining steady employment, poor work or school performances, on-the-job injuries; verbalization of inability to cope or ask for help.

Powerlessness may be related to substance addiction with or without periods of abstinence, episodic compulsive indulgence, attempts at recovery, and lifestyle of helplessness, possibly evidenced by ineffective recovery attempts, statements of inability to stop behavior, requests for help, constantly thinking about drug and/or obtaining drug, alteration in personal, occupational, and social life.

imbalanced Nutrition: less than body requirements may be related to insufficient dietary intake to meet metabolic needs for psychological, physiological, or economic reasons, possibly evidenced by weight less than normal for height and body build; decreased subcutaneous fat or muscle mass; reported altered taste sensation; lack of interest in food; poor muscle tone; sore, inflamed buccal cavity; laboratory evidence of protein or vitamin deficiencies.

Sexual Dysfunction may be related to altered body function (neurological damage and debilitating effects of drug use), possibly evidenced by progressive interference with sexual functioning, a significant degree of testicular atrophy, gynecomastia, impotence or decreased sperm counts in men; and loss of body hair; thin, soft skin; spider angiomas; amenorrhea; and increase in miscarriages in women.

dysfunctional Family Processes may be related to abuse and history of alcoholism or drug use, inadequate coping skills, lack of problem-solving skills, genetic predisposition or biochemical influences, possibly evidenced by feelings of anger, frustration, or responsibility for alcoholic's behavior; suppressed rage, shame, embarrassment, repressed emotions, guilt, vulnerability, disturbed family dynamics or deterioration in family relationships, family denial or rationalization, closed communication systems, triangulating family relationships, manipulation, blaming, enabling to maintain substance use, inability to accept or receive help.

OB

risk for fetal Injury: risk factors may include drug or alcohol use, exposure to teratogens.*

deficient Knowledge [Learning Need] regarding condition, effects on pregnancy, prognosis, treatment needs may be related to lack or misinterpretation of information, lack of recall, cognitive limitations, interference with learning, possibly evidenced by statements of concern, questions, misconceptions, inaccurate follow-through of instructions, development of preventable complications, continued use in spite of complications.

compromised/disabled Family Coping may be related to codependency issues, situational crisis of pregnancy and drug abuse, family disorganization, exhausted supportive capacity of family members possibly evidenced by denial or belief that all problems are due to

---

*A risk diagnosis is not evidenced by signs and symptoms, as the problem has not occurred; rather, nursing interventions are directed at prevention.

substance use, financial difficulties, severely dysfunctional family, codependent behaviors.

Surgery, general   MS

Also refer to Postoperative recovery period

deficient Knowledge [Learning Need] regarding surgical procedure, expectations, postoperative routines, therapy, and self-care needs may be related to lack of information or recall, misinterpretation, possibly evidenced by statements of concern, questions, and misconceptions.

Anxiety [specify level]/Fear may be related to situational crisis, unfamiliarity with environment, change in health status, threat of death and separation from usual support systems, possibly evidenced by increased tension, apprehension, decreased self-assurance, fear of unspecific consequences, focus on self, sympathetic stimulation, and restlessness.

risk for perioperative-positioning Injury: risk factors may include disorientation, sensory and perceptual disturbances due to anesthesia, immobilization, musculoskeletal impairments, obesity, emaciation, edema.*

risk for Injury: risk factors may include wrong client, procedure, site, implants, equipment or materials; interactive conditions between individual and environment; external environment—physical design, structure of environment, exposure to equipment, instrumentation, positioning, use of pharmaceutical agents; internal environment—tissue hypoxia, abnormal blood profile or altered clotting factors, broken skin.*

risk for Infection: risk factors may include broken skin, traumatized tissues, stasis of body fluids; presence of pathogens or contaminants, environmental exposure, invasive procedures.*

risk for imbalanced body Temperature: risk factors may include exposure to cool environment, use of medications, anesthetic agents; extremes of age, weight; dehydration.*

ineffective Breathing Pattern may be related to chemically induced muscular relaxation, perception or cognitive impairment, decreased lung expansion, energy; tracheobronchial obstruction.

risk for deficient Fluid Volume: risk factors may include preoperative fluid deprivation, nausea, blood loss, and excessive gastrointestinal losses (vomiting or gastric suction), extremes of age and weight.*

Synovitis (knee)   CH

acute Pain may be related to inflammation of synovial membrane of the joint with effusion, possibly evidenced by verbal reports, guarding or distraction behaviors, self-focus, and changes in vital signs.

impaired Walking may be related to pain and decreased strength of joint, possibly evidenced by reluctance to attempt movement, inability to move about environment as desired.

Syphilis, congenital   PED

Also refer to Sexually transmitted disease (STD)

acute Pain may be related to inflammatory process, edema formation, and development of skin lesions, possibly evidenced by irritability

---

*A risk diagnosis is not evidenced by signs and symptoms, as the problem has not occurred; rather, nursing interventions are directed at prevention.

or crying that may be increased with movement of extremities and changes in vital signs.

impaired Skin/Tissue Integrity may be related to exposure to pathogens during vaginal delivery, possibly evidenced by disruption of skin surfaces and rhinitis.

delayed Growth and Development may be related to effect of infectious process, possibly evidenced by altered physical growth and delay or difficulty performing skills typical of age group.

deficient Knowledge [Learning Need] regarding pathophysiology of condition, transmissibility, therapy needs, expected outcomes, and potential complications may be related to caretaker/parental lack of information, misinterpretation, possibly evidenced by statements of concern, questions, and misconceptions.

Syringomyelia   MS

disturbed Sensory Perception (specify) may be related to altered sensory perception (neurological lesion), possibly evidenced by change in usual response to stimuli and motor incoordination.

Anxiety [specify level]/Fear may be related to change in health status, threat of change in role functioning and socioeconomic status, and threat to self-concept, possibly evidenced by increased tension, apprehension, uncertainty, focus on self, and expressed concerns.

impaired physical Mobility may be related to neuromuscular and sensory impairment, possibly evidenced by decreased muscle strength, control, and mass; and impaired coordination.

Self-Care Deficit [specify] may be related to neuromuscular and sensory impairments, possibly evidenced by statement of inability to perform care tasks.

Tay-Sachs disease   PED

delayed Growth and Development may be related to effects of physical condition, possibly evidenced by altered physical growth, loss of or failure to acquire skills typical of age, flat affect, and decreased responses.

disturbed visual Sensory Perception may be related to neurological deterioration of optic nerve, possibly evidenced by loss of visual acuity.

CH

[family] Grieving may be related to expected eventual loss of infant/child, possibly evidenced by expressions of distress, denial, guilt, anger, and sorrow; choked feelings; changes in sleep and eating habits; and altered libido.

[family] Powerlessness may be related to absence of therapeutic interventions for progressive and fatal disease, possibly evidenced by verbal expressions of having no control over situation or outcome and depression over physical and mental deterioration.

risk for Spiritual Distress: risk factors may include challenged belief and value system by presence of fatal condition with racial or religious connotations and intense suffering.*

---

*A risk diagnosis is not evidenced by signs and symptoms, as the problem has not occurred; rather, nursing interventions are directed at prevention.

compromised family Coping may be related to situational crisis, temporary preoccupation with managing emotional conflicts and personal suffering, family disorganization, and prolonged and progressive nature of disease, possibly evidenced by preoccupations with personal reactions, expressed concern about reactions of other family members, inadequate support of one another, and altered communication patterns.

Thrombophlebitis CH/MS/OB

ineffective peripheral tissue Perfusion may be related to interruption of venous blood flow, venous stasis, possibly evidenced by changes in skin color and temperature over affected area, development of edema, pain, diminished peripheral pulses, slow capillary refill.

acute Pain/impaired Comfort may be related to vascular inflammation and irritation, edema formation, accumulation of lactic acid, possibly evidenced by verbal reports, guarding or distraction behaviors, restlessness, and self-focus.

risk for impaired physical Mobility: risk factors may include pain and discomfort and restrictive therapies or safety precautions.*

deficient Knowledge [Learning Need] regarding pathophysiology of condition, therapy/self-care needs, and risk of embolization may be related to lack of information, misinterpretation, possibly evidenced by statements of concern, questions, inaccurate follow-through of instructions, and development of preventable complications.

Thrombosis, venous MS
Refer to Thrombophlebitis

Thrush CH

impaired Oral Mucous Membrane may be related to presence of infection as evidenced by white patches or plaques, oral discomfort, mucosal irritation, bleeding.

Thyroidectomy MS
Also refer to Hyperthyroidism; Hypoparathyroidism; Hypothyroidism

risk for ineffective Airway Clearance: risk factors may include tracheal obstruction—edema, hematoma formation, laryngeal spasms.*

impaired verbal Communication may be related to tissue edema, pain or discomfort, and vocal cord injury or laryngeal nerve damage, possibly evidenced by impaired articulation, does not or cannot speak, and use of nonverbal cues and gestures.

risk for Injury [tetany]: risk factors may include chemical imbalance—hypocalcemia, increased release of thyroid hormones; excessive CNS stimulation.*

risk for [head/neck] Trauma: risk factors may include loss of muscle control and support, and position of suture line.*

acute Pain may be related to presence of surgical incision and manipulation of tissues and muscles, postoperative edema, possibly evidenced by verbal reports, guarding or distraction behaviors, narrowed focus, and changes in vital signs.

T

---

*A risk diagnosis is not evidenced by signs and symptoms, as the problem has not occurred; rather, nursing interventions are directed at prevention.

Thyrotoxicosis   MS
Also refer to Hyperthyroidism

risk for decreased Cardiac Output: risk factors may include uncontrolled
    hypermetabolic state increasing cardiac workload, changes in venous
    return and systemic vascular resistance, and alterations in rate,
    rhythm, and electrical conduction.*

Anxiety [specify level] may be related to physiological factors or CNS
    stimulation—hypermetabolic state and pseudocatecholamine effect
    of thyroid hormones; possibly evidenced by increased feelings of
    apprehension, shakiness, loss of control, panic, changes in cognition,
    distortion of environmental stimuli, extraneous movements, restless-
    ness, and tremors.

risk for disturbed Thought Processes: risk factors may include physio-
    logical changes—increased CNS stimulation, accelerated mental ac-
    tivity, and altered sleep patterns.*

deficient Knowledge [Learning Needs] regarding condition, treatment
    needs, and potential for complications or crisis situation may be re-
    lated to lack of information or recall, misinterpretation, possibly ev-
    idenced by statements of concern, questions, and misconceptions,
    and inaccurate follow-through of instructions.

TIA   CH
Refer to Transient ischemic attack

Tic douloureux   CH
Refer to Neuralgia, trigeminal

Tonsillectomy   PED/MS
Anxiety [specify level]/Fear may be related to separation from sup-
    portive others, unfamiliar surroundings, and perceived threat of in-
    jury or abandonment, possibly evidenced by crying, apprehension,
    trembling, and sympathetic stimulation (pupil dilation, increased
    heart rate).

risk for ineffective Airway Clearance: risk factors may include sedation,
    collection of secretions and blood in oropharynx, and vomiting.*

risk for deficient Fluid Volume: risk factors may include operative
    trauma to highly vascular site, hemorrhage.*

acute Pain may be related to physical trauma to oronasopharynx, pres-
    ence of packing, possibly evidenced by restlessness, crying, and fa-
    cial mask of pain.

Tonsillitis   PED
acute Pain may be related to inflammation of tonsils and effects of
    circulating toxins, possibly evidenced by verbal reports, guarding or
    distraction behaviors, reluctance or refusal to swallow, self-focus,
    and changes in vital signs.

Hyperthermia may be related to presence of inflammatory process, hy-
    permetabolic state and dehydration, possibly evidenced by increased
    body temperature; warm, flushed skin; and tachycardia.

deficient Knowledge [Learning Need] regarding cause, transmission,
    treatment needs, and potential complications may be related to lack

---

*A risk diagnosis is not evidenced by signs and symptoms, as the problem has
not occurred; rather, nursing interventions are directed at prevention.

of information, misinterpretation, possibly evidenced by statements of concern, questions, inaccurate follow-through of instructions, and recurrence of condition.

Total joint replacement   MS
Also refer to Surgery, general

risk for Infection: risk factors may include inadequate primary defenses (broken skin, exposure of joint), inadequate secondary defenses or immunosuppression (long-term corticosteroid use), invasive procedures, surgical manipulation, implantation of foreign body, and decreased mobility.*

impaired physical Mobility may be related to pain and discomfort, musculoskeletal impairment, and surgery and restrictive therapies, possibly evidenced by reluctance to attempt movement, difficulty purposefully moving within the physical environment, reports of pain or discomfort on movement, limited range of motion, and decreased muscle strength and control.

risk for ineffective peripheral tissue Perfusion: risk factors may include reduced arterial or venous blood flow, direct trauma to blood vessels, tissue edema, improper location or dislocation of prosthesis, and hypovolemia.*

acute Pain may be related to physical agents (traumatized tissues, surgical intervention, degeneration of joints, muscle spasms) and psychological factors (anxiety, advanced age), possibly evidenced by verbal reports, guarding or distraction behaviors, self-focus, and changes in vital signs.

risk for Constipation: risk factors may include insufficient physical activity, decreased mobility, weakness, insufficient fiber or fluid intake, dehydration, poor eating habits, decreased gastrointestinal motility, effects of medications—anesthesia, opiate analgesics; environmental changes, inadequate toileting.*

Toxemia of pregnancy   OB
Refer to Pregnancy-induced hypertension

Toxic shock syndrome   MS
Also refer to Septicemia

Hyperthermia may be related to inflammatory process, hypermetabolic state and dehydration, possibly evidenced by increased body temperature; warm, flushed skin; and tachycardia.

deficient Fluid Volume [isotonic] may be related to increased gastric losses (diarrhea, vomiting), fever and hypermetabolic state, and decreased intake, possibly evidenced by dry mucous membranes; increased pulse; hypotension; delayed venous filling; decreased, concentrated urine; and hemoconcentration.

acute Pain may be related to inflammatory process, effects of circulating toxins, and skin disruptions, possibly evidenced by verbal reports, guarding or distraction behaviors, self-focus, and changes in vital signs.

T

---

*A risk diagnosis is not evidenced by signs and symptoms, as the problem has not occurred; rather, nursing interventions are directed at prevention.

impaired Skin/Tissue Integrity may be related to effects of circulating toxins and dehydration, possibly evidenced by development of desquamating rash, hyperemia, and inflammation of mucous membranes.

Traction   MS
Also refer to Casts; Fractures

acute Pain may be related to direct trauma to tissue/bone, muscle spasms, movement of bone fragments, edema, injury to soft tissue, traction or immobility device, anxiety, possibly evidenced by verbal reports, guarding or distraction behaviors, self-focus, alteration in muscle tone, and changes in vital signs.

impaired physical Mobility may be related to neuromuscular and skeletal impairment, pain, psychological immobility, and therapeutic restrictions of movement, possibly evidenced by limited range of motion, inability to move purposefully in environment, reluctance to attempt movement, and decreased muscle strength and control.

risk for Infection: risk factors may include invasive procedures–including insertion of foreign body through skin and bone; presence of traumatized tissue, and reduced activity with stasis of body fluids.*

deficient Diversional Activity may be related to length of hospitalization or therapeutic intervention and environmental lack of usual activity, possibly evidenced by statements of boredom, restlessness, and irritability.

Transfusion reaction, blood   MS
Also refer to Anaphylaxis

risk for imbalanced Body Temperature: risk factors may include infusion of cold blood products, systemic response to toxins.*

Anxiety [specify level] may be related to change in health status and threat of death, exposure to toxins, possibly evidenced by increased tension, apprehension, sympathetic stimulation, restlessness, and expressions of concern.

risk for impaired Skin Integrity: risk factors may include immunological response.*

Transient ischemic attack (TIA)   CH
ineffective cerebral tissue Perfusion may be related to interruption of blood flow (e.g., vasospasm), possibly evidenced by altered mental status, behavioral changes, language deficit, change in motor or sensory response.

Anxiety/Fear may be related to change in health status, threat to self-concept, situational crisis, interpersonal contagion, possibly evidenced by expressed concerns, apprehension, restlessness, irritability.

risk for ineffective Denial risk factors may include change in health status requiring change in lifestyle, fear of consequences, lack of motivation.

---

*A risk diagnosis is not evidenced by signs and symptoms, as the problem has not occurred; rather, nursing interventions are directed at prevention.

Traumatic brain injury (TBI) CH

ineffective cerebral tissue Perfusion may be related to interruption of blood flow—hemorrhage, hematoma, cerebral edema (localized or generalized response to injury, metabolic alterations, drug or alcohol overdose), decreased systemic BP—hypovolemia, cardiac dysrhythmias; hypoxia, possibly evidenced by altered level of consciousness, memory loss, changes in motor or sensory responses, restlessness, changes in vital signs.

risk for decreased Intracranial Adaptive Capacity: risk factors may include brain injuries, systemic hypotension with intracranial hypertension.*

risk for ineffective Breathing Pattern: risk factors may include neuromuscular dysfunction—injury to respiratory center of brain; perception or cognitive impairment, tracheobronchial obstruction.*

disturbed Sensory Perception (specify) may be related to altered sensory reception, transmission and/or integration—neurological trauma or deficit, possibly evidenced by disorientation to time, place, person; change in usual response to stimuli, motor incoordination, altered communication patterns, visual or auditory distortions, altered thought processes or bizarre thinking, exaggerated emotional responses, change in behavior pattern.

risk for Infection: risk factors may include traumatized tissues, broken skin, invasive procedures, decreased ciliary action, stasis of body fluids, nutritional deficits, suppressed inflammatory response—steroid use; altered integrity of closed system—cerebrospinal fluid leak.*

risk for imbalanced Nutrition: less than body requirements: risk factors may include altered ability to ingest nutrients—decreased level of consciousness; weakness of muscles for chewing or swallowing, hypermetabolic state.*

CH

impaired physical Mobility may be related to perceptual or cognitive impairment, decreased strength and endurance, restrictive therapies or safety precautions possibly evidenced by inability to purposefully move within physical environment—bed mobility, transfer, ambulation; impaired coordination, limited range of motion, decreased muscle strength or control.

disturbed Thought Processes may be related to changes, psychological conflicts possibly evidenced by memory deficits, distractibility, altered attention span or concentration, disorientation to time, place, person, circumstances, or events; impaired ability to make decisions, problem-solve, reason, or conceptualize; personality changes, inappropriate social behavior.

interrupted Family Processes may be related to situational transition and crisis, uncertainty about ultimate outcome, expectations possibly evidenced by difficulty adapting to change or dealing with traumatic experience constructively, family not meeting needs of all members, difficulty accepting or receiving help appropriately, inability to express or to accept feelings of members.

T

---

*A risk diagnosis is not evidenced by signs and symptoms, as the problem has not occurred; rather, nursing interventions are directed at prevention.

Health Conditions and Client Concerns **1057**

Self-Care Deficit (specify) may be related to neuromuscular or musculoskeletal impairment, weakness, pain, perceptual or cognitive impairment possibly evidenced by inability to perform desired or appropriate ADLs.

Trichinosis   CH

acute Pain may be related to parasitic invasion of muscle tissues, edema of upper eyelids, small localized hemorrhages, and development of urticaria, possibly evidenced by verbal reports, guarding or distraction behaviors (restlessness), and changes in vital signs.

deficient Fluid Volume [isotonic] may be related to hypermetabolic state (fever, diaphoresis), excessive gastric losses (vomiting, diarrhea), and decreased intake (difficulty swallowing), possibly evidenced by dry mucous membranes; decreased skin turgor; hypotension; decreased venous filling; decreased, concentrated urine; and hemoconcentration.

ineffective Breathing Pattern may be related to myositis of the diaphragm and intercostal muscles, possibly evidenced by resulting changes in respiratory depth, tachypnea, dyspnea, and abnormal ABGs.

deficient Knowledge [Learning Need] regarding cause and prevention of condition, therapy needs, and possible complications may be related to lack of information, misinterpretation, possibly evidenced by statements of concern, questions, and misconceptions.

Tuberculosis (pulmonary)   CH

risk for Infection [spread/reactivation]: risk factors may include inadequate primary defenses (decreased ciliary action and stasis of secretions, tissue destruction with extension of infection), lowered resistance, suppressed inflammatory response, malnutrition, environmental exposure, insufficient knowledge to avoid exposure to pathogens, or inadequate therapeutic intervention.*

ineffective Airway Clearance may be related to thick, viscous, or bloody secretions; fatigue with poor cough effort, and tracheal or pharyngeal edema, possibly evidenced by abnormal respiratory rate, rhythm, and depth; adventitious breath sounds (rhonchi, wheezes), stridor, and dyspnea.

risk for impaired Gas Exchange: risk factors may include decrease in effective lung surface, atelectasis, destruction of alveolar-capillary membrane, bronchial edema, thick, viscous secretions.*

Activity Intolerance may be related to imbalance between O_2 supply and demand, possibly evidenced by reports of fatigue, weakness, and exertional dyspnea.

imbalanced Nutrition: less than body requirements may be related to inability to ingest adequate nutrients (anorexia, effects of drug therapy, fatigue, insufficient financial resources), possibly evidenced by weight loss, reported lack of interest in food/altered taste sensation, and poor muscle tone.

risk for ineffective self Health Management: risk factors may include complexity of therapeutic regimen, economic difficulties, family

---

*A risk diagnosis is not evidenced by signs and symptoms, as the problem has not occurred; rather, nursing interventions are directed at prevention.

patterns of healthcare, perceived seriousness or benefits (especially during remission), side effects of therapy.*

Tympanoplasty   MS
Refer to Stapedectomy

Typhus (tick-borne/Rocky Mountain
spotted fever)   CH/MS
Hyperthermia may be related to generalized inflammatory process (vasculitis), possibly evidenced by increased body temperature; warm, flushed skin; and tachycardia.

acute Pain may be related to generalized vasculitis and edema formation, possibly evidenced by verbal reports, guarding or distraction behaviors, self-focus, and changes in vital signs.

ineffective tissue Perfusion (specify) may be related to reduction or interruption of blood flow (generalized vasculitis, thrombi formation), possibly evidenced by reports of headache or abdominal pain, changes in mentation, and areas of peripheral ulceration or necrosis.

Ulcer, decubitus   CH/MS
impaired Skin/Tissue Integrity may be related to altered circulation, nutritional deficit, fluid imbalance, impaired physical mobility, irritation of body excretions or secretions, and sensory impairments, evidenced by tissue damage or destruction.

acute Pain may be related to destruction of protective skin layers and exposure of nerves, possibly evidenced by verbal reports, distraction behaviors, and self-focus.

risk for Infection: risk factors may include broken or traumatized tissue, increased environmental exposure, and nutritional deficits.*

Ulcer, peptic (acute)   MS/CH
risk for Shock: risk factors may include hypovolemia, hypotension.*

Fear/Anxiety [specify level] may be related to change in health status and threat of death, possibly evidenced by increased tension, restlessness, irritability, fearfulness, trembling, tachycardia, diaphoresis, lack of eye contact, focus on self, verbalization of concerns, withdrawal, and panic or attack behavior.

acute Pain may be related to caustic irritation and destruction of gastric tissues, reflex muscle spasms in stomach wall possibly evidenced by verbal reports, distraction behaviors, self-focus, and changes in vital signs.

deficient Knowledge [Learning Need] regarding condition, therapy and self-care needs, and potential complications may be related to lack of information, recall, misinterpretation, possibly evidenced by statements of concern, questions, misconceptions; inaccurate follow-through of instructions; and development of preventable complications or recurrence of condition.

Ulcer, venous stasis   CH
impaired Skin/Tissue Integrity may be related to altered venous circulation, edema formation, inflammation, decreased sensation possibly evidenced by destruction of skin layers, invasion of body structures.

U

---

*A risk diagnosis is not evidenced by signs and symptoms, as the problem has not occurred; rather, nursing interventions are directed at prevention.

ineffective peripheral tissue Perfusion may be related to interruption of venous flow—small-vessel vasoconstrictive reflex, possibly evidenced by skin discoloration, edema formation, altered sensation, delayed healing.

Unconsciousness   MS
Refer to Coma

Urinary diversion   MS/CH
risk for impaired Skin Integrity: risk factors may include absence of sphincter at stoma, character and flow of urine from stoma, reaction to product or chemicals, and improperly fitting appliance or removal of adhesive.*

disturbed Body Image related factors may include biophysical factors (presence of stoma, loss of control of urine flow), and psychosocial factors (altered body structure, disease process and associated treatment regimen, such as cancer), possibly evidenced by verbalization of change in body image, fear of rejection or reaction of others, negative feelings about body, not touching or looking at stoma, refusal to participate in care.

acute Pain may be related to physical factors (disruption of skin or tissues, presence of incisions and drains), biological factors (activity of disease process, such as cancer, trauma), and psychological factors (fear, anxiety), possibly evidenced by verbal reports, self-focusing, guarding or distraction behaviors, restlessness, and changes in vital signs.

impaired Urinary Elimination may be related to surgical diversion, tissue trauma, and postoperative edema, possibly evidenced by loss of continence, changes in amount and character of urine, and urinary retention.

Urolithiasis   MS/CH
Refer to Calculi, urinary

Uterine bleeding, dysfunctional   GYN/MS
Anxiety [specify level] may be related to perceived change in health status and unknown etiology, possibly evidenced by apprehension, uncertainty, fear of unspecified consequences, expressed concerns, and focus on self.

Activity Intolerance may be related to imbalance between O_2 supply and demand/decreased O_2-carrying capacity of blood (anemia), possibly evidenced by reports of fatigue or weakness.

Uterus, rupture of, in pregnancy   OB
deficient Fluid Volume [isotonic] may be related to excessive vascular losses, possibly evidenced by hypotension, increased pulse rate, decreased venous filling, and decreased urine output.

decreased Cardiac Output may be related to decreased preload (hypovolemia), possibly evidenced by cold, clammy skin; decreased peripheral pulses; variations in hemodynamic readings; tachycardia; and cyanosis.

---

*A risk diagnosis is not evidenced by signs and symptoms, as the problem has not occurred; rather, nursing interventions are directed at prevention.

acute Pain may be related to tissue trauma and irritation of accumulating blood, possibly evidenced by verbal reports, guarding or distraction behaviors, self-focus, and changes in vital signs.

Anxiety [specify level] may be related to threat of death of self or fetus, interpersonal contagion, physiological response (release of catecholamines), possibly evidenced by fearful, scared affect; sympathetic stimulation, stated fear of unspecified consequences, and expressed concerns.

Vaginismus   GYN/CH

acute Pain may be related to muscle spasm and hyperesthesia of the nerve supply to vaginal mucous membrane, possibly evidenced by verbal reports, distraction behaviors, and self-focus.

Sexual Dysfunction may be related to physical and/or psychological alteration in function (severe spasms of vaginal muscles), possibly evidenced by verbalization of problem, inability to achieve desired satisfaction, and alteration in relationship with SO.

Vaginitis   GYN/CH

impaired Tissue Integrity may be related to irritation and inflammation and mechanical trauma (scratching) of sensitive tissues, possibly evidenced by damaged or destroyed tissue, presence of lesions.

acute Pain may be related to localized inflammation and tissue trauma, possibly evidenced by verbal reports, distraction behaviors, and self-focus.

deficient Knowledge [Learning Need] regarding hygienic and therapy needs and sexual behaviors and transmission of organisms may be related to lack of information, misinterpretation, possibly evidenced by statements of concern, questions, and misconceptions.

VAP (ventilator-aquired pneumonia)   MS

Refer to Bronchopneumonia

Varices, esophageal   MS

Also refer to Ulcer, peptic (acute)

risk for Bleeding/deficient Fluid Volume [isotonic]: risk factors may include presence of varices, reduced intake, and gastric losses (vomiting), vascular loss.*

Anxiety [specify level]/Fear may be related to change in health status and threat of death, possibly evidenced by increased tension, apprehension, sympathetic stimulation, restlessness, focus on self, and expressed concerns.

Varicose veins   CH

chronic Pain may be related to venous insufficiency and stasis, possibly evidenced by verbal reports.

disturbed Body Image may be related to change in structure (presence of enlarged, discolored tortuous superficial leg veins), possibly evidenced by hiding affected parts and negative feelings about body.

risk for impaired Skin/Tissue Integrity: risk factors may include altered circulation, venous stasis, and edema formation.*

V

*A risk diagnosis is not evidenced by signs and symptoms, as the problem has not occurred; rather, nursing interventions are directed at prevention.

Venereal disease   **CH**
Refer to Sexually transmitted disease (STD)

Ventricular fibrillation   **MS**
Also refer to Dysrhythmias
decreased Cardiac Output may be related to altered electrical conduc-
    tion and reduced myocardial contractility possibly evidenced by ab-
    sence of measurable cardiac output, loss of consciousness, no pal-
    pable pulses.

Ventricular tachycardia   **MS**
Also refer to Dysrhythmias
risk for decreased Cardiac Output: risk factors may include altered elec-
    trical conduction and reduced myocardial contractility.*

West Nile fever   **CH/MS**
Hyperthermia may be related to infectious process, possibly evidenced
    by elevated body temperature, skin flushed and warm to touch, tachy-
    cardia, increased respiratory rate.
acute Pain may be related to infectious process and circulating toxins,
    possibly evidenced by reports of headache, myalgia, eye pain, ab-
    dominal discomfort.
risk for deficient Fluid Volume: risk factors may include hypermeta-
    bolic state, decreased intake, anorexia, nausea, losses from normal
    routes (vomiting, diarrhea).*
risk for impaired Skin Integrity: risk factors may include hyperthermia,
    decreased fluid intake, alterations in skin turgor, bedrest, circulating
    toxins.*

Wilms' tumor   **PED**
Also refer to Cancer; Chemotherapy
Anxiety [specify level]/Fear may be related to change in environment
    and interaction patterns with family members and threat of death with
    family transmission and contagion of concerns, possibly evidenced
    by fearful or scared affect, distress, crying, insomnia, and sympa-
    thetic stimulation.
risk for Injury: risk factors may include nature of tumor (vascular,
    mushy with very thin covering) with increased danger of metastasis
    when manipulated.*
interrupted Family Processes may be related to situational crisis of life-
    threatening illness, possibly evidenced by a family system that has
    difficulty meeting physical, emotional, and spiritual needs of its
    members, and inability to deal with traumatic experience effectively.
deficient Diversional Activity may be related to environmental lack of
    age-appropriate activity (including activity restrictions) and length
    of hospitalization and treatment, possibly evidenced by restlessness,
    crying, lethargy, and acting-out behavior.

W

Wound, gunshot   **MS**
(Depends on site and speed/character of bullet.)
risk for deficient Fluid Volume: risk factors may include excessive vas-
    cular losses, altered intake or restrictions.*

---

*A risk diagnosis is not evidenced by signs and symptoms, as the problem has
not occurred; rather, nursing interventions are directed at prevention.

acute Pain may be related to destruction of tissue (including organ and musculoskeletal), surgical repair, and therapeutic interventions, possibly evidenced by verbal reports, guarding or distraction behaviors, self-focus, and changes in vital signs.

impaired Tissue Integrity may be related to mechanical factors (yaw of projectile and muzzle blast), possibly evidenced by damaged or destroyed tissue.

risk for Infection: risk factors may include tissue destruction and increased environmental exposure, invasive procedures, and decreased Hb.*

CH

risk for Post-Trauma Syndrome: risk factors may include nature of incident (catastrophic accident, assault, suicide attempt) and possibly injury or death of other(s) involved.*

---

*A risk diagnosis is not evidenced by signs and symptoms, as the problem has not occurred; rather, nursing interventions are directed at prevention.

NANDA-I's Taxonomy II

The 13 domains and their classes are:

Domain 1 Health Promotion: The awareness of well-being or normality of function and the strategies used to maintain control of and enhance that well-being or normality of function

Class 1 Health Awareness: Recognition of normal function and well-being

Class 2 Health Management: Identifying, controlling, performing, and integrating activities to maintain health and well-being

Domain 2 Nutrition: The activities of taking in, assimilating, and using nutrients for the purposes of tissue maintenance, tissue repair, and the production of energy

Class 1 Ingestion: Taking food or nutrients into the body

Class 2 Digestion: The physical and chemical activities that convert foodstuffs into substances suitable for absorption and assimilation

Class 3 Absorption: The act of taking up nutrients through body tissues

Class 4 Metabolism: The chemical and physical processes occurring in living organisms and cells for the development and use of protoplasm, production of waste and energy, with the release of energy for all vital processes

Class 5 Hydration: The taking in and absorption of fluids and electrolytes

Domain 3 Elimination and Exchange: Secretion and excretion of waste products from the body

Class 1 Urinary Function: The process of secretion, reabsorption, and excretion of urine

Class 2 Gastrointestinal Function: The process of absorption and excretion of the end products of digestion

Class 3 Integumentary Function: The process of secretion and excretion through the skin

Class 4 Respiratory Function: The process of exchange of gases and removal of the end products of metabolism

Domain 4 Activity/Rest: The production, conservation, expenditure, or balance of energy resources

> **Class 1 Sleep/Rest: Slumber, repose, ease, or inactivity**
>
> **Class 2 Activity/Exercise: Moving parts of the body (mobility), doing work, or performing actions often (but not always) against resistance**
>
> **Class 3 Energy Balance: A dynamic state of harmony between intake and expenditure of resources**
>
> **Class 4 Cardiovascular/Pulmonary Responses: Cardiopulmonary mechanisms that support activity/rest**
>
> **Class 5 Self-Care: Ability to perform activities to care for one's body and bodily functions**

Domain 5 Perception/Cognition: The human information-processing system including attention, orientation, sensation, perception, cognition, and communication

> **Class 1 Attention: Mental readiness to notice or observe**
>
> **Class 2 Orientation: Awareness of time, place, and person**
>
> **Class 3 Sensation/Perception: Receiving information through the senses of touch, taste, smell, vision, hearing, and kinesthesia and the comprehension of sense data resulting in naming, associating, and/or pattern recognition**
>
> **Class 4 Cognition: Use of memory, learning, thinking, problem-solving, abstraction, judgment, insight, intellectual capacity, calculation, and language**
>
> **Class 5 Communication: Sending and receiving verbal and nonverbal information**

Domain 6 Self-Perception: Awareness about the self

> **Class 1 Self-Concept: The perception(s) about the total self**
>
> **Class 2 Self-Esteem: Assessment of one's own worth, capability, significance, and success**
>
> **Class 3 Body Image: A mental image of one's own body**

Domain 7 Role Relationships: The positive and negative connections or associations between people or groups of people and the means by which those connections are demonstrated

> **Class 1 Caregiving Roles: Socially expected behavior patterns by people providing care who are not healthcare professionals**
>
> **Class 2 Family Relationships: Associations of people who are biologically related or related by choice**

Class 3 Role Performance: Quality of functioning in socially expected behavior patterns

Domain 8 Sexuality: Sexual identity, sexual function, and reproduction

Class 1 Sexual Identity: The state of being a specific person in regard to sexuality and/or gender

Class 2 Sexual Function: The capacity or ability to participate in sexual activities

Class 3 Reproduction: Any process by which human beings are produced

Domain 9 Coping/Stress Tolerance: Contending with life events/life processes

Class 1 Post-Trauma Responses: Reactions occurring after physical or psychological trauma

Class 2 Coping Responses: The process of managing environmental stress

Class 3 Neurobehavioral Stress: Behavioral responses reflecting nerve and brain function

Domain 10 Life Principles: Principles underlying conduct, thought, and behavior about acts, customs, or institutions viewed as being true or having intrinsic worth

Class 1 Values: The identification and ranking of preferred mode of conduct or end states

Class 2 Beliefs: Opinions, expectations, or judgments about acts, customs, or institutions viewed as being true or having intrinsic worth

Class 3 Value/Belief/Action Congruence: The correspondence or balance achieved among values, beliefs, and actions

Domain 11 Safety/Protection: Freedom from danger, physical injury, or immune system damage; preservation from loss; and protection of safety and security

Class 1 Infection: Host responses following pathogenic invasion

Class 2 Physical Injury: Bodily harm or hurt

Class 3 Violence: The exertion of excessive force or power so as to cause injury or abuse

Class 4 Environmental Hazards: Sources of danger in the surroundings

Class 5 Defensive Processes: The processes by which the self protects itself from the non-self

Class 6 Thermoregulation: The physiological process of regulating heat and energy within the body for purposes of protecting the organism

Domain 12 Comfort: Sense of mental, physical, or social well-being or ease

Class 1 Physical Comfort: Sense of well-being or ease and/or freedom from pain

> **Class 2 Environmental Comfort: Sense of well-being or ease in/with one's environment**
> **Class 3 Social Comfort: Sense of well-being or ease with one's social situations**

Domain 13 Growth/Development: Age-appropriate increases in physical dimensions, maturation of organ systems, and/or progression through the developmental milestone[s]

> **Class 1 Growth: Increases in physical dimensions or maturity of organ systems**
> **Class 2 Development: Progression or regression through a sequence of recognized milestones in life**

Definitions of Taxonomy II Axes

AXIS 1 DIAGNOSTIC CONCEPT: Defined as the principal element or the fundamental and essential part, the root, of the diagnostic statement.

AXIS 2 SUBJECT OF THE DIAGNOSIS: The person(s) for whom a nursing diagnosis is determined. Values are:

Individual: A single human being distinct from others, a person.

Family: Two or more people having continuous or sustained relationships, perceiving reciprocal obligations, sensing common meaning, and sharing certain obligations toward others; related by blood and/or choice.

Group: A number of people with shared characteristics.

Community: A group of people living in the same locale under the same governance, such as neighborhoods, cities, census tracts. When the unit of care is not explicitly stated, it becomes the individual by default.

AXIS 3 JUDGMENT: A descriptor or modifier that limits or specifies the meaning of the diagnostic concept. Values are:

Complicated: Intricately involved, complex

Compromised: Damaged, made vulnerable

Decreased: Lessened (in size, amount, or degree)

Defensive: Used or intended to defend or protect

Deficient: Insufficient, inadequate

Delayed: Late, slow, or postponed

Disabled: Limited, handicapped

Disorganized: Not properly arranged or controlled

Disproportionate: Too large or too small in comparison with norm

Disturbed: Agitated, interrupted, interfered with

Dysfunctional: Not operating normally

Effective: Producing the intended or desired effect

Enhanced: Improved in quality, value, or extent

Excessive: Greater than necessary or desirable

Imbalanced: Out of proportion or balance

Impaired: Damaged, weakened

Ineffective: Not producing the intended or desired effect

Interrupted: Having its continuity broken

Low: Below the norm

Organized: Properly arranged or controlled

Perceived: Observed through the senses

Readiness for: In a suitable state for an activity or situation

Situational: Related to a particular circumstance

AXIS 4 LOCATION: Consists of parts/regions of the body and/or their related functions—all tissues, organs, anatomical sites or structures. Values are:

Auditory	Intracranial	Skin
Bladder	Kinesthetic	Tactile
Bowel	Mucous membranes	Tissue
Cardiac	Olfactory	Vascular
Cardiopulmonary	Oral	Visual
Cerebral	Peripheral neurovascular	Urinary
Gastrointestinal	Peripheral vascular	
Gustatory	Renal	

AXIS 5 AGE: The age of the person who is the subject of the diagnosis. Values are:

Fetus	School-age child
Neonate	Adolescent
Infant	Adult
Toddler	Older adult
Preschool child	

AXIS 6 TIME: The duration of the diagnostic concept. Values are:

Acute: Lasting less than 6 months

Chronic: Lasting more than 6 months

Intermittent: Stopping or starting again at intervals, periodic, cyclic

Continuous: Uninterrupted, going on without stop

AXIS 7 STATUS OF THE DIAGNOSIS: The actuality or potentiality of the problem or the catagorization of the diagnosis as a wellness/health promotion diagnosis. Values are:

Actual: Existing in fact or reality, existing at the present time

Health Promotion: Behavior motivated by the desire to increase well-being and actualize human health potential (Pender, Murdaugh, & Parsons, 2006)

Risk: Vulnerability, especially as a result of exposure to factors that increase the chance of injury or loss

Wellness: The quality or state of being healthy

Permission from NANDA International. (2009). *NANDA-I Nursing Diagnoses: Definitions & Classification 2009–2011.* Philadelphia: NANDA-I.

Bibliography

Books

Aacovou, I: The Role of the Nurse in the Rehabilitation of Patients with Radical Changes in body Image due to Burn Injuries. Psychiatric Department, Makarios Hospital, Nicosia, Cyprus, 2004.

Ackley, BJ, and Ladwig, GB: Nursing Diagnosis Handbook: A Guide to Planning Care, ed. 7. Mosby Elsevier, St. Louis, MO, 2006.

Acute Pain Management: Operative or Medical Procedures and Trauma: Clinical Practice Guideline. US Department of Health and Human Services, Public Health Service Agency for Health Care Policy and Research, Rockville, MD, Feb 1992.

Adams, L: Be Your Best (rev. ed.). Perigee Trade, New York, 1989.

Adams, S: Shock, systemic inflammatory response and multiple organ dysfunction. In Brooker, C, and Nicol, M (eds): Nursing Adults: The Practice of Caring. Mosby, Edinburgh, Scotland, 2003.

Alberte, R, and Emmons, M: Your Perfect Right. Impact, San Luis Obispo, CA, 1970.

American Nurses Association: Nursing's Social Policy Statement. Washington, DC, 1995.

American Nurses Association: Nursing's Social Policy Statement, ed. 2. Washington, DC, 2003, p 6.

American Nurses Association: Social Policy Statement. Kansas City, MO, 1980.

American Nurses Association: Standards of Clinical Nursing Practice. Kansas City, MO, 1991.

Androwich, I, Burkhart, L, and Gettrust, KV: Community and Home Health Nursing. Delmar, Albany, NY, 1996.

Asp, AA: Diabetes mellitus. In Copstead, LC, and Banasik, JL (eds): Pathophysiology, ed. 3. Elsevier Saunders, Philadelphia, 2005.

Banasik, JL and Copstead, LEC (eds): Pathophysiology, ed. 3. Elsevier Saunders, St. Louis, MO, 2005.

Bastable, SB: Essentials of Patient Education. Jones and Bartlett, Sudbury, MA, 2005.

Beers, MH, and Berkow, R: The Merck Manual of Diagnosis and Therapy, ed. 17. Merck Research Laboratories, Whitehouse Station, NJ, 1999.

Bellis, TJ: When the Brain Can't Hear: Unraveling the Mystery of Auditory Processing Disorder. Atria Books, New York, 2002.

Blach, DA, and Ignatavicius, DD: Interventions for clients with vascular problems. In Ignatavicius, DD, and Workman, ML: Medical-Surgical Nursing: Critical Thinking for Collaborative Care, ed. 5. Elsevier Saunders, St. Louis, MO, 2006.

Branden, N: Healthy Relationships. Bantam Books, New York, 1994.

Branden, N: The Six Pillars of Self-Esteem. Bantam Books, New York, 1995.

Carey, CF, Lee, HH, and Woeltje, KF (eds): The Washington Manual of Medical Therapeutics, ed. 29. Lippincott-Raven, Philadelphia, 1998.

Cassileth, BR: The Alternative Medicine Handbook: The Complete Reference Guide to Alternative and Complementary Therapies. WW Norton, New York, 1998.

Cataract in Adults: Management of Functional Impairment. AHCPR Pub. 93-0542, US Department of Health and Human Services, Public Health Agency for Health Care Policy and Research, Rockville, MD, 1993.

Condon, RE, and Nyhus, LM (eds): Manual of Surgical Therapeutics, ed. 9. Little, Brown., Boston, 1996.

Cox, H, Saidaromont, K, King, M, et al: Clinical Applications of Nursing Diagnosis: Adult, Child, Women's Psychiatric, Gerontic, and Home Health Considerations, ed. 4. FA Davis, Philadelphia, 2002.

Cummings, B: Managing stress: Coping with life's challenges. In Health: The Basics, ed. 5. Pearson Education, Upper Saddle River, NJ, 2003.

Deglin, JH, and Vallerand, AH: Davis's Drug Guide for Nurses, ed. 9. FA Davis, Philadelphia, 2005.

Depression in Primary Care, Vol. 1, Detection and Diagnosis. AHCPR Pub. 93-0550, US Department of Health and Human Services, Public Health Service Agency for Health Care Policy and Research, Rockville, MD, April 1993.

Depression in Primary Care, Vol. 2, Treatment of Major Depression. AHCPR Pub. 93-0551, US Department of Health and Human Services, Public Health Service Agency for Health Care Policy and Research, Rockville, MD, April 1993.

Dietzen, KK: Assessment of the gastrointestinal system. In Ignatavicius, DD, and Workman, ML: Medical-Surgical Nursing: Critical Thinking for Collaborative Care, ed. 5. Elsevier Saunders, St. Louis, MO, 2006.

Doenges, M, and Moorhouse, M: Maternal/Newborn Plans of Care, ed. 3. FA Davis, Philadelphia, 1999.

Doenges, M, Moorhouse, M, and Murr, A: Nursing Care Plans Across the Life Span, ed. 8. FA Davis, Philadelphia, 2010.

Doenges, M, Moorhouse, M, and Murr, A: Nursing Diagnosis Manual: Planning, Individualizing, and Documenting Client Care, ed. 2. FA Davis, Philadelphia, 2008.

Doenges, M, Townsend, M, and Moorhouse, M: Psychiatric Care Plans: Guidelines for Planning and Documenting Client Care, ed. 3. FA Davis, Philadelphia, 1998.

Early Identification of Alzheimer's Disease and Related Dementias: Clinical Practice Guideline, US Department of Health and Human Services, Public Health Service Agency for Health Care Policy and Research, Rockville, MD, November 1996.

Editorial Staff: Complications and high-risk conditions of the prenatal period. In Straight A's in Maternal-Neonatal Nursing, ed. 2. Wolters Kluwer, Lippincott Williams & Wilkins, Philadelphia, 2008.

Editorial Staff: Cultural Childbearing Practices. Monograph in Lippincott Manual of Nursing Practice Pocket Guides: Maternal-Neonatal Nursing. Lippincott Williams & Wilkins, Philadelphia, 2007.

Editorial Staff: RDAs for Pregnant Women. Monograph in Lippincott Manual of Nursing Practice Pocket Guides: Maternal-Neonatal Nursing. Lippincott Williams & Wilkins, Philadelphia, 2007.

Editorial Staff: Renal system. In Pathophysiology Made Incredibly Easy! ed. 3. Lippincott Williams & Wilkins, Philadelphia, 2006.

Engel, J: Pocket Guide to Pediatric Assessment, ed. 4. Mosby, St. Louis, MO, 2002.

Felver, L, and Kirkhorn, MJ: Fluid, electrolyte, and acid-base homeostasis. In Copstead, LEC, and Banasik, JL, (eds): Pathophysiology, ed. 3. Elsevier Saunders, St. Louis, MO, 2005.

Floyd, JA: Sleep enhancement. In Ackley, BJ, et al: Evidence-Based Nursing Care Guidelines: Medical-Surgical Interventions. Mosby Elsevier, St. Louis, MO, 2008.

Goleman, D: Emotional Intelligence: Why It Can Matter More than IQ. Bantam Books, New York, 1995.

Goleman, D: Emotional Intelligence: Why It Matters More than IQ (10th Anniversary ed). Bantam, New York, 2006.

Gordon, M: Manual of Nursing Diagnosis. Mosby, St. Louis, MO, 1997.

Gordon, T: Family Effectiveness Training. Gordon Training International, Solana Beach, CA, 1997.

Gordon, T: Parent Effectiveness Training. Three Rivers Press, New York, 2000.

Gordon, T: Teaching Children Self-Discipline: At Home and at School. Random House, New York, 1989.

Gorman, L, Sultan, D, and Raines, M: Davis's Manual of Psychosocial Nursing for General Patient Care. FA Davis, Philadelphia, 1996.

Gorski, LA: Intravenous therapy. In Ackley, BJ, et al: Evidence-Based Nursing Care Guidelines: Medical-Surgical Interventions. Mosby Elsevier, St. Louis, MO, 2008.

Harkulich, JT, et al: Teacher's Guide: A Manual for Caregivers of Alzheimer's Disease in Long-Term Care. Embassy Printing, Cleveland Heights, OH, Copyright pending.

Higgs, ZR, and Gustafson, DD: Community as a Client: Assessment and Diagnosis. FA Davis, Philadelphia, 1985.

Hogstel, MO, and Curry, LC: Health Assessment Through the Life Span, ed. 4. FA Davis, Philadelphia, 2005.

Holloway, B, Moredich, C, and Aduddell, K: OB Peds Women's Health Notes: Nurse's Clinical Pocket Guide. FA Davis, Philadelphia, 2006.

Ignatavicius, DD, and Workman, ML (eds): Medical-Surgical Nursing: Critical Thinking for Collaborative Care. Elsevier Saunders, St. Louis, MO, 2006.

Jaffe, MS, and McVan, BF: Laboratory and Diagnostic Test Handbook. FA.Davis, Philadelphia, 1997.

Johnson, M, and Maas, M: Nursing Outcomes Classification (NOC), ed. 2. Mosby, St. Louis, MO, 2000.

King, L: Toward a Theory for Nursing: General Concepts of Human Behavior. Wiley, New York, 1971.

Kuhn, MA: Pharmacotherapeutics: A Nursing Process Approach, ed. 4. FA Davis, Philadelphia, 1998.

Kuriansky, J: The Complete Idiot's Guide to a Healthy Relationship. Alpha Books, Indianapolis, IN, 2002.

Lampe, S: Focus Charting, ed. 7. Creative Healthcare Management, Minneapolis, MN, 1997.

Lauderdale, J: Transcultural perspectives in childbearing. In Andrews, MM, and Boyle, JS. (eds): Transcultural Concepts in Nursing Care, ed. 5. Philadelphia, Wolters Kluwer Health, Lippincott Williams & Wilkins, 2007.

Lee, D, Barrett, C, and Ignatavicius, D: Fluids and Electrolytes: A Practical Approach, ed. 4. FA Davis, Philadelphia, 1996.

Leeuwen, AM, Kranpitz, TR, and Smith, L: Davis's Comprehensive Handbook of Diagnostic Tests with Nursing Implications, ed. 2. FA Davis, Philadelphia, 2006.

Leiniger, MM: Transcultural Nursing: Theories, Research and Practices, ed. 3. McGraw-Hill, Hilliard, OH, 1996.

Lipson, JG, Dibble, S, and Minarik, P (eds): Culture and Nursing Care: A Pocket Guide. UCSF Nursing Press, University of California, San Francisco, 1996.

Maier, RV: Approach to the patient with shock. In Kasper, DL, et al (eds): Harrison's Principles of Internal Medicine, ed. 16. McGraw-Hill, New York, 2005.

Management of Cancer Pain. AHCPR Pub. 93-0592, US Department of Health and Human Services, Public Health Agency for Health Care Policy and Research, Rockville, MD, 1994.

Manning, JE: Fluid and blood resuscitation. In Tintinalli, JE (ed): Emergency Medicine: A Comprehensive Study Guide. McGraw-Hill, New York, 2004.

McCance, KL, and Huether, SE: Pathophysiology: The Biologic Basis for Disease in Adults and Children, ed. 3. Mosby, St. Louis, MO, 1997.

McCloskey, JC, and Bulechek, GM (eds): Nursing Interventions Classification, ed. 3. Mosby, St. Louis, MO, 2000.

McCormack B, and Yorkey, M: Ten great things that exercise can do for you. Chapter 24 in Fit Over 40 for Dummies. Wiley, Hoboken, NJ, 2000.

McIlvoy, LH, and Meyer, K: Cerebral perfusion promotion. In Ackley, BJ, et al: Evidence-Based Nursing Care Guidelines: Medical-Surgical Interventions. Mosby Elsevier, St. Louis, MO, 2008.

McLeod, ME: Interventions for clients with diabetes mellitus. In Ignativicius, DD, and Workman, ML (eds): Medical-Surgical Nursing: Critical Thinking for Collaborative Care, ed. 5. Elsevier Saunders, Philadelphia, 2006.

Meek, J (ed): The American Academy of Pediatrics New Mother's Guide to Breastfeeding. Bantam Books, New York, 2002.

Mentgen, J, and Bulbrook, MJT: Healing Touch, Level I Notebook. Healing Touch, Lakewood, CO, 1994.

Murray-Swank, A, et al: Religiosity, Psychosocial Adjustment, and Subjective Burden of Persons Who Care for Those with Mental Illness. Psychiatric Services, American Psychiatric Association, Arlington, VA, 2006.

NANDA Nursing Diagnoses: Definitions and Classification 2005–2006. NANDA International, Philadelphia, 2005.

Olds, SB, London, ML, Ladewig, PW, and Davidson, MR: Maternity-Newborn Nursing: A Family-Centered Approach, ed. 7. Prentice Hall, Upper Saddle River, NJ, 2003.

Pender, NJ, Murdaugh, CC, and Parsons, MA: Health Promotion in Nursing Practice, ed. 5. Prentice Hall, Upper Saddle River, NJ, 2006.

Peplau, HE: Interpersonal Relations in Nursing: A Conceptual Frame of Reference for Psychodynamic Nursing. Putnam, New York, 1952.

Phillips, CR: Family-Centered Maternity Care. Jones & Bartlett, Sudbury, MA, 2003.

Post-Stroke Rehabilitation: Assessment, Referral, and Patient Management. AHCPR Pub. 95-0663, US Department of Health and Human Services, Public Health Service Agency for Health Care Policy and Research, Rockville, MD, 1995.

Pressure Ulcers in Adults: Prediction and Prevention. AHCPR Pub. 92-0047, US Department of Health and Human Services, Public Health Service Agency for Health Care Policy and Research, Rockville, MD, 1992.

Purnell, LD, and Paulanka, BJ: Transcultural Health Care: A Culturally Competent Approach, ed. 3. FA Davis, Philadelphia, 2008.

Ricci, SS, and Kyle, T: (2008). Maternity and Pediatric Nursing. Lippincott Williams & Wilkins, Philadelphia, 2008.

Rimmer, JH: Aging, Mental Retardation and Physical Fitness. Center on Health Promotion Research for Persons with Disabilities. University of Illinois at Chicago, 1996.

Sartin, JS: Gastrointestinal disorders. In Copstead, LEC, and Banasik, JL: Pathophysiology, ed. 3. Elsevier Saunders, St. Louis, MO, 2005.

Seligman, M, Reivich, K, Jaycox, LH, and Gillham, J: The Optimistic Child. Houghton Mifflin, Boston, 1995.

Shore, LS: Nursing Diagnosis: What It Is and How to Do It: A Programmed Text. Medical College of Virginia Hospitals, Richmond, 1988.

Sickle Cell Disease: Screening, Diagnosis, Management, and Counseling in Newborns and Infants. AHCPR Pub 93-0562, US Department of Health and Human Services, Public Health Service Agency for Health Care Policy and Research, Rockville, MD, April 1993.

Singer Kaplan, H: Sexual Desire Disorders Dysfunctional Regulation of Sexual Motivation. Routledge, London, 1995.

Sommers, MS, Johnson, SA, and Beery, TA: Diseases and Disorders: A Nursing Therapeutics Manual, ed. 3. FA Davis, Philadelphia, 2007.

Sparks, SM, and Taylor, CM: Nursing Diagnoses Reference Manual, ed. 5. Springhouse, Springhouse, PA, 2001.

Springhouse (ed): Phototherapy. In Lippincott's Nursing Procedures, ed. 5. Lippincott Williams & Wilkins, Philadelphia, 2008.

Stanley, M, Blair, KA, and Beare, PG: Gerontological Nursing: Promoting Successful Aging with Older Adults, ed. 3. FA Davis, Philadelphia, 2005.

Stark, J: The renal system. In Alspach, JG (ed): Core Corriculum for Critical Care Nursing. Saunders, St. Louis, MO, 2006.

Tabloski, PA (ed): Gerontological Nursing. Pearson Prentice-Hall, Upper Saddle River, NJ, 2006.

Townsend, M: Nursing Diagnoses in Psychiatric Nursing: Care Plans and Psychotropic Medications, ed. 6. FA Davis, Philadelphia, 2004.

Townsend, M: Psychiatric Mental Health Nursing Concepts of Care, ed. 5. FA Davis, Philadelphia, 2006.

Traumatic Brain Injury Medical Treatment Guidelines. State of Colorado Labor and Employment, Division of Worker's Compensation, Denver, March 15, 1998.

Urinary Incontinence in Adults: Clinical Practice Guideline. AHCPR Pub. 92-0038, US Department of Health and Human Services, Public Health Service Agency for Health Care Policy and Research, Rockville, MD, March 1992.

Venes, D (ed): Taber's Cyclopedic Medical Dictionary, ed. 21. FA Davis, Philadelphia, 2009.

Viscovsky, C: Interventions for clients with hematologic problems. In Ignatavicius, DD, and Workman, LM (eds): Medical-Surgical Nursing: Critical Thinking for Collaborative Care, ed. 5. Elsevier Saunders, St. Louis, MO, 2006.

Winkleman, C. Assessment of the renal/urinary system. In Ignatavicius, DD, and Workman, ML (eds): Medical-Surgical Nursing: Critical Thinking for Collaborative Care, ed. 5. Elsevier Saunders, St. Louis, MO, 2006.

Workman, ML: Interventions for clients with electrolyte imbalances. In Ignatavicius, DD, and Workman, ML (eds): Medical-Surgical Nursing: Critical Thinking for Collaborative Care, ed. 5. Elsevier Saunders, St. Louis, MO, 2006.

Workman, ML: Interventions for clients with shock. In Ignatavicius, DD, and Workman, ML (eds): Medical-Surgical Nursing: Critical Thinking for Collaborative Care, ed. 5. Elsevier Saunders, St. Louis, MO, 2006.

Yura, H, and Walsh, MB: The Nursing Process: Assessing, Planning, Implementing, Evaluating, ed. 5. Appleton & Lange, Norwalk, CT, 1988.

Articles

Abrams, RC, et al: Predictors of self-neglect in community-dwelling elders. Am J Psychiatry 159:1724–30, 2002.

Ackerman, MH, and Mick, DJ: Instillation of normal saline before suctioning patients with pulmonary infections: A prospective randomized controlled trial. Am J Crit Care 7(4):261, 1998.

Acute Confusion/Delirium. Research Dissemination Core, University of Iowa Gerontological Nursing Interventions Research Center (GNIRC). Iowa City, IA, 1998.

Albert, N: Heart failure: The physiologic basis for current therapeutic concepts. Crit Care Nurse 19(3 Suppl):2–13, 1999.

Allen, LA: Treating agitation without drugs. Am J Nurs 99(4):36, 1999.

American Academy of Pediatrics, Task Force on Sleep Position and SIDS: Changing concepts of sudden infant death syndrome: Implications for infant sleeping environment and sleep position. Pediatrics 105:650, 2000.

American College of Obstetricians and Gynecologists (ACOG). Committee on Obstetric Practice: Exercise during pregnancy and the postpartum period. ACOG Committee Opinion 267. Obstetrics & Gynecology 99:171–73, 2002.

Anderson, NR: The role of the home healthcare nurse in smoking cessation: Guidelines for successful intervention. Home Healthcare Nurse 24(7):424–31, 2006.

Angelucci, PA: Caring for patients with benign prostatic hyperplasia. Nursing 27(11):34, 1997.

AORN latex guideline: 2004 standards, recommended practices, and guidelines. AORN J 79(3):653–72, 2004.

Armstrong, ML, and Murphy, KP: A look at adolescent tattooing. School Health Reporter, Summer 1999.

Astle, SM: Restoring electrolyte balance. RN 68(5):31–34, 2005.

Augustus, LJ: Nutritional care for patients with HIV. Am J Nurs 97(10): 62, 1997.

Ayers, DM, and Montgomery, M: Putting a stop to dysfunctional uterine bleeding, Nursing 39(1):44–50, 2009.

Baldwin, K: Stroke: It's a knock-out punch. Nursing Made Incredibly Easy! 4(2):10–23, 2006.

Baranoski, S: Skin tears: Staying on guard against the enemy of frail skin. Nursing 2003, 33(10 Suppl-Travel Nursing):14–20, 2003.

Barry, J, McQuade, C, and Livingstone, T: Using nurse case management to promote self-efficiency in individuals with rheumatoid arthritis. Rehabil Nurs 23(6):300, 1998.

Bartley, MK: Keep venous thromboembolism at bay. Nursing2006 36(10):36–41, 2006.

Barton-Burke, M: Cancer-related fatigue and sleep disturbances: Further research on the prevalence of these two symptoms in long-term cancer survivors can inform education, policy, and clinical practice. AJN 106(3 Suppl):72–77, 2006.

Bates, B, Choi, JY, Duncan PW, et al: Veterans Affairs/Department of Defense Clinical Practice Guidelines for the Management of Adult Stroke Rehabilitation Care: An executive summary. Stroke 36(9): 2049–56, 2005.

Bauer, J, and Steinhauer, R: A readied response: The emergency plan. RN 65(6):40, 2002.

Bauldoff, GS, and Diaz, PT: Improving outcomes for COPD patients. Nurse Practitioner: Am J Primary Care 31(8):26–43, 2006.

Beattie, S: Bedside emergency: Hemorrhage. RN 70(8): 30–34, 2007.

Beattie, S: In from the cold. RN 69(11):22–27, 2006.

Beatty, GE: Shedding light on Alzheimer's. The Nurse Practitioner: The American J of Primary Health Care 31(9):32–43, 2006.

Beauchamp-Johnson, BM: Scale down bariatric surgery risks, Nurs Management 37(9):27–32, 2006.

Becker, B: To stand or not to stand. Rehab Management 18(2):28–34, 2005.

Belza, B: The impact of fatigue on exercise performance. Arthritis Care and Research 7(4), 176–80, 1994.

Bergen, AF: Heads up: A 20-year tale in several parts. Team Rehabilitation Report 9(9):45, 1998.

Berkowitz, C: Epidural pain control: Your job, too. RN 60(8):22, 1997.

Bermingham, J: Discharge planning: Charting patient progress. Contin Care 16(1):13, 1997.

Bernardi, L, Saviolo, R, Sodick, DH, et al: Do hemodynamic responses to the Valsalva maneuver reflect myocardial dysfunction? Chest 95(5):986–91, 1989.

Birkett, DP: What is the relationship between stroke and depression? Harv Ment Health Lett 14(12):8, 1998.

Blank, CA, and Reid, PC: Taking the tension out of traumatic pneumothoraxes. Nursing 29(4):41, 1999.

Blank-Reid, C: Abdominal trauma: Dealing with the damage. Nursing 37(4 Suppl: ED Insider):4–11, 2007.

Blann, LE: Early intervention for children and families with special needs. MCN, Am J Maternal/Child Nurs 30(4):263–67, 2005.

Boesch, C, Myers, J, Habersaat, A, et al: Maintenance of exercise capacity and physical activity patterns after cardiac rehabilitation. J Cardiopulm Rehab 25(1):14–21, 2005.

Bonanno, G, et al: "What predicts psychological resilience after disaster?" The role of demographics, resources, and life stress. J Consulting Clinical Psychology 75(5):671–82, 2007.

Bone, LA: Restoring electrolyte balance: Calcium and phosphorus. RN 59(3):47, 1996.

Bonner, SM: TKO knee pain with total knee replacement. Nursing Made Incredibly Easy! 5(2):30–39, 2007.

Boon, T: Don't forget the hospice option. RN 61(2):32, 1998.

Borbasi, S, Jones, J, Lockwood, C, et al: Health professionals' perspective of providing care to people with dementia in the acute setting: Toward better practice. Geriatric Nurs 27(5):300–308, 2006.

Borton, D: Isolation precautions: Clearing up the confusion. Nursing 27(1):49, 1997.

Boucher, MA: When laryngectomy complicates care. RN 59(88):40, 1996.

Bowman, A, Breiner, JE, Doerschug, KC, et al: Implementation of an evidence-based feeding protocol and aspiration risk reduction algorithm. Crit Care Nurs Q 28(4):324–33, 2005.

Bradley, M, and Pupiales, M: Essential elements of ostomy care. Am J Nurs 97(7):38, 1997.

Branski, SH: Delirium in hospitalized geriatric patients. Am J Nurs 97(4):161, 1998.

Bray, B, Van Sell, SL, and Miller-Anderson, M: Stress incontinence: It's no laughing matter. RN 70(4):25–29, 2007.

Breakey, James W: Body Image: The Inner Mirror. J Prosthetics Orthotics 9(3):107, 1997.

Breitenbach, JE: Putting an end to perfusion confusion. Nursing Made Incredibly Easy! 5(3):50–60, 2007.

Bright, L: Strategies to improve the patient safety outcome indicator: Preventing or reducing falls. Home Healthcare Nurse 23(1):29–36, 2005.

Brown, KA: Malignant hyperthermia. Am J Nurs 97(10):33, 1997.

Buckle, J: Alternative/complementary therapies. Crit Care Nurse 18(5):54, 1998.

Burgio, KL, et al: Behavioral training for post-prostatectomy urinary incontinence. J Urol 141(2):303, 1989.

Burkhart, I, and Solari-Twadell, PA. Spirituality and religiousness: Differentiating the diagnosis through a review of the nursing literature. Nurs Diag Int J Nurs Lang Class 12, 45–54, 2001.

Burns, SM: Mechanical ventilation of patients with acute respiratory distress syndrome and patents requiring weaning: The evidence guiding practice. Crit Care Nurse 25(4):14–24, 2005.

Burt, S: What you need to know about latex allergy. Nursing 28(10):33, 1998.

Butcher, HK, and McGonigal-Kenney, M: Depression & dispiritedness in later life. Am J Nurs 105(12):52–61, 2005.

Butler, AC, and Beck, AT: Cognitive therapy for depression. Clinical Psychologist 48(3):3–5, 1995.

Calamaro, C, and Waite, R: Cultural proficiency, research, and evidence-based practice: Implications for the nurse practitioner. J Pediatric Health Care 23(1):69–72, 2008.

Calcium in kidney stones. Harv Health Lett 22(8):8, 1997.

Calianno, C, and Holton, SJ: Fighting the triple threat of lower extremity ulcers. Nursing 37(3):57–63, 2007.

Campbell, H, et al: Diogenes syndrome: Frontal lobe dysfunction or multi-factorial disorder. Geriatr Med 35(3):77–79, 2005.

Canales, MAP: Asthma management, putting your patient on the team. Nursing 27(12):33, 1997.

Capili, B, and Anastasi, JK: A symptom review: Nausea and vomiting in HIV. JANAC 9(6):47, 1998.

Carbone, IM: An interdisciplinary approach to the rehabilitation of open-heart surgical patients. Rehabil Nurs 24(2):55, 1999.

Carlson, EV, Kemp, MG, and Short, S: Predicting the risk of pressure ulcers in critically ill patients. Am J Crit Care 8(4):262, 1999.

Carroll, P: Closing in on safer suctioning. RN 61(5):22, 1998.

Carroll, P: Preventing nosocomial pneumonia. RN 61(6):44, 1998.

Carroll, P: Pulse oximetry: At your fingertips. RN 60(2):22, 1997.

Cataldo, R: Decoding the mystery: Evaluating complementary and alternative medicine. Rehab Manag 12(2):42, 1999.

Catania, K, Huang, C, James, P, and Ohr, M: PUPPI: The pressure ulcer prevention protocol interventions. AJN 107(4):44–51, 2007.

Cavendish, R: Clinical snapshot: Periodontal disease. Am J Nurs 99(3): 36, 1999.

Cayley, WE: Diagnosing the cause of chest pain. Am Fam Physician (72):2012–21, 2005.

Centers for Disease Control and Prevention: Recommended immunization schedules for persons aged 0–18 years—United States. MMWR, 55(51–52):Q1–Q4, 2006.

Chatters, IM, Taylor, RJ, and Lincoln, KD. Advances in the measurement of religiosity among older African Americans: Implications for health and mental health researchers. J Ment Health Aging 8(1):181–200, 2001.

Chatterton, R, McTaggart, P, Baum, K, et al: Suicides in an Australian inpatient environment. J Psychosoc Nurs Ment Health Serv 37(6): 34, 1999.

Cheever, KH: An overview of pulmonary arterial hypertension: Risks, pathogenesis, clinical manifestations, and management. J Cardiovasc Nurs 20(2):108–16, 2005.

Chilton, BA: Recognizing spirituality. Image: J Nurs Scholarship 30(4): 400, 1998.

Cirolia, B: Understanding edema: When fluid balance fails. Nursing 26(2):66, 1996.

Clark, CC: Posttraumatic stress disorder: How to support healing. Am J Nurs 97(8):26, 1996.

Cleary-Goldman, J, et al: Impact of maternal age on obstetric outcome. Obstet & Gynecol 105(5):983–90, 2005.

Cochran, H: Diagnose and treat primary insomnia. Nurse Pract: Am J Primary Health Care 28(9):13–27, 2003.

Cohen, D: Optional but necessary. Rehab Manage 18(10):26–29, 2005.

Cole, C, and Richards, K: Sleep disruption in older adults. Am J Nurs, 107 (5):40–49, 2007.

Consult Stat: Chest tubes: When you don't need a seal. RN 61(3):67, 1998.

Cook, L: The value of lab values. Am J Nurs 99(5):66, 1999.

Cook, LS: Choosing the right intravenous catheter. Home Healthcare Nurse 25(8):523–31, 2007.

Cormier, M: The role of hepatitis C support groups. Gastroenterol Nurs 28(3 Suppl): S4–S9, 2005.

Creswell, C, and Chalder, T: Defensive coping styles in chronic Fatigue syndrome. J Psychosom Res 51(4): 607–10, 2001.

Crigger, N, and Forbes, W: Assessing neurologic function in older patients. Am J Nurs 97(3):37, 1997.

Crow, S: Combating infection: Your guide to gloves. Nursing 27(3): 26, 1997.

Dahlin, C: Oral complications at the end of life. Am J Nurs 104(7):40–47, 2004.

Day, MW: Fight back against inflammatory bowel disease. Nursing 38(11):34–40, 2008.

D'Arcy, Y: Conquering PAIN: Have you tried these new techniques? Nursing2005 35(3):36–41, 2005.

D'Arcy, Y: Eye on capnography. Men in Nursing 2(2):25–29, 2007.

D'Arcy, Y: Managing pain in a patient who's drug-dependent. Nursing2007 37(3):36–40, 2007.

Dellinger, RP, et al: Surviving sepsis campaign: Guidelines for management for severe sepsis and septic shock. Crit Care Med 32(3): 858–73, 2004.

DeJong, MJ: Emergency! Hyponatremia. Am J Nurs 98(12):36, 1998.

Denison, B: Touch the pain away: New research on therapeutic touch and persons with fibromyalgia syndrome. Holist Nurs Pract 18(3): 142–51, 2004.

Dennison, RD: Nurse's guide to common postoperative complications. Nursing 27(11):56, 1997.

De Olazabal, JR, et al: Disordered breathing and hypoxia during sleep in coronary artery disease. Chest 1378(5):548–52,1982.

Diel-Oplinger, L, and Kaminski, MF: Choosing the right fluid to counter hypovolemic shock. Nursing2004 34(3):52–54, 2004.

diMaria-Ghalili, RA and Amelia, E: Nutrition in older adults: Interventions and assessment can help curb the growing threat of malnutrition. Am J Nurs 105(3):4050, 2005.

Dionne, M: This bed is just right. Rehab Manage 18(1):32–39, 2005.

Dossey, BM: Holistic modalities and healing moments. Am J Nurs 98(6):44, 1998.

Dossey, BM, and Dossey, L: Body-Mind-Spirit: Attending to holistic care. Am J Nurs 98(8):35, 1998.

Drugs that bring erections down. Sex & Health Institute, p 5, May 1998.

Ducharme, S: Autonomic dysreflexia (sexuality and SCI). Paraplegia News, Nov 1, 2006.

Dunn, D: Age-smart care: Preventing perioperative complications in older adults. Nursing 2006 4(3):30–39, 2006.

Dunn, D: Preventing perioperative complicatons in special populations. Nursing2005 35(11):36–43, 2005.

Dunne, D: Common questions about ileoanal reservoirs. Am J Nurs 97(11):67, 1997.

Durston, S: What you need to know about viral hepatitis. Nursing2005 35(8):3641, 2005.

Dutton, RP: Current concepts in hemorrhagic shock, Anesthesiol Clin North Am 25(1):23, 2007.

Dworak, PA, and Levy, A: Strolling along. Rehab Manage 18(9):26–31, 2005.

Editorial Staff: Patho Puzzler: Don't let your head explode over increased ICP. Nursing Made Incredibly Easy! 5(2):21–25, 2007.

Edmond, M: Combating infection: Tackling disease transmission. Nursing 27(7):65, 1997.

Edwards-Beckett, J, and King, H: The impact of spinal pathology on bowel control in children. Rehabil Nurs 21(6):292, 1996.

Eisenhauer, C: Media review: The new glucose revolution: The authoritative guide to the glycemic index—The dietary solution for lifelong health. Fam Community Health 30(1):86, 2007.

Eldar-Avidan, D, Haj-Yahia, M, and Greenbaum, C: Divorce is a part of my life . . . resilience, survival, and vulnerability: Young adults' perception of the implications of parental divorce. J Marital Fam Ther 35(1):30–46, 2009.

Elgart, HN, Johnson, KL, and Munro, N: Assessment of fluids and eletrolytes. AACN Adv Crit Care 15(4):607–21, 2004.

Elpern, EH, Covert, B, and Kleinpell, R: Moral distress of staff nurses in a medical intensive care unit. Am J Crit Care 14:523–39, 2005.

Epps, CK: The delicate business of ostomy care. RN 5(11):32, 1996.

Epstein, CD, and Peerless, JR: Weaning readiness and fluid balance in older critically ill surgical patients. Am J Crit Care 15(1):54–64, 2006.

Erickson, EH: Reflections on the dissent of contemporary youth. Int JPsychoanal 51:11–22, 1970.

Estes, K, and Thomure, J: Aspirin for the primary prevention of adverse cardiovascular events. Crit Care Nurs Q 31(4):324–39, 2008.

Fagring, AJ, Gaston-Johansson, F, and Danielson, E: Description of unexplained chest pain and its influence on daily life in men and women. Eur J Cardiovasc Nurs (4):337–44, 2005.

Faries, J: Easing your patient's postoperative pain. Nursing 28(6):58, 1998.

Feigenbaum, K: Update on gastroparesis. Gastroenterol Nurs 29(3):239–44, 2006.

Feldman, R, Eidelman, AI, Sirota, L, and Weller, A: Comparison of skin-to-skin (kangaroo) and traditional care: Parenting outcomes and preterm infant development. Pediatr 110(1):16–26, 2002.

Ferrin, MS: Restoring electrolyte balance: Magnesium. RN 59(5):31, 1996.

Fish, KB: Suicide awareness at the elementary school level. J Psychosoc Nurs Ment Health Serv 38(7):20, 2000.

Fishman, TD, Freedline, AD, and Kahn, D: Putting the best foot forward. Nursing 26(1):58, 1996.

Flannery, J: Using the levels of cognitive functioning assessment scale with traumatic brain injury in an acute care setting. Rehabil Nurs 23(2):88, 1998.

Focazio, B: Clinical snapshot: Mucositis. Am J Nurs 97(12):48, 1997.

Frost, KL, and Topp, R: A physical activity RX for the hypertensive patient. Nurse Pract: Am J Primary Health Care 31(4):29–37, 2006.

Fry, VS: The creative approach to nursing. Am J Nurs 53:301, 1953.

Galea, S, Nandi, A, and Vlahov, D: The epidemiology of post-traumatic stress disorders after disasters. Epidemiol Rev 27(1):78–91, 2005.

Gance-Cleveland, B: Motivational interviewing as a strategy to increase families' adherence to treatment regimens. J Specialists Pediatr Nurs 10(3):151–55, 2005.

Garnett, LR: Is obesity all in the genes? Harv Health Lett 21(6):1, 1996.

Giasson, M, and Bouchard, L: Effect of therapeutic touch on the well-being ofpersons with terminal cancer. J Holistic Nurs 16(3):383–98, 1998.

Gibbons, S, Lauder, W, and Ludwick, R: Self-neglect: A proposed new NANDA diagnosis. Int J Nurs Terminologies Classifications 17(1): 10–18, 2006.

Goertz, S: Eye of diagnostics: Gauging fluid balance with osmolality. Nursing2006 36(10):70–71, 2006.

Goldberg, SM: Identifying intestinal obstruction: Better safe than sorry. Nurs Crit Care 3(5):18–23, 2008.

Goldrich, G: Understanding the 12-lead ECG, part I. Nursing2006 36(11):36–41, 2006.

Goldrick, BA, and Goetz, AM: 'Tis the season for influenza. Nurse Pract: Am J Primary Health Care 31(12):24–33, 2006.

Good, KK, Verble, JA, Secrest, J, et al: Postoperative hypthermia—The chilling consequences. AORN 83(5):1055–66, 2006.

Gorman, D, et al: Take a rapid treatment approach to cardiogenic shock. Nurs Crit Care 3(4):18–27, 2008.

Goshorn, J: Clinical snapshot: Kidney stones. Am J Nurs 96(9):40, 1996.

Graf, C: Functional decline in hospitalized older adults. Am J Nurs 106(1):58–67, 2006.

Grandjean, CK, and Gibbons, SW: Assessing ambulatory geriatric sleep complaints. Nurse Pract: Am J Primary Health Care, 25(9):25, 2000.

Gray, M: Assessment and management of urinary incontinence. Nurse Pract: Am J Primary Health Care 30(7):32–43, 2005.

Gray, M: Overactive bladder: An overview. JWound, Ostomy Continence Nurs 32(3): Suppl 1–5, 2005.

Gray, M, Bliss, DZ, Doughty, DB, et al: Incontinence-associated dermatitis: A consensus. J Wound, Ostomy Continence Nurs 34(1):45–54, 2007.

Gregory, CM: Caring for caregivers: Proactive planning eases burdens on caregivers. Lifelines 1(2):51, 1997.

Greifzu, S: Fighting cancer fatigue. RN 61(8):41, 1998.

Gritter, M: The latex threat. Am J Nurs 98(9):26, 1998.

Grzankowski, JA: Altered thought processes related to traumatic brain injury and their nursing implications. Rehabil Nurs 22(1):24, 1997.

Hadaway, LC: Reopen the pipeline for IV therapy. Nursing 35(8):54–61, 2005.

Hadaway, LC: Targeting therapy with central venous access devices. Nursing 38(6):34–40, 2008.

Hadaway, LC, and Millam, DA: On the road to successful IV starts. Nursing 37(8) Suppl:1–14, 2007.

Hahn, J: Cueing in to client language. Reflections 25(1):8–11, 1999.

Halpin-Landry, JE, and Goldsmith, S: Feet first: Diabetes care. Am J Nurs 99(2):26, 1999.

Hankins, J: The role of albumin in fluid and electrolyte balance. J Infusion Nurs 29(5):260–65, 2006.

Hanley, C: Delirium in the acute care setting: MEDSURG Nurs 13(4): 217–25, 2004.

Hanneman, SK, and Gusick, M: Frequency of oral care and positioning of patients in critical care: A replication study. Am J Crit Care 14(5): 378–86, 2005.

Bibliography

Hanson, MJS: Caring for a patient with COPD. Nursing 27(12):39, 1997.

Harvey, C, Dixon, M, and Padberg, N: Support group for families of trauma patients: A unique approach. Crit Care Nurs 15(4):59, 1995.

Hayes, DD: Bradycardia. Keeping the current flowing. Nursing 27(6):50, 1997.

Hayn, MA, and Fisher, TR: Stroke rehabilitation: Salvaging ability after the storm. Nursing 27(3):40, 1997.

Hedges, ST, et al: Evidence-based treatment recommendations for uremic bleeding. Nat Clin Pract Nephrol 3(3):138–53, 2007.

Held-Warmkessel, J, and Schiech, L: Responding to 4 gastrointestinal complications in cancer patients. Nursing 38(7):3238, 2008.

Hernandez, D: Microvascular complications of diabetes: Nursing assessment and interventions. Am J Nurs 98(6):16, 1998.

Herson, L, Hart, K, Gordon, M, et al: Identifying and overcoming barriers to providing sexuality information in the clinical setting. Rehabil Nurs 24(4):148, 1999.

Hess, CT: Caring for a diabetic ulcer. Nursing 29(5):70, 1999.

Hess, CT: Wound care. Nursing 28(3):18, 1998.

Hill, R: Don't let constipation stop you up. Nursing Made Incredibly Easy! 5(5):40–47, 2007.

Hoffman, J: Tuning in to the power of music. RN 60(6):52, 1997.

Holcomb, SS: Acute abdomen: What a pain! Nursing 38(9):34–40, 2008.

Holcomb, SS: Understanding the ins and outs of diuretic therapy. Nursing 27(2):34, 1997.

Holm, K, and Foreman, M: Analysis of measures of functional and cognitive ability for aging adults with cardiac and vascular disease. J Cardiovasc Nurs 21(5 Suppl 1):S40–S45, 2006.

Honkus, VL: Sleep deprivation in critical care units. Crit Care Nurs Q, 26(3), 179–91, 2003.

Houghton, D: HAI prevention: The power is in your hands. Nurs Manage 37(5):Suppl: 1–7, 2006.

Hughes, L. Physical and psychological variables that influence pain in patients with fibromyalgia. Orthop Nurs 25(2):112–19, 2006.

Hunt, R: Community-based nursing. Am J Nurs 98(10):44, 1998.

Hunter, A, Denman-Vitale, S, and Garzon, L: Global infections: Recognition, management, and prevention. Nurse Pract: Am J Primary Health Care 32(2):34–41, 2007.

Huston, CJ: Emergency! Dental luxation and avulsion. Am J Nurs 97(9):48, 1997.

Hutchison, CP: Healing touch: An energetic approach. Am J Nurs 99(4):43, 1999.

Infusion Nurses Society: Infusion nursing standards of practice. J Infusium Nurs 29(1 Suppl):S1–S92, 2006.

Isaacs, A: Depression and your patient. Am J Nurs 98(7):26, 1998.

Iscoe, KE, Campbell, JE, Jamnik, V, et al: Efficacy of continuous real-time blood glucose monitoring during and after prolonged high-intensity cycling exercise: Spinning with a continuous glucose monitoring system. Diabetes TechnolTher 8(6):627–35, 2006.

It's probably not Alzheimer's: New insights on memory loss. Focus on Healthy Aging 2(7):1, 1999.

Iyasu, S, Randall, L, Welty, K, et al: Risk factors for sudden infant death syndrome among Northern Plains Indians. JAMA 288(21): 2717, 2002.

Jaempf, G, and Goralski, VJ: Monitoring postop patients. RN 59(7):30, 1996.

Jennings, LM: Latex allergy: Another real Y2K issue. Rehabil Nurs 24(4):140, 1999.

Jirovec, MM, Wyman, JF, and Wells, TJ: Addressing urinary incontinence with educational continence-care competencies. Image: J Nurs Scholarship 30(4):375, 1998.

Johnson, CV, and Hayes, JA: Troubled spirits: Prevalence and predictors of religious and spiritual concerns among university students and counseling center clients. J Counseling Psychol 50:409–19, 2003.

Johnson, J, Pearson, V, and McDivitt, L: Stroke rehabilitation: Assessing stroke survivors' long-term learning needs. Rehabil Nurs 22(5): 243, 1997.

Kachourbos, MJ: Relief at last: An implanted bladder control system helps people control their bodily functions. Team Rehabil Rep, p 31, August 1997.

Kalvemark S, Hoglund AAT, Hansson MG, et al: Living with conflicts—Ethical dilemmas and moral distress in the health care system. Soc Sci Med, 58(6):1075–84, 2004.

Kanachki, L: How to guide ventilator-dependent patients from hospital to home. Am J Nurs 97(2):37, 1997.

Kania, DS, and Scott, CM: Postexposure prophylaxis considerations for occupational and nonoccupational exposures. Adv Emerg Nurs J 29(1):20–32, 2007.

Kaplow, R: AACN synergy model for patient care: A framework to optimize outcomes. Crit Care Nurse (Suppl):27–30, February 2003.

Katerndahl, D: Panic and plaques: Panic disorder and coronary artery disease in patients with chest pain. J Am Board Fam Pract 17(2): 114–26, 2004.

Kearney, PM, and Griffin, T: Between joy and sorrow: Being a parent of a child with a developmental disability. JAdv N 34:582–92, 2001.

Keegan, L: Getting comfortable with alternative and complementary therapies. Nursing 28(4):50, 1998.

Kehl-Pruett, W: Deep vein thrombosis in hospitalized patients: A review of evidence-based guidelines for prevention. Dimens Crit Care Nurs 25(2):53–59, 2006.

Kelso, LA: Cirrhosis: Caring for patients with end-stage liver failure, Nurs Pract: Am J Primary Health Care, 33(7):24–30, 2008.

Kersting, K: A new approach to complicated grief. Monitor on Psych 35(10):51, 2004.

King, B: Preserving renal function. RN 60(8):34, 1997.

Kinloch, D: Instillation of normal saline during endotracheal suctioning: Effects on mixed venous oxygen saturation. Am J Crit Care 8(4): 231, 1999.

Kirshblum, S, and O'Connor, K: The problem of pain: A common condition of people with SCI. Team Rehab Rep, p 15, August 1997.

Kirton, C: The HIV/AIDS epidemic: A case of good news/bad news. Nursing Made Incredibly Easy! 3(2):28–40, 2005.

Klonowski, EI, and Masodi, JE: The patient with Crohn's disease. RN 62(3):32, 1999.

Klotter, J: Latex allergy prevention. Townsend Letter for Doctors and Patients, May 1, 2006.

Kolcaba, K, and DiMarco, MA: Comfort theory and its application to pediatric nursing. Pediatr Nurse 31(3):187–94, 2005.

Kolcaba, KY, and Fisher EM: A holistic perspective on comfort care as an advance directive. Crit Care Nurs Quarterly 18(4):66–67, 1996.

Kopala, B, and Burkhart, L: Ethical dilemma and moral distress: Proposed new NANDA diagnoses. Int J Nurs Terminologies Classifications 16(1): 3–13, 2005.

Korinko, A, and Yurick, A: Maintaining skin integrity during radiation therapy. Am J Nurs 97(2):40, 1997.

Kouch, M: Managing symptoms for a "good death" Nursing2006 36(11):58–63, 2006.

Kumasaka, L, and Miles, A: "My pain is God's will." Am J Nurs 96(6): 45, 1996.

Kurtz, MJ, Van Zandt, DK, and Sapp, LR: A new technique in independent intermittent catheterization: The Mitrofanoff catheterizable channel. Rehabil Nurs 21(6):311, 1996.

Lai, SC, and Cohen, MN: Promoting lifestyle changes. Am J Nurs 99(4):63, 1999.

Lambing, A: Bleeding disorders: Patient history key to diagnosis. Nurse Pract: Am J Primary Health Care 32(12):16–24, 2007.

Lamblass, M: Treating Ppediatric overweight through reductions in sedentary behavior: A review of the literature. J Pediatr Health Care, 23(1):29–36, 2008.

Lapointe, LA: Coagulopathies in trauma patients. AACN Adv Pract in Acute Crit Care 13(2):192–203, 2002.

Larden, CN, Palmer, ML, and Janssen, P: Efficacy of therapeutic touch in treating pregnant inpatients who have a chemical dependency. J Holist Nurs 22(4):320–32, 2004.

Lark, S: The 21-day arthritis and pain miracle. Article for the Lark Letter: A Woman's Guide to Optimal Health and Balance, Special Report, 2005.

Larsen, LS: Effectiveness of a counseling intervention to assist family caregivers of chronically ill relatives. J Psychosoc Nurs Ment Health Serv 36(8):26, 1998.

Laskowski-Jones, L: Responding to trauma: Your priorities in the first hour. Nursing2006 36(9):52–58, 2006.

Lauder, W, Anderson, I, and Barclay, A: A framework for good practice in interagency interventions with cases of self-neglect. J Psychiatr Ment Health Nurs 12(2):192–98, 2005.

Lauder, W, Anderson, I, and Barclay, A: Housing and self-neglect: The responses of health, social care and environmental health agencies. J Interprof Care 19(4):317–25, 2005.

Lewis, ML, and Dehn, DS: Violence against nurses in outpatient mental health settings. J Psychosoc Nurs Ment Health Serv 37(6):28, 1999.

Linch, SH: Elder abuse: What to look for, how to intervene. Am J Nurs 97(1):26, 1997.

Livneh, H, and Antonak, RF: Psychosocial adaptation to chronic illness and disability: A primer for counselors (practice & theory). J Counseling Dev 83(1):12–20, 2005.

Loeb, JL: Pain management in long-term care. Am J Nurs 99(2):48, 1999.

Lorente L, Lecuona M, Jimenez A, et al: Ventilator-associated pneumonia using a heated humidifier or a heat and moisture exchanger:
A randomized controlled trial. Crit Care 10:4, 2006.

Lorio, AK: Transfer dependent. Rehab Management 18(7):2226, 2005.

Loughrey, L: Taking a sensitive approach to urinary incontinence.
Nursing 29(5):60, 1999.

Lyman, B: Metabolic complications associated with parenteral nutrition. J Infusium Nurs 25(1):36–44, 2002.

MacNeill, D, and Weis, T: Case study: Coordinating care. Continuing
Care 17(4):78, 1998.

Malinowski, A, and Stamler, LL: Comfort: Exploration of the concept
in nursing. JAN 39(6):599–606, 2002.

Mann, AR: Manage the power of pain. Men in Nurs 1(4):20–28, 2006.

Manoguerra, AS, and Cobaugh, DJ: Guideline on the use of ipecac
syrup in the out-of-hospital management of ingested poisons. Clin
Toxicol 43(1):1–10, 2005.

Matthews, PJ: Ventilator-associated infections. I. Reducing the risks.
Nursing 27(2):59, 1997.

Mauk, KL: Medications for management of overactive bladder. ARN
Network, June/July, 3–7, 2005.

McAllister, M: Promoting physiologic-physical adaptation in chronic
obstructive pulomonary disease: Pharmacotherapeutic evidence-
based research and guidelines. Home Healthcare Nurse 23(8):523–
31, 2005.

McCaffery, M: Pain management handbook. Nursing 27(4):42, 1997.

McCaffery, M, and Ferrell, BR: Opioids and pain management: What
do nurses know? Nursing 29(3):48, 1999.

McCaffrey, R, and Rozzano, L: The effect of music on pain and acute
confusion in older adults undergoing hip and knee surgery. Holistic
Nurs Pract 20(5):218–24, 2006.

McCain, D, and Sutherland, S: Nursing essentials: Skin grafts for patients with burns. Am J Nurs 98(7):34, 1998.

McClave, SA, Lowen, CC, Kleber, MJ, et al: Are patients fed appropriately according to their caloric requirements? JPEN 22(6):375–
81, 1998.

McClave, SA, Lukan, JK, Lowen, JA, et al: Poor validity of residual
volumes as a marker for risk of aspiration in critically ill patients.
Crit Care Med 33(2):324–30, 2005.

McConnel, E: Preventing transient increases in intracranial pressure.
Nursing 28(4):66, 1998.

McCool, FD, and Rosen, MJ: Nonpharmacologic airway clearance therapies. Chest 129(250S–259S), 2006.

McCullagh, MC: Home modification. Am J Nurs 106(10):54–63, 2006.

McHale, JM, Phipps, MA, Horvath, K, et al: Expert nursing knowledge
in the care of patients at risk of impaired swallowing. Image: J Nurs
Scholarship 30(2):137, 1998.

McKinley, LL, and Zasler, CP: Weaving a plan of care. Continuing
Care 17(7):38, 1998.

McLean, SE, Jensen, LA, Schroeder, DG, et al: Improving adherence
to a mechanical ventilation weaning protocol for critically ill adults:
Outcomes after an implementation program. Am J Crit Care 15(3):
299–309, 2006.

Mendez-Eastman, S: When wounds won't heal. RN 51(1):20, 1998.

Metheny, N, et al: Testing feeding tube placement: Auscultation vs pH method. Am J Nurs 98(5):37, 1998.

Michael, KM, Allen, JK, and Macko, RE: Fatigue after stroke: Relationship to mobility, fitness, ambulatory activity, social support, and falls efficacy. Rehabil Nurs 31(5):210–17, 2006.

Miller, CK, Ulbrecht, JS, Lyons, J, et al: A reduced-carbohydrate diet improves outcomes in patients with metabolic syndrome: A transitional study. Top Clin Nutr 22(1):82–91, 2007.

Miller, D: Is advanced maternal age an independent risk factor for uteroplacental insufficiency? Am J Obstet Gynecol 192(6):1974–82, 2005.

Miller, SK, and Alpert, PT: Assessment and differential diagnosis of abdominal pain. Nurse Pract: Am J Primary Health Care 31(7):39–47, 2006.

Milne, JL, and Krissovich, M: Behavioral therapies at the primary care level: The current state of knowledge. J Wound, Ostomy Continence Nurs 31(6):367–76, 2004.

Mintz, TG: Relocation stress syndrome in older adults. Social Work Today 5(6):38, 2005.

Moe, SM: Disorders involving calcium, phosphorus, and magnesium. Primary Care 35(2):215–37, 2008.

Mohr, WK: Cross-ethnic variations in the care of psychiatric patients: A review of contributing factors and practice considerations. J Psychosoc Nurs Ment Health Serv 36(5):16, 1998.

Moshang, J: The growing problem of type 2 diabetes. LPN2005 1(3):26–34, 2005.

Mosocco, D: Clipboard: Childhood vaccines. Home Healthcare Nurse 25(1):7–8, 2007.

Muller, AC, and Bell, AE: Diagnostic update: Electrolyte update: Potassium, chloride and magnesium. Nurs Crit Care 3(1):5–7, 2008.

Murphy, K: Anxiety: When is it too much? Nursing Made Incredibly Easy! 3(5):22–31, 2005.

Nadolski, M: Getting a good night's sleep: Diagnosing and treating insomnia. Plast Surg Nurs 25(4):167–73, 2005.

Naylor, MD, Stephens, C, Bowles, KH, et al: Cognitively impaired older adults. Am J Nurs 105(2):52–61, 2005.

Neal-Boylan, L: Health assessment of the very old person at home. Home Healthcare Nurse 25(6):388–98, 2007.

Nelson, DP, et al: Recognizing sepsis in the adult patient. Am J Nurs 109(3):40–50, 2009.

Newman, DK: Assessment of the patient with an overactive bladder. JWound, Ostomy Continence Nurs 32(3 Suppl):5–10, 2005.

Nieves, J, and Capone-Swearer, D: The clot that changes lives. Nursing2006 Critical Care 1(3):18–28, 2006.

No author listed: The changing concept of sudden infant death syndrome: Diagnostic coding shifts, controversies regarding the sleeping environment, and new variations to consider in reducing risk. Pediatr 116(5):1245–55, 2005.

No author listed: Changing concepts of sudden infant death syndrome: Implications for infant sleeping environment and sleep position. Task Force on Infant Sleep Position and Sudden Infant Death Syndrome. Pediatr 105(3):650–56, 2000.

No author listed: Defensive Functioning Scale, Brandeis University Psychological Counseling Center, Waltham, MA, 2002.

No author listed: Smog—Who does it hurt? What you need to know about ozone and your health. Public information brochure. US Environmental Protection Agency, Washington, DC, 1999.

No author listed: Taking Control of Stress. Harvard Health Publications: Big Sandy, TX, Special Supplement, 2007.

No author listed: Understanding transcultural nursing. Nursing2005 35(1):14–23. Supplement Career Directory, 2005.

Nunnelee, JD: Healing venous ulcers. RN 60(11):38, 1997.

Nusbaum, N: Safety versus autonomy: Dilemmas and strategies in protection of vulnerable community-dwelling elderly. Annals Long-Term Care 12(5):50–53, 2004.

Oddy WH, Li J, Landsborough L, et al: The association of maternal overweight and obesity with breastfeeding duration. J Pediatr 149(2): 185–91, 2006.

Odom-Forren, J: Preventing surgical site infections. Nursing2006 36(6): 59–63, 2006.

O'Donnell, M: Addisonian crisis. Am J Nurs 97(3):41, 1997.

Okan, K, Woo, K, Ayello, EA et al: The role of moisture balance in wound healing. Advances for skin & wound care. J Prev Healing 20(1):39–53, 2007.

Olansky, S: Chronic sorrow: A response to having a mentally defective child. Social Casework 43:190–93, 1962.

Olsen, DM, et al: Quiet time: A nursing intervention to promote sleep in neurocritical care units. Am J Crit Care, 10(2):74–78, 2001.

O'Neil, C, Avila, JR, and Fetrow, CW: Herbal medicines, getting beyond the hype. Nursing 29(4):58, 1999.

Palmer, JL, and Metheny, NA: How to try this: Preventing aspiration in older adults with dysphagia. Am J Nurs 108:1–40, 2008.

Parkman, CA, and Calfee, BE: Advance directives, honoring your patient's end-of-life wishes. Nursing 27(4):48, 1997.

Parsons, KS, Galinsky, TL, and Waters, T: Suggestions for preventing musculoskeletal disorders in home healthcare workers, Part 1: Lift and transfer assistance for partially weight-bearing home care patients. Home Healthcare Nurse 24(3):158–64, 2006.

Parsons, KS, Galinsky, TL, and Waters, T: Suggestions for preventing musculoskeletal disorders in home healthcare workers. Part 2: Lift and transfer assistance for non-weight-bearing home care patients. Home Healthcare Nurse 24(4):227–33, 2006.

Pasero, C, and McCaffrey, M: No self-report means no pain-intensity rating. Am J Nurs 105(10):50–53, 2005.

Patel, M, et al: Sleep in the intesnsive care setting. Crit Care Nurs Q 31(4):309–18, 2008.

Pearsen, OR, Busse, ME, van Deursen, RWM, et al: Quantification of walking mobility in neruological disorders. QJM: Int J Med 97:463–75, 2004.

Perry, A: Quality of life. Rehabil Manage 18(7):18–21, 2005.

Phillips, JK: Actionstat: Wound dehiscence. Nursing 28(3):33, 1998.

Pieper, B, Sieggreen, M, Freeland, B, et al: Discharge information needs of patients after surgery. J Wound, Ostomy Continence Nurs 33(3): 281–90, 2006.

Pierce, LL: Barriers to access: Frustrations of people who use a wheelchair for full-time mobility. Rehabil Nurs 23(3):120, 1998.

Pignone, MP, Ammerman, A, Fernandez, L, et al: Counseling to promote a healthy diet in adults: A summary of the evidence for the US
Preventive Services Task Force. Am J Prev Med 24(1):75, 2003.

Poe, SS, Cvach, MM, Gartrell, DG, et al: An evidence-based approach
to fall risk assessment, prevention, and management: Lessons
learned. J Nurs Care Quality 20(2):107–16, 2005.

Powers, J, and Bennett, SJ: Measurement of dyspnea in patients treated
with mechanical ventilation. Am J Crit Care 8(4):254, 1999.

Pringle-Specht, JK: Nine myths of incontinence in older adults. Am J
Nurs, 105(6):58–68, 2005.

Pronitis-Ruotolo, D: Surviving the night shift: Making Zeitgeber work
for you. Am J Nurs 101(7):63, 2001.

Pruitt, B: Weaning patients from mechanical ventilation. Nursing2006
36(9):36–41, 2006.

Purgason, K: Broken hearts: Differentiating stress-induced cardiomyopathy from acute myocardial infarction in the patient presenting
with acute coronary syndrome. Dimensions Crit Care Nurs 25(6):
247–53, 2006.

Ragsdale, JA: Hereditary hemorrhagic telangiectasia from epistaxis to
life-threatening GI bleeding. Gastroenterol Nurs 30(4):293–99,
2007.

Raina, P, O'Donnell, M, Rosenbaum, P, et al: The health and well-
being of caregivers of children with cerebral palsy. Pediatr 115(6):
e626–e636, 2005.

Rawsky, E: Review of the literature on falls among the elderly. Image:
J Nurs Scholarship 30(1):47, 1998.

Reddy, L: Heads up on cerebral bleeds. Nursing2006 3(5 Suppl E D):
4–9, 2006.

Richards, KC: Sleep promotion. Crit Care Clin North Am 8(1):39–52,
1996.

Ried, S, and Dassen, T: Chronic confusion, dementia, and impaired
environmental interpretation syndrome: A concept comparison. Nurs
Diagn 11(2):45–59, 2000.

Riggs, JM: Manage heart failure. Nursing2006 Crit Care 1(4):18–28,
2006.

Robertson, RG, and Montagnini, M: Geriatric failure to thrive. Am Fam
Physician 70(2):343–50, 2004.

Robinson, AW: Getting to the heart of denial. Am J Nurs 99(5):38,
1999.

Rogers, S, Ryan, M, and Slepoy, L: Successful ventilator weaning: A
collaborative effort. Rehabil Nurs 23(5):265, 1998.

Romero, DV, Treston, J, and O'Sullivan, AL: Hand-to-hand combat:
Preventing MRSA infection: Advances in skin & wound care: J Prev
Healing 19(6):328–33, 2006.

Rosen, L: Sit on it. Rehabil Manage 18(2):36–41, 2005.

Rosenthal, K: Guarding against vascular site infection. Nurs Manage
37(4):54–66, 2006.

Rosenthal, K: Tailor your IV insertion-techniques for special populations. Nursing 35(5):36–41, 2005.

Sacks, FM, and Katan, M: Randomized clinical trials on the effects of
dietary fat and carbohydrate on plasma proteins and cardiovascular
disease. Am J Med 113(Suppl 9B):13–24, 2002.

Sallis, JF: The role of behavioral science in improving health through
physical activity. Summary of presentation. Science Writers

Briefing. Sponsored by OBSSR and the American Psychological Association, December 1996.

Salmon, DA, Moulton, LH, Omer, SB, et al: Factors associated with refusal of childhood vaccines among parents of school-aged children: A case-control. Arch Pediatr Adolesc Med 159(5):470–76, 2005.

Samarel N, Fawcett J, Davis MM, and Ryan FM: Effects of dialogue and therapeutic touch on preoperative and postoperative experiences of breast cancer surgery: An exploratory study. Oncol Nurs Forum 25(8):1369–76, 1998.

Sampselle, CM: Behavioral interventions in young and middle-age women. Am J Nurs 103(3):9, 2003. (Suppl) State of the Science on Urinary Incontinence.

Sateia, MJ, et al: Evaluation of chronic insomnia: An American Academy of Sleep Medicine review. Sleep 23(2):243–308, 2000.

Sauerbeck, LR: Primary stroke prevention. Am J Nurs 106(11):40–49, 2006.

Scanlon, C: Defining standards for end-of-life care. Am J Nurs 97(11): 58, 1997.

Schaffer, DB: Closed suction wound drainage. Nursing 27(11):62, 1997.

Scharer, K, and Brooks, G: Mothers of chronically ill neonates and primary nurses in the NICU: Transfer of care. Neonatal Network 13(5):37–46, 1994.

Scheck, A: Therapists on the team: Diabetic wound prevention is everybody's business. Rehabil Nurs 16(7):18, 1999.

Schiffman, RF: Drug and subtance use in Adolescents MCN, Am J Maternal/Child Nurs 29(1):21–27, 2004.

Schiweiger, JL, and Huey, RA: Alzheimer's disease. Nursing 29(6):34, 1999.

Schmelling, S: Home, adapted home. Rehabil Manage 18(6):12–19, 2005.

Schraeder, C, et al: Community nursing organizations: A new frontier. Am J Nurs 97(1):63, 1997.

Schulman, A: Staff Working Paper. The President's Council on Bioethics. Bioethics and Human Dignity, 2005.

Schulman, C: End points of resuscitation: Choosing the right parameters to monitor. Dimensions Crit Care Nurs 21(1):2–10, 2002.

Schulmeister, L: Pacemakers and environmental safety: What your patient needs to know. Nursing 28(7):58, 1998.

Schumacher, K, Beck, CA, and Marren, JM: Family caregivers: Caring for older adults, working with their families. Am J Nurs 106(8):40–49, 2006.

Schwebel, DC, and Barton, BK: Contributions of multiple risk factors to child injury. J Pediatr Psychol 30(7):553–61, 2005.

Short stature and growth hormone: A delicate balance. Practice Update (newsletter). The Children's Hospital, Denver, Summer 1999.

Sieggreen, M: A contemporary approach to peripheral arterial disease. Health Pract: Am J of Primary Health Care 31(7):14–25, 2006.

Sieggreen, M: Understanding critical limb ischemia. Nursing 38(10): 50–55, 2008.

Sieggreen, MY: Getting a leg up on managing venous ulcers. Nursing Made Incredibly Easy! 4(6):52–60, 2006.

Sinacore, DR: Managing the diabetic foot. Rehabil Manag 11(4):60, 1998.

Singh, H, et al: Gastrointestinal prophylaxis in critically ill patients. Crit Care Nurs Q 31(4):291–301, 2008.

Smatlak, P, and Knebel, AR: Clinical evaluation of noninvasive monitoring of oxygen saturation in critically ill patients. Am J Crit Care 7(5):370, 1998.

Smith, AM, and Schwirian, PM: The relationship between caregiver burden and TBI survivors' cognition and functional ability after discharge. Rehabil Nurs 23(5):252, 1998.

Smith, DH: Managing acute acetaminophen toxicity. Nursing2007 37(1):58–63, 2007.

Smith, DW, Arnstein, P, Rosa, KC, and Wells-Federman, C: Effects of integrating therapeutic touch into a cognitive behavioral pain treatment program. Report of a pilot clinical trial. J Holist Nurs 20(4): 367–87, 2002.

Smith Hammond, CA, and Goldstein, LB: Cough and aspiration of food and liquids due to oral-pharyngeal dysphagia: AACP evidence-based clinical practice guidelines. Chest 129(1 Suppl):154S–168S, 2006.

Smochek, MR, Oblaczynsk, C, Lauck, DL, et al: Interventions for risk for suicide and risk for violence. Nurs Diagn. Int J Nurs Lang Class 11(2):60, April–June 2000.

Sommer, KD, and Sommer, NW: When your patient is hearing impaired. RN 65(12):28–32, 2002.

Sonnenblick, M, Friedlander, Y, and Rosin, AJ: Diuretic-induced severe hyponatremia: Review and analysis of 129 reported patients. Chest 103(2):601–606, 1993.

Spahn, DR: Management of bleeding following major trauma: A European guideline. Crit Care 11(1):17, 2006.

Spaniol, JR, et al: Fluid resuscitation therapy for hemorrhagic shock. J Trauma Nurs 14(3):152–60, 2007.

Spenceley, SM: Sleep inquiry: A look with fresh eyes. Image: J Nurs Scholarship 25(3), 249–55, 1993.

Spurlock, WR: Spiritual well-being and caregiver burden in Alzheimer's caregivers. Geriatr Nurs 26(3):154–61 2005.

Stabin, MG, and Breitz, H: Breast milk secretion of radiopharmaceuticals; mechanisms, findings, and radiation dosimetry. J Nuclear Med 41(5):863–73, 2000.

Stegeman, CA: Oral manifestations of diabetes. Home Healthcare Nurse 23(4):233–40, 2005.

Steiner, ME, and Despotis, GJ: Transfusion algorithims and how they apply to blood conservation: The high-risk cardiac surgical patient. Oncol Clin North Am 21(1):177, 2007.

Stockert, PA: Getting UTI patients back on track. RN 62(3):49, 1999.

Stockman, J: In too deep: Understanding deep vein thrombosis. Nursing Made Incredibly Easy! 6(2):29–38, 2008.

Strimike, CL, Wojcik, JM, and Stark, BA: Incision care that really cuts it. RN 60(7):22, 1997.

Sullivan, CS, Logan, J, and Kolasa, KM: Medical nutrition therapy for the bariatric patient. Nutrition Today 41(5):207–12, 2006.

Summer, CH: Recognizing and responding to spiritual distress. Am J Nurs 98(1):26, 1998.

Szymanski, L, and King, B: Practice parameters for the assessment and treatment of children, adolescents, and adults with mental retardation and comorbid mental disorders. American Academy of Child and

Adolescent Psychiatry Working Group on Quality Issues. J Am Acad Child Adolesc Psychiatry 38(12 Suppl):5S–31S, 1999.

Tablan, OC, Anderson, LJ, Besser, R, et al: Guidelines for preventing health-care associated pneumonia, 2003—Recommendations of CDC and Healthcare Infection Control Practices Advisory Committee. MMWR March 26, 53(RRO3):1–36, 2004.

Thom, T, et al: Heart disease and stroke statistics—2006 update: A report from the American Health Association Committee and Stroke Statistics Subcommittee. Circulation 113:e85–e151, 2006.

Tierney, M, et al: Risk factors for harm in cognitively impaired seniors who live alone: A prospective study. J Am Geriatr Society 52(9): 1435–41, 2004.

Travers, PL: Autonomic dysreflexia: A clinical rehabilitation problem. Rehabil Nurs 24(1):19, 1997.

Travers, PL: Poststroke dysphagia: Implications for nurses. Rehabil Nurs 24(2):69, 1999.

Travis, S: "Caring for you, caring for me": A ten-year caregiver educational initiative of the Rosalynn Carter Institute for Human Development. Health and Social Work, May 1, 2006.

Trendall, J: Concept analysis: Chronic fatigue. J AdvNurs 32(5):1126–31, 2005.

Turkowski, BB: Managing insomnia. Orthop Nurs 25(5):339–45, 2006.

Turnbough, L, and Wilson, L: Take your medicine: Nonadherence issues in patients with ulcerative colitis. Gastroenterol Nurs 30(3): 212–17, 2007.

Ufema, J: Reflections on death and dying. Nursing 29(6):96, 1999.

Vacca, VM, and Vilolett, S: Teamwork integral to treating cerebral arteriovenous malformation. Nurs Crit Care 3(3):20–27, 2008.

Vigilance pays off in preventing falls. Harv Health Lett 24(6):1, 1999.

Walker, BL: Preventing falls. RN 61(5):40, 1998.

Walker, D: Back to basics: Choosing the correct wound dressing. Am J Nurs 96(9):35, 1996.

Wallhagen, MI, Pettengill, E, and Whiteside, M: Sensory impairment in older adults. Part 1: Hearing loss. Am J Nurs 106(10):40–49, 2006.

Wallston, BS, and Wallston, KA: Locus of control and health: A review of the literature. Health Education Monographs, University of South Florida, Spring 1978, 107–17 (rev Jan 11. 1999).

Warms, CA, Marshal, JM, Hoffman, AJ, et al: There are a few things you did not ask about my pain: Writing in the margins of a survey questionnaire. Rehabil Nurs 30(6):248–56, 2006.

Watson, R, Modeste, N, Catolico, O, et al: The relationship between caregiver burden and self-care deficits in former rehabilitation patients. Rehabil Nurs 23(5):258, 1998.

Waugh, KG: Measuring the right angle. Rehabil Manage 18(1):40–47, 2005.

Weeks, SM: Caring for patients with heart failure. Nursing 26(3):52, 1996.

Wehling-Weepie, AK, and McCarthy, A: A healthy lifestyle program: Promoting child health in schools. J School Nurs 18(6):322, 2002.

Weinhouse, GL, and Schwab, RJ: Sleep in the critically ill patient. Sleep, 29:707–15, 2006.

Weiss, B: When a family member requires your care. RN 68(4):63–65 2005.

Wheeler, MS: Pain assessment and management in the patient with mild to moderate cogntive impairement. Home Healthcare Nurse 24(6): 354–59, 2006.

Wheeler, SL, and Houston, K: The role of diversional activities in the general medical hospital setting. Holistic Nurs Practice 19(2):67–69, 2005.

Whetstone, L, and Morrissey, S: Children at risk: The association between perceived weight status and suicidal thoughts and attempts in middle school youth. J School Health 77(2): 59–66, 2007.

Whiteman, K and McCormick, C: When your patient is in liver failure. Nursing2005 35(4):58–63, 2005.

Whiteside, MM, Wallhagen, MI, and Pettengill, E: Sensory impairment in older adults Part 2: Vision loss. Am J Nurs 106 (11):52–61, 2006.

Whitfield, W: Research in religion and mental health. Naming of parts—Some reflections. Int J Psychiatr Nurs Res 8(1), 891–96, 2002.

Whittle, H, et al: Nursing management of pressure ulcers using a hydrogel dressing protocol: Four case studies. Rehabil Nurs 21(5):237, 1996.

Williams, AM, and Deaton, SB: Phantom limb pain: Elusive, yet real. Rehabil Nurs 22(2):73, 1997.

Wipke-Tevis, DD, and Sae-Sia, W: Caring for vascular leg ulcers. Home Healthcare Nurse 22(4):237–47, 2004.

Woods, DL, Craven, RF, and Whitney, J: The effect of therapeutic touch on behavioral symptoms of persons with dementia. Altern Ther Health Med 11(1):66–74, 2005.

Woods, DL, and Dimond, M: The effect of therapeutic touch on agitated behavior and cortisol in persons with Alzheimer's disease. Biol Res Nurs 4(2):104–14, 2002.

Wooten, JM: OTC laxatives aren't all the same. RN 69(9):78, 2006.

Wung, S, and Kozik, T: Electrocardiographic evaluation of cardiovascular status. J Cardiovasc Nurs 23(2):169–74, 2008.

Wyman, JF: Behavioral interventions for the patient with overactive bladder. J Wound, Ostomy Continence Nurs 32(3 Suppl):11–15, 2005.

Wyman, JF: Treatment of urinary incontinence in men and older women: The evidence shows the efficacy of a variety of techniques. Am J Nurs 103(3 Suppl):26–35, 2003.

Wyman, JF, Fantl, JA, McClish, DK, et al: Comparative efficacy of behavioral interventions in the management of female urinary incontinence. Am J Obstet Gynecol 179(4):999, 1998.

Yawn, B, et al: Identification of women's coronary heart disease risk factors prior to first myocardial infarction. J Women's Health 13(10): 1087–96, 2004.

Zimmario, D, et al: Supplementation with dietary fiber improves fecal incontinence. Nurs Res 50(4):203–13, 2001.

Zink, EK, and McQuillan, K: Managing traumatic brain injury. Nursing2005 35(9):36–43, 2005.

Electronic Resources

Aazer, SA. (2005). Constipation in adults. Retrieved January 2007, from http://www.emedicinehealth/com.

Adams, L. (2008). How to deal with adversity. Retrieved February 2009, from http://www.gordontraining.com/How_Do_You_Deal _With_Adversity.html

Adams, L. (no date). Taking personal responsibility. Retrieved February 2009, from http://www.gordontraining.com/Taking_Personal _Responsibility.html

Adams, L. (2006, December). Working together: Climate—The emotional one that is Retrieved March 2007, from http://www .gordontraining.com/pdf/wt-200612-climate-the-emotional-one-that-is.pdf

Adams, L. (no date). Working together: The language of love. Retrieved April 2007, from http://www.gordontraining.com/pdf/wt-200702 -the-language-of-love.pdf

Adams, L. (no date). Working together: Paying attention to children. Retrieved April 2007, from http://www.gordontraining.com/pdf/wt -200603-paying-attention-to-children.pdf

Adams, L. (no date). Working together: The power of P.E.T. Retrieved April 2007, from http://www.gordontraining.com/pdf/wt-200607 -the-power-of-pet.pdf

Agency for Healthcare Research and Quality (AHRQ). (2003). Pharmacologic management of heart failure and left ventricular systolic dysfunction: Effect in female, black, and diabetic patients, and cost-effectiveness. Summary, Evidence Report/Technology Assessment. Rockville, MD. Retrieved March 2009, from http://www.ahrq.gov/ clinic/epcsums/hrtfailsum.htm

Albo, M, and Richter, HE. (2006). Urodynamic testing. Fact sheet for National Kidney and Urologic Diseases Information Clearinghouse. Retrieved May 2007, from http://kidney.niddk.nih.gov/kudiseases/ pubs/urodynamic/index.htm

Allergy testing. (no date). Retrieved February 2007, from http:// www.labtestsonline.com

ALR Technologies, Inc. (no date). Human medication noncompliance. Retrieved April 2007, from http://www.alrt.com/humnonc.html

Amaragiri, SV, and Lees TA (2000). Elastic compression stockings for prevention of deep vein thrombosis. Cochrane Database Syst Rev. CD001484. Retrieved March 2009, from http://www.mrw .inter-science.wiley.com/cochrane/clsysrev/articles/CD001484/ frame.html

American Academy of Clinical Toxicology. (no date). Position statement—Ipecac syrup. Retrieved April 2007, from http://www .clintox.org/Pos_Statements/Ipecac.html

American Academy of Family Physicians. (no date). Breastfeeding, family physicians supporting (Position paper). Retrieved February 2009, from http://www.aafp.org/online/en/home/policy/policies/b/ breastfeedingpositionpaper.html

American Academy of Pediatrics. (Revised 2003, May). Ten steps to support parents' choice to breastfeed their baby. Retrieved February 2007, from http://www.aap.org/breastfeeding/tenSteps.pdf

American Academy of Pediatrics. (2004). Treatment of hyperbilirubinema in the newborn infant 35 or more weeks of gestation. Pediatrics 114(1):297–316. Retrieved February 2009, from http:// aappolicy.aappublications.org/cgi/content/full/pediatrics;114/1/297

American Geriatrics Society Foundation for Health in Aging. (2004). Incontinence. In Eldercare at Home, Chapter 10. Retrieved May

2007, from http://healthinaging.org/public_education/eldercare/10.xml

American Heart Association. (no date). AHA scientific position: Risk factors and coronary heart disease. Retrieved February 2009, from http://www.americanheart.org/presenter.jhtml?identifier=4726

American Heart Association. (no date). AHA scientific position: Smoking cessation, citing 2004 Surgeon General's Report, The Health Consequences of Smoking. Retrieved February 2009, from http://www.americanheart.org/presenter.jhtml?identifier=4731

American Heart Association. (1998). American Heart Association journal report: Researchers discover how cocaine use may cause heart attacks. Retrieved February 2009, from http://www.sciencedaily.com/releases/1998/08/980807104412.htm

American Heart Association. (2009). What is peripheral vascular disease? Retrieved March 2009, from http://www.americanheart.org/presenter.jhtml?identifier=4692

American Pediatric Surgical Association. (no date). Necrotizing enterocolitis (NEC). Adapted from O'Neill, JA, et al: Principles of Pediatric Surgery, ed. 2. Mosby, St Louis, MO, 2003. Retrieved February 2009, from http://www.eapsa.org/parents/resources/NEC.cfm

American Psychological Association. (2004). The road to resilience. Retrieved February 2009, from http://apahelpcenter.org/featuredtopics/feature.php?id=6&ch;=1

American Society of Health-System Pharmacists Fact Sheet. (no date). Medications and you. Retrieved January 2007, from http://www.safemedication.com

American Speech-Language-Hearing Association (ASHA). (no date). Noise. Information sheet. Retrieved June 2003, from http://www.asha.org

American Speech-Language-Hearing Association (ASHA). (no date). Questions/answers about voice problems. Information sheet. Retrieved June 2003, from http://www.asha.org

American Speech-Language-Hearing Association (ASHA). (no date). Speech for clients with tracheostomies or ventilators. Information sheet. Retrieved June 2003, from http://www.asha.org

American Speech-Language-Hearing Association (ASHA). (no date). What is language? What is speech? Information sheet. Retrieved August 2003, from http://www.asha.org/public/speech/development

Amitai, A, and Sinert, D. (2006). Ventilator management. Retrieved May 2007, from http://www.emedicine.com/emerg/topic788.htm

Arnold, JL. (2006). Personal protective equipment. Article for patient education, eMedicineHealth Web site. Retrieved February 2007, from http://www.emedicinehealth.com

Assertiveness Training. (no date). Retrieved April 2007, from http://www.csusm.edu/caps/Assertiveness.html

Ballas, P. (2006). Sexual problems overview. Retrieved May 2007, from MedlinePlus at http://www.nlm.nih.gov/medlineplus/ency/article/001951.htm

Barclay, L. (2009). Hospital-supervised exercise may prevent need for surgery in patients with claudication. Retrieved March 2009, from http://cme.medscape.com/viewarticle/587997

Barclay, L, and Lie, D. (2007). New guidelines issued for family support in patient-centered ICU. CME/CE for Medscape Web site.

Retrieved February 2009, from http://www.medscape/viewarticle/551738

Barclay, L, and Vega, C. (2009). Severe adverse effects of smoking may be reversible if mothers quit early in pregnancy. Retrieved April 2009, from http://cme.medscape.com/viewarticle/590543?src=cmemp

Bates, B. (2007, February 15). Simple questions can help uncover urinary incontinence. Family Practice News. Retrieved May 2007, from http://www.highbeam.com/

Beckett, C. (2000). Family theory as a framework for assessment. Retrieved April 2007, from http://jan.ucc.nau.edu/~nur350-c/class/2_family/theory/lesson2-1-3.html

Behrman, AJ, and Howarth, M. (2005). Latex allergy. Retrieved February 2007 from http://www.emedicine.com/emerg/topic814.htm

Beland, N. (2005, April/May). Special report: The pursuit of happiness. Women's Health. Retrieved April 2007, from http://womenshealthmag.com/article/0,6176,s1-3-72-111-2,00.html

Berczi, I. (1994). Stress and disease: The contributions of Hans Selye to neuroimmunology, in Advances in Psychoneuroimmunology. Plenum Press, New York, pp 1-15. Retrieved March 2009, from http://home.cc.umanitoba.ca/~berczii/page2.htm

Boyles, S. (2005). Hope for people stuck in grief. Article for WebMD. Retrieved March 2007, from http://www.webmd.com/depression/news/20050531/

Boyles, S. (2005). Spouse caregivers most likely to be abusive. Retrieved February 2007 from http://www.webmd.com/content/Article/100/105831.htm

Brain Trauma Foundation, Inc. (2007). American Association of Neurological Surgeons. Guidelines for the management of severe traumatic brain injury: Blood pressure and oxygenation. Retrieved March 2009, from http://www.guideline.gov

Brandler, ES, Sinert, R, and Hostetler, MA. (2006). Shock, cardiogenic. Retrieved January 2007, from http://www.emedicine.com/emerg/topic530.htm

Breastfeeding guidelines following radiopharmaceutical administration. (no date). Retrieved February 2007, from http://nuclearpharmacy.uams.edu/resources/breastfeeding.asp

Breazeale, T. (2007). Attachment parenting: A practical approach for the reduction of attachment disorders and the promotion of emotionally secure children. A master's thesis submitted to the Faculty of Bethel College. Retrieved February 2007, from http://www.visi.com/~jib/thesis.html

Bridges, LJ, and Moore, KA. (2002, September). Religious involvement and children's well-being: What research tells us (and what it doesn't), Child Trends Research Brief. Child Trends Data Bank, Washington, DC. Retrieved from http://www.childstrendsdatabank.org/Files/religiosityRB.pdf

Brown, SE. (2009). Bone health: The calcium myth. Retrieved January 2009, from http://www.womentowomen.com/bonehealth/calciummyth.aspx

Buck, ML. (1998). Treatment of intravenous extravasations. Adapted from Pediatric Pharm 4(1). Retrieved March 2009, from http://www.medscape.com/viewarticle/416651/

Buse, JB. (2003). Normal A1C but unstable blood glucose. Article for Medscape Diabetes and Endocrinology site. Retrieved January 2007, from http://www.medscape.com/viewarticle/46302

Callen, J, and Pinelli, J. (2005). A review of the literature examining the benefits and challenges, incidence and duration, and barriers to breastfeeding in preterm infants. Adv Neonatal Care 5(2):72–88. Retrieved February 2007, from http://www.medscape.com/viewarticle/502591

Calver, P, Braungardt, T, Kupchik, N, et al. (2005). The big chill: Improving the odds after cardiac arrest. CE Home Study Program for RNweb. Retrieved March 2007, from http://www.rnweb.com

Campagnolo, DI. (2006). Autonomic dysreflexia in spinal cord injury. Retrieved January 2007, from http://www.emedicine.com

Canadian Paediatric Society. (2007). Position statement. Guidelines for detection, management and prevention of hyperbilirubinemia in term and late preterm newborn infants (35 or more weeks' gestation). Paediatr Child Health 12(Suppl B):1B–12B. Retrieved March 2009, from http://www.cps.ca/english/statements/FN/FN07-02.pdf

Carls, C. (2007). The prevalence of stress urinary incontinence in high school and college-age female athletes in the Midwest: Implications for education and prevention. Urol Nurs 27(1):21–24, 39. Retrieved May 2007, from http://www.medscape.com/viewarticle/555700?src=mp

Center for Ethics and Advocacy in Healthcare. (no date). Retrieved March, 2007 from http://www.healthcare-ethics.org/about/

Centers for Disease Control and Prevention. (2003). What would happen if we stopped vaccinations? Fact sheet for National Immunization Program. Retrieved March 2007, from http://www.cdc.gov/nip

Centers for Disease Control and Prevention. (2006, August). When should a mother avoid breastfeeding. Retrieved February 2007, from http://www.cdc.gov/breastfeeding/disease/contraindicators.htm

Centers for Disease Control and Prevention. (2006). Adult immunization schedule. Fact sheet for National Immunization Program. Retrieved March 2007, from http://www.cdc.gov/nip

Centers for Disease Control and Prevention. (2008). STDs & pregnancy. CDC fact sheet. Retrieved March 2009, from http://www.cdc.gov/std/STDFact-STDs&Pregnancy.htm

Centers for Disease Control and Prevention. (reviewed 2009). Violence and reproductive health. Retrieved April 2009, from http://www.cdc.gov/reproductivehealth/violence/index.htm

Champion Aspirations for Human Dignity. (no date). The White House. Retrieved March 2007, from http://www.whitehouse.gov/nsc/nss2.html

Cheshire, Jr. WP. (2007). Grey matters when eloquence is inarticulate. An article for Ethics & Medicine: An International Journal of Bioethics 22(3). Retrieved March 2007, at the Center for Bioethics Human Dignity, from http://www.cbhd.org/resources/neuroethics/cheshire_2007-01-26.htm

Child Trends Data Bank. (no date). Religiosity. Retrieved November 2005, from http://www.childrtrendsdatabank.org

Children's Hospital Boston. (no date). Fact sheet, Poisons. Retrieved April 2007, from http://www.childrenshospital.org/az/Site868

Clinical Manual for Management of the HIV-infected Adult, 2006 ed. Section 3: Antiretroviral therapy adherence, pp 3–11. Retrieved

April 2007, from http://www.aidsetc.org/aetc/pdf/AETC-CM
_092206.pdf

Cody, T, and Zieroff, V. (2005). Autonomic dysreflexia. Fact sheet for Northeast Rehabilitation Health Network. Retrieved January 2007, from http://www.northeastrehab.com

Connecticut Poison Control Center. (no date). Fact sheet about poisons. Retrieved March 2007, from http://www.poisoncontrol.uchc.edu/ poisons/medications.htm

Cooper, S. (no date). Sylvia's inquiry into violence and the brain. Retrieved May 2007, from http://serendip.brynmawr.edu/local/suminst/ bbi01/projects/cooper/

Counseling Center at University of Illinois Urbana–Champaign. (no date). Self-help brochures: Assertiveness. Retrieved April 2007, from http://www.couns.uiuc.edu/Brochures/assertiv.htm

Cultural awareness self concept. (no date). Retrieved April 2007, from http://academic.cuesta.edu/atorrey/culture.pdf

Cunha, JP, and Shiel, WC. (2007). Medical shock. Retrieved March 2009, from http://www.medicinenet.com/shock/article.htm

Darby, F, and Brown, D. (2003). Nice work if you can get it. Retrieved April 2007, from http://www.pocket-stress.com/articles/nice %20work.php

Davis, JL. (2006). New type 2 diabetes treatment options. Retrieved January 2007, at http://www.webmd.com/content/Article/129/ 117304.htm

Davis, N. (2003). (Short online summaries from): Multi-Sensory Trauma Processing, A Manual for Understanding and Treating PTSD and Job-Related Trauma. Retrieved April 2007, from http:// www.rescue-workers.com/1.htm

dbS Productions. (2000–2007). Alzheimer's disease and related disorders SAR research: Wandering overview. Excerpt from book in progress available at Source of Search & Rescue Research, Publications and Training. http://www.dbs-sar.com/SAR_Research/ wandering.htm

De Broe, ME. (1999). Renal injury due to environmental toxins, drugs, and contrast agents. In Berl, T, and Bonventre, JV: Atlas of Diseases of the Kidney, Vol. 1, Chap. 12. Retrieved March 2009, from http://www.kidneyatlas.org/book1/adk1_11.pdf

de Graef, A, Kyper, MB, and Hesselmann, GM. (2006). Nausea and vomiting. National Guideline Clearinghouse. Retrieved January 2009, from http://www.guideline.gov

DeNoon, D. (2006). C. Diff: New threat from old bug: Epidemic gut infection causing rapid rise in life-threatening disease. Retrieved February 2007, from http://www.medicinenet.com

Deshpande, PG. (2008 update). Breast milk jaundice. Retrieved March 2009, from http://emedicine.medscape.com/article/973629-overview

Dharan, VB, and Parvianen, ELK. (2009). Psychosocial and environmental pregnancy risks. Retrieved March 2009, from http://emedicine.medscape.com/article/259346-overview

Diego, R. (2003). Man in denial. Retrieved February 2007, from http://www.insmkt.com/myhome.htm

Dion, R. (2005). Overcoming relocation stress. Article provided by Military OneSource, PTSD Support Services. Retrieved April 2007, from http://www.ptsdsupport.net/relocation_stress.html

Dire, DJ. (2005). Biological warfare. Article for patient education, eMedicineHealth Web site. Retrieved February 2007, from http://www.emedicinehealth.com

Diskin, A. (2006). Gastroenteritis. Retrieved February 2007, from http://www.emedicine.com/emerg/topic213.htm

Diversional therapy. (2006). Article for the Diversional Therapy Association of New South Wales. Retrieved February 2007, from http://www/diversionaltherapy.com.au

Doheny, K. (2006). Adults with children at home consume more fat, study shows. Article for WebMD Medical News. Retrieved January 2007, from http://www.webmd.com/content/Article/131/117923.htm

Dowshen, S. (2005). Kids and dangerous "suffocation games." Article for KidsHealth Web site. Retrieved April 2007, from http://www.kidshealth.org/research/suffocation.html

Dunai, J. (2003). Assessment of unilateral neglect (update). (Patient behavior pattern after stroke). Article for HighBeam Research. Retrieved December 2006, from http://www.highbeam.com/

Eby, N, and Car, M. (2004, Spring). Violence and brain injuries. Quality Matters. Retrieved May 2007, at Brain Injury Association of Montana, from http://www.biamt.org/publications/violence.htm

Editorial staff. (2006): Fitness at any age. Article for MedicineNet Web site. Retrieved March 2007, from http://www.medicinenet.com

Ehrenberg, HM (2009): Maternal obesity, uterine activity, and the risk of spontaneous preterm birth. Obstet & Gynecol 113(1):48–52. Retrieved March 2009, from http://www.ncbi.nlm.nih.gov/pubmed/19104359

Ellis, A. (1994 update). Showing people, they are not worthless individuals. Voices: The Art and Science of Psychotherapy, 1(2):74–77, 1965. Retrieved March 2009, from http://www.geocities.com/rebtus/worthless.html

Enslein, J, et al. (2002). Evidence-based protocol. Interpreter facilitation for persons with limited English proficiency. University of Iowa Gerontological Nursing Interventions Research Center. Retrieved from National Guidelines Clearinghouse, June 2003, from http://www.guideline.gov.

Evans, M. (no date). Loneliness. Self-Help Information Counseling and Testing Center, University of Oregon Counseling Center. Retrieved March 2007, from http://darkwing.uoregon.edu/~counsel/loneliness.htm

Ferry, RJ, and Shim, M. (2006). Gigantism and acromegaly. Retrieved March 2007, from http://www.emedicine.com/ped/toipic2634.htm

Finch, Alison. (2007). Fed up with feeling alone? Self-esteem eZine "Touching Half the World." Retrieved February 2007, from http://www.selfesteem4women.com

Focus Adolescent Services. (2000). Self-injury. Retrieved April 2007, from http://www.focusas.com/SelfInjury.html

Fong, T. (2002). Acetaminophen (Tylenol) liver damage. Retrieved December 2006, from http://www.medicinenet.com

Forrette, TL. (2006). Transitioning from mechanical ventilation. CE article for Medscape Web site. Retrieved May 2007, from http://www.medscape.com/viewprogram/5230_pnt

Frey, R. (2006, December). Self-mutilation. Gale Encyclopedia of Medicine. Retrieved April 2007, from http://www.healthatoz

.com/healthatoz/Atoz/common/standard/transform.jsp?requestURI=/
healthatoz/Atoz/ency/self-mutilation.jsp

Fulmer, T. (2003). Elder abuse and neglect assessment. Gerontal Nurs
29(1):8–9. Retrieved March 2009, from http://www.hartfordign.org/
uploads/File/Fulmer_EM_EAL_Short_Printable.pdf

Fulop, T, et al. (2007 update). Hypomagnesemia. Retrieved January
2009, from http://emedicine.medscape.com/article/246366-overview

Gardner, BM. (2002). Current approaches to type 2 diabetes mellitus.
Article for Medscape CME. American Academy of Family Physicians (AAFP) 2002 Annual Scientific Assembly Common Clinical
Problem Update and Family Medicine Research. Retrieved December 2006, from http://www.medscape.com/viewarticle/444348

Gettinger-Dinner, L. (2007). Suicide risk assessment: What providers
need to know. Retrieved May 2007, from http://news.nurse.com/
apps/pbcs.dll/article?AID=/20070430/CA09/
304300012&SearchID=73281745058190

Gibson, P, and Carson, MP. (2007). Hypertension and pregnancy. Retrieved March 2009, from http://emedicine.medscape.com/article/
261435-overview

Gisbert, JP. (2004). H. pylori eradication therapy vs. antisecretory non-
eradication therapy (with or without long-term maintenance antisecretory therapy) for the prevention of recurrent bleeding from peptic
ulcer. Retrieved March 2009, from http://www.cochrane.org/
reviews/en/ab004062.html

Gladwell, M. (2006). Blink, snap decision making. Retrieved February
2007, from http://www.talentsmart.com

Goldstein, S. (no date). Risk, resilience and futurists: Changing the
lives of our children. Retrieved 2009, from http://www
.raisingresilientkids.com/resources/articles/futurists.html

Goleman, D. (1995, October 3). Early violence leaves its mark on the
brain. New York Times. Retrieved May 2007, from http://www.cirp
.org/library/psych/goleman/

Gordon Training International. (no date). Retrieved April 2007, at
newsletter@gordontraining.com

Gore, TA, and Richards-Reid, GM. (2006). Posttraumatic stress disorder. Retrieved April 2007, from http://www.emedicine.com/med/
topic1900.htm

Gourley, GR, et al. (2005). A controlled, randomized, double-blind trial
of prophylaxis against jaundice among breastfed newborns. Pediatr
116(2):385–91. Retrieved March 2009, from http://pediatrics
.aappublications.org/cgi/reprint/116/2/385

Grenz, K, Bynum, G, Pine, D. et al. (update version 2005). Preventive
services for children and adolescents. Institute for Clinical Systems
Improvement [ICSI]. Article for National Guideline Clearinghouse.
Web site. Retrieved February 2007, from http://www.guideline.gov.

Haines, C. (2005). Heart failure: Recognizing caregiver burnout. Retrieved February 2007, from http://www.webmd.com/content/
Article/51/40695.htm

Haines, C. (2006). Diabetes: Treating diabetes with insulin. Retrieved
January 2007, from http://www.webmd.com/content/Article/46/
1667_50931.htm

Haines, C. (2006). Digestive diseases: Swallowing problems. Retrieved
April 2007, from http://www.medicinetnet.com/swallowing/

Haines, C. (2006). Learning about allergies to latex. Retrieved February 2007, from http://www.webmd.com/content/pages/10/1625.htm

Hallenbeck, J, and Weissman, D. (2007). Treatment of nausea and vomiting. Retrieved April 2007, from http://www.jasonprogram.org/nausea_treatment.htm

Harvard Health Publications. (2007). Coping with anxiety and phobias. Retrieved January 2007, from http://www.health.harvard.edu/special_health_reports/Coping_with_Anxiety_and_Phobias.htm

Hansen, TWR. (2007 update). Neonatal jaundice. Retrieved March 2009, from http://emedicine.medscape.com/article/974786-overview

Headsets911. (no date). Actively cope with stress. Retrieved March 2007, from http://www.headsets911.com/activecoping.htm

Healthcommunities.com, Inc. (2003). Female sexual dysfunction: Overview, incidence, female sexual response. Retrieved May 2007, from http://www.womenshealthchannel.com/fsd/index.shtml

Health Resources, Services Administration (HRSA) Maternal, and Child Health Bureau. (no date). What is SIDS? Public information of the National SIDS/Infant Death Resource Center. Retrieved February 2007, from http://www.hrsa.gov

Health Sciences Centre. (2007). Suffocation. Fact sheet for IMPACT Web site. Retrieved April 2007, from http://www.hsc.mb.ca/impact/suffocation.htm

Hertz, G, and Cataletto, ME. (2006). Sleep dysfunction in women. Retrieved December 2006, from http://www.emedicine.com/med/topic656.htm

Hingley, AT. (2007). Preventing accidental poisoning. Article for Pregnancy Weekly Web site. Retrieved April 2007, from http://www.pregnancyweekly.com

Hobdell, E. (2004). Chronic sorrow and depression in parents of children with neural tube defects. J Neurosci Nurs 36(2):82–88, 94. Retrieved May 2007, from http://www.medscape.com/viewarticle/474596_1

Hollister, WG, and Edgerton, JW. (1974). Teaching relationship building skills. Am J Public Health 64(1):41–46. Retrieved March 2009, at http://www.pubmedcentral.nih.gov/articlerender.fcgi?artid=1775361

Holson, D, and Gathers, S. (2006). Constipation. Retrieved January 2007, from http://www.emedicine.com/emerg/topic111.htm

Homeir, BP. (2004). Household safety: Preventing suffocation. Article for KidsHealth Web site. Retrieved April 2007, from http://www.kidshealth.org/parent/positive/family/safety_suffocation.html

Hope for Today Al-Anon Group. (no date). Available at http://health.groups.yahoo.com/group/HopeForTodayGroup/

Hoppe, J, and Sinert, R. (2006). Heat exhaustion and heatstroke. Retrieved March 2007, from http://www.emedicine.com/emert/topic236.htm

Hopper, J. (2008 update). Mindfulness and kindness, inner sources of freedom and happiness. Retrieved March 2009, from http://www.jimhopper.com/mindfulness/

Hospital and Palliative Nurses Association. (2005). Spiritual distress. Patient/Family Teaching Sheets. Retrieved May 2007, from http://www.hpna.org/pdf/PatientSheet_SpiritualDistress.pdf

House, J. (2001). Social isolation kills, but how and why? Psychosom Med 63:273–74. Retrieved May 2007, from http://www.psychosomaticmedicine.org/cgi/content/full/63/2/273

Hubbynet. (2000). Coping with stress. (2000). Retrieved March 2007, from http://www.hubbynet.com/stresscoping,htm

Hyman, SE. (1998). Thinking about violence in our schools, Discussion at the White House. National Institute of Mental Health. Retrieved May 2007, from http://www.medhelp.org/NIHlib/GF-376.html

Institute of Medicine. (2006). Preterm birth: Causes, consequences, and prevention. Retrieved April 2009, from http://books.nap.edu/openbook.php?record_id=11622=R1

International Lactation Consultant Association. (1999, April). Evidenced-based guidelines for breastfeeding management during the first fourteen days. Retrieved February 2007, from http://www.ilca.org/pubs/ebg.pdf

Jacobs, DH. (2005). Aphasia. Retrieved February 2007, from http://www.emedicine.com/NEURO/topic437.htm

Jacobs, DH. (2006). Confusional states and acute memory disorders. Retrieved January 2007, from http://www.emedicine.com/neuro/topic435.htm.

Jagminas, L. (2005). CBRN—Evaluation of a biological warfare victim. Retrieved February 2007, from http://www.emedicine.com/emerg/topic891.htm

Jagminas, L, and Erdman, DP. (2006). CBRNE—Chemical decontamination. Retrieved February 2007, from http://www.emedicine.com/emerg/topic893.htm

Johns Hopkins Vasculitis Center. (no date). Buerger's disease. Retrieved March 2009, from http://vasculitis.med.jhu.edu/typesof/buergers.html

Kanaparthi, LK, and Lessnau, KD. (2009). Shock, distributive. Retrieved March 2009, from http://emedicine.medscape.com/article/168689/

Kater, K. (2006). Building healthy body esteem in a body toxic world. Retrieved April 2007, from http://www.BodyImageHealth.org

Kearl's Guide to the Sociology of the Family. (no date). Marriage and family processes. Retrieved April 2007, at http://www.trinity.edu/~mkearl/family.html

Kearney, P. (updated 2006). Chronic grief (or is it periodic grief?) Grief in a family context. Retrieved May 2007, from http://www.indiana.edu/~famlygrf/units/chronic.html

Keepnews, D, and Mitchell, PH. (2003). Health systems' accountability for patient safety. Online Journal of Issues in Nursing, 8(2). Manuscript 2. Retrieved March 2007, from http://nursingworld.org/ojin/topic22/tpc22_2.htm

Keim, SM, and Kent, M. (2005). Nausea and vomiting. Retrieved April 2007, from http://www.emedicinehealth.com/vomiting_and_nausea/article_em.htm

Kemp, S, and Gungor, N. (2005). Growth failure. Retrieved March 2007, from http://www.emedicine.com/ped/topic902.htm

Klimes, R. (2007). Managing stress: Living without stress overload. CE offering for LearnWell.org Web site. Retrieved April 2007, from http://www.learnwell.org/stress.htm

Kolcaba, K. (2006). FAQs (frequently asked questions). On the Comfort Line. Web site devoted to the concept of comfort in nursing.

Retrieved February 2009, from http://www.thecomfortline.com/FAQ.htm

Lafreniere, R, Berguer, R, Seifert, PC, et al. (2005). Preparation of the operating room. Retrieved March 2007, from http://www.medscape.com/viewarticle/503004

Lamemeh, T, Shah, AM, and Hsu, K. (2006). Anxiety. Retrieved January 2007, from http://www.emedicine.com/emerg/topic35.htm

Lashley, FR. (2006). Emerging infectious diseases at the beginning of the 21st century. Online Journal of Issues in Nursing, 11(1). Retrieved March 2007, from http://www.nursingworld.org.ojin/topic 29_1.htm

Lauer, T. (no date). Rape trauma. American Association for Marriage and Family Therapy Consumer Update. Retrieved April 2007, from http://www.aamft.org/families/Consumer_Updates/RapeTrauma.asp

Lawrence, S. (2005). When health fears are overblown. Article for WebMD Health and Balance feature stories. Retrieved February 2007, from http://www.webmd.com/balance/features

Lederer, E, et al. (2008 update). Hyperkalemia. Retrieved January 2009, from http://emedicine.medscape.com/article/240903-overview

Lederer, E, Ouseph, R, and Yazel, L. (2007 update). Hypokalemia. Retrieved January 2009, from http://emedicine.medscape.com/article/242008-overview

Lehrer, JK. (2006). Bowel incontinence. Article for MedlinePlus, a service of National Library of Medicine and National Institutes of Health. Retrieved January 2007, from http://www.nlm.nih.gov/medlineplus.

Li, J, and Decker, W. (2005). Hypothermia. Retrieved March 2007, from http://www.emedicine.com/emerg/topic279.htm

Lien, CA. (no date). Thermoregulation in the elderly. Syllabus on Geriatric Anesthesiology. American Society of Anesthesiologists Web site. Retrieved January 2007, from http://www.asahq.org/clinical/geriatrics/thermo.htm

Llewellyn-Thomas, H (2004). Helping patients make health care decisions. Center for the Evaluative Clinical Sciences, Dartmouth Medical School. Retrieved March 2007, from http://www.dartmouthatlas.org

Lubit, R. (2005). Acute treatment of disaster survivors. Retrieved March 2007, from http://www.emedicine.com/med/topic3540.htm

Lyons, SS, and Specht, JKP. (1999). Prompted voiding for persons with urinary\incontinence. University of Iowa Gerontological Nursing Interventions Research Center Web site. Retrieved from the National Guidelines Clearinghouse [NGC: 950], June 2003, from http://www.guideline.gov

Male Sexual Health. (2005). Retrieved May 2007, from http://www.moderntherapy.com/male/sexual-health.html

Marano, HE. (2003). Procrastination: Ten things to know. Retrieved March 2009, from http://www.psychologytoday.com/rss/pto-2003 0823-000001.html

March of Dimes. (2006). Fact sheets: Illicit drug use during pregnancy. Retrieved March 2009, from http://www.marchofdimes.com/professionals/14332_1169.asp

March of Dimes. (no date). Work and pregnancy. Retrieved April 2009, from http://www.marchofdimes.com/pnhec/159_11488.asp

Marks, JW. (2006). Constipation. Retrieved January 2007, from http://www.medicinenet.com.

Marks, JW, and Lee, D. (2004). Diarrhea. Retrieved February 2007, from http://www.medicinenet.com

Mathur, R. (2007). Obesity. Retrieved April 2007, from http://www.medicinenet.com

Mayo Clinic—Rochester. (2006, April 4). Mild cognitive impairment prevalent in elderly population: Risk increases as age goes up and education goes down. Retrieved January 2007, from http://www.mayoclinic.org/news2006-rst/3306.html

Mayo Clinic Staff. (2005). Alzheimer's: Understand and control wandering. Retrieved May 2007, from http://www.mayoclinic.com/health/alzheimers/HQ00218

Mayo Clinic Staff. (2007). Childbirth education: Get ready for labor and delivery. Retrieved April 2009, from http://www.mayoclinic.com/health/pregnancy/PR00119

Mayo Clinic Staff. (2007). Dehydration. Retrieved February 2007, from http://www.mayoclinic.com/health/dehydration/DS0056/DSECTION=1

McElgunn, V. (1990). Environmental hazards and child health and development: Advances in research and policy. Presentation in the Linking Research to Practice: Second Canadian Forum Proceedings Report; published by the Canadian Child Care Federation. Retrieved February 2007, from http://www.cfc-efc.ca/cccf

McPherson, M, Smith-Lovin, L, and Brashears, M. (2006, June). Social isolation in US: Changes in core discussion networks over two decades. American Sociological Review, 71:353–75. Retrieved May 2007, from http://www.asanet.org/galleries/default-file/June06ASRFeature.pdf

Meadows, M. (2006). Nutrition: Healthy eating. Retrieved April 2007, from http://www.medicinenet.com

Menna, A. (no date). Rape trauma syndrome: The journey to healing belongs to everyone. Retrieved April 2007, from http://www.giftfromwithin.org/html/journey.html

Messina, J, and Messina, C. (no date). Tools for coping with life's stressors. Retrieved March 2007, from http://www.coping.org/control/manipul.htm

Miller, L, et al (1999). Religiosity as a protective factor in depressive disorder. Am J Psychiatry 156:808A–809. Retrieved January 2007, from http://ajp.psychiatryonline.org

Mills, J. (2006). The ontology of religiosity: The oceanic feeling and the value of the lived experience. HUUmanists. Retrieved April 2007, from http://www.huumanists.org/rh/mills.html

Moore, A. (2008). Hedonism. The Stanford Encyclopedia of Philosophy (Fall 2008 ed.), Edward N Zalta (ed). Retrieved March 2009, from http://plato.stanford.edu/archives/fall2008/entries/hedonism

Morrissey, P. (2005). Noncompliance after transplantation. A newsletter from the transplant team at Rhode Island Hospital. Retrieved March 2007, from http://www.lifespan.org/rih/services/transplant/news/02-07.htm

Moses, S. (2008). Unna's boot. Family Practice Notebook. Retrieved March 2009, from http://www.fpnotebook.com/Surgery/Pharm/UnsBt.htm

Muche, JA, and McCarty, S. (2006). Geriatric rehabilitation. Retrieved April 2007, from http://www.emedicine.com/pmr/topic164.htm

Muller, C (1996): Dealing with the modern crisis of religiosity: Reflections from the Aum case. Retrieved from http://www.hm.tyg.jp/~acmuller/articles/dayori1.htm

Murry, M (2008). What is a birth plan and why do I need one? Retrieved April 2009, from http://www.mayoclinic.com/health/birth-plan/MY00052

National Ag Safety Database (NASD). (2002). Sleep deprivation: Cause and consequences. Fact sheet for Nebraska Rural Health and Safety Coalition. Retrieved January 2007, from http://www.cdc.gov.nasd/

National Center on Elder Abuse, Administration on Aging. (Updated 2007). Self-neglect: An update of the literature, 2000–2005. Retrieved March 2009, from http://www.ncea.aoa.gov/NCEAroot/Main_Site/Library/CANE/CANE_Series/CANE_Selfneglectupdate.aspx

National Coalition for Cancer Survivors. (no date). Palliative care & management: Nausea & vomiting. Retrieved April 2007, from http://www.canceradvocacy.org/resources/essential/effects/nausea.aspx

National Comprehensive Cancer Network. (2005). Nausea and vomiting: Treatment guidelines for patients with cancer. Vol 3. Retrieved April 2007, from http://www.cancer.org/downloads/CRI/NCCN_Nausea.pdf

National Guideline Clearinghouse (AHRQ). (2003, June). Management of breastfeeding for healthy full term infants. Retrieved February 2007, from http://www.guideline.gov/summary/summary.aspx?view_id=1&doc_id=3624

National Heart, Lung, and Blood Institute. (2008). Rh incompatibility. Retrieved April 2009, from http://www.nhlbi.nih.gov/health/dci/Diseases/rh/rh_what.html

National Institute of Aging (1996, August). Exercise can boost cardiac fitness in conditioned and out of shape people. Public information article. Retrieved July 2005, from http://www.nia.nih.gov

National Institute of Child Health and Human Development. (2006). High-risk pregnancy. Retrieved March 2009, from http://www.nichd.nih.gov/health/topics/high_risk_pregnancy.cfm

National Institute of Child Health and Human Development. (2009). Care before and during pregnancy—Prenatal care. Retrieved March 2009, from http://www.nichd.nih.gov/womenshealth/research/pregbirth/prenatal_care.cfm

National Institute on Deafness and Other Communication Disorders (NIDCD). (2006). Strategic plan: Plain language version FY 2003–2005. Retrieved April 2007, from http://www.nidcd.nih/

National Institute of Neurological Disorders and Stroke (NINDS). (2007 update). Brain basics. Understanding sleep. Retrieved March 2009, from http://www.ninds.nih.gov/disorders/brain_basics/understanding_sleep.htm

National Institute of Neurological Disorders and Stroke (NINDS). (2007). Swallowing disorders information page. Retrieved April 2007, from http://www.ninds.nih.gov/

National Stroke Association (NSA). (2009 update). Various public information monographs regarding stroke risk reduction. Retrieved March 2009, from http://www.stroke.org/site/PageServer ?pagename=RISKRED

National Women's Health Resource Center Fact Sheet. (2005). Medication safety. Retrieved April 2007, from http://www .healthywomen.org

Nauert, R. (2007). Coke and speed increase risk of stroke. Article reporting result of study at UT Southwestern. Retrieved March 2009, from http://psychcentral.com/news/2007/04/05/coke-and-speed -increase-stroke-risk

Newman, DK. (2006). Using the BladderScan for bladder volume assessment. Retrieved May 2007, from http://www.seekwellness.com/ incontinence/using_the_bladderscan.htm

Newton, E. (2005). Hyperventilation syndrome. Retrieved January 2007, from http://www.emedicine.com/emerg/topic270.htm.

No author listed. (no date). Anticipatory grief. Featured columns under Life Topics/Grief & Loss for Psychologist 4therapy web site. Retrieved March 2007, from http://www.4therapy.com

No author listed. (no date). The development of social skills. Retrieved May 2007, from http://www.incrediblehorizons.com/ socialskills.htm

No author listed. (no date). Health maintenance evaluation: Replacing the "annual physical." Fact sheet for Palo Alto Medical Foundation website. Retrieved March 2007, from http://www.pamf.org/children/ maintenance/healtheval.html

No author listed. (no date). Monitoring diabetes control. Diabetes Manual. Royal Children's Hospital. Retrieved January 2007, from http://www.rch.org.au/diabetesmanual.cfm

No author listed. (no date). Older Americans Month. Food & nutrition information. American Dietetic Association Web site. Retrieved June 2003, from http://www.eatright.org/Public/Nutritioninformation/ 92_12402.cfm

No author listed. (no date). Overview: Intra-abdominal hypertension and abdominal compartment syndrome. Retrieved February 2009, from http://www.abdominalcompartmentsyndrome.org

No author listed. (no date). Sometimes grief becomes complicated, unresolved or stuck. Featured columns under Life Topics/Grief & Loss for Psychologist 4therapy Web site. Retrieved March 2007, from http://www.4therapy.com

No author listed. (no date). Symptom: Walking symptoms. Retrieved May 2007, from http://wrongdiagnosis.com/sym/walking _symptoms.htm

No author listed. (1990, April 1). Bag the brown paper bag. (Bag rebreathing as a treatment for hyperventilation.) Newsletter—People's Medical Society. Retrieved January 2007, from http:// www.highbeam.com/doc/1G1-9094801.html

No author listed. (1999). Chemical toxins safety. Fact sheet for Resources for Child Care Givers. All Family Resources Web site. Retrieved February 2007, from http://familymanagement.com/ childcare/facility/chemical.toxins.safety.html

No author listed. (2000–2004). Diabetes and healthy eating. Better Health Channel Fact Sheet, Victoria, Australia. Retrieved January 2007, from http://www.betterhealth.vic.gov.au

No author listed. (2005). Hyperthermia: Too hot for your health. Article for National Institute on Aging Web site. Retrieved March 2007, from http://www.niapublications/org/agepages/hyperther.asp

No author listed. (2005). Liver blood enzymes. Retrieved December 2006, from http://www.medicinenet.com

No author listed. (2006). Oral cancer. Retrieved April 2007, from http://www.medicinenet.com

No author listed. (2007). The causes, effects and dangers of sleep deprivation. Article for Sleep Deprivation Web site. Retrieved April 2007, from http://www.sleep-deprivation.com/

No author listed. (Updated 2007). Tooth decay—Prevention. Article for WebMD health topics Web site. Retrieved September 2009, from http://www.webmd.com/oral-health/tc/tooth-decay-prevention

No author listed. (1995–2007). Urinary incontinence. The Merck Manual of Health & Aging (online), Section 3, Chap. 57. Retrieved May 2007, from http://www.merck.com/pubs/mmanual_ha/sec3/ch57/ch57a.html

Novello, NP, and Blumstein, HA. (2007 update). Hypermagnesemia. Retrieved January 2009, from http://emedicine.medscape.com/article/7666604-overview

Null, J. (2007). Hyperthermia deaths of children in vehicles. Fact sheet for San Francisco State University department of Geosciences Web site. Retrieved March 2007, from http://ggweather.com/heat/

Olade, R, Safi, A, and Kesari, S. (2006). Cardiac catheterization (left heart). Retrieved January 2007 from http://www.emedicine.com/emerg/topic2958,htm

Olson, ET. (Revised 2008). Personal identity. Stanford Encyclopedia of Philosophy. Retrieved September 2009, from http://plato.stanford.edu/entries/identity-personal/

Oncology Nursing Society (ONS). (2004). Access device guidelines: Recommendations for nursing practice and education, ed. 2. ONS, Pittsburgh, PA. Retrieved March 2009, from http://www.guideline.gov/summary/summary.aspx?ss=15&doc_id=8338&nbr;=4666

Oommen, K. (2006). Neurological history and physical examination. Retrieved April 2007, from http://www.emedicine.com/neuro/topic632.htm

Owens, TA. (2005). Medical Encyclopedia: Delayed growth. Retrieved March 2007, from http://nim.nih.gov/medlineplus/ency/aritcle/003021.htm

Palmer, RM. (2006). Management of common clinical disorders in geriatric patients: Delirium. Retrieved May 2007, from http://www.medscape.com/viewarticle/53466

Panzera, AK. (2007). Interstitial cystitis/painful bladder syndrome. Urol Nurs 27(1):13–19. Retrieved May 2007, from http://www.medscape.com/viewarticle/555699?src=mp

Pasley, J. (2004). Introduction to gastrointestinal physiology. University of Arkansas Medical School Lecture. Retrieved February 2009, from http://www.uams.edu/m2008/notes/phys/pdf/April%2016%20Intro%20to%20GI%20Phys.pdf

Paula, R (2006). Compartment syndrome, abdominal. Retrieved April 2009, from http://www.emedicine.medscape.com/article/829008

Planned Parenthood. (2006). Sexual health—Sexuality. Retrieved May 2007, from http://plannedparenthood.org/sexual-health/sexual-health-relationship/sexuality.htm

Pham, TQ. (2007 update). Hypernatremia. Retrieved January 2009, from http://emedicine.medscape.com/article/241094-overview

Pickhardt, C. (no date). Role conflict of the single parent. Retrieved September 2009, from http://www.carlpickhardt.com/page48.html

Pisacane, A, Continisio, G, et al. (2005). A controlled trial of the father's role in breastfeeding promotion. Pediatr 116(4):e494–e498. Retrieved February 2007, from http://www.sidsalliance.org/research/Fathers%20Role%20in%20Successful%20Breastfeeding.pdf

Policastro, MA, Sinert, R, and Guerrero, P. (2007). Urinary obstructio. Retrieved May 2007, from http://www.emedicine.com/emerg/topic624.htm

Porter, ML, and Dennis, BL (2002). Hyperbilirubinemia in the term newborn. Am Fam Physician, 65(4):599–606, 613–14. Retrieved March 2009, from http://organizedwisdom.com/helpbar/index.html?return=http://organizedwisdom.com/Hyperbilirubinemia and http://www.aafp.org/afp/20020215/599.html

Providence Health System. (2000). Ethical decision making. Retrieved February 2007, from http://www.providence.org/phs/ethics/resources/decision_managers.htm

Rackley R, and Vasavada, SP. (2006). Incontinence, urinary: Nonsurgical therapies. Retrieved May 2007, from http://www.emedicine.com/med/topic3085.htm

Rajen, M. (2006). Toxins everywhere. Article for New Straits Times on HighBeam Research Web site. Retrieved February 2007, from http://www.highbeam.com

Rape, Abuse, & Incest National Network (RAINN). (no date). Prevention. Retrieved April 2007, from http://www.rainn.org/

Rasul, AT. (2005). Compartment syndrome. Retrieved May 2007, from http://www.emedicine.com/pmr/topic33.htm

Reasoner, R. (no date). The true meaning of self-esteem. National Association for Self-Esteem. Retrieved April 2007, from http://www.self-esteem-nase.org/whatisselfesteem.shtml

Rehabilitation Institute of Chicago—Spinal Cord Injury Team. (2006). Complications: Autonomic dysreflexia. Rehabilitation Institute of Chicago Life Center Web site. Retrieved January 2007, from http://lifecenter.ric.org.

Renter, TA. (no date). Upper extremity positioning injuries during operative/other invasive procedures. Article for Anesthesia Consulting Web site. Retrieved March 2007, from http://www.anesthesia-consulting.com

Robert, P. (2007). Sleeplessness clouds moral choices. American Academy of Sleep Medicine. Retrieved March 2007, from http://www.healthday.com/printer.asp?AID=602367

Robinson, K. (2007). Loneliness. Counseling Services, University of NewYork at Buffalo. Retrieved March 2007, from http://ub-counseling.buffalo.edu/loneliness.shtml

Saglimbeni, AJ. (2005). Exercise-induced asthma. Retrieved January 2007, from http://www.emedicine.com

Salinas, P, and Hanbali, F. (2006). Closed head trauma. Retrieved March 2007, from http://www.emedicine.com/med/topic3403.htm

Santos, A, and Hunt, M. (2005). Managing incontinence: Once a cause of isolation and embarrassment, incontinence does not have to limit quality of life. Paraplegia News, 59(11). Retrieved September 2009, from http://www.pvamagazines.com/pnnews/magazine/article.php ?art=1687

Sarici, SU, et al. (2004). Incidence, course, and prediction of hyperbilirubinemia in near-term and term newborns. Pediatr 113(4):775–80. Retrieved March 2009, from http://pediatrics.aappublications.org/cgi/reprint/113/4/775

Savrock, J. (2006): Counseling distressed students may be improved by religious discussion. Retrieved May 2007, from http://www.ed.psu.edu/news/spiritual.asp

Scheinfeld, NS, and Mokashi, A. (2007). Protein-energy malnutrition. Retrieved April 2007, from http://www.emedicine.com/derm/topic797.htm

Schmidt, RJ, and Somam, SS. (2008). Renovascular hypertension. Retrieved March 2009, from http://emedicine.medscape.com/article/245140/

Schoenborn, C (2004, December 15). Marital status and health: United States, 1999–2002. Advance Data from Vital and Health Statistics, no 351. Retrieved March 2007, from http://www.cdc.gov/nchs/data/ad/ad351.pdf

Schuman, W. (no date). Keeping your sunny side up. Retrieved April 2007, from http://www.beliefnet.com/story/147/story_14745_1.html

Scott M, et al. (2006). Nutritional status is altered in the self-neglecting elderly. Journal of Nutrition Online, 136:2534–41. Retrieved March 2009, from http://jn.nutrition.org/cgi/content/full/136/10/2534

Scott-Conner, CEH, and Ballinger, B. (2007). Abdominal angina. Retrieved May 2009, from http://www.emedicine.medscape.com/article/188618

Searle, J. (no date). Eating and swallowing. Fact sheet regarding Huntington's disease. Retrieved April 2007, from http://www.kumc.edu/hosp/huntingtons/swallowing.htm

Seepersad, S. Critical analysis paper. Understanding loneliness using attachment and systems theories and Developing an applied intervention. Retrieved March 2007, from http://www.webofloneliness.com/publications/critical/pubintro.htm

Segal, J, Segal, R, and Smith, M. (2008 update). Relationship help: Building great relationships using emotional intelligence. Retrieved March 2009, from http://www.helpguide.org/mental/improve_relationships.htm

Sexuality Information and Education Council of the United States (SIECUS). (no date). Sexuality education Q & A. Retrieved September 2009, from http://www.siecus.org/pubs/fact/fact0007.html

Sharma, S. (2007). Septic shock. Retrieved March 2009, from http://emedicine.medscape.com/article/168402/

Sharma, S, and Hayes, JA. (2006). Hypoventilation syndromes. Retrieved May 2007, from http://www.emedicine.com/emerg/topic3470.htm

Sharma, VP. (1996). Normal mourning and "complicated grief." Article for Mind Publications Web site. Retrieved March 2007, from http://www.Mindpub.com/art045.htm

Sherman, C. (2002). Antisuicidal effect of psychotropics remains uncertain. Clin Psychiatry News 30(8). Retrieved May 2007, from http://www.namiscc.org/Research/2002/AntipsychoticSuicideRisk.htm

Simon, EE, and Hamrahian, SM. (2007 update). Hyponatremia. Retrieved January 2009, from http://emedicine.medscape.com/article/242166-overview

Simon, JH. (2004). Schizophrenia. CME article for Hardin Memorial Hospital web site. Retrieved May 2007, from http://www.hmh.net/adam/patientreports/000047.htm

Singleton, JK, (no date). Nurses' perspectives of encouraging client's care-of-self in a short-term rehabilitation unit within a long-term care facility. CE offering for ARN Web site. Retrieved April 2007, from http://www.rehabnurse.org/ce/010200/010200_a.htm

Society for Neuroscience. (2007). What is neuroscience? Retrieved May 2007, from http://www.sfn.org/index.cfm?pagename=whatIsNeuroscience

Spader, C. (2006). Post-MI cooldown. Article for Nursing Spectrum Web site. Retrieved March 2007, from http://www.community.nursingspectrum.com

Spinowitz, BS, and Rodriguez, J. (2008). Renal artery stenosis. Retrieved March 2009, from http://emedicine.medscape.com/article/245023/

Stephens, E. (2009 update). Peripheral vascular disease. Retrieved March 2009, from http://www.emedicine.com/emerg/topic862.htm

Stotts, NA, Wipke-Tevis, DD, and Hopf, HW. (2007): Cofactors in impaired wound healing (excerpts). In Chronic Wound Care, ed. 4. Retrieved February 2007, from http://www.chronicwoundcarebook.com/

Suneja, M, and Muster, HA. (2008 update). Hypocalcemia. Retrieved January 2009, from http://emedicine.medscape.com/article/241893-overview

Surgeon General. (2007 update). Surgeon General's advisory on alcohol use in pregnancy. February 21, 2005. Retrieved March 2009, from http://www.surgeongeneral.gov/pressreleases/sg02222005.html

Swan, L. (2001). Unilateral spatial neglect. Article for HighBeam Research. Retrieved December 2006, from http://www.highbeam.com/

Tan WA, and Makaroun, MS. (2007). Abdominal aortic aneurysm, rupture. Retrieved March 2009, from http://emedicine.medscape.com/article/416397

Texas Medical Association. (2009). Effective and ineffective coping: The process of stress. Retrieved September 2009, from http://www.texmed.org/Template.aspx?id=4479

Tufts University. (2002). Organizational development & training tip sheet. Retrieved March 2007, from http://www.tufts.edu/hr/tips/assert.html

US Department of Health and Human Services. (2008). HIV during pregnancy, labor and delivery, and after birth. Retrieved March 2009, from http://aidsinfo.nih.gov/ContentFiles/Perinatal_FS_en.pdf

US Department of Health and Human Services, Office on Women's Health. (2005, August). Coping with breastfeeding challenges. Retrieved February 2007, from http://www.4woman.gov/Breastfeeding/index.cfm?page=229

Vij, S, and Gentili, A. (2005). Sleep disorder, geriatric. Retrieved December 2006, from http://www.emedicine.com/med/topic3179.htm

Vinik, AI, Freeman, R, and Erbas, T. (2004). Diabetic autonomic neuropathy. Retrieved April 2007, from http://www.medscape.com/viewarticle/43205

Von Wager, K. (no date). Identity crisis—Theory and research. Retrieved March 2007, from http://psychology.about.com/od/theoriesofpersonality/a/identitycrisis.htm

Weiss, BD. (1998). Diagnostic evaluation of urinary incontinence in geriatric patients. Am Fam Physician 57(11). Retrieved May 2007, from http://www.aafp.org/afp/980600ap/weiss.html

Wilson, L, and Kolcaba, K. (2004). Practical application of comfort theory in the perianesthesia setting. Journal of Perianesthesia Nursing Online. Retrieved February 2007, from http://www.aspan.org/JOPAN/comfort_theory.htm

terWolbeek, M vanDoormen, LJ Kavelaars, A, Heijnen, CJ. (2006). Severe fatigue in adolescents: A common phenomenon? Pediatr 117(6):e1078–e1086. Retrieved February 2007, from http://pediatrics.aappublications.org/cgi/content/abstract/117/6/e1078

Wolfe, TR, and Gallagher, J (2006): Intra-abdominal hypertension: Pitfalls, prevalence and treatment options. AACN News. Algorithm retrieved March 2009, from http://www.wolfetory.com/pdf/Pocketalgorithm.pdf

Woolston, C (2006). Stress and aging. Article for Caremark Health Resources. Retrieved April 2007, from http://www.healthresources.caremark.com

World Health Organization (WHO). (2002). World Health Report. Reducing risks, promoting healthy life. Report of the WHO. Retrieved March 2007, from http://www.who.int/whr/2002/en/whr02_en.pdf

World Health Organization (WHO). (2007). Preventing leading causes of premature death, disease and disability. Fact sheet of the WHO. Retrieved March 2007, from http://www.who.int/school_youth_health/en/

World Health Organization (WHO). (2007). Sedentary lifestyle: A global public health problem. "Move for health" information sheet. Retrieved from WHO Web site March 2007, at http://www.who.int

Yale Medical Group. (no date). High-risk pregnancy. Retrieved March 2009, from http://ymghealthinfo.org/content.asp?page=p02461

Yale Medical Group. (no date). High-risk pregnancy: Hyperemesis gravidarum. Retrieved March 2009, from http://ymghealthinfo.org/content.asp?pageid=P02457

Yale Medical Group. (no date). High-risk pregnancy: Maternal and fetal testing. Retrieved March 2009, from http://ymghealthinfo.org/content.asp?pageid=P02469

Yale Medical Group. (no date). High-risk pregnancy: Pregnancy and medical conditions. Retrieved March 2009, from http://ymghealthinfo.org/content.asp?pageid=P02483

Yale Medical Group. (no date). High-risk pregnancy: Prenatal counseling. Retrieved March 2009, from http://ymghealthinfo.org/content.asp?pageid=P02493

Zuger, A. (2001). Adherence by any measure still matters. Journal Watch. Retrieved April 2007, from http://aids-clinical-care.jwatch.org/cgi/content/full/2001/701/1

Index

A

Abdominal hysterectomy. *See* Hysterectomy
Abdominal perineal resection, 926
Abortion
  elective termination, 926
  spontaneous termination, 926–927
Abruptio placentae, 927
Abscess
  brain, 927
  skin/tissue, 927
Abuse
  physical, 927–928
  psychological, 928
Acgalasia (cardiospasm), 928
Acidosis
  metabolic. *See* Diabetic ketoacidosis
  respiratory, 929
Acne, 929
Acquired immune deficiency syndrome. *See* AIDS
Acromegaly, 929
Activity intolerance, 69–73
  risk for, 73–76
Activity planning, ineffective, 76–79
Acute alcohol withdrawal, 969
Acute confusion, 211–215
Acute pain, 586–591
Acute polyneuritis, 989–990
Acute respiratory distress syndrome. *See* Respiratory distress
  syndrome, acute
Adams-Stokes syndrome. *See* Dysrhythmia
ADD. *See* Attention deficit disorder
Addiction. *See* Substance abuse
Addison's disease, 929–930
Adenoidectomy. *See* Tonsillectomy
Adjustment disorder. *See* Anxiety disorders
Adoption/loss of child custody, 930
Adrenal crisis, acute, 930–931
Adrenal insufficiency. *See* Addison's disease
Adrenalectomy, 931
Adult failure to thrive, 329–333
Adult medical/surgical assessment tool, 22–33
Affective disorder, seasonal, 931
Agoraphobia, 931–932
Agranulocytosis, 932
AIDS (acquired immunodeficiency syndrome), 932–933
AIDS dementia, 933
Airway clearance, ineffective, 80–84
Alcohol intoxication, acute, 933–934
Aldosteronism, primary, 934

Alkalosis
   metabolic, 934
   respiratory, 934
Allergy response
   latex, 84–88, 1005
   risk for latex, 89–91
Alopecia, 934
ALS. *See* Amytrophic lateral sclerosis
Alzheimer's disease, 934–935
American Nurses Association (ANA)
   Social Policy Statement, 1, 5
   Standards of Clinical Nursing Practice, 1
Amputation, 935–936
Amyotropic lateral sclerosis (ALS), 936
ANA. *See* American Nurses Association (ANA)
Anaphylaxis, 936–937. *See also* Shock
Anemia, 937
   sickle cell, 937–938
Angina pectoris, 938–939
Anorexia nervosa, 939
Antisocial personality disorder, 939–940
Anxiety, 91–98
   death, 98–101
Anxiety disorders, 941
   generalized, 940–941
Aortic aneurysm, abdominal (AAA), 941
   repair, 942
Aortic stenosis, 942
Aplastic anemia, 942
Appendicitis, 942
ARDS. *See* Respiratory distress syndrome, acute
Arterial occlusive disease, peripheral, 943
Arthritis
   juvenile rheumatoid, 943
   osteoarthritis, 1020
   rheumatoid, 943
   septic, 943–944
Arthroplasty, 944
Aspiration, risk for, 102–106
Assessment tools for choosing nursing diagnoses, 21–29
Asthma, 944
Atherosclerosis, 1025–1026
Athlete's foot, 944–945
Athroscopy, knee, 944
Atrial fibrillation, 945
Attachment, risk for impaired, 106–109
Attention deficit disorder (ADD), 945
Autistic disorder, 945–946
Autonomic dysreflexia, 109–113
   risk for, 113–116

B
Battered child syndrome, 946–947
Behavior, risk-prone health, 116–120

Benign prostatic hyperplasia, 947
Bipolar disorder, 947–948
Bleeding, risk for, 120–124
Blood glucose level, risk for unstable, 391–395
Body image, disturbed, 125–130
Body temperature, risk for imbalanced, 130–133
Bone cancer, 948
Borderline personality disorder, 948
Botulism (food-borne), 949
Bowel incontinence, 134–137
Brain
    abscess, 927
    concussion, 964
    traumatic brain injury, 1057–1058
    tumor, 949
Breast cancer, 949–950
Breastfeeding
    effective, 137–141
    ineffective, 141–147
    interrupted, 147–151
Breathing pattern, ineffective, 151–155
Bronchitis, 950
Bronchopneumonia, 950
Bulimia nervosa, 950–951
Burns, 951
Bursitis, 952

C
Calculi, urinary, 952
Cancer, 952–953
Candidiasis, 953
Cardiac catheterization, 953
Cardiac output, decreased, 156–162
Cardiac surgery, 953–954
Cardiac tissue perfusion, risk for decreased, 614–618
Cardiomyopathy, 954
Caregiver role strain, 162–169
    risk for, 169–173
Carotid endarterectomy, 954
Carpal tunnel syndrome, 954–955
Casts, 955
Cat scratch disease, 955
Cataract, 955
Cellulitis, 956
Cerebral palsy, 1021
Cerebral tissue perfusion, risk for ineffective, 618–622
Cerebrovascular accident (CVA), 956–957
Cervix, premature dilation, 975
Cesarean birth, 957
    postpartal, 957–958
    unplanned, 958
Charting formats, 64–68
Chemotherapy, 958–959

Childbearing process, readiness for enhanced, 173–182
Cholecystectomy, 959
Cholelithiasis, 959
Chronic confusion, 215–219
Chronic fatigue syndrome, 983
Chronic low self-esteem, 718–722
Chronic obstructive lung disease, 959–960
Chronic pain, 591–596
Chronic sorrow, 787–791
Circumcision, 960
Cirrhosis, 960–961
Client database, 2
Client diagnostic statement, 2
Client situation, 46
Cocaine hydrochloride poisoning, acute, 961
Coccidioidimycosis (San Joaquin/Valley Fever), 962
Colitis, ulcerative, 962
Colostomy, 963
Coma, 963, 1019
    diabetic. *See* Diabetic ketoacidosis
Comfort
    impaired, 182–188
    readiness for enhanced, 188–193
Communication
    impaired verbal, 193–198
    readiness for enhanced, 198–203
Complex regional pain syndrome, 964
Complicated grieving, 399–404
    risk for, 404–407
Compromised family coping, 246–249
Concussion, brain, 964
Conduct disorder, 964–965
Conflict
    chronic, 215–219
    decisional, 203–207
    parental role, 207–210
Confusion
    acute, 211–215
    risk for acute, 219–223
Congestive heart failure. *See* Heart failure
Constipation, 223–228, 965
    perceived, 228–230
    risk for, 230–233
Contamination, 233–241
    risk for, 241–246
Coping
    compromised family, 246–249
    defensive, 250–253
    disabled family, 253–257
    ineffective, 257–262
    ineffective community, 262–265
    readiness for enhanced, 265–268
    readiness for enhanced community, 268–271
    readiness for enhanced family, 271–274

Coronary artery bypass surgery, 965–966
Crohn's disease, 966
Croup, 966
    membranous, 966–967
C-section. *See* Cesarean birth
Cushing's syndrome, 967
CVA. *See* Cerebrovascular accident
Cystic fibrosis, 967–968
Cystitis, 968
Cytomegalovirus (CMV) infection, 968

D

Death anxiety, 98–101
Death of child, 1025
Decision making, readiness for enhanced, 278–281
Decisional conflict, 203–207
Decreased cardiac output, 156–162
Decreased intracranial adaptive capacity, 485–489
Deep vein thrombosis. *See* Thrombophlebitis
Defensive coping, 250–253
Deficient diversional activity, 308–312
Deficient fluid volume
    hyper/hypotonic, 367–371
    isotonic, 372–375
    risk for, 379–382
Deficient knowledge, 495–500
Degenerative joint disease, 1020
Dehiscence, abdominal, 968
Dehydration, 969
Delayed growth and development, 411–417
Delayed surgical recovery, 817–821
Delirium tremens, 969
Delivery, precipitous/out of hospital, 969
Delusional disorder, 969–970
Dementia, presenile/senile, 970
Denial, ineffective, 281–284
Dentition, impaired, 284–287
Depressant abuse, 971
Depression, postpartum, 972
Depressive disorders, 971–972
Dermatitis, 972, 980
Development, risk for delayed, 288–291
Diabetes mellitus, 972–973
    plan of care, 54–61
Diabetic ketoacidosis, 973
Diagnostic divisions, 40–45
Dialysis
    general, 973–974
    peritoneal, 974
Diarrhea, 291–296, 974–975
Digitalis toxicity, 975
Dignity, risk for compromised, 296–298
Dilation and curettage (D and C), 975

Dilation of cervix, premature, 975
Disabled family coping, 253–257
Dislocation/subluxation of joint, 976
Disorganized infant behavior, 456–463
   risk for, 466–467
Disseminated intravascular coagulation (DIC), 976
Dissociative disorders, 976–977
Distress, moral, 299–302
Disturbed body image, 125–130
Disturbed energy field, 320–324
Disturbed personal identity, 449–452
Disturbed sensory perception, 738–743
Disturbed sleep pattern, 775–778
Disturbed thought processes, 838–843
Disuse syndrome, risk for, 302–308
Diversional activity, deficient, 308–312
Diverticulitis, 977
Documentation techniques, 64–68
Down syndrome, 977–978
Drug overdose, acute, 978
Drug withdrawal, 978
Dysfunctional family processes, 338–342
Dysfunctional gastrointestinal motility, 535–540
   risk for, 541–545
Dysfunctional ventilatory weaning process, 904–909
Dysmenorrhea, 978–979
Dysrhythmia, cardiac, 979
Dysthymia, 971–972

E
Eating disorders, 950–951
Eclampsia, 979
Ectopic pregnancy, 979–980
Eczema, 980
Edema, pulmonary, 980, 1035
Effective breastfeeding, 137–141
Effective therapeutic regimen management, 827–830
Electrolyte imbalance, risk for, 312–320
Elimination
   urinary, impaired, 860–866
   urinary, readiness for enhanced, 866–869
Emphysema, 980–981
Encephalitis, 981
Endocarditis, 981
End-of-life care, 995–996
Endometriosis, 981
Energy field, disturbed, 320–324
Enteral feeding, 981–982
Environmental interpretation syndrome, impaired, 324–328
Epididymitis, 982
Epilepsy. *See* Seizure disorder
Erectile dysfunction, 982
Excess fluid volume, 376–379

F

Failure to thrive
adult, 329–333
infant/child, 982–983
Falls, risk for, 333–337
Family processes
dysfunctional, 338–342
interrupted, 343–346
readiness for enhanced, 346–350
Fatigue, 351–356
Fatigue syndrome, chronic, 983
Fear, 356–360
Feeding pattern, ineffective infant, 360–363
Fetal alcohol syndrome, 983–984
Fetal demise, 984
Fibromyalgia syndrome, primary, 984
Fluid balance, readiness for enhanced, 364–367
Fluid volume
deficient, 367–375
excess, 376–379
hyper/hypotonic, 367–371
isotonic, 372–375
risk for deficient, 379–382
risk for imbalanced, 383–386
Focus Charting system, 64, 67–68
Fractures, 984–985
Frostbite, 985
Functional urinary incontinence, 869–872

G

Gallstones. *See* Cholelithiasis
Gangrene, dry, 985
Gas exchange, impaired, 386–390
Gas, lung irritant, 985–986
Gastrenteritis, 986
Gastritis
acute, 986
chronic, 986
Gastroesophageal reflux disease (GERD), 986–987
Gastrointestinal motility
dysfunctional, 535–540
risk for dysfunctional, 541–545
Gastrointestinal perfusion, risk for ineffective, 622–626
Gender identity disorder, 987
Genetic disorder, 987–988
GERD. *See* Gastroesophageal reflux disease (GERD)
Glaucoma, 988
Glomerulonephritis, 988
Glucose level, risk for unstable blood, 391–395
Goiter, 988–989
Gonorrhea, 989
Gout, 989

Grieving, 395–399
  complicated, 399–404
  risk for complicated, 404–407
Growth
  delayed, 411–417
  risk for disproportionate, 407–411
Guillain-Barré syndrome, 989–990
Gunshot wound, 1062–1063

H

Hallucinogen abuse, 990
Hay fever, 990
Health conditions, nursing diagnoses, 925–1063
Health maintenance, ineffective, 417–422
Health management
  ineffective self, 422–425
  readiness for enhanced, 425–428
Heart failure, chronic, 990–991
Heatstroke, 991
Hemodialysis, 991
Hemophilia, 991–992
Hemorrhoidectomy, 992
Hemorrhoids, 992
Hemothorax, 992
Hepatitis, acute viral, 992–993
Hernia, hiatal, 993
Herniated nucleus pulposus, 993
Heroin withdrawal, 993–994
Herpes simplex, 994
Herpes zoster (shingles), 994
High-altitude pulmonary edema (HAPE), 994
HIV infection, 994–995
Hodgkin's disease, 995
Home maintenance, impaired, 428–431
Hope, readiness for enhanced, 432–435
Hopelessness, 435–439
Hospice, 995–996
Hydrocephalus, 996
Hyperactivity disorder, 996–997
Hyperbilirubinemia, 997
Hyperemesis gravidarum, 997
Hyper/hypotonic fluid volume, 367–371
Hypertension, 997–998
  pulmonary, 1036
Hyperthermia, 439–444
Hyperthyroidism, 998
Hypoglycemia, 998–999
Hypoparathyroidism (acute), 999
Hypothermia, 444–448, 999
Hypothyroidism, 999
Hysterectomy, 1000

I

Identity, disturbed personal, 449–452
Ileocolitis. *See* Crohn's disease
Ileostomy. *See* Colostomy
Ileus, 1000
Imbalanced nutrition
  less than body requirements, 564–569
  more than body requirements, 570–574
  risk for, 574–577
Immunization status, readiness for enhanced, 452–456
Impaired bed mobility, 524–527
Impaired comfort, 182–188
Impaired dentition, 284–287
Impaired environmental interpretation syndrome, 324–328
Impaired gas exchange, 386–390
Impaired home maintenance, 428–431
Impaired individual resilience, 690–694
Impaired memory, 521–524
Impaired oral mucous membrane, 581–586
Impaired parenting, 597–602
  risk for, 606–608
Impaired physical mobility, 528–532
Impaired religiosity, 673–677
  risk for, 680–683
Impaired skin integrity, 757–763
  risk for, 763–767
Impaired social interaction, 778–783
Impaired spontaneous ventilation, 898–904
Impaired swallowing, 821–827
Impaired tissue integrity, 843–848
Impaired transfer ability, 848–851
Impaired urinary elimination, 860–866
Impaired verbal communication, 193–198
Impaired walking, 917–920
Impaired wheelchair mobility, 532–535
Impetigo, 1000
Incontinence
  bowel, 134–137
  urinary, 869–881
Ineffective activity planning, 76–79
Ineffective adherence, 559–564
Ineffective airway clearance, 80–84
Ineffective breastfeeding, 141–147
Ineffective breathing pattern, 151–155
Ineffective community coping, 262–265
Ineffective community therapeutic regimen management, 830–832
Ineffective coping, 257–262
Ineffective denial, 281–284
Ineffective family therapeutic regimen management, 833–835
Ineffective health maintenance, 417–422
Ineffective infant feeding pattern, 360–363
Ineffective peripheral tissue perfusion, 608–614
Ineffective protection, 660–662

Ineffective role performance, 701–705
Ineffective self health management, 422–425
Ineffective sexuality pattern, 748–752
Ineffective thermoregulation, 835–838
Infant behavior
    disorganized, 456–463
    readiness for enhanced organized, 463–466
Infection
    prenatal, 1000–1001
    risk for, 467–471
Infertility, 1001
Inflammatory bowel disease. *See* Colitis; Crohn's disease
Influenza, 1001
Injury
    risk for, 472–477
    risk for perioperative positioning, 477–480
Insomnia, 480–485
International Classification of Diseases, 15
Interrupted breastfeeding, 147–151
Interrupted family processes, 343–346
Intracranial adaptive capacity, decreased, 485–489
Intrapartal assessment tool, 38–39
Irritable bowel syndrome, 1001–1002

J
Jaundice, neonatal, 489–495
Joint, dislocation/subluxation, 976

K
Kawasaki disease, 1002
Kidney stones. *See* Calculi, urinary
Knowledge
    deficient, 495–500
    readiness for enhanced, 500–503

L
Labor
    induced/augmented, 1002
    precipitous, 1003
    preterm, 1003
    stage 1 (active), 1003
    stage 2 (expulsion), 1003–1004
Laminectomy, lumbar, 1004
Laryngectomy, 1004–1005
Latex allergy, 1005
Latex allergy response, 84–88
Lead poisoning
    acute, 1005–1006
    chronic, 1006
Leukemia
    acute, 1006–1007
    chronic, 1007

Lifestyle, sedentary, 503–507
Liver function, risk for impaired, 507–511
Loneliness, risk for, 511–514
Long-term care, 1007–1008
Lupus erythematosus, systemic (SLE), 1008
Lyme disease, 1008

M

Macular degeneration, 1008–1009
Major depression, 971–972
Mallory-Weiss syndrome, 1009
Mastectomy, 1009
Mastitis, 1009–1010
Mastoidectomy, 1010
Maternal/fetal dyad, risk for disturbed, 514–521
Measles, 1010
Memory, impaired, 521–524
Meningitis, acute meningococcal, 1010–1011
Meniscectomy, 1011
Menopause, 1011
Mental retardation, 1011–1012
Metabolic syndrome, 1012
Mind mapping, 19, 62–63
Miscarriage, 926–927
Mitral stenosis, 1013
Mobility
    impaired bed, 524–527
    impaired physical, 528–532
    impaired wheelchair, 532–535
Mononucleosis, infectious, 1013
Mood disorders. See Depressive disorders
Moral distress, 299–302
Motility
    dysfunctional gastrointestinal, 535–540
    risk for dysfunctional gastrointestinal, 541–545
Mountain sickness, acute (AMS), 1013
Multiple sclerosis, 1014
Mumps, 1014
Muscular dystrophy, 1015
Myasthenia gravis, 1015–1016
Myeloma, multiple, 1016
Myocardial infarction, 1016
Myocarditis, 1016–1017
Myxedema, 1017

N

NANDA International (NANDA-I), 2, 15
Nausea, 545–550
Neglect. See also Abuse
    self, 550–554
    unilateral, 554–559

Neonatal
   normal newborn, 1017
   premature newborn, 1017–1018
Neonatal jaundice, 489–495
Nephrectomy, 1018
Nephrotic syndrome, 1018–1019
Neuralgia, trigeminal, 1019
Neuritis, 1019
Neurovascular dysfunction, risk for peripheral, 630–634
Noncompliance, 559–564
Nonketotic hyperglycemic-hyperosmolar coma, 1019
Nurse Practice Acts, 1
Nursing diagnoses
   definition, 7, 14
   by health condition, 925–1063
   selection of, 14
   for use/research, 8–13
Nursing Interventions Classification (NIC), 15
Nursing Outcomes Classification (NOC), 15
Nursing process, 1–6
   application of, 7–17
Nutrition
   imbalanced, less than body requirements, 564–569
   imbalanced, more than body requirements, 570–574
   readiness for enhanced, 578–581
   risk for imbalanced, 574–577

O
Obesity, 1019–1020
Obsessive-compulsive disorder, 1020
Oral mucous membrane, impaired, 581–586
Osteoarthritis, 1020
Osteomalacia, 1041
Osteomyelitis, 1021
Osteoporosis, 1021
Other-directed violence, actual/risk for, 909–910
Overflow urinary incontinence, 872–875

P
Pain
   acute, 586–591
   chronic, 591–596
Palsy, cerebral, 1021
Pancreatitis, 1022
Panic, 91–98
Paranoid personality disorder, 1022–1023
Paraplegia, 1023
Parathyroidectomy, 1023
Parental role conflict, 207–210
Parenteral feeding, 1023–1024

Parenting
   impaired, 597–602
   readiness for enhanced, 602–606
   risk for impaired, 606–608
Parkinson's disease, 1024
Pelvic inflammatory disease, 1024–1025
Perceived constipation, 228–230
Perfusion
   ineffective peripheral tissue, 608–614
   risk for decreased cardiac tissue, 614–618
   risk for ineffective cerebral tissue, 618–622
   risk for ineffective gastrointestinal, 622–626
   risk for ineffective renal, 626–630
Pericarditis, 1025
Perinatal loss, 1025
Perioperative positioning injury, risk for, 477–480
Peripheral arterial occlusive disease. *See* Arterial occlusive disease,
   peripheral
Peripheral neurovascular dysfunction, risk for, 630–634
Peripheral tissue perfusion, ineffective, 608–614
Peripheral vascular disease, 1025–1026
Peritonitis, 1026
Pheochromocytoma, 1026
Phlebitis. *See* Thrombophlebitis
Physical abuse, 927–928
Physical mobility, impaired, 528–532
Placenta previa, 1027
Plan of care, 2–3, 7, 15–16
   prototype, 46–61
Pleurisy, 1027
PMS. *See* Premenstrual tension syndrome (PMS)
Pneumothorax, 1027–1028
Poisoning, risk for, 635–639
Polyarteritis (nodosa), 1028
Polycythemia vera, 1028
Polyradiculitis. *See* Guillain-Barré syndrome
Postoperative recovery period, 1028–1029
Postpartal period, 1029–1030
Post-trauma syndrome, 639–645
   risk for, 646–649
Posttraumatic stress disorder, 1030
Power, readiness for enhanced, 649–652
Powerlessness, 653–657
   risk for, 657–660
Preeclampsia, 1033
Pregnancy
   1st trimester, 1030–1031
   2nd trimester, 1031–1032
   3rd trimester, 1032
   adolescent, 1032–1033
   high-risk, 1033
Pregnancy-induced hypertension, 1033
Premature newborn, 1017–1018
Premenstrual tension syndrome (PMS), 1034

Prenatal assessment tool, 36–37
Pressure ulcer or sore, 1034
Preterm labor. *See* Labor, preterm
Problem-sensing, 14
Progress notes, 20
Prostatectomy, 1034–1035
Protection, ineffective, 660–662
Pruritus, 1035
Psoriasis, 1035
Psychiatric nursing assessment tool, 34–35
Psychological abuse, 928
PTSD. *See* Posttraumatic stress disorder
Pulmonary edema, 1035
   high-altitude, 994
Pulmonary embolus, 1035–1036
Pulmonary hypertension, 1036
Purpura, idiopathic thrombocytopenic, 1036
Pyelonephritis, 1036

Q
Quadriplegia, 1037

R
Rape, 1037–1038
Rape-trauma syndrome, 663–669
Raynaud's syndrome, 1038
Readiness for enhanced childbearing process, 173–182
Readiness for enhanced comfort, 188–193
Readiness for enhanced communication, 198–203
Readiness for enhanced community coping, 268–271
Readiness for enhanced coping, 265–268
Readiness for enhanced decision making, 278–281
Readiness for enhanced family coping, 271–274
Readiness for enhanced family processes, 346–350
Readiness for enhanced fluid balance, 364–367
Readiness for enhanced hope, 432–435, 467–471
Readiness for enhanced immunization status, 452–456
Readiness for enhanced knowledge, 500–503
Readiness for enhanced nutrition, 578–581
Readiness for enhanced organized infant behavior, 463–466
Readiness for enhanced parenting, 602–606
Readiness for enhanced power, 649–652
Readiness for enhanced relationship, 669–673
Readiness for enhanced religiosity, 677–680
Readiness for enhanced resilience, 694–697
Readiness for enhanced self-care, 705–708
Readiness for enhanced self-concept, 714–718
Readiness for enhanced self health management, 425–428
Readiness for enhanced sleep, 767–770
Readiness for enhanced spiritual well-being, 800–803
Readiness for enhanced urinary elimination, 866–869

Reflex sympathetic dystrophy. *See* Complex regional pain syndrome
Reflex urinary incontinence, 875–879
Regional enteritis. *See* Crohn's disease
Relationship, readiness for enhanced, 669–673
Religiosity
    impaired, 673–677
    readiness for enhanced, 677–680
    risk for impaired, 680–683
Relocation stress syndrome, 683–687
    risk for, 688–690
Renal failure
    acute, 1038
    chronic, 1038–1039
Renal perfusion, risk for ineffective, 626–630
Renal transplantation, 1039
Resilience
    impaired individual, 690–694
    readiness for enhanced, 694–697
    risk for compromised, 697–701
Respiratory distress syndrome
    acute, 1039–1040
    premature infant, 1040
Retinal detachment, 1040–1041
Reye's syndrome, 1041
Rheumatic fever, 1041
Rickets, 1041
Ringworm, tinea, 1041–1042
Risk for activity intolerance, 73–76
Risk for acute confusion, 219–223
Risk for aspiration, 102–106
Risk for autonomic dysreflexia, 113–116
Risk for bleeding, 120–124
Risk for caregiver role strain, 169–173
Risk for complicated grieving, 404–407
Risk for compromised human dignity, 296–298
Risk for compromised resilience, 697–701
Risk for constipation, 230–233
Risk for contamination, 241–246
Risk for decreased cardiac tissue perfusion, 614–618
Risk for deficient fluid volume, 379–382
Risk for delayed development, 288–291
Risk for disorganized infant behavior, 466–467
Risk for disproportionate growth, 407–411
Risk for disturbed maternal/fetal dyad, 514–521
Risk for disuse syndrome, 302–308
Risk for dysfunctional gastrointestinal motility, 541–545
Risk for electrolyte imbalance, 312–320
Risk for falls, 333–337
Risk for imbalanced body temperature, 130–133
Risk for imbalanced fluid volume, 383–386
Risk for imbalanced nutrition, more than body requirements,
    574–577
Risk for impaired attachment, 106–109
Risk for impaired liver function, 507–511

Risk for impaired parenting, 606–608
Risk for impaired religiosity, 680–683
Risk for impaired skin integrity, 763–767
Risk for ineffective cerebral tissue perfusion, 618–622
Risk for ineffective gastrointestinal perfusion, 622–626
Risk for ineffective renal perfusion, 626–630
Risk for infection, 467–471
Risk for injury, 472–477
Risk for latex allergy response, 89–91
Risk for loneliness, 511–514
Risk for perioperative positioning injury, 477–480
Risk for peripheral neurovascular dysfunction, 630–634
Risk for poisoning, 635–639
Risk for post-trauma syndrome, 646–649
Risk for powerlessness, 657–660
Risk for relocation stress syndrome, 688–690
Risk for self-mutilation, 733–738
Risk for shock, 752–757
Risk for situational low self-esteem, 726–729
Risk for spiritual distress, 796–800
Risk for sudden infant death syndrome, 274–278
Risk for suffocation, 808–812
Risk for suicide, 812–817
Risk for trauma, 851–856
Risk for unstable blood glucose level, 391–395
Risk for urge urinary incontinence, 879–881
Risk or vascular trauma, 856–860
Risk-prone health behavior, 116–120
Rocky Mountain spotted fever, 1059
Role performance, ineffective, 701–705
Rubella, 1042
Ruptured intervertebral disk, 993

S
San Joaquin/Valley Fever, 962
Scabies, 1042
Scarlet fever, 1042
Schizophrenia, 1042–1043
Sciatica, 1043
Scleroderma, 1043–1044
Scoliosis, 1044
Sedentary lifestyle, 503–507
Seizure disorder, 1044–1045
Self-care, readiness for enhanced, 705–708
Self-care deficit, bathing, dressing, feeding, toileting, 708–714
Self-concept, readiness for enhanced, 714–718
Self-directed violence, actual/risk for, 910–917
Self-esteem
    chronic low, 718–722
    risk for situational low, 726–729
    situational low, 723–726
Self-mutilation, 729–733
    risk for, 733–738

Self neglect, 550–554
Sensory perception, disturbed, 738–743
Sepsis, 1045
    puerperal, 1045
Serum sickness, 1045–1046
Sexual dysfunction, 743–748
Sexuality pattern, ineffective, 748–752
Sexually transmitted disease (STD), 1046
Shingles, 994
Shock, 1046
    cardiogenic, 1046
    hypovolemic/hemorrhagic, 1046
    risk for, 752–757
    septic. *See* Sepsis
Sick sinus syndrome, 1046–1047
Sickle cell anemia, 937–938
SIDS. *See* Sudden infant death syndrome (SIDS)
Situational low self-esteem, 723–726
    risk for, 726–729
Skin integrity
    impaired, 757–763
    risk for impaired, 763–767
SLE. *See* Lupus erythematosus, systemic (SLE)
Sleep, readiness for enhanced, 767–770
Sleep deprivation, 770–774
Sleep pattern, disturbed, 775–778
Smallpox, 1047
Snow blindness, 1047
SOAP/SOAPIER charting, 64–66
Social interaction, impaired, 778–783
Social isolation, 783–787
Social Policy Statement (American Nurses Association), 1, 5
Somatoform disorders, 1048
Sorrow, chronic, 787–791
Spinal cord injury. *See* Paraplegia; Quadriplegia
Spiritual distress, 791–796
    risk for, 796–800
Spiritual well-being, readiness for enhanced, 800–803
Sprain of ankle or foot, 1048
Standards of Clinical Nursing Practice (American Nurses
    Association), 1
Stapedectomy, 1048–1049
STD. *See* Sexually transmitted disease (STD)
Stimulant abuse, 1049
Stress overload, 804–808
Stress urinary incontinence, 882–885
Substance dependence/abuse rehabilitation, 1049–1051
Sudden infant death syndrome (SIDS), risk for, 274–278
Suffocation, risk for, 808–812
Suicide, risk for, 812–817
Surgery, general, 1051
Surgical recovery, delayed, 817–821
Swallowing, impaired, 821–827
Synovitis (knee), 1051

Syphilis, congential, 1051–1052
Syringomyelia, 1052
Systemized Nomenclature of Medicine (SNOMED), 15

T

Tay-Sachs disease, 1052–1053
Therapeutic regimen management
    effective, 827–830
    ineffective community, 830–832
    ineffective family, 833–835
Thermoregulation, ineffective, 835–838
Thought processes, disturbed, 838–843
Thrombophlebitis, 1053
Thrush, 1053
Thyroidectomy, 1053
Thyrotoxicosis, 1054
TIA. *See* Transient ischemic attack
Tissue integrity, impaired, 843–848
Tonsillectomy, 1054
Tonsillitis, 1054–1055
Total joint replacement, 1055
Total urinary incontinence, 885–889
Toxemia of pregnancy. *See* Pregnancy-induced hypertension
Toxic shock syndrome, 1055–1056
Traction, 1056
Transfer ability, impaired, 848–851
Transfusion reaction, blood, 1056
Transient ischemic attack (TIA), 1056
Trauma
    risk for, 851–856
    risk for vascular, 856–860
Traumatic brain injury (TBI), 1057–1058
Trichinosis, 1058
Tubal pregnancy, 979–980
Tuberculosis, 1058–1059
Tympanoplasty. *See* Stapedectomy
Typhus, 1059

U

Ulcer
    decubitus, 1059
    peptic, 1059
    pressure, 1034
    venous stasis, 1059–1060
Unilateral neglect, 554–559
Urinary diversion, 1060
Urinary elimination
    impaired, 860–866
    readiness for enhanced, 866–869
Urinary incontinence
    functional, 869–872
    overflow, 872–875

   reflex, 875–879
   risk for urge, 879–881
   stress, 882–885
   total, 885–889
   urge, 889–893
Urinary retention, acute/chronic, 893–898
Uterine bleeding, dysfunctional, 1060
Uterus, rupture of, in pregnancy, 1060–1061

V
Vaginismus, 1061
Vaginitis, 1061
Varices, esophageal, 1061
Varicose veins, 1061
Vascular trauma, risk for, 856–860
Venereal disease. *See* Sexually transmitted disease (STD)
Ventilation, impaired spontaneous, 898–904
Ventilatory weaning process, dysfunctional, 904–909
Ventricular fibrillation, 1062
Ventricular tachycardia, 1062
Violence
   other-directed, 909–910
   self-directed, 910–917

W
Walking, impaired, 917–920
Wandering, 920–924
West Nile fever, 1062
Wheelchair mobility, impaired, 532–535
Wilms' tumor, 1062
Wound, gunshot, 1062–1063